David Emmans, Arto Laihinen (Eds.)

Comparative Neuropsychology and Brain Imaging

Neuropsychologie – interdisziplinär

Neuropsychology:
An Interdisciplinary Approach

herausgegeben von
edited by

Prof. Dr. Ulrike Halsband
(Universität Freiburg)

Band / Volume 2

LIT

Comparative Neuropsychology and Brain Imaging

edited by

David Emmans and Arto Laihinen

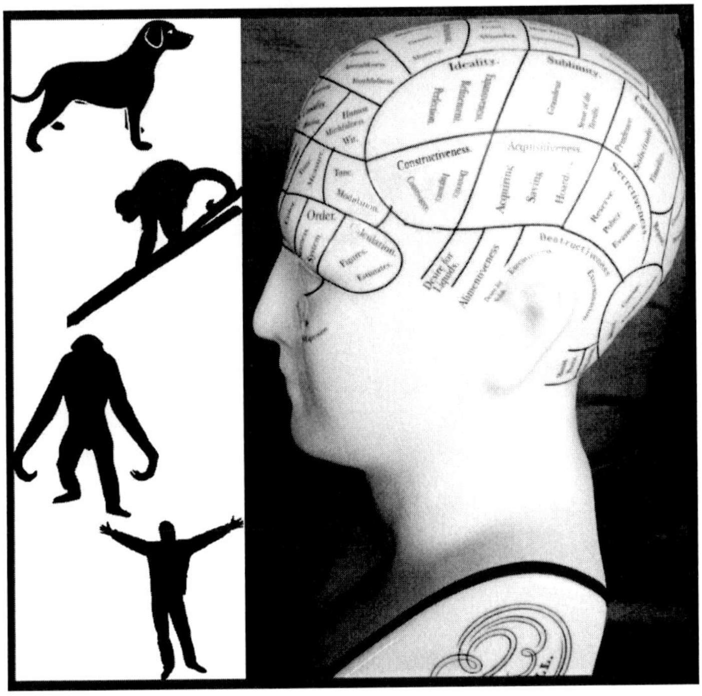

LIT

Cover picture / mammals in collage with "Phrenology" by L. N. Fowler,
© photo by Eva Luckenbach, Freiburg

This book is printed on acid-free paper.

Bibliographic information published by the Deutsche Nationalbibliothek
The Deutsche Nationalbibliothek lists this publication in the Deutsche Nationalbibliografie; detailed bibliographic data are available in the Internet at http://dnb.d-nb.de.

ISBN 978-3-643-90653-3

A catalogue record for this book is available from the British Library

Klosbachstr. 107
CH-8032 Zürich
Tel. +41 (0) 44-251 75 05 Fax +41 (0) 44-251 75 06
E-Mail: zuerich@lit-verlag.ch http://www.lit-verlag.ch
Distribution:
In the UK: Global Book Marketing, e-mail: mo@centralbooks.com
In North America: International Specialized Book Services, e-mail: orders@isbs.com
In Germany: LIT Verlag Fresnostr. 2, D-48159 Münster
Tel. +49 (0) 2 51-620 32 22, Fax +49 (0) 2 51-922 60 99, E-mail: vertrieb@lit-verlag.de
In Austria: Medienlogistik Pichler-ÖBZ, e-mail: mlo@medien-logistik.at
e-books are available at www.litwebshop.de

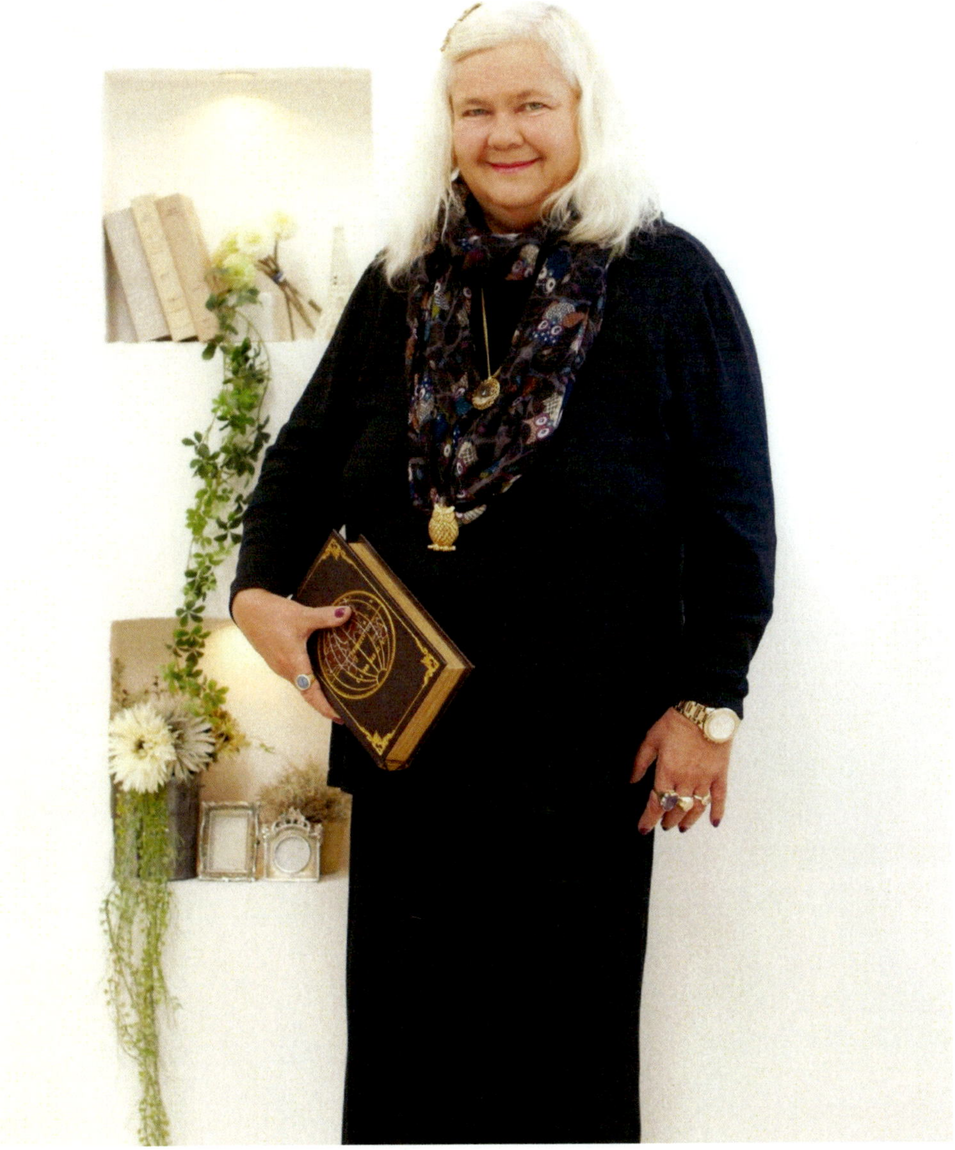

Festschrift in honour of
Prof. Dr. Ulrike Halsband
on the occasion of her 60th birthday

The Authors

DMD PhD student Anita Beck
Clinic of Pediatric Dentistry and Orthodontics
Faculty of Dentistry
Semmelweis University Budapest
Hungary

Univ.-Prof. Dr. med. Ferdinand C. Binkofski
Universitätsklinikum Aachen (AöR)
Pauwelsstraße 30
D-52074 Aachen
Germany
Tel.: 0241 80-88426
fbinkofski@ukaachen.de

Prof. Dr. Dr. hc. mult. Niels Birbaumer
Institute for Medical Psychology and Behavioural Neurobiology
University Tübingen
Silcherstr. 5
D-72076 Tübingen
Germany
Tel. +49 7071 29-74219 (Secretariat)
Fax +49 7071 29-5956
niels.birbaumer@uni-tuebingen.de

Corinna Buderer
Master Student
Department of Psychology
University of Freiburg
Engelbergerstr. 41, D-79085 Freiburg
Germany

PD Dr. Dr. Svenja Caspers
Institut für Neurowissenschaften und Medizin (INM-1)
Forschungszentrum Jülich
D-52425 Jülich
Phone: +49 2461 61-1742
Fax: +49 2461 61-3483
email: s.caspers@fz-juelich.de

Ujwal Chaudhary
Universitätsklinikum Tübingen
Geissweg 3, D-72076 Tübingen
Germany
Tel. 07071/29-0
Fax 07071/29-3966

Dr. Arun D'Souza
Neuropsychology, Department of Psychology
University of Freiburg
Engelbergerstr. 41, D-79085 Freiburg
Germany
dsouza@psychologie.uni-freiburg.de

Dr. Ann Dowker
Department of Experimental Psychology,
Oxford University
Oxford OX1 3UD, UK
GB-England
+44 (0)1865 271407
ann.dowker@psy.ox.ac.uk

David Emmans
Parkinson-Clinic Wolfach
Kreuzbergstraße 12-24
D-77709 Wolfach
Germany
d.emmans@parkinson-klinik.de

Associate Prof. Dr. Gábor Fábián
Clinic of Pediatric Dentistry and Orthodontics
Faculty of Dentistry
Semmelweis University Budapest
1088 Budapest VIII., Szentkirályi u. 47.
Hungary

DMD PhD Tibor Károly Fábián
Private practitioner
Ludvigsmindevej 14
DK-5600 Faaborg
++#-Local-22878198
Denmark
fabiantiborkaroly@gmail.com

Prof. (em.) Dr. Jochen Fahrenberg
Waldhofstrasse 42, D-79117 Freiburg
Germany
jochen.fahrenberg@psychologie.uni-freiburg.de
http://www.jochen-fahrenberg.de

Prof. DMD Pál Fejérdy
Clinic of Prosthetic Dentistry
Faculty of Dentistry
Semmelweis University Budapest
1088 Budapest VIII., Szentkirályi u. 47.
Hungary

Prof. Dr. Herta Flor
Work address: Institut für Neuropsychologie und Klinische Psychologie
Bernstein Center for Computational Neuroscience
Heidelberg/Mannheim
D-68159 MannheimGermany
herta.flor@zi-mannheim.de...

Prof. Dr.med. Hans-Joachim Freund
Moorenstr. 5 D-40225 Düsseldorf
Germany
Telefon: ++-49-(0)211-3117880
Hans-Joachim.Freund@uni-duesseldorf.de

Prof. Péter Hermann
Clinic of Prosthetic Dentistry
Faculty of Dentistry
Semmelweis University
Budapest
Hungary

Prof. Dr. Thilo Hinterberger
Forschungsbereich Angewandte Bewusstseinswissenschaften
Abteilung für Psychosomatische Medizin
Universitätsklinikum Regensburg
Albertstr. 2, 93047 Regensburg
Germany
Tel.: +49 941 944 2748
Thilo.Hinterberger@ukr.de
www.ab-wissenschaften.de

Dr. Juliane Klann MA
Deputy Professor
Chair of German Linguistics
Department of German Studies
Comparative Literature and Cultural Studies
University of Bonn
Am Hof 1d , D- 53113 Bonn
Germany
Phone: +49 228 73-7367
jklann@ukaachen.de
www.germanistik.uni-bonn.de/institut/abteilungen/germanistische-linguistik/abteilung/personal/klann-juliane

Prof. Dr. Boris Kotchoubey
Institute of Medical Psychology and Behavioral Neurobiology
University of Tuebingen
Silcherstr. 5, 72076 Tuebingen
Germany
Phone #49 7071 29 74221 Fax #49 7071 29 5956
boris.kotchoubey@uni-tuebingen.de

MD Chefarzt Wolf-Rainer Krause
Harzklinikum Dorothea Christiane Erxleben
Klinik für Psychiatrie, Psychotherapie und Psychosomatik
Blankenburg
Germany

Prof. Dr. Arní Kristjánsson
Laboratory of Vision, Faculty of Psychology, School of Health Sciences,
University of Iceland,
Reykjavik, Iceland
ak@hi.is
Institute of Cognitive Neuroscience,
University College London,
London, UK

PD Dr. med. Arto Laihinen
Neurologist, a special expertise in rehabilitation is acknowledged
Medical Director / Rehamed Neuro – out-patient neurological rehabilitation
Industriestrasse 3
D-70565 Stuttgart
Germany
Tel (Mobile): +49-173 378 72 75, Tel (Office) +49-711-8569803
Fax (Office): +49-711-8569806
arto.laihinen@gmx.de

Prof. Dr. Martin Lotze
University of Greifswald, Germany
Functional Imaging Unit
Center for Diagnostic Radiology and Neuroradiology; University of Greifswald
Walther-Rathenau-Str.46, D-17475 Greifswald
Germany
Phone: +49-3834 866899 Fax: +49-3834 866898
mail: martin.lotze@uni-greifswald.de
webside: www.baltic-imaging-center.de

Mohammadsaeid Marandi
26 Kavian St.
Chaharbaghebala Ave.
Isfahan, Iran
Postal code: 81739-85341
msmarandi@yahoo.com

PhD Psychologist Dr. Patric Meyer
Department of Cognitive and Clinical Neuroscience
Central Institute of Mental Health
Medical Faculty Mannheim / Heidelberg University
Square J5
D-68159 Mannheim / Germany
phone: +49-(0)621-1703-6314
Fax: +49-(0)621-1703-6305
patric.meyer@zi-mannheim.de
http://www.zi-mannheim.de

Francesco Piccione
Institute of Medical Psychology and Behavioral Neurobiology
University of Tuebingen
Otfried-Müller-Straße 25, D- 72076 Tübingen
Germany

Denise Potthoff, born **Prochnow**
Department of Neurology,
University Hospital Düsseldorf
Bergische Landstrasse 2, 40629 Düsseldorf
Germany

Prof. Dr. Dirk Revenstorf
Universität Tübingen
Biesingerstr. 14
D-72070 Tübingen
Germany
Tel 07071-410915
mobil 01728653720
drevenstor@aol.com

Dipl.-Psych. Hans Riebensahm
Humboldtallee 24, D-37073 Göttingen
Germany
phone: 0551-486279
mobile 0176-90788089
riebensahm@aol.com

Prof. Dr. Juha O. Rinne
MD, PhD, Neurologist, Professor of neurotransmission
University of Turku and Turku University Hospital
Kiinamyllynkatu 4-8, FI-20520 Turku
Finland
Tel. +358-2-3131866
fax +358-2-2318191
juha.rinne@tyks.fi

Dr. Styrmir Saevarsson
(Dr.phil, Freiburg; PhD, Reykjavík; MSc, Utrecht; & BA, Reykjavík)
Städtisches Klinikum München GmbH
Klinikum Schwabing - EKN
Haus 19, 2. Stock
Kölner Platz 1, 80804 München
Germany
Tel. 0049 - (0) 89 30 68 58 13
Fax: 0049 - (0) 89 30 68 75 61
styrmir.saevarsson@gmail.com
http://www.ekn-muenchen.de/index.php/de/mitarbeiter/styrmir-saevarsson

Dr. Francesca Scarpinato-Hirt
Psychologische Psychotherapeutin
Dozentin bei der GAP (Göttinger Akademie für Psychotherapie)
Dozentin bei der WSPP (Weiterbildender Studiengang Psychologische Psychotherapie, Georg-August-Universität Göttingen)
Lehrperson bei APAW
APAW
Akademie für Psychotherapeutische Aus- und Weiterbildung
Rosdorfer Weg 70, D-37081 Göttingen
Germany

Verena Schreiner
Master Student
Department of Psychology
University of Freiburg
Engelbergerstr. 41, D-79085 Freiburg
Germany

Prof. Dr. med. Rüdiger Seitz
Professor and Head
Department of Neurology
Centre of Neurology and Neuropsychiatry
Heinrich-Heine-University Dusseldorf
Bergische Landstrasse 2, D-40629 Dusseldorf
Germany
Phone: +49-211-922-4600
Fax: +49-211-922-4603
seitz@neurologie.uni-duesseldorf.de
Florey Neuroscience Institutes, Melbourne, Victoria, Australia

Prof. Dr. Jun Tanji
Neuroscience Center, Tohoku University
2-chome, Katahira, Aoba-Ku, Sendai 980-8577
Japan
jtanji@m.tohoku.ac.jp

Dr. Jana Uher
Research Group Leader
Comparative Differential and Personality Psychology
Freie Universität Berlin
Habelschwerdter Allee 45, D-14195 Berlin
Germany
mail: jana.uher@fu-berlin.de
fax: +49-(0)321-2117 4699
web: www.primate-personality.net
www.comparativepersonalityresearch.org

Dr. Rainer Wohlfarth
Freiburger Institut für tiergestützte Therapie
Brandbach 4, D-77887 Sasbachwalden
Germany
T. 0151-53525118
Mail: rainer@tiere-begleiten-leben.de

Table of Contents

Part 3 Neuropsychology- A Bridge to the Sciences, Arts and Education

Part 4 Animal Behaviour and Pet Ownership Relationships

Part 5 Altered States of Conciousness

Part 6 History of Experimental Psychology and Clinical Neuroscience

PREFACE

By David Emmans and Arto Laihinen

One of the truly great pleasures of working in research, whether in an academic, clinical or private institutional setting, is the opportunity to meet other highly capable and motivated scholars throughout the years. But when our work at the home office does become demanding at times, combining masses of teaching, research and administrative duties, direct contacts can thin out at times, something which is only somewhat bridged over with the help of emails, in international conferences or even the rare and far-between joint vacations and the even scarcer sabbaticals.

After a long period of time spent in research in different settings and in places spread out across the world, we sometimes look for a convincing reason to work again in some kind of joint seminal project or at least to bring some of these old friendships back together with a common target.

The occasion of Professor Dr. Ulrike Halsband's upcoming 60th birthday and her celebration of 40 years of university life (in the UK, Germany, Finland and Japan) offer one such opportunity to bring together a large number of scholars in the fields of psychology, neuropsychology, neurology, anatomy, animal psychology, functional imagery, medicine and psychotherapy, truly spread out throughout the world representing fields of research for over several decades. Considering the broad fields of research that Professor Halsband herself has been actively involved in, it is only appropriate that her colleagues not only live widely apart, but also that they represent the vastly different fields of basic and applied research, animal and human behavior, biology and psychology, neurology and neuropsychology, diagnostics and therapy. The array of authors contributing to this volume represent the recent convergence of the sciences.

Professor Ulrike Halsband herself grew up in an academic family. Both of her parents were biologists specializing within the area of marine biology and environmental protection. They received several academic rewards and the Federal Cross of Merits for their struggle against pollution and the protection of our animal life. Ulrike Halsband grew up in Hamburg as the only child of her father, Prof. Dr. Egon Halsband and her mother Dr. Ingeborg Halsband. From early childhood onwards she lived together with any number of animals which she learned to love. But she also remembers many weekends which she spent in her parents´ Institute while they prepared for their weekly Monday morning lectures in Biochemistry and Sea Biology.

Ulrike Halsband earned her first degree, in Experimental Psychology, but, typical for her, in the School of Biological Sciences in Sussex, England. Thereafter she received her doctorate from the University of Oxford; her supervisor was Prof. Dr. Richard Passingham. Thereafter she returned to her home-country of Germany and earned her most advanced academic post-doctoral degree, in Germany termed a Habilitation, in the Department of Neurology, at the Medical School of the University of Düsseldorf. Her mentor was Prof. Dr. Hans-Joachim Freund. She worked on deficits in motor learning and apraxia in patients with circumscribed brain lesions within the premotor, supplementary motor and parietal cortices in man, a highly anatomical-functional topic. During this period she accepted a two year visiting professorship in Japan (Tohoku University and Okazaki National Research Institute); her host-professor was Prof. Dr. Jun Tanji.

Ulrike Halsband has continued to make use of state of the art neuroscientific methods (imaging techniques such as fMRT, PET and EEG) in researching not only primarily neurological phenomena (such as apraxias, amnesias, neglect, Parkinson´s disease, dementias, lesions in the hippocampus, frontal, parietal and temporal lobes) but also psychological topics in the healthy brain , such as learning and memory, multilingualism, planning and problem solving, interhemispheric communication, and emotional processing in music production. She conducted research and teaching at the German Universities of Bielefeld, Kiel and Tübingen. She obtained the Alexander von Humboldt Research Award to work on multilingual processing in the brain at the Univerity of Turku in Finland.

In recent years her research has dealt more and more with the brain mechanisms of altered states of consciousness in hypnosis and meditation. She was awarded the Milton Erickson prize for her research in hypnosis and since 2000 she has been the president of the Scientific Advisory Board of the German speaking societies of hypnosis. At the same time she has kept up a vital interest in teaching psychology students in the use of hypnosis, and combines her teaching with research projects on the efficiacy of hypnosis and meditation in subjects with specific phobias and anxieties.

Just to round off her broad interests: She never gave up her interests in animal psychology. A recent book of hers on the anatomy, evolution and behavior in dogs has caused some excitement: One of the few examples of what we call "readable scholarship", the book concerned itself not just with dogs as a subject in its own right, but dogs as unique companions of us humans. Her research on the emotional binds between dogs and humans, and what living together means for both species is continuing and making us curious about the upcoming results. With such a broad background in basic sciences, it is no wonder when it is difficult for some to tell whether she is a psychologist for humans or animals, a neurologist or a neuroanatomist.

The authors contributing to this volume reflect Professor Halsband's scientific convergence: Their chapters cover functional neuroanatomy, clinical neuropsychology specifically related to the brain and neuropsychology related to arts, education and as a bridge to the exact sciences, animal behavior and pet ownership, altered states of consciousness and the history of experimental psychology and clinical neurosciences.

One of the texts reflects Professor Halsband's academic work in the Federal Republic of Germany: Professor Fahrenberg wrote his text in German and we have kept it that way due to his central orientation on German texts and the history of psychology in that country. Scholars interested in such historical themes will most probably have no ptoblems with this text.

As we said at the start of the preface, one of the pleasures of our work is to meet or at least work with such scholars as our contributors are. And throughout working on this volume we enjoyed another pleasure: Hearing how much they had enjoyed their working period with Professor Halsband and her commitment to keeping up high standards of research and teaching, in spite of the ever more demanding load of administrative duties.

We all of us join together in wishing her the best for her birthday and for all her future productive years ahead: Happy birthday and keep up the good work!

David Emmans and Arto Laihinen

P.S.: A word of thanks to Mrs. Eva Luckenbach, our secretary: Without her command of English, her professional command of computers and especially her insistence on organizing texts, emails and people, we would never have completed this volume. In addition, two students helped us essentially from the very start to the very end: Mrs. Miriam Matysik, Mr. Maximilian Wertz and Mrs, Eva Gußmann: They combined hard work, computer expertise with the best of a working atmosphere. To all of you: Thanks!

Part 1:

Functional Neuroanatomy

1 Higher-Order Motor Areas in the Frontal Cortex: How do We Use Them?

Jun Tanji

Key Words:
higher-order motor areas, primary motor cortex, premotor cortex, supplementary motor area, pre-supplementary motor area, cingulate, motor areas, voluntary movement, action selection, action planning, spatial coding, temporal coding

1. Facts, Current Understandings, and Remaining Problems

Motor areas rostral to the primary motor cortex develop greatly in primates. It is generally agreed that at least five motor areas exist medially (SMA, pre-SMA, SEF, CMAr, and CMAc; Fig. 1), and three areas laterally (PMd, PMv, and FEF; Fig. 2), constituting the higher-order motor areas. First and foremost, it is of great importance to scrutinize the anatomical connectivity characterizing the eight areas (Dum & Strick, 2002; Morecraft et al., 2004; Passingham et al., 2002) as a basis of understanding the roles played by individual areas. Despite the facts that some afferent inputs are distributed to several of these areas and efferent projections from multiple areas converge into common target areas, each of the eight areas is characterized by unique combinations of both cortico-cortical and cortico-subcortical connections. Differences in afferent and efferent connectivity provide plausible explanations for area-unique lesion effects reported in animal studies and as clinical signs among brain-damaged patients.

Although all of these areas influence limb or oculomotor actions, roles in selecting muscles and in determining the magnitudes of muscle activity are much less significant than for the primary motor cortex. Conversely, premotor areas are more important in the selection of action based on sensory information, memorized information, and on behavioral context. Electrical stimulation is by no means suitable for detecting functional roles played by each of higher-order motor areas; stimulus artifacts are totally remote from the workings of any areas in naturally occurring behavior. There is no point in torturing subjects by passing formidable electrical currents in the brain to blindly activate or suppress immense, unknown expanses of the brain to induce bizarre and unnatural behaviors. Indeed, it is now established that functional properties characterizing each area can be revealed only under behavioral conditions specifically calling for the use of individual areas. The accumulation of analytical studies has clarified aspects of the preferential roles played by each area in controlling motor behavior, albeit operations of cortical areas based on neural circuits involving multiple cortical and subcortical areas. Furthermore, recent studies have begun to discover the hitherto unknown and surprising reality of their participation in temporal, spatial, motivational, and even social aspects of behavioral control. Future studies will reveal the involvement of higher-order motor areas in an even broader spectrum of complex behaviors. In the following sections, highlights of past history and current knowledge on the workings of higher-order motor areas are described; the oculomotor fields were excluded from this review because of space limitations.

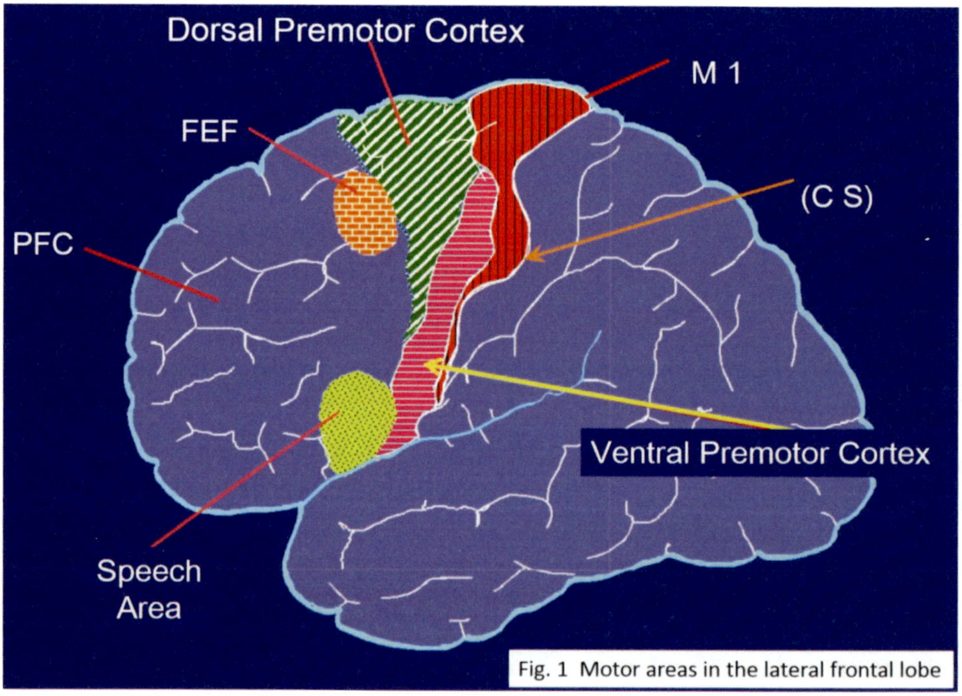

Figure 1: *Motor areas in the lateral frontal lobe.*

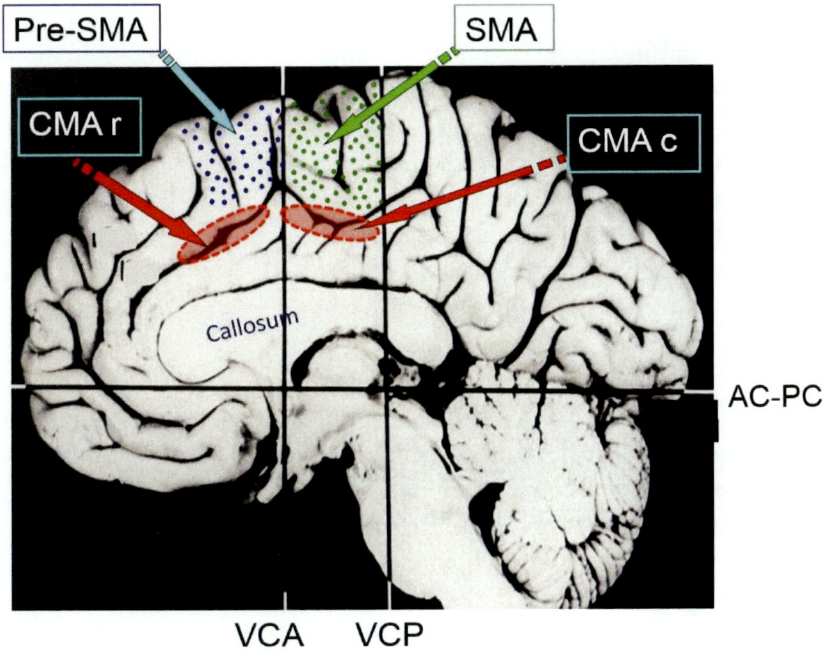

Figure 2: *Motor areas in the medial frontal lobe, drawn on a surface view of the mesial cortex. SMA, supplementary motor area; pre-SMA, pre-supplementary motor area; CMAr, rostral cingulate motor area; CMAc, caudal cingulate motor area; VCA, VCP, and AC-PC are stereotaxic coordinates.*

2. What is Known about the Primary Motor Cortex?

The primary motor cortex (M1) of primates is unique in its anatomical connectivity (Phillips & Porter, 1977). Its descending projections to the brain stem and spinal cord are much more powerful than those from other cortical areas. The density of spinal projections is by far thicker than that of the secondary motor areas (Maier et al., 2002). Only the M1 has potent direct connections to spinal motoneurons with effective synaptic linkages (Porter & Lemon, 1993). Reciprocal connections with the somatosensory cortex constitute a powerful neural circuit providing means for sensorimotor adjustments in motor acts. In contrast, M1 is remote from cortical visual or auditory centers, and is connected only indirectly to the prefrontal cortex.

Much is known about the synaptic connectivity of M1 descending projections (Phillips & Porter, 1977) and neural circuits formed with cortical areas and subcortical structures (Dum & Strick, 2005). Microstructures within the M1 have also been investigated extensively. Despite these understandings, however, the functional roles played by the M1 are understood only partially. Corticospinal projections from M1 are thought to be organized in a way that enables the selection of muscle groups to be activated or inhibited in such combinations to be suitable for purposeful limb movements (Porter & Lemon, 1993). As such, M1 outputs are useful to specify directions of limb movements (Georgopoulos et al., 1982) on the one hand, and to adjust muscle activity to cope with changes in the load of moving objects on the other (Kalaska et al., 1989). Parameters of limb movements are viewed as effectively controlled by the magnitudes of M1 output neurons: Firing rates of pyramidal tract neurons (Evarts, 1968) or corticospinal neurons (Chiney & Fetz, 1980) regulate the magnitudes of force produced in voluntary arm movements.

However, many questions concerning the operations of M1 neural structures remain unanswered. First, functional roles played by individual neurons sending outputs to cortical or subcortical target structures are largely unknown, except for some limited knowledge about the role of corticospinal neurons. Little is known about the functions of corticothalamic, cortico-basal ganglia, corticorubral, corticopontine, and corticobulbar neurons. Nor is the function of the corticocortical neurons projecting to other cortical areas understood. The workings of cortico-cerebellar loops and cortico-basal ganglia loops need to be clarified. Furthermore, it is not known what type of information processing is taking place upon receipt of the massive inputs from the higher-order motor areas. Thus, the M1, despite the substantial knowledge accumulated to date, remains a site for extensive research to reveal the operations of its structural elements in actual motor control.

3. Premotor Cortex in the Lateral Hemisphere

In the lateral surface of the frontal lobe of humans and subhuman primates, in common, lies the premotor cortex, just rostral to the M1 (Wise, 1986). Based on an architectonic concept of cortical evolution proposed by Sanides (1964) and also on the anatomical organization of neural circuits (Rizzolatti & Luppino, 2001), the premotor cortex is divided into two distinct areas: the ventral premotor cortex (PMv) and dorsal premotor cortex (PMd). Studies on the effects of ablation of or lesions in the PM substantiate the concept of areal differentiation within the PM (Passingham, 1993). PMv lesions lead to impairments in attending to peripersonal space (Rizzolatti et al., 1983), in grasping objects (Fogassi et al., 2001), in visual tracking with wrist movements (Kurata & Hoffman, 1994), and in remapping of visual and motor space after prism adaptation (Kurata & Hoshi, 1999). In contrast, PMd lesion studies have emphasized the effects on learning and executing conditional motor behavior (Halsband & Passingham, 1985; Petrides et al., 1986; Kurata & Hoffman, 1994). Subsequent functional studies have revealed that the use of each area differs in a number of respects, under a variety of conditions imposing demands on subjects with respect to different aspects of behavioral factors (Hoshi & Tanji, 2007).

3.1. The Role of the PMv

Anatomically the PMv, a potent frontal lobe source of input to the M1, is characterized as the premotor cortex that receives and processes multi-modal sensory information: visual, auditory, and somatosensory. Above all, potent visual inputs originating from the inferior parietal cortex provide the basis for visuomotor control, informing the shape of objects on the one hand, and the location of objects to be approached on the other. The anterior intraparietal cortex (AIP), connected to the rostral PMv (area F5), carries information necessary for hand grasping of objects, whereas the ventral intraparietal cortex (VIP) informs on the location of reach-target objects to the caudal PMv (area F4, Rizzolatti & Matelli, 2003). Information as to the performance of an action in both sectors of the PMv is fed back to the parietal cortex, and the sensory-motor information is transmitted back and forth in the reciprocal parietofrontal circuit, forming the basis for perception-action cycles recognizing an action target and regulating the action (Jeannerod et al., 1995; Sakata et al., 1995).

Viewed from a different perspective, the PMv could be a site providing the affordance for action (Gibson, 1979; Rizzolatti & Luppino, 2001), and also action perception (Gallese et al., 1996). Many reports on 'mirror neurons' stress the presence of activity in the PMv during observations of actions performed by others: neuronal activity during observation and performance alike (Rizzolatti et al., 1996). Despite the enthusiasm in interpreting this interesting neural activity, which has resulted in limitless speculation on its role in a broad spectrum of cognitive function, the exact nature and functional significance of this mirror-like activity remains uncertain. Given that this mirror-like activity is also found in many other areas in cortical and subcortical structures (Kraskov et al., 2014), it seems reasonable to view the mirror-like activity from the perspective of neural circuit operations that include top-down and bottom-up signaling. Furthermore, before discussing its relevance to cognitive mechanisms of conceptual significance, a much simpler interpretation should first be considered, of its involvement in sensorimotor processes of preparing for or withholding intended actions (Kilner & Lemon, 2013).

Subsequent functional studies have revealed neuronal activity in the PMv actually taking place in the processes of the sensorimotor matching and sensory guidance of motion. The followings summarize the behavioral procedures reported as involving PMv activity.

1. Attention for an action toward an object (Boussaoud & Wise, 1993)
2. Acquisition of the shape of an object of interest (Murata et al., 1997)
3. Matching of an object and action (Fogassi et al., 2001)
4. Retrieval of an action from an action repertoire (Rizzolatti et al., 1988)
5. Buffering information for perception-action cycles (Jeannerod et al., 1995)
6. Transformation of information: visuospatial to somatomotor (Kurata & Hoshi 2002; Hoshi & Tanji, 2006)
7. Action initiation via M1 (Kakei et al., 2001; Shimazu et al., 2004).

3.2. The Role of the PMd

Involvement in motor preparation and execution

Early functional studies focused on its role in motor execution and preparation. Because the PMd is intimately connected anatomically to M1, with reciprocal projections, there is no surprise that PMd neuronal activity at the behavioral stage of motor execution often appears similar to M1 activity. PMd neurons are found to exhibit properties specifying spatiotemporal forms of movement just as M1 neurons do (Caminiti et al., 1991; Scott et al., 1997). However, differences are apparent too; PMd neurons represent movements in a more abstract or task-dependent and effector-independent manner than M1 neurons (Cisek et al., 2003).

Involvement of the PMd in motor preparation was first described as motor-set-related activity, defined as neuronal activity that starts once a forthcoming movement is instructed and continues until the movement is executed (Weinrich & Wise, 1982). If a visual cue is used to instruct motor preparation to capture a target in space, PMd activity reflects the motor significance of the instructional cue rather than its sensory or attentional significance (di Pellegrino & Wise, 1993). Subsequently, it was shown that the preparatory activity reflects such movement parameters as direction, amplitude, and speed of arm movements (*e.g.*, Kurata, 1993; Messier & Kalaska, 2000; Churchland et al., 2006). A report on the effects of microstimulation of the PMd provided evidence that the preparatory activity facilitated the initiation of arm movements according to predetermined motor parameters (Churchland & Shenoy, 2007). Another study that dissociated three motor variables required for preparing arm-reaching motion (motor target location and the starting positions of the hand and eye) found that PMD neurons encoded the relative positions of the target, hand, and eye, during the reach planning, as do neurons in the medial intraparietal cortex (Pesaran et al., 2006).

Conditional motor task: arbitrary association of sensory signals and actions

In 1982, Halsband and Passingham trained monkeys to select limb movements on a conditional motor task. They presented a color cue on a central panel that the monkey pushed aside to gain access to a handle. The monkeys were taught to pull the handle if the panel was blue, and to turn it if the panel was yellow. Removal of the dorsal premotor cortex led to the impairment of this conditional motor task. After the premotor lesion, however, monkeys were able to perform the reaching movements themselves, and they were not impaired in choosing one object given one color, and another object given another color (Halsband & Passinghan, 1985). Essentially the same effects of a PMd lesion were reported from the laboratory of Petrides (1986). In a subsequent clinical study in human subjects, it was reported that the premotor cortex played a role in sensory conditional motor learning (Halsband & Freund, 1990). These reports established that the PMd is essential for the learning and performance of conditional motor tasks where an association of sensory signals and actions are required. One should note that the arbitrary use of non-spatial visual cues to produce actions has fundamental importance in human behavior; without this ability, drivers could not operate cars in accordance with traffic signals.

Integration of multiple information items to formulate a motor plan

The process of planning motor acts often requires the selection of more than two motor variables (*e.g.,* direction, amplitude), and the determination of each variable could be performed in steps with intervening time intervals. Under such a behavioral condition, what is the role of the premotor cortex? In the first attempt to answer this question, Requin and Riehle (1989) found that PMd neurons were engaged in preparing either amplitude or direction alone before using each piece of information to initiate a particular wrist movement. Subsequently, Kurata (1993) found that PMd neurons take part in selecting each of two variables in two steps (amplitude first and direction next, or *vice versa*) at the stage of motor planning.

To plan an action to reach to a target object, we need to select a reach target and a body part (e.g., right or left arm, or mouth) to accomplish the reach. Hoshi and Tanji (2000) explored how the two sets of information for selecting the target and body part are obtained and integrated in the premotor cortex. Monkeys were required to gather the two sets of information by receiving two sets of visual instruction signals given in two steps, and then prepare for a reaching action by combining the two. PMd neurons were found to retrieve information for the target or body part from visual instructions, keep hold of either information for subsequent use, and then combine them to formulate a motor plan to reach;

PMv neurons tended to reflect more of the visuospatial features of instruction signals (Hoshi & Tanji, 2006). Thus, the PMd plays an essential part in retrieving multiple information items for the planning of an intended motor act, and then integrating them to prepare a reaching movement. This aspect of PMd use has been confirmed in human subjects (Beurze et al., 2007).

Several studies have examined the involvement of the PMd in the process of selecting an appropriate motor act from multiple options. Ohbayashi et al. (2003) studied the role of rostral PMd on selecting two saccades in an order determined by later instructions. Cisek and Kalaska (2005) reported that PMd neurons initially represented more than one potential reach direction, and subsequently represented the direction of actually selected reach target. They proposed that multiple reach options are initially specified in the PMd, and then gradually eliminated in competition for overt execution. Wallis and Miller (2003) found that PMd neurons initially reflected whether the behavioral rule was for matching or non-matching and, thereafter, represented the selected motor response.

Transformation of an abstract action plan into an actual motor plan

A behavioral action plan can be formulated at an abstract level before an actual motor act is planned in the presence of motor targets. When communicating with phones or letters, one can specify a behavioral action intended, even when no motor target is in view or no motor effectors are specified. For instance, with a remark such as "Come into my room, approach the desk on your right, and pick up the book placed on the left of the two books on the desk", we can specify an action plan. The action plan could be transformed into actual motor plan when the motor target and motor effectors are available. With this in mind, the following question is inevitable: Are action plans represented in the PMd, and if so, does the PMd take part in transforming the action plan into an actual motor plan?

Hoshi and colleagues (2008, 2009) trained monkeys to receive visual cues that instructed a behavioral action plan to select the right or left objects that would appear seconds later. They found that PMd neurons retrieved information about the action plan from the visual cue at the behavioral stage when no motor targets existed. Thereafter, when monkeys started to prepare a reaching motion to reach to a motor target, PMd neurons ceased to reflect the action plan, and, in turn, began to represent the actual motor plan. Thus, individual PMd neurons actively take part in transforming the action plan to the motor plan.

4. Supplementary Motor Area

4.1. Starting Point

As stated in the previous section, the supplementary motor area (SMA) is characterized as a somatotopically organized cortical area having a unique combination of afferent and efferent corticocortical and cortico-subcortical connections (Goldberg, 1985; Tanji, 1994). Effects of lesion or inactivation of the SMA differ greatly from those of M1 lesions (Passingham, 1993). SMA ablation gave rise to no apparent paralysis (Brinkman, 1984), in accordance with the effects of SMA lesions in human subjects (Luria, 1966; Laplane et al., 1977). SMA inactivation by cooling or with chemical means resulted in little alteration in motor initiation or execution, as indicated by negative effects on subjects' reaction time or motor time (Tanji et al., 1985; Shima & Tanji 1998). Thus, lesion studies provided evidence that the SMA is not essential for the initiation or execution of limb movements, although necessary for other aspects of motor behavior, such as selecting actions without external cues (Thaler & Passingham, 1989) or performing bimanual coordination (Brinkman, 1984).

Although the analysis of SMA neurons has detected activity closely related to motor execution (irrespective of whether self-initiated or signal-triggered), such peri-movement activity does not necessarily signify a vital contribution to movement initiation or a role in specifying motor parameters (Tanji & Kurata, 1982). Rather, the activity should be regarded as being used in various aspects of motor or behavioral control other than movement initiation (Tanji, 1996; Nachev et al., 2008; Scangos & Stuphorn, 2010). It could play a role in specifying actions rather than movements (Tanji et al., 1987), detecting or monitoring motor events, suppressing unwanted movements (Schall et al., 2002), or in signaling the occurrence of individual components in a sequential action.

4.2. Action Selection Without External Prompts and Temporal Ordering of Multiple Actions

Thaler and Passingham (1989) trained monkeys to select a correct action (pull or turn a handle when presented) based on a context. On any day only one of the two actions was correct, but if the animal reached a criterion level of performance the other action was correct (reversal). At the start of a trial, a screen was raised to give the animal access to the handle and then the monkeys made a selection. In this task requirement, there was no sensory instruction telling the animal what to do; the animal had to select an action according to the success of its previous actions. They found that the learning of this task was impaired after a medial premotor cortex lesion.

The selection of action could be harder if multiple selections must be made in a correct order, with no external instructions. Halsband (1987) trained monkeys to perform multiple actions in a correct order without external cues. A T-shaped manipulandum (plastic plate) was presented for use repeatedly, each time with an intervening interval of several seconds. To obtain a food reward, monkeys learned to first push it up, then twist it, and finally lift it up. After the removal of the medial premotor cortex, including the SMA, monkeys failed to relearn the sequence at all in 1,000 trials. Examination of the activity of single neurons performed years later (Halsband et al., 1994) revealed that the SMA, indeed, is a focus of activity when the selection of multiple actions (push, pull, or turn a handle, each with intervening intervals) must be performed without external instructions. Subsequently, Tanji and colleagues set up a behavioral condition in which the complexity of the multiple-selection task was greatly enhanced in a way that each of the three action components could appear as any of the first, second, or third action. Consequently, the number of action sequences amounted to six, excluding repetitions. Specifically, the monkeys had to select actions to arrange in any of the orders of push-pull-turn, push-turn-pull, pull-turn-push, pull-push-turn, turn-push-pull, or turn-pull-push. After the training period of 12-16 months, the monkeys performed the temporal-ordering task in full accordance with the requirements. Then, 1-2 μL of muscimol (GABA agonist) was injected into the forelimb part of the physiologically identified SMA (Shima & Tanji, 1998). The effect was devastating. Within 10 min, the monkeys started committing sequencing errors with increasing frequency. After 20 min, the sequential selection of action had mostly deteriorated. Even at that stage, it was confirmed that the monkeys could perform the sequential task if individual actions were instructed with visual signals.

These studies revealed that the SMA is essential for the selection of actions based on memorized or internally generated information. The need for the participation of SMA is more apparent if the selection requires temporal ordering. Such results of animal studies also provide explanations for findings reported in clinical studies of patients with lesions in the SMA and the adjoining medial premotor cortex. Laplane et al. (1977) proposed that focal damage produced impairment of "intentional" action arising primarily out of an internal context as opposed to an environmentally contingent "responsive" action. Luria (1966) reported disturbance in organizing smooth, integrated sequences of limb movements. Goldberg et al. (1981) also interpreted the patient's greatest difficulty as an inability in the assembly of component movements into a smooth and continuous sequence.

4.3. How is the Orderly Selection of Action Achieved with Neural Elements?

Brain imaging studies measuring regional cerebral blood flow have reported the participation of the medial premotor cortex in the elaboration of motor subroutines that specified the sequence of actions (Roland et al., 1982), in the selection of action sets (Rushworth et al., 2004), and in the self-generation of action (Passingham et al., 2010). These and many other human-brain imaging studies inquired ***where*** the active foci appeared when confronted with the need to select an action without an external prompt. We now proceed to deal with the next question of ***how*** the brain works for the adequate selection of multiple actions (Tanji, 2001). For this inquiry, we need to explore the workings of neural elements and their dynamic behavior with high temporal resolution; time-dependent analysis of neuronal activity currently appears to be the most effective means to achieve that purpose.

Consider the behavioral condition for the temporal ordering of action components A, B, and C, as introduced in the previous section concerning the ordering of push, pull, and turn (Shima & Tanji, 1998). Chronologically, the first requirement for achieving the multiple selection is the retrieval of temporal-sequence information, based on behavioral context or memory, and its retention until the use of that information. We found neuronal activity that met such requirements during the period of preparation for the sequential selection of A, B, and C (Fig. 3). As can be seen, the activity is selective, appearing only when the monkey holds the information that the selection in that trial will be in the order A, B, and C. Given this activity, subjects could prepare to perform the sequential selection of action in that particular order. Using this information, it should be easy to decode that the first action will be A. Interestingly, however, the sequence-selective preparatory activity ceased after the first action A was performed. Then, what kind of neural elements could take over the temporal control of sequential selection? We next found the activity starting at the end of action A that continued to be active until the initiation of the second action, B (Fig. 4). The activity appeared only during that interval and not during intervals of other actions. This activity holds the information that the second action B follows the first action A. This type of activity is useful as an element linking the occurrence of A to B. Subsequently, in the next step of the behavioral-task performance, we found neuronal activity that started at the end of the second action B, which lasted until the selection of the third action C (Fig. 5). This type of activity is useful as an element linking the second action B to the third action C.

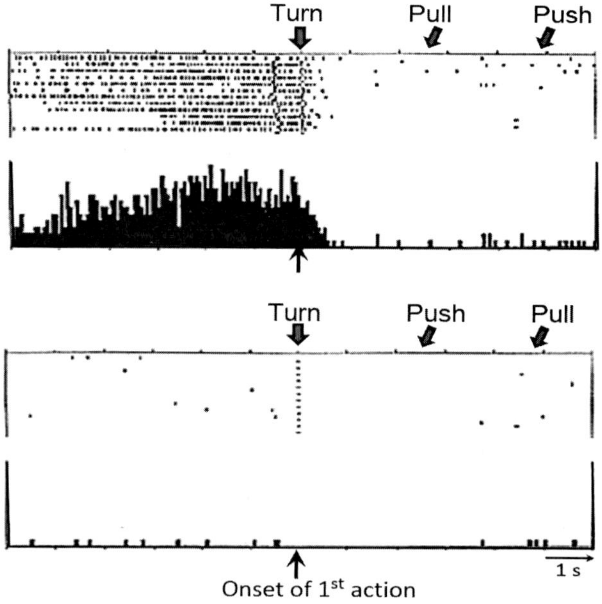

Figure 3: *Cellular activity in the SMA, representing a sequence of planned actions. Discharges of this cell build up markedly, specifically when planning to select three actions in the order of Turn, Pull, and Push, with time intervals. In the raster displays, individual dots indicate the time of occurrence of cell discharges aligned on the onset of the first action. Each row of dots represent individual behavioral trials. The histograms at the bottoms sum the numbers of discharges in a time-dependent manner over 12 trials of the task performance.*

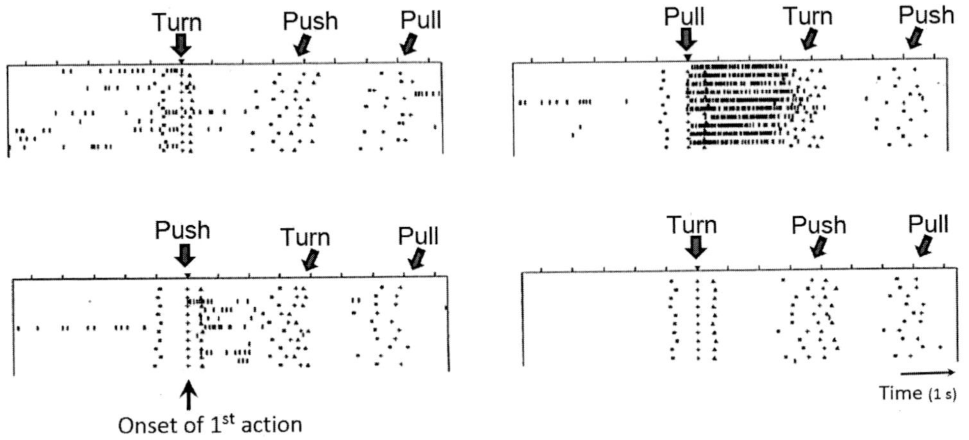

Figure 4: *Cellular activity in the SMA representing a particular transition of two actions. This cell is active specifically after the first action of Pull, and the activity continues until the second action Turn is signaled. Thus, the activity time-links the occurrences of the two actions in the order of Pull – Turn.*

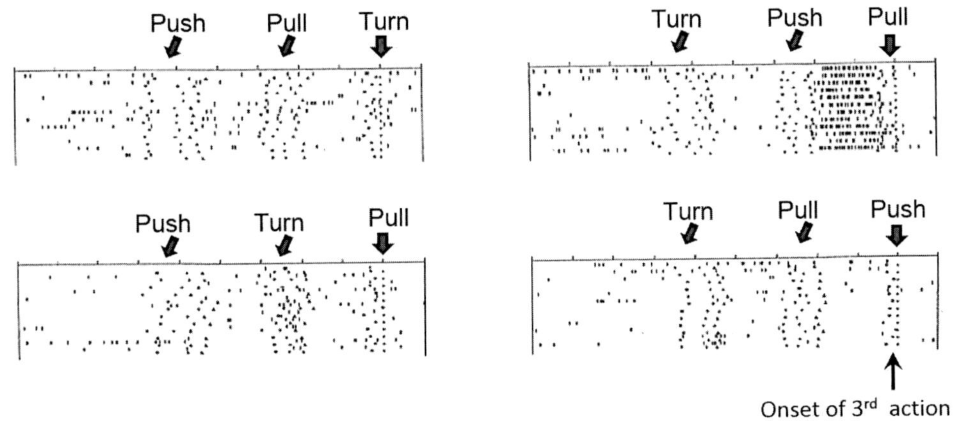

Figure 5: *SMA cell activity representing the time-linking of a specific set of second and third actions. The tonic activity begins after the second action Push and continues until the selection of the third action Pull (top right panel). Thus, the activity exclusively time-links the selections of second Push and third Pull.*

We found that all of the time sequences (six permutations for A, B, and C) were represented during the sequence planning period among a large number of SMA and pre-SMA neurons. We also found the time-linking elements for all combinations of actions in either the second or third step of the sequence control period. We propose that these two categories of neuronal activity, one representing preparation for the sequential action selection and the other for time-linking of two specific actions, are useful as building blocks of neuronal circuits that enable the selection of actions in an appropriate time series. We also found neuronal representation of the rank-order of the behavioral components. This type of neuronal activity selectively predicted that the action selection will be the first, second, or third in a series of selections. Such activity was prevalent among neurons in the SMA and pre-SMA. In total, these findings indicate that neural elements useful for constructing neural circuits required for the development of sequential selection are represented with neuronal activity in the SMA and pre-SMA. The question of whether and to what extent such neural elements could be found in other cortical or subcortical areas is the matter for future investigation, with the exception of the finding that they occur only infrequently in the M1 (Shima & Tanji, 2000).

5. Pre-Supplementary Motor Area (Pre-SMA)

5.1. SMA and Pre-SMA are Two Separate Areas

It is now established that two motor areas exist in the medial area 6, corresponding to area 6aα (SMA) and 6aβ (pre-SMA, Matsuzaka et al., 1992). These two areas constitute largely separate neural circuits in the brain with distinct anatomical connectivity (Fig. 6).

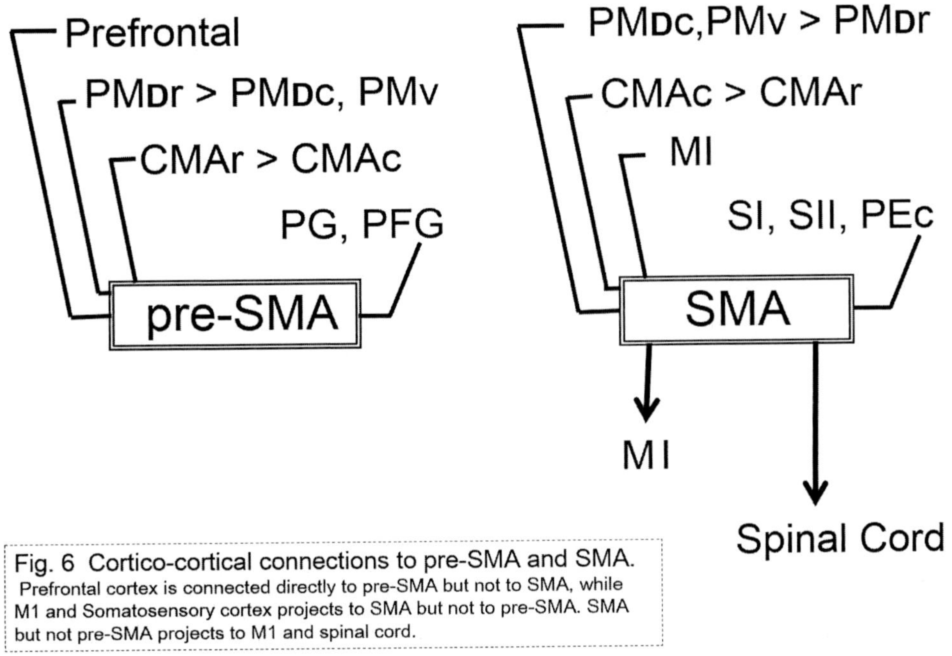

Figure 6: *Cortico-cortical connections to pre-SMA and SMA. The prefrontal cortex is connected directly to the pre-SMA but not to the SMA, while M1 and the somatosensory cortex project to the SMA but not to the pre-SMA. The SMA, but not the pre-SMA, projects to M1 and the spinal cord. Connections of the two areas with subareas of the premotor cortex and the cingulate motor areas also differ greatly.*

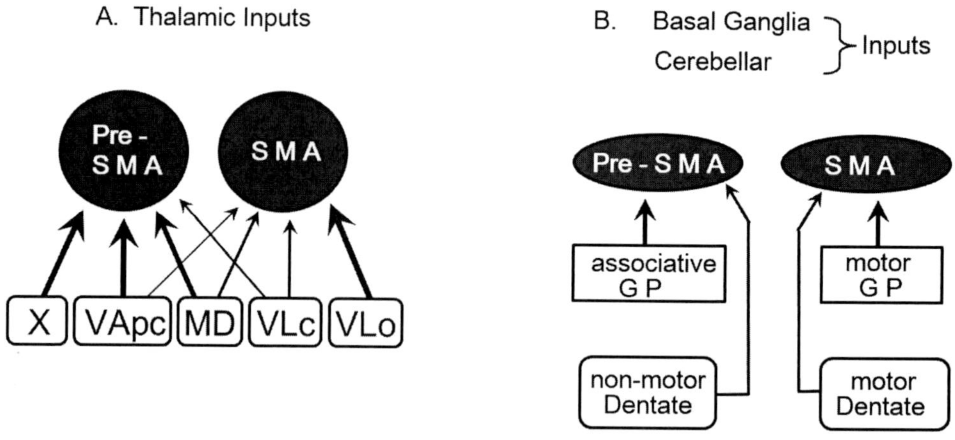

Figure 7: *Thalamic and trans-thalamic inputs to the pre-SMA and SMA. A. Distribution of inputs from thalamic nuclei. B. Contrasting trans-thalamic inputs from the basal ganglia and the cerebellum. The associative part of GPi and non-motor part of dentate nucleus reach the pre-SMA, while the motor part of GPi and the motor part of dentate reach the SMA.*

The prefrontal cortex projects directly to the pre-SMA, but not to the SMA. The M1 and somatosensory cortex project to the SMA but not to the pre-SMA. Distributions of inputs from the premotor and cingulate motor cortex to the two areas differ in many ways. The SMA projects to the M1 and spinal cord, whereas the pre-SMA lacks these outputs. On the other hand, subcortical connections also provide unique combinations of input sources to the two areas. The density distributions of inputs from the thalamic nuclei to the SMA and pre-SMA differ greatly (Fig. 7A). By way of these thalamic nuclei, different parts of the basal ganglia and cerebellar nuclei preferentially reach to either of these areas (Strick & Akkal, 2007). The associative territory of GPi and the non-motor part of the dentate nucleus get access to the pre-SMA, whereas the motor part of GPi and the motor part of dentate reach to the SMA (Fig. 7B). These findings of anatomical connectivity point to different uses of the two motor areas.

Indeed, the physiological properties of neurons in the two areas differ profoundly with respect to various behavioral factors, although they may appear similar on casual observation during motor preparation. Generally, the activity of pre-SMA neurons becomes more evident when subjects face behavioral conditions that require temporal organization or selection of an action, or the purposeful use of environmental or memorized information for appropriate action initiation or action planning (Tanji 1996; Nachev et al., 2008; Passingham et al., 2010).

Numerous reports of studies on the activity of medial motor areas in human subjects, measuring rCBF changes under a variety of behavioral settings, are consistent with the views on the use of the pre-SMA based on animal studies (Picard & Strick 1996; Tanji, 1996: Rushworth et al., 2004; Passingham et al., 2010).

5.2. Neuronal Activity Characterizing the Pre-SMA

1. Effecter-independent action specification

In contrast to the existence of apparent somatotopy in the SMA, somatotopic organization in the pre-SMA is not the basic principle governing the pre-SMA. Instead, effector-independent action specification has been reported. A group of pre-SMA neurons specify a spatial target to be captured with either eye movements or arm-reach (Fujii et al., 2002). Specification of the right or left of spatial targets to be reached with either right or left arm was also reported to be most abundant in the pre-SMA (Hoshi & Tanji, 2004).

Intention is central to the concept of voluntary action. Using fMRI, Lau et al. (2004) compared conditions in which human subjects made self-paced actions and attended either to their intention to move or to the actual movement. When they attended to their intention rather than their movement, there was enhanced activity in the pre-SMA. This finding invites studies at the single-cell level to seek spatial and temporal precision.

2. Switching motor tasks

Matsuzaka and Tanji (1996) found that pre-SMA neurons were active in association with motor task switching; this was evident when monkeys switched from performing a visually triggered arm-reach task based on a current routine to performing the task on an alternative stimulus-response combination. Such behavioral switch-related activity was much less among SMA neurons. Recently, Merten and Nieder (2013) found that pre-SMA neurons responded to visual signals that instructed a rule to switch between a pair of stimulus-response combinations for two forthcoming response signals. Rushworth et al. (2002) studied human subjects by measuring pre-SMA activity with fMRI, and found that the activity was enhanced when subjects switched between different rules for response selection and had to choose between competing visual stimuli. They also found that the pre-SMA is essential for task switching with the technique of repetitive transcranial magnetic stimulation.

3. Learning of spatially based motor sequence

When subjects follow and reach multiple spatial targets that appear at a predetermined, fixed spatial location, the reaction time and motor time shorten considerably upon repetition of a particular spatial sequence: learning effects that facilitate spatial following. Nakamura et al. (1998) found that pre-SMA neurons were particularly active during performance of an orderly spatial-target reach task when spatial arrangements of targets were renewed. Subsequently, in parallel with the animal's learning of a new spatial sequence, the task-related neuronal activity underwent gradual changes in a learning-dependent manner. They found further that chemical inactivation of the pre-SMA led to impairment in performing the target-following task with the newly arranged spatial targets, but not with familiarized targets (Nakamura et al., 1999). Thus, the pre-SMA was involved in acquiring the spatial sequence of target-following or in learning spatial trajectories of continuous target-following procedures.

4. Numerical representation of action and updating of current action routine

Apart from information concerning sensorimotor events occurring in the past, present, or future, we need a variety of information of an abstract nature to cope with a high degree of behavioral demands. One such example is numerical information. If the temporal structuring of multiple actions is required to be arranged in multiple orders, we need numerical information on the actions to be performed. Specifically, if required to select three actions in multiple orders, we need to keep track of a behavioral sequence by specifying the exact rank order of actions to be performed; the first, second, or third in a sequence. Such numerical representation, in the form of rank-order of each action, is found most abundantly in the pre-SMA (Shima & Tanji, 2000).

If a series of actions is repeated in a certain routine sequence and completed before initiating the next series, the sequential pattern should be discarded and updated. This requires cancellation of the current information to proceed to the acquisition of the next action-series information. When confronted with this requirement, pre-SMA neurons are found to be active during the time interval exactly corresponding to that behavioral epoch (Shima et al., 1994).

5. Switching from automatic to controlled action

A considerable part of our actions in daily life is habitual and is performed in automatic fashion, without much conscious control. When in need, neuronal circuits in the brain should be geared to incorporate controlled operation of action-generating system, especially when automatic action becomes invalid.

Isoda and Hikosaka (2007) found that pre-SMA neurons became active when subjects were successful in switching from an automatic unwanted action to a controlled desired action. They found further that the pre-SMA enabled switching by first suppressing an automatic unwanted action and then facilitating a desired action.

5.3. Novel Aspects of Pre-SMA Use

Recent research on the medial frontal cortex is coming to a stage where we can discuss the most challenging directions of inquiry into the workings of the medial motor cortex. Examples of advanced attempts to explore novel aspects of pre-SMA use will be discussed.

1. Motor initiation based on time estimation:

Both humans and animals are able to initiate an action after a specific time period in the range of seconds or more, by generating the appropriate time internally without an external time device. Studies in humans have suggested that a corticostriatal network that includes the pre-SMA and SMA is activated during time production (Macar et al., 1999) or during internal generation of motor timing (Coull et al., 2004). To explore the role of the pre-SMA in the time estimation-based motor initiation, monkeys were trained to perform an interval generation task requiring them to determine pre-motion waiting periods of three different durations (Mita et al., 2009). It was found that (i) visual color signals were converted into time-instruction signals represented in the pre-SMA neurons, (ii) pre-SMA neurons signaled the initiation of action in a time-specific manner, and (iii) the passage of time is expressed preferentially among separate groups of pre-SMA neurons as the time-dependent changes in neuronal activity, with a time course following an exponential function. These results indicate how the pre-SMA take part in initiating actions on the basis of self-generated time estimates.

2. Social aspects of behavioral control

Although much behavioral learning is based on information as to the outcome of self-generated behavior, we can also learn successful achievement of motor behavior by observing and judging the outcome of actions performed by others. Such social-interaction based learning constitutes considerable part of our behavioral learning. Subhuman primates can also learn by observing the behavioral outcomes of other individuals. Isoda and colleagues trained a pair of monkeys together to make use of information obtained while observing each other's actions for adaptive behavioral planning. They found first that neurons in the medial frontal cortex including the pre-SMA encode actions performed by the opponent monkey (Yoshida et al., 2011). Second, they found neuronal activity that specifically encoded the occurrence of behavioral errors committed by an opponent individual (Yoshida et al., 2012), indicating that the pre-SMA takes part in action correction, based on error monitoring of an opponent player.

6. Cingulate Motor Areas (CMAs)

6.1. Where are the CMAs?

The cingulate motor areas (CMAs) in subhuman primates reside in the banks of the cingulate sulcus but do not extend into the cingulate gyrus on the interhemispheric surface. The cingulate gyrus has few anatomical projections to the cortical motor areas and no reported projections to subcortical motor areas. This part of the cortex is not excitable with microstimulation, and cells are not active with movement execution. Thus, the cingulate gyrus, rather than being involved in motor functions, appears to be involved primarily in other higher-order behaviors, such as the control of autonomic functions, the expression of emotions or inner drives, and the affective response to noxious stimuli.

The CMAs can be defined on the basis of anatomical and physiological criteria. A good starting point is the identification of the regions of cingulate cortex directly projecting to the primary motor cortex (Morecraft & Van Hoesen 1992; Muakkassa & Strick 1979). A rostral projection site is situated on the dorsal and ventral banks of the cingulate sulcus at levels caudal to the genu of the corpus callosum, and rostral to the genu of the arcuate sulcus. This region, called the rostral cingulate motor area (CMAr), lies within a subfield of area 24 (24c,d). A second major projection site is located on the dorsal bank of the cingulate sulcus at the levels caudal to the genu of the arcuate sulcus. This region, termed CMAd, lies within a subfield of area 6 (6c). The third region is located in the ventral bank of the cingulate sulcus at levels slightly caudal to the CMAd. This region, termed CMAv, lies within a subfield of area 23 (23c,d). The CMAd and CMAv are often treated as a single area, situated caudally in the cingulate sulcus and termed the caudal cingulate motor area (CMAc). The demonstration of regions projecting directly to the spinal cord (Dum & Strick 2002) supports the delineation of CMAr and CMAc. Physiological studies have confirmed the existence of these motor areas by demonstrating cellular activity during the performance of limb movements (Shima et al., 1991) and by revealing that intracortical microstimulation evokes limb movements (Luppino et al., 1991). Each of CMAr and CMAc are somatotopically organized in such a way that the face, forelimb, and hind-limb regions are arranged approximately rostrocaudally. Regions projecting to the frontal eye field are located in the rostral-most part of each of the CMAr and CMAc (Wang et al., 2004).

6.2. Exploring Functions of Cingulate Motor Areas: Animal Studies

Motor Control Functions

The CMAs are known to have anatomical connectivity with cortical motor areas, the brain stem, and the spinal cord, with somatotopical arrangements. Based on this, it is reasonable to investigate how these areas contribute to specific aspects of motor control. However, physiological studies examining cellular activity during the execution of motor behavior have been few in number, due mainly to the location of the CMAs, buried in the cingulate sulcus in the medial hemisphere. Shima et al. (1991) demonstrated that cells in both CMAr and CMAc do, indeed, change their activity before and during a key-press movement with a hand. The activity was readily observable when movements were initiated in response to visual, auditory, or somatosensory signals, or initiated internally. CMAc cells change their activity more intensely than CMAr cells. CMAr cells, on the other hand, tended to be more active when the hand movement was self-initiated than signal-triggered. Some CMAr cells exhibited activity long before the initiation of self-paced movement. Subsequently, Cadoret and Smith (1995) reported activity modulations of CMAc cells during grasping, lifting, and holding an object with the contralateral thumb and index fingers.

How then are the CMAs involved in aspects of motor control? One issue of high importance is awareness of how sensorimotor variables are represented in the CMAs. Regarding this, recent studies have revealed striking differences in the properties of cellular activity in the CMAr and CMAc. Russo et al. (2002) studied activity in the CMAc during visually guided arm-shoulder movements destined to eight directions. They assessed cellular activity associated with the onset of a visual cue, delay (motor-set), and motor responses for directional tuning. As many as 24% of cue responses, 46% of motor-set activity, and 66% of movement-related activity were directionally tuned. They also found that the directional tuning appeared similar in the CMAd and CMAv.

In contrast, studies in the CMAr showed very different results. Akkal et al. (2002) studied activity during performance of a sequential reaching task with delay. They found no CMAr cells that were influenced by the spatial location of targets during the visual cue or delay periods. For the activity during movement, only 5% of cells showed selectivity to the spatial location of four targets to reach. Isomura et al. (2003) studied activity in the CMAs during performance of a

GO/NO-GO task. Despite the abundance of CMA activity selectively coding a GO or NO-GO response by the animal, only a small number of CMAr cells showed selectivity for spatial or color cues. Subsequently, Hoshi et al. (2005) examined cellular activity in the CMAr with respect to multiple behavioral factors that ranged from the retrieval and processing of associative visual signals to the planning and execution of instructed actions. Cellular activity was analyzed while monkeys performed a behavioral task in which two visual instruction cues were given, each followed by a delay: one cue for the location of the target to be reached and the other for the arm to be used. The activity of cells in the CMAr changed profoundly throughout the behavioral task, in each epoch of the behavioral task. However, the activity was only modestly selective for the spatial location of the visual cues or for the instructional information delivered with the signals (target location or arm use). The activity during the period of motor planning or movement execution, although robust and intense, also exhibited modest selectivity for motor parameters.

These reports indicate that the CMAr and CMAc take part in controlling different aspects of motor behavior. The CMAc is intimately involved in preparing and controlling movements, by specifying the parameters thereof. In contrast, CMAr does not seem to play a major role in selecting or regulating specific details of movements. Rather, the CMAr is more useful in delineating individual phases of behavior that has complex temporal structures, by monitoring individual behavioral events to keep track of the progress of required behavioral tasks. However, CMAr activity during delay or a motor set period is likely to reflect the emergence of a general intention for action, or decisions as to whether to initiate action.

Cognitive Aspects of Behavioral Control

The cingulate motor areas are positioned in the cortex at a pivotal position between input sources from the limbic and association cortex and motor areas to which the cingulate outputs are targeted. This unique anatomical connectivity invites physiological studies examining participation of CMAs in motivational or emotional aspect of behavioral control on the one hand, and in integrative regulation of perceptual or memorized information for behavioral regulation on the other. Although animal studies in search of such aspects of cingulate function are still at an early stage, reported findings suggest that the CMAs are part of a medial frontal network involved in supervisory control of action.

Reward-Based Control of Behavior

The relationship between the CMAr and its adjacent areas to the occurrence of reward was reported initially by Niki and Watanabe (1979). It is now generally accepted that cells in the cingulate motor areas respond to the occurrence of reward (Shima & Tanji, 1998; Akkal et al., 2002). Importantly, however, cellular responses to the occurrence of reward vary greatly depending on the nature of behavioral conditions. Hoshi et al. (2005) examined reward-related activity in the CMAr of monkeys that were highly trained for more than two years, and found that few cells responded to reward delivery. This finding suggests that CMAr response to reward is greatly attenuated if motor behavior is automatized, depending little on reward information (Koechlin et al., 2002).

More interesting is the question of how the reward information captured with CMAr cells is used for behavioral planning or modification. Shima and Tanji (1998) trained monkeys to select and perform two different arm movements triggered with a visual signal. The selection of the motor task was made by the monkeys themselves, based on the amount of reward. During a series of constant-reward trials, monkeys had to keep selecting a particular movement. If they detected reduction of the reward, they chose to perform the alternate movement, because, if they did, the reward returned to its full amount. Muscimol injection revealed that CMAr inactivation resulted in the impairment of proper selection based on the reward amount. Furthermore, CMAr cells were found to exhibit changes in activity during the interval between the detection of the reduced reward and the initiation of a newly selected movement (Fig. 8). A group of cells responded shortly after the occurrence of the reduced reward (cell A), but did not respond to the ordinary, non-reduced reward. Other groups of cells responded to the reduced reward progressively later (cells B and C). Still others exhibited activity that was gradually building up until the selection of the alternate movement (cell D). These findings support a view that CMAr cells take part in selecting action based on the reward obtained as a result of action. In a subsequent study, the effect of ablation of the CMAr and its adjacent region was examined in monkeys performing a reward-conditional response selection task (Hadland et al., 2003). The results of this study led the authors to conclude that (1) the CMAr was concerned with action-reward associations and not only with detecting when actions resulted in errors, and (2) the role of the CMAr was limited to action-reinforcer associations and it was not concerned with stimulus-reward associations.

A different aspect of CMAr involvement in reward-based behavioral control was proposed by Shidara and Richmond (2002) who trained monkeys to perform a color-discrimination response. To obtain a reward, monkeys had to complete a set of trials that was scheduled to vary from one to four. A set of visual signals told the animal the progress of the trial schedule; *i.e.,* proximity to the reward. They found that anterior cingulate cells had responses that changed strength progressively with reward expectancy. Interestingly, cells of this type were recorded from the ventral bank of the CMAr, a region that receives strong inputs from limbic structures.

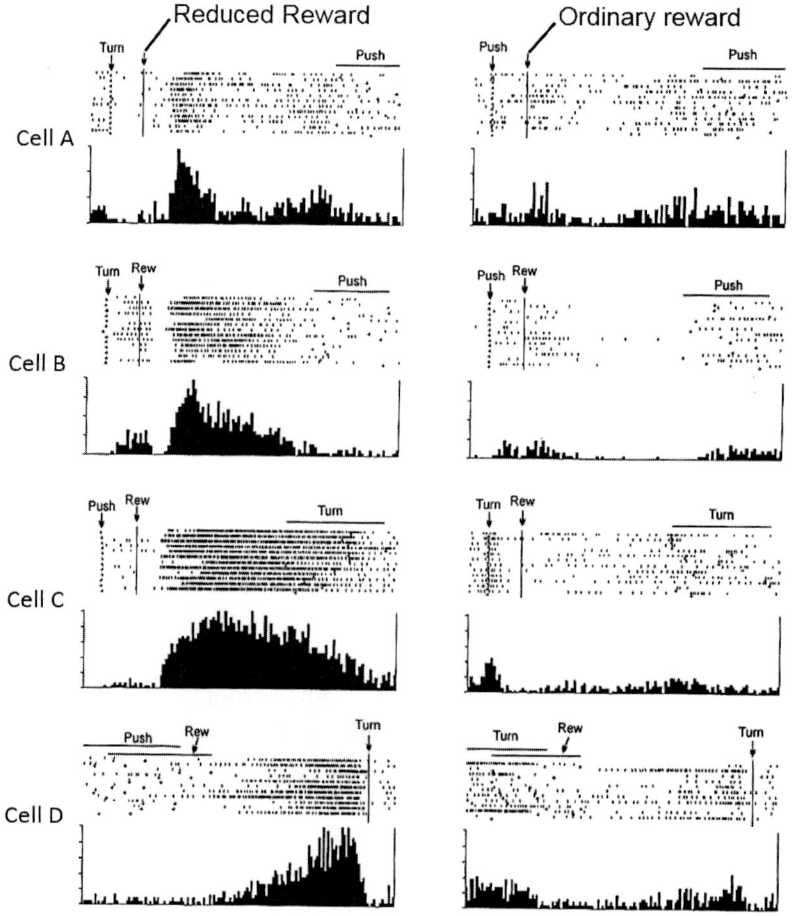

Figure 8: *Activity of CMAr cells responding to a reduced reward before switching to select an alternative action. Four types of cell (cells A to D) respond selectively to the reduced reward with characteristic temporal patterns, with phasic or sustained activity (left panels). The activity of each type of cell appear as if to relay in time the occurrence of the reduced reward and the preparation for the selection of the next action. For Cell A and Cell B, the activity is markedly enhanced when the selection of Turn resulted in the reduced reward, inducing the animal to select the action Push for the next trial. For Cells C and D, activity appeared when the selection of Push caused the reduction of reward that led to the next selection of Turn. Note the absence of cellular responses to the reward with the ordinary, constant amount (right panels).*

Error Detection, Behavioral Monitoring, and Conflict Monitoring

Although a role for CMAs in error detection had long been inferred from animal studies, interpretation of error-related activity is problematic because the occurrence of error causes the animals to get excited or frustrated, resulting in a number of confounding behavioral responses. Ito et al. (2003) avoided this problem by designing an oculomotor behavioral task. Monkeys were trained to perform an eye-movement countermanding task. In trials with no stop signal, the monkeys were rewarded following a saccade to a target. On trials with a stop signal, the monkeys earned reinforcement when the partially prepared saccade to the target was cancelled and fixation was maintained. Under this behavioral condition, they found error-related cells that were active 180 ms after the initiation of incorrect saccades; they were not active during correct saccades or at the delivery of reward. Interestingly, Ito et al. did not find any cells monitoring conflict during performance of that behavioral task, despite the fact that they found such cells in the supplementary eye field. In a subsequent report (Nakamura et al., 2005), conflict-monitoring cells were not found in the CMAr, although the authors designed an oculomotor task in which conflict was evident in behavioral measures.

How can these reports be reconciled with several human studies reporting apparent conflict-related activity in the anterior cingulate (Botvinik et al. 2001)? One explanation may be that these studies employed oculomotor tasks. As mentioned above, an oculomotor part of the CMA in monkeys is located in small regions rostral to the forelimb regions of CMAr and CMAc. It is possible that the oculomotor CMA was not penetrated with electrodes in both studies. Another possibility may be that conflict monitoring is achieved in the region of the anterior cingulate outside of the CMAr. This possibility should be tested with studies in subhuman primates where exact localization of relevant activity is possible. In the prefrontal cortex rostral to the CMAr, Matsumoto et al. (2003) found that cellular responses to color cues or delay activity appeared strongly, with specific action-reward combinations. It remains possible that cells monitoring behavioral conflict may reside in the anterior cingulate region, belonging to the medial prefrontal cortex.

6.2. Exploring Functions of Cingulate Motor Areas: Studies on Human Subjects

Motor Control Functions

The nature of CMA involvement in specific aspects of motor control is not well understood. Due to the morphological complexity of the cingulate cortex and technical difficulties in approaching each of its sub-regions, even a simple question of the spatial localization of cingulate motor areas has not been satisfactorily answered, and not enough is known about the issue of somatotopy. Paus et al. (1993) measured changes in rCBF during performance of manual, oculomotor, and verbal motor tasks. With motor tasks performed with a hand, two foci of activity increase were found close to the cingulate sulcus anterior to and posterior to the vertical plane that passes through the anterior commissure (Paus, 2001). Their oculomotor task yielded two activation foci: rostrally within the most anterior part of the anterior cingulate cortex, just above the genu of the corpus callosum, and caudally in an area rostral to the forelimb focus. Furthermore, their verbal task yielded activations in the paracingulate gyrus and the peri-genual aspect of the cingulate sulcus, with an additional focus just anterior to the caudal oculomotor focus. These findings suggest the existence of somatotopic organization for cingulate motor areas, basically similar to that found in subhuman primates. Studies on deficits after localized lesions in the cingulate cortex (Paus et al., 1991; Stephan et al., 1999) lend support to this view of somatotopic organization. One possibility is that the caudal focus for the forelimb task corresponds to the caudal cingulate zone (CCZ, Picard & Strick, 1996), and the rostral focus may reside in the rostral cingulate zone (RCZ). Although the CCZ has been viewed as involved in the execution of simple motor tasks (Fink et al., 1997), no reported study has attempted to look into its contribution to the control of parameters for motor outputs, such as direction or force. This seems to be because deficits caused by cingulate lesions, in general, do not include apparent paralysis or motor ataxia.

Published reports point to the role of the anterior cingulate cortex in response initiation and maintaining a state of motor readiness (Turken & Swick 1999; Hoshi et al. 2005). For the rostral activation foci, the magnitude of activation varies greatly depending on the nature of the behavioral task, being greater during unlearned motor tasks, and in the presence of stimulus-response conflict (Paus et al., 1993). Human studies on the rostral cingulate zone, thus, have been focused primarily on exploring its role in cognitive aspects of motor behavior.

Executive Control, Conflict/Error Detection, and Action-Outcome Association

Brain imaging studies have suggested that the anterior cingulate cortex (ACC) has a role in the executive control of behavior, together with the lateral prefrontal cortex (Cohen et al., 1997; Courtney et al., 1998; Duncan & Owen, 2000). Behavioral conditions requiring working memory (Petit et al., 1998) or requiring task interference or task switching (Botvinick et al., 2001; Kerns et al., 2004), activate both areas. A subsequent study, however, revealed that the lateral prefrontal cortex is more involved in maintaining the attentional demands, while the ACC is more involved in evaluative processes (Macdonald et al., 2000). It was also found that the ACC is more active when there is a change in response set or when there is a conflict between possible responses, and less active when stimulus selection is at issue (Van Veen et al., 2001; Rushworth et al., 2002). Lesion studies also suggest different behavioral roles of the two areas. ACC lesions had little effect on working memory tasks (Murray et al., 1989; Rushworth et al., 2003), but resulted in impairment of response preparation tasks with response conflict, but not of selective-attention or divided-attention tasks (Turken & Swick, 1999). Taken together, the ACC appears more involved in behavioral adjustments, based on an assessment of an individual's own actions or the outcome, rather than exerting top-down regulation of behavior in accordance with information on stimulus-outcome association.

A combination of ERP and fMRI measurements revealed an error-associated activity centered on the anterior cingulate region (Ullsperger & Cramon, 2001). Although the error-related activity may reflect the detection of an error, an alternative interpretation suggests that the activity may reflect response conflict (Botvinik et al., 2001). One possibility is that the source of error- and conflict-detecting activity may reside in different portions in the ACC. From a different perspective arose the view that the ACC has a role in encoding the relationship between an action and the reinforcement value of its outcome. Two reports support this view; an fMRI study (Bush et al., 2002) found that dorsal ACC is active when subjects performed reward-based decision making, and analysis of single-cells in the dACC pointed to its role in linking reward information with alternative actions (Williams et al., 2004; see Shima & Tanji, 1998). Moreover, ACC cells encode the values of action outcomes in terms of their probability, payoff, and cost (Kennerley et al., 2009). It seems reasonable to summarize the relevant literature to indicate that the ACC, including human analog of CMAr, is concerned with the evaluation of behavioral outcomes and the association between action and outcome (Rushworth et al., 2004); the monitoring of response conflict might be subsumed under the more general description of the evaluation of outcomes (Botvinick et al., 2007). Future work will reveal the validity of a more recent proposal that the ACC is involved in self-reflection on actions (Passingham et al., 2010).

7. Concluding remarks

When exploring the raisons d'être for the existence of multiple higher-order motor areas, one should first establish the anatomical framework of the neural circuits in which each area is uniquely situated. The ultimate goal of the inquiry, then, is to understand how individual areas are used for behavioral control in the midst of dynamic, multilevel operations of structures encompassing the entire part of the central nervous system. To reach this goal, it is essential to investigate mechanisms of operations of each area with experimental studies adequately planned to look into area-unique involvement in behavioral control; we have learned enough that ill-posed questions or inadequately performed studies can easily misdirect the understanding of motor areas. It is fortunate to conclude this chapter with a remark that we have finally begun to witness the fascinating reality of operations taking place in each of the multiple areas, with prospects of future studies revealing a great deal more.

2 Hand and Face Observation and the Role of Frontal Areas for Emotional Appraisal

Martin Lotze

Key Words: Gesture, Mirror neuronal System, dopaminergic, temporo-frontal Interaction, emotional Face Recognition, social Interaction, superior temporal Gyrus, Putamen, BA 47

1. Instead of a Preface - Some Personal Comments on the Work Together with Ulrike

In 2000/2001, Ulrike and I were preparing an application as a contribution to the Sonderforschungsbereich SFB 550 "Erkennen-Lokalisieren-Handeln" at the Institute of Niels Birbaumer in Tübingen who brought us together. I was highly interested in the neuropsychology of apraxia and gesture recognition and therefore I knew Ulrike Halsband´s work and felt honoured to do research together. The idea was to joint our knowledge in neuropsychology, emotional research and functional imaging. In addition, we intended to integrate Arto Laihinen´s knowledge about PET and Parkinson's Disease (PD). At that time not much had been published about emotional perceptive disturbances in Parkinson patients. The aim was to develop a combination of gestural and emotional presentation material to separate different aspects of hand movement processing, hand motor performance in relation to the body (in an emotional neutral context) and expressive gestures. In the absence of a proper presentation set (we were eager to present videos and not only pictures), we developed video material on emotional expressive gestures and applied them to healthy participants and dopamine restricted Parkinson patients. Arto Laihinen presented us with some emotional expressive video sets from Finland, but for a European located farther south it was hard to find any emotional expression in the faces of the Finnish performers, especially when we asked our Italian researchers at the institute. For conducting the studies and investigating patients we received considerable help from Ulrike Heymans, who worked as a Ph.D. student in the project. In addition, all the investigations on dopamine availability in the patients were done by Matthias Reimold of the PET-Centre in Tübingen, who was interested to test a new dopamine tracer for our project.

2. Important Findings our Work was Based on

When we started our investigation most of the models on movement observation were drawn from research in monkeys. Ungerleider and Mishkin (1982) differentiated a ventral pathway for object recognition and a dorsal pathway for additionally needed visual guidance of actions towards the object. Based on observations in neurological impaired patients, Milner and Goodale (1995). postulated that both streams process information about object features and their spatial localization, but differ in their preferential functions, which is the recognition and categorization for the ventral pathway, and the location of objects in relation to the observer for the dorsal pathway. Whereas the dorsal stream refers to rapid transformations of sensory input into motor commands, the ventral stream uses cognitive cues for generating actions (Jeanerod, 1994). In 1999, Decety and Grézes published a functional imaging study in humans and differentiated the two streams: the ventral pathway projects from V1 through V2 and V4 to the inferior temporal cortex and the anterior section of the superior temporal sulcus (STS), whereas the dorsal pathway projects from V1 through V2 and V3 to the middle temporal area (V5/MT) and into the superior temporal and parietal cortex.

If moving hands are presented to monkeys (Fadiga et al., 1995) or humans (Hari et al., 1998; Grézes et al., 1998), the dorsal pathway is particularly active: an internal repetition of the observed hand movements leads to an activation in the premotor cortex (PMC) and the primary motor cortex (M1). With activation of premotor areas during hand and face movement observation, a close relation of a simple internal repetition in a motor region and the recognition of signals, which can then be used for communication, was shown by Rizzolatti and co-workers (e.g. Gallese et al., 1996). Additional activation in the supplementary motor area (SMA), present only during meaningful movement observation, may be internally generated by a participation of programs of action plans (Decety & Grézes, 1999).

Expressive gestures can be differentiated from conversational gestures (gestures accompanying speech; Zinnober & Martlew, 1985), since they are performed without additional articulation. The evolvement of spoken language from hand gestures has a long history in speech theory (e.g., Piaget, 1930). In monkeys, the perception of hand gestures activates area F5, which is thought to be a homologue of Brodmann's area (BA) 45. Along the pars opercularis (BA 44) it constitutes Broca's area (Rizzolatti & Arbib, 1998).

Expressive gestures do not only share a common cognitive representation with language (Goldin-Meadow, 1999) but also show a high emotional involvement. Together with the existence of gestic communication in monkeys this leads to the assumption that gestures activate phylogenetically older brain areas than spoken language.

Thus based on the studies on movement observation in monkeys, we postulated that the observation of meaningful hand movements and gestures should both involve left BA 44, but only expressive gestures were supposed to evoke activation in BA 45 and 47, which are involved in the recognition of semantic and emotional aspects of speech. The internal motor repletion and the interaction of gestures and language are not only highly interesting but also a common poly-sensory area for both, the ventral and the dorsal pathway, the superior temporal sulcus (STS). Here, form and motion interact (Oram & Perrett, 1996) and both facial and hand movements are recognized with regard to the relevance in the social context (Allison et al., 2000).

3. Interaction of Temporal and Frontal Areas and the Basal anglia Loops

It has been shown in macaque monkeys that non-spatial visual information recognition processed in the inferior temporal lobe is conveyed to the frontal cortex via direct cortico-cortical connections and indirectly through the basal ganglia (Wise & Murray, 2000). Therefore the basal ganglia may be important for facial recognition involved in gesture understanding, too. In humans, activations in the right putamen and insula were shown to be specific for the perception of the facial expression of disgust (Phillips et al., 1997). Lesion data in humans support findings that the putamen and insula are crucial for the perception of disgust in facial recognition and vocal expression recognition (Calder et al., 2001). These data are especially interesting, because they describe interactions between the different networks for gestural and emotional detection. However, little was known about moving facial or gestural stimuli demonstrating the loop between the STS, the basal ganglia and the fronto-basal structures in man.

In our first study, we compared possible differences between fMRI activation maps during the observation of different types of meaningful movements: isolated hand movements of the right dominant side, body referred movements and expressive gestures. We hypothesized that the cerebral representation of the observation of hand and body referred movements should differ in relevant cerebral regions for face and body movement recognition whereas expressive gestures should involve additional emotional relevant areas. Differences in movements in relation to the actor's face and trunk compared to isolated hand movements should be reflected in an increased STS activation, since more relevant information of the social context integrating hand face and trunk movements are given.

4. The Role of Dopamine: Why Investigate Parkinson Patients?

Parkinson´s disease (PD) is predominantly associated with motor production impairment, resulting in reduced facial and gesture expression as one of the key symptoms (Smith et al., 1996). Motor impairment is often accompanied by neuropsychological deficits (Dubois & Pillon, 1997) including impaired recognition of emotional (e.g. Breitenstein et al., 1998) and non-emotional faces (Dewick et al., 1991). Selective deficits in the recognition of facial expressions of disgust are observed in symptomatic PD patients as well as pre-symptomatic

Huntington's disease patients, an illness associated with neuronal loss in the striatum (Suzuki et al., 2006).

The most important pathology in PD is the loss of dopaminergic neurons in the substantia nigra, resulting in substantially reduced dopamine availability predominantly in the striatum. The striatum, including the caudate nucleus and the putamen, is critically involved in involuntary emotional responses such as facial expressions during the execution of expressive gestures (Yin & Knowlton, 2006). In addition, the striatum has an important function for the recognition of emotional faces. For the putamen, it has been demonstrated that it is critically involved in the perception of facial expression in both monkey (Logothetis et al., 1999) and man (Calder et al., 2000). Therefore, probably in humans as well, the putamen is part of a perceptive system involved in both higher order visual processing and presumably in the recognition of emotional facial expression.

In this context the structural connectivity of the basal ganglia is of high interest: In addition to the motor loops, the striatum is interconnected via the dorsal caudate nucleus to the dorsolateral prefrontal cortex (BA 46) and via the ventral striatum (ventral caudate and putamen) to the lateral orbitofrontal lobe and via the ventral striatum to the anterior cingulate cortex and the medial orbitofrontal lobe (Alexander & Crutcher, 1990). In addition, Middleton and Strick (Middleton & Strick, 1996) described a projection from the ventral striatum to the temporal lobe (fusiform gyrus up to the superior temporal sulcus: STS), which might be extremely important for facial expression recognition.

Temporal higher visual recognition areas involved in facial (fusiform gyrus; Haxby et al., 2000), and social perception (STS; Allison et al., 2000) are connected to limbic areas and the ventrolateral prefrontal cortex (VLPFC; BA 47; Sprengelmeyer et al., 1998) engaged in emotional processing via dopamine sensitive structures in the putamen and caudate. In addition, more unspecific influences might also contribute to altered emotional expression perception in PD patients: for instance severe neuropathological changes in the amygdala in these patients (Braak et al., 1994) might alone result in deficits in emotional facial recognition.

We intended to test whether PD patients show a specific decrease in cerebral activation in response to expressive (rated with different emotional valence) and other body and face referred meaningful gestures. We expected that, due to decreased striatal dopamine, a reduced fMRI-activation should be present in areas known to be involved in the processing of emotional facial expression. In order to investigate possible associations between striatal dopamine transporter availability (DTA) and functional activation during expressive gesture recognition including emotional facial expression we used a combination of a positron emission tomography (PET) and fMRI approach.

For PET, new dopamine ligands, such as $[^{11}C]$d-threo-methylphenidate, both seem specific to accurately estimate DTA in regions with high DTA density (i.e. striatum) (Volkow et al., 1995), and also correlate highly positively with the severity of motor symptoms in idiopathic PD patients (Breit et al., 2006). We expected to detect correlations between the fMRI-response to specific gestures and DTA in the putamen or caudate.

5. Results for the Main Effects of the Different Type of Gestures

All conditions showed occipital (V1/V2), occipitotemporal (V5), left superior parietal (SPL), superior temporal sulcus (STS), bilateral inferior frontal gyrus (especially in BA 44), premotor cortex (PMC) and cerebellar activation when compared to rest (see Figure 1). Observed hand movements performed in extrapersonal space showed additional activation in the left M1 and the bilateral thalamus. Body referred movements including presentation of the actor's face showed bilateral activation in M1, bilateral thalamus, anterior part of the SMA (pre-SMA), right SPL and right gyrus fusiformis. Gestures showed additional activation in the right putamen, right amygdala, pre-SMA, anterior inferior frontal gyrus (predominantly BA 45), bilateral orbitofrontal cortex (BA 47), left medial temporal lobe and right gyrus fusiformis. Cerebellar activation sites differed within conditions: expressive gestures activated the posterior hemisphere whereas isolated hand movements activated the anterior hemisphere bilaterally.

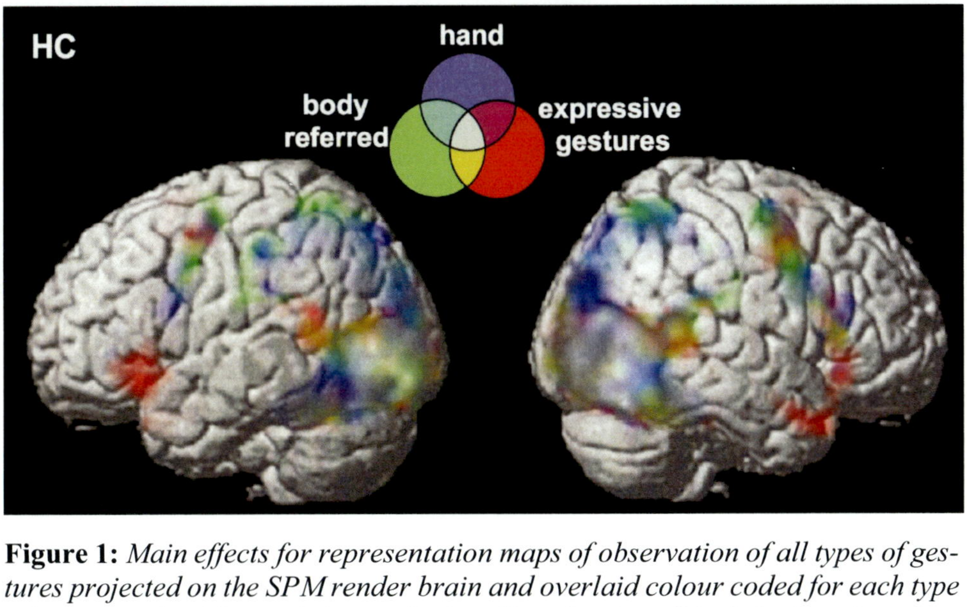

Figure 1: *Main effects for representation maps of observation of all types of gestures projected on the SPM render brain and overlaid colour coded for each type of gesture in healthy participants. Isolated hand actions (blue), body-referred actions (green), expressive gestures (red). Overlay is coded in additive colouring demonstrated with colour circles (Figure from Lotze et al., 2006).*

6. Results of the Comparisons Between Different Types of Meaningful Gestures in Healthy Participants

We found that isolated hand movements showed increased activation in primary and secondary motor areas, possibly implying an internal repetition of the movement (Lotze et al., 2006). Body referred movements with presentation of the actor's face, contrasted with hand movements, showed increased activation in the left STS. The putamen showed the highest significance level if expressive gestures were compared to hand movements. By direct comparison of observed movements (hand and body referred) with emotional relevant expressive gestures activation in the "dorsal pathway" was present, whereas observation of emotional expressive gestures showed higher activation in the "ventral pathway" including the putamen and the basal areas of the frontal lobes.

7. PET-and Performance Characteristics for the PD Patients

Dopamine transporter availability (DTA) of PD patients was reduced (to 22% in the left putamen and to 30% in the left caudate) a finding which is comparable to previous reports (Breit et al., 2006). PD patients made more gesture recognition mistakes (24% incorrect) than HCs (5% incorrect) but valence ratings did not differ between subject groups. Cognitive screening (Mini Mental State) scores did not differ between patient and control group.

8. fMRI Differences Between PD Patients and Matched Controls

In contrast to HC, PD patients showed lower fMRI-activation during observation of all presented gestures in the bilateral occipito-temporal junction including visual motion area (V5), the fusiform gyrus, around the bilateral parietal sulcus, the right dorsal premotor cortex, SMA and cerebellar hemispheres, right STS, right temporal pole and left putamen. Therefore, for the observation of hand gestures only, a decrease of activation both in the dorsal stream (M1, SPL, dPMC, SMA) but also in parts of the ventral stream (V5, STS, fusiform gyrus, occipito-temporal junction) was present (Figure 2A).

Representation during observation of body referred movements showed predominantly decreased activation in PD patients in inferior parietal and occipito-temporal areas and the right anterior pole. These are areas of the ventral stream.

When brain activation during observation of expressive gestures was compared between groups, PD patients showed additionally lower activation in the left BA 47, left STS, bilateral sensorimotor cortex, bilateral putamen, medial cingulate gyrus, midbrain and in the bilateral amygdala. Again, except for the sensorimotor cortex, these are areas of the ventral stream, but also areas processing emotional response (amygdala, BA 47) and social recognition (STS).

The contrast patients minus HC revealed no significant effect for any of the observed gestures. Results of the comparison HC minus PD are shown in Figure 2 for all three types of gestures investigated.

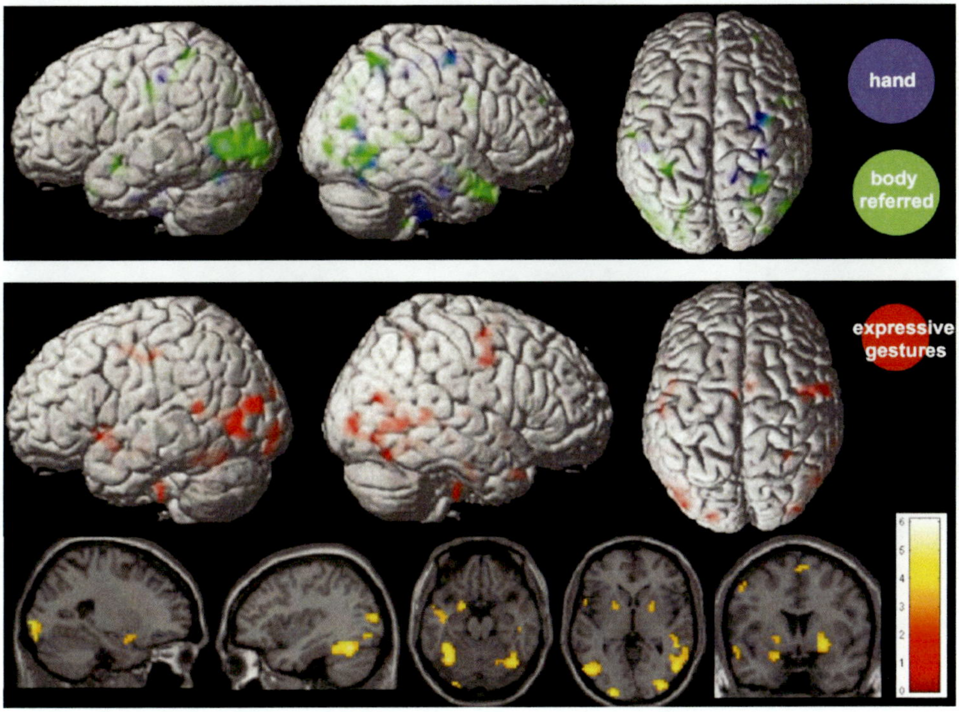

Figure 2: *Contrast of activation patterns HC minus PD. Top: comparison for hand movements (blue) and body referred movements (green). Bottom:* comparison for expressive gestures (red; partially taken from Lotze et al., 2009).

9. Correlation Analysis of DTA in Patients and fMRI and Behavioural Measures

The Hoehn and Yahr score (Hoehn & Yahr, 1967), the most frequently used score to measure impairment in PD increasing with more impairment, was inversely associated to striatal DTA. In addition, DTA in the right caudate correlated negatively with the total number of mistakes of expressive gesture recognition. During observation of expressive gestures, bilateral BA 47 fMRI-activation showed a positive association with left putamen DTA (see Figure 3).

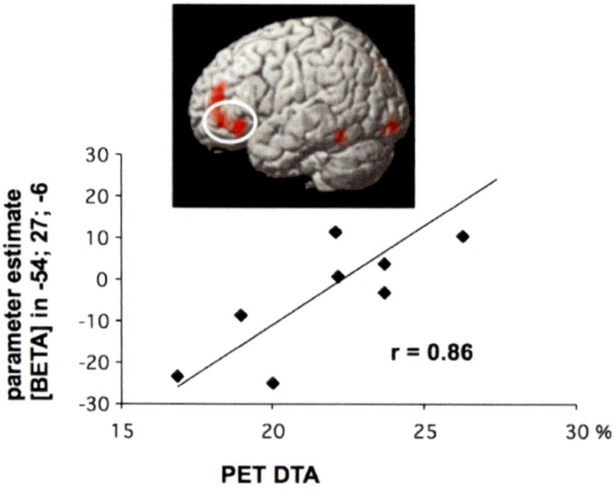

Figure 3: *Positive association between left putamen DTA and left BA 47 fMRI-activation magnitude during observation of emotional gestures minus observation of non-emotional body referred gestures. Brain image shows the results for regression analysis uncorrected for multiple comparisons ($p<0.001$). The white circle depicts BA 47 left.*

For non-emotional body referred movements an increasing number of mistakes in gesture recognition correlated positively with activation in left STS, left putamen and right BA 46. Therefore the frontal evaluation areas in BA 46 and the putamen on the dominant hemisphere were increasingly involved together with right hemispheric observation areas discriminating social relevance of gestures in the STS.

10. Discussion: What was New for Our Understanding of Gestural Processing?

Our data from the studies conducted together in Tübingen are in good accordance with more recent reports about gesture observation in imaging and large lesion mapping studies. A recent overview and further differentiation of the dorsal stream in a dorso-dorsal and a ventro-dorsal was provided by Binkofski and Buxbaum (2013). Here, the ventro-dorsal stream comprises the ventral premotor cortex (vPMC), the inferior frontal gyrus, the inferior parietal lobe (IPL) and V5, V5, whereas the dorso-dorsal includes the dorsal PMC (dPMC) and superior parietal lobe (SPL). Lesion mapping studies showed that inferior frontal and insula lesions are associated more with transient gestures, which are those involving tools and pantomimes, whereas IPL and SPL lesions are more associated with intransient gestures (semantic meaning such as applauding) (Hoeren et al., 2014).

In our study, during the observation of hand movements an apparent internal repetition was present, which activated left M1, bilateral PMC and areas involved in sensorimotor integration (left superior parietal cortex, anterior cerebellar hemisphere). Motor activation during movement observation might therefore enable a direct recruitment of relevant regions for motor learning important for short and long term motor training (Lotze et al., 2003; Pau et al., 2013).

Apart from the described inferior frontal gyrus (in our study more precisely located in BA 44 or pars opercularis) being involved in all three types of movements observed, we found activation in the anterior part of the left inferior frontal gyrus (BA 45; pars triangularis) during expressive gesture observation. Together with the activation in left BA 47 this area is important for semantic evaluation (Dapretto & Bookheimer, 1999).

In the parietal cortex the most pronounced activation was observed when body referred movements were presented. These findings are in agreement with clinical brain lesion studies, suggesting that a basic deficit in patients with apraxia concerns the ability to code and comprehend movements in relation to the body-scheme (e.g. Halsband et al., 2001).

The left STS region was activated during all conditions, since it is relevant for the perception of hand, body and face movements. Grézes et al. (1999) showed that especially the left STS region is activated during the observation of meaningful hand movements. In the present study, the left STS had significantly higher activation when body referred movements were compared to isolated hand movements. The increased STS activation during body related movements may be explained by a higher amount of socially relevant objects. In a review of 15 different studies evaluating face, body and hand representation in the right and left STS (Allison et al., 2000), the face and body are represented more posterior than the hand, in the same location which showed activation after contrasting body referred to isolated hand movements. The STS receives feedback and sends feed-forward projections from and to the amygdala, that assigns emotional valence to sensory input together with the orbitofrontal cortex (Puce et al., 1999).

The putamen has been described as important for facial expression in monkeys, since it conveys information of face perception represented in the inferior temporal lobe to the frontal lobe (Logothetis, 1999; Wise & Murray, 2000). In our study comparing gestures to hand movements, the only significant activation was observed in the right putamen underlining its relevance for the evaluation of emotion in facial stimuli.

11. What was New in Our Understanding of the Dopamine Modulation of Emotional Gestures?

In line with other studies that reported impaired emotional recognition in PD-patients (e.g. Suzuki et al., 2006), we found a significant decrease of recognition of emotional, but not non-emotional gestures in the PD patients. With respect to the specific recognition deficits of emotional gestures, we hypothesized that a decrease in left BA47-activation should correlate with decreased left putamen DAT, which indeed was the case; access to BA 47 seems to be modulated by left putamen DAT.

Facial and social recognition areas in the temporal lobe are connected to the ventral striatum (Middleton & Strick, 1996), and the ventral striatum projects into the VLPFC (Alexander & Crutcher, 1990). Loss of ventral striatal dopamine might therefore specifically modulate the interconnection between analytic temporal facial recognition areas (fusiform gyrus and STS) and an area of prefrontal appraisal such as the VLPFC. This is supported by the findings that representation maps during emotional minus non-emotional gestures reveal only VLPFC activation in HC, left VLPFC activation was increased in HC, if compared to PD, and DAT in the left putamen and left VLPFC BOLD magnitude was associated in PD.

12. Insula Activation in Response to Emotional Gestures is Altered in PDA

The bilateral anterior insula showed increased activation with an increasing amount of errors in emotional gesture recognition in PD patients. Together with the bilateral amygdala, the anterior cingulate cortex (ACC) and the medial and lateral ventral prefrontal cortex (mPFC/vPFC), this area is involved in emotional processing of pictures (Phan et al., 2002). The insula is associated with the subjective feeling of emotional states. The anterior insula seems to reflect the self-conscious aspect of the rated valence of a given emotion (Anders et al., 2004) and is highly associated with anticipation of emotional response (Büchel & Dolan, 2000). For PD patients, it seems plausible that with increasing problems in the recognition of emotional gestures, the insula is increasingly involved, possibly compensating for a loss of dopamine in the putamen.

13. STS Activation and the Processing of Gestures in PD

Bilateral MT and left STS activation correlated with problems in recognizing non-emotional gestures. These data underline that areas involved in the analysis of movements and gestures are increasingly active when having trouble in the appropriate assignment of the non-emotional gestures. Correlates of recognition mistakes in non-emotional material are restricted on these analytic areas and do not include prefrontal regions or regions involved in emotional processing. In the patient group, BOLD magnitude specific to emotional gestures was not only decreased in the left VLPFC, but also in the right STS. The STS receives axons from and sends projections into the amygdala and the VLPFC cortex (e.g. Ethofer et al., 2013). This tight interconnection and the highly important role of the STS for the recognition of emotional facial expressions (e.g. Breiter et al., 1996) make this region a key area for the recognition of emotional gestures. In our pre-study (Lotze et al., 2006), we observed a highly positive correlation between the activation in the right STS and the negative valence of emotional gestures. In this context, a reduced activation in PD patients may underlie the substantial deficit in the recognition of emotional gestures.

14. Outlook: New Plans and Current Protocols

There are several new investigations, since we performed and published our studies on gesture observation. Dirk Wildgruber's group in Tübingen continued to conduct remarkable studies on emotional facial and prosodic recognition and some of their latest studies were performed together with our group in Greifswald (Brück et al., 2011; Jacob et al., 2014; Kreifelts et al., 2014). Cornelius Weiller's group in Freiburg carried out lesion mapping studies that demonstrated specific lesion locations for the imitation of hand movements or pantomimes (Hoeren et al., 2014): Imitation deficits were observed in areas specifically related to the dorso-dorsal stream, such as the posterior intraparietal sulcus and superior parietal lobule. Pantomime deficits were associated with ventro-dorsal regions, such as the supramarginal gyrus, as well as brain structures belonging to the ventral stream. They also combined diffusion weighted imaging studies with fMRI in healthy participants and showed different pathways between areas involved in gesture imitation (Vry et al., 2015). These authors concluded, that "abstract, meaningless as well as previously unknown gestures can be imitated via a direct sensorimotor route encompassing dorsal visuo-motor pathways (dorso-dorsal route), whereas object-associated actions involving semantic processing are established by interactions with the ventral stream, anatomically implemented in the ventro-dorsal route. Object effects can be assigned to the ventro-dorsal route and are anatomically separable from pantomime-specific effects. Pantomime additionally implicates a symbolic gesture involving a functional interaction with an absent object, requiring an additional cognitive process to guide movement planning."

In a recent principal component analysis of fMRI measurements during observation of co-speech gestures showed that co-speech gesture production engages areas of both the language and gesture production networks (Marstaller & Burianová, 2015). In a group of patients with white matter lesions due to encephalitis disseminata, we performed a lesion mapping study and found that white matter lesions associated with deficits in facial emotional recognition were located in regions that interconnect the temporal and the frontal lobe (Krause et al., 2009). Interestingly, in children with obesity, who exhibit impaired emotional response and psychophysiological deficits in emotional pictures might well be associated with a dopamine deficit discussed for people with obesity (Davids et al., 2010; Kinder et al., 2014). It is tempting to associate these findings with PD patients with dopamine deficits. It might also be appealing to investigate the recognition of facial expression, emotional gestures and body related gestures in a group of Parkinson patients who are freshly diagnosed before and after a Dopamine provocation. Here the modulation of emotional recognition can be demonstrated in the same patient and might be combined again with mapping data during observation.

3 Towards a Representational Understanding of Medial Temporal Lobe Processing

Patric Meyer and Herta Flor

Key Words: *Recognition memory, hippocampus, perirhinal cortex, fMRI, ERPs, VBM, contextual conditioning, semantics, aMCI, neuropsychological assessment*

Memory is not a unitary construct but can be subdivided into different functional categories. Therefore the psychological term "memory" refers to a large set of distinct cognitive abilities. Encoding refers to the acquisition of new information. Storage reflects the maintenance of this information over an extended time period. The duration of this maintenance delineates short-term memory from long-term memory (James, 1890; Atkinson & Shifrin, 1968). Retrieval captures the access to this stored information. Reports by Scoville and Milner (1957) on the famous patient H.M., who showed a deep amnesia for all events that occurred after the bilateral resection of his medial temporal lobes (MTL) but at the same time displayed an intact ability to acquire several skills and habits, raised the question whether long-term memory can be seen as a unitary system. Subsequently, long-term memory has been subdivided into implicit (non-declarative) and explicit (declarative) memory. Implicit memory refers to the fact that experiences of an event can affect later behaviour in the absence of conscious retrieval. This may encompass procedural memories, simple forms of conditioning or priming (see Schacter, 1994, for a review). It can be assessed by indirect tasks in which memory for studied information is expressed by speeded reaction times or identification accuracy like word stem or word fragment completions. Explicit memory instead is accompanied by the awareness of remembering, for example, when people bring to mind an event from the past and figuratively relive it. This form of remembrance can be further divided into episodic memory, i.e. memory for events that compose a unique personal experience, and semantic memory, i.e. factual information that is independent of the specific episodes in which that information was acquired (Tulving, 1973). These two components of declarative memory can be shown to dissociate if one tries to remember the episode that led to the learning of a particular fact. We know that Paris is the capital of France but are unlikely to remember the episode that led to the learning of this fact. Explicit memory can be assessed by direct tasks such as free recall, cued recall or recognition.

Recognition memory describes the mental capacity of becoming aware that a particular event has been encountered before, for example when one recognizes a person one knows in a crowd of strangers. Recognition can be compared with various forms of recall memory where specific content information is retrieved from memory. However, recognition does not require the recall of specific details (e.g., one can recognize a person as being familiar without being able to recall who exactly they are or where you know them from). Nevertheless, recognition can certainly benefit from recall of specific information, if one can recall that the person one recognized at the supermarket is in fact one's doctor. The observation that recognition memory can be subserved by these two qualitatively different types of memory signals - recollection and familiarity - is the fundamental idea of dual-process theories of recognition memory (Mandler, 1980; Yonelinas, 2002). Recollection generally refers to retrieval of contextual information; familiarity refers to a feeling attributed to recent exposure to an item, in the absence of retrieval of contextual information and can vary from a weak intuition to a strong belief. Others, however, have argued that behavioural data from the recognition memory paradigm can be explained by assuming only a single continuum of memory strength (usually within the context of signal detection theory: Dunn, 2004; Heathcote, 2003). Under such a notion the sense of familiarity only reflects a weaker trace strength than recollection of prior information, i.e. these two processes differ only quantitatively.

The difference between these two kinds of subjective experiences that occur during recognition is easily demonstrated in everyday life by the example of meeting a person one recognizes on the street. Sometimes we can specifically place where, or when in the past, we had met the person. This is a recollective process. In contrast, we sometimes gain a strong sense that we have met the person before, but cannot identify where or when we originally encountered the individual. The person is familiar to us, despite the fact that we cannot recollect unique details of the initial meeting event. This is a familiarity process.

Past cognitive and neuropsychological research suggests that recollection and familiarity are functionally distinct processes, with different experimental manipulations producing different effects on recollection and familiarity (for reviews see Diana et al., 2006; Yonelinas, 2002). For example, levels of processing manipulations (Gregg & Gardiner, 1994), division of attention (Gardiner & Parkin, 1990), and benzodiazepine administration (Hirshman et al., 2002) during study affect recollection estimates more so than familiarity. In contrast, speeded responding experiments suggest that familiarity processes are present earlier than recollection processes (Yonelinas & Jacoby, 1995). Moreover, familiarity is supposed to be restricted to single or unitized items detached from additional contextual information (although there are cases where familiarity can contribute to contextual memory (Montaldi & Mayes, 2010; Addante et al., 2012a). By this, familiarity-supporting representations share important characteristics with semantic long-term memory. Recollection instead allows the retrieval of associations between arbitrary events and hence is seen as a core feature of episodic memory.

A considerable number of electrophysiological studies suggested that the two processes of recognition are distinct in showing that familiarity and recollection can be mapped onto two qualitatively distinguishable event-related potential (ERP) components. In recognition memory tasks, a robust ERP difference between correctly judged old and new items, the so-called old/new effect, has been found that starts around 300 ms after item onset and takes the form of more positive waveforms for correctly recognized old compared to correctly rejected new items. Moreover, distinct spatiotemporal aspects of these old/new effects have been linked to different subcomponents of recognition memory. An early old/new effect between 300 and 500 ms can be dissociated from a later effect with a more parietal topography between 400 and 800 ms (e.g. Mecklinger, 2000). The early component has been associated with the assessment of the overall similarity between study and test items, a form of memory that is accompanied by a subjective feeling of familiarity or knowing. This effect is assumed to arise from the attenuation of a frontally focused N400-like component (Curran, 1999) presumably reflecting the facilitated access to conceptual and perceptual information related to the test item (Mecklinger, 2006). Moreover, it has been dissociated from ERP correlates of pure implicit memory processes (Nessler et al., 2005) and was shown to be insensitive to levels of processing (Rugg et al., 1998) and perceptual manipulations (Curran & Cleary, 2003). The assumed memory process reflected in this effect permits to discriminate between old and new items but does not support a further differentiation between studied items and perceptually or semantically similar lures (Nessler et al., 2001). However, the exact functional meaning of the early old/new effect is still under debate. Yovel and Paller (2004) investigated recognition memory for pre-experimentally unfamiliar face stimuli. They showed that familiarity and recollection were associated with topographically similar ERP correlates. Both memory processes elicited parietally accentuated brain potentials, merely with smaller amplitudes and a shorter duration for familiarity than for recollection. This finding led the authors to assume that familiarity may arise by virtue of a subset of the neural processing responsible for recollection and that the mid-frontal old/new effect, generally observed in studies using highly overlearned stimulus material, may not reflect familiarity, but verbally mediated conceptual priming.

Performance in associative memory tests is commonly thought to necessitate recollection while familiarity cannot support memory for associations. However, familiarity may contribute to associative memory when the to-be-associated stimuli are unitized during learning. We investigated the electrophysiological correlates of retrieval of word pairs after two different encoding conditions (Bader et al., 2010). Semantically unrelated word pairs were presented as distinct lexical units in a sentence frame (nonunitized word pairs) or together with a definition that allows to combine word pairs to a new concept (unitized word pairs). At test, participants discriminated between word pairs that appeared in the identical pairing during study, recombined, or new pairs. Memory processes were examined by mean ERPs. An early old/new effect with a parietal maximum was found for unitized word pairs while a qualitatively different late old/new effect was elicited by non-unitized word pairs. These findings suggest that one-trial-unitized word pairs are recognized in a different way than non-unitized word pairs suggesting that unitization leads to the engagement of specific forms of familiarity— conceptual fluency and absolute familiarity.

In contrast, the parietal old/new effect that can be observed in situations where participants are capable of remembering detailed information about studied items is related to recollection (Wilding & Herron, 2006). For instance, this component was shown to be larger for remember than for know responses (Düzel et al., 1997), was associated with the successful retrieval of stimulus features (Wilding & Rugg, 1996) and was shown to be selectively impaired in hippocampal amnesia (Düzel et al., 2001).

While item memory tasks are solvable by relying on familiarity-based processes, subjects usually have to engage in recollective processing to perform accurately in source memory tasks. Numerous behavioural studies report that in comparison to younger adults, memory performance in older adults is associated with an impairment of recollection while familiarity seems to be unaffected. To isolate brain activity related to item and context memory in real-time resolution and to determine the neuronal basis underlying memory alterations due to ageing, we established an EEG source memory paradigm, in which pictures had to be learned together with one of four screen positions (Hoppstädter et al., unpublished data). Retrieval of items and item-context associations was tested in a cross-sectional sample of 16 young and 16 healthy elderly subjects. Behavioural measures of accuracy for contextual retrieval were strongly reduced in seniors relative to young adults whereas item recognition was comparable. The ERP data indicated an early frontal old/new effect independent of source memory accuracy in both age groups suggesting intact familiarity-based item memory processes. In younger adults, a later left parietal old/new effect was evident when source memory success was taken into account. This effect was absent in healthy seniors suggesting impaired recollection. A later old/new effect emerged over frontal areas and might indicate the evaluative contribution of prefrontal areas to memory decisions. This effect was also missing in the older subjects implying a lack of strategic monitoring processes. In the young adults, ERP effects conclude with a late posterior effect independent of source memory accuracy, which presumably indicates the reinstatement of study details as part of response monitoring. In addition, results from oscillatory analyses suggest that differences in alpha and theta band power might explain the success of source memory decisions as well as the discrepancies observable between age groups in the ERP and on a behavioural level.

Taken together, ERP studies provide strong support that dissociable brain processes underlie recognition memory, although they do not establish the anatomical basis of these processes with any great precision due to the low spatial resolution of this method.

However, the processes underlying recognition memory have also been examined with functional neuroimaging techniques. Although this growing number of neuroimaging studies does not yield completely unequivocal findings, there seems to be converging evidence that recollection relies critically on the hippocampus proper, whereas familiarity-based recognition seems to be instantiated by computations in the anterior medial temporal lobe cortex (AMTL) comprising the entorhinal, parahippocampal and perirhinal cortices (see Henson, 2005, for a review). In sum, the hippocampus and the posterior parahippocampal cortex appear particularly important for encoding and retrieving source information and associations between distinct items. The AMTL on the other hand seems more involved in item information. For instance, using event-related functional magnetic resonance imaging (fMRI), Eldrige et al. (2000) demonstrated that activity in the hippocampus increased only when memory retrieval was accompanied by conscious recollection of the learning episode. Hippocampal activity did not increase for items recognized based on familiarity or for unrecognized items. It was argued that these results indicate that the hippocampus selectively supports the retrieval of episodic memories.

Other event-related fMRI studies have shown suppression effects of AMTL activity related to non-contextual item recognition which resembles decreased firing rates associated with familiarity in perirhinal neurons in animals (Brown & Xiang, 1998). For instance, Henson et al. (2003) reported a meta-analysis of data obtained in four experiments that used visually presented words, pictures of everyday objects, or faces as stimuli. When contrasting brain activity to experimentally familiar and unfamiliar items, a decrease of AMTL activity for familiar as opposed to unfamiliar items was found in all four datasets.

By contrasting brain activity for trials classified as 'misses' with brain activity for trials classified as 'hits', Weis et al. (2004) showed that the AMTL activity decrease is associated with the success of recognition and specifically with the success of non-contextual item recognition. To introduce context during study, stimuli (photographs of buildings and natural landscapes) were transformed into one of four single-color-scales. In the subsequent old/new recognition memory test, all stimuli were presented as grey scale photographs, and old-responses were followed by a four-alternative source judgment referring to the colour in which the stimulus was presented during study. While successful retrieval of contextual information was accompanied with an activity increase in the hippocampus, an activity decrease in the AMTL provided a familiarity signal sufficient for successful item recognition. Interestingly, also false alarms displayed a significant activity decrease which might be due to feature overlap between items actually studied and new, inducing a feeling of familiarity.

Subsequently, Gonsalves et al. (2005) revealed that the suppression of AMTL activity parametrically tracked levels of perceived item memory strength supporting the notion that this activity decrease is associated with non-contextual item recognition memory and represents a familiarity signal.

Parametric analyses of levels of felt familiarity-based responses could confirm that activity in the AMTL linearly decreased with the amount of perceived familiarity (Daselaar et al., 2006; Montaldi et al., 2006).

However, the mapping of ERPs on fMRI data remains difficult as scalp electroencephalography (EEG) is assumed to be largely insensitive to deep brain structures. Simultaneous recordings of EEG and fMRI might be helpful in reconciling surface ERPs with hemodynamic activations in medial temporal lobe (MTL) structures related to recognition memory. For this reason, we assessed EEG and fMRI simultaneously during a recognition memory paradigm to investigate which brain activations are modulated in relation to the ERP old/new effects (Hoppstädter et al., unpublished data). To this end we examined 17 participants in a yes/no recognition task with word stimuli. Single-trial amplitudes of ERP old/new effects were related to the haemodynamic signal in an EEG-informed fMRI analysis for a subset of 12 subjects. FMRI activation in the right dorsolateral prefrontal cortex and the right intraparietal sulcus was associated with the amplitude of the early frontal old/new effect (350-550 ms), and activation in the right posterior hippocampus, parahippocampal cortex and retrosplenial cortex was associated with the amplitude of the late parietal old new effect (580-750 ms). These results provide a direct link between electrophysiological and haemodynamic correlates of familiarity and recollection. Moreover, these findings in healthy subjects complement data from intracranial ERP recordings in epilepsy patients and lesion studies in hypoxia patients (Addante et al., 2012b; Grunwald et al., 2003) .

Although distinct parts of the MTL have been shown to be crucial for memory retrieval, controversy remains on how the specific subregions within the MTL contribute to the acquisition of memories. Encoding refers to those neural processes by which an event is transformed into a lasting neural representation that can later be used to adaptively guide behaviour. From a cognitive viewpoint encoding is not assumed as a singular process but rather built on a variety of operations such as perceiving, attending to, and working with internal and external events (Craik et al., 2007). From a neural perspective, successful encoding encompasses the formation of an engram or mnemonic trace that results from the brain mechanisms supporting the above-mentioned cognitive operations (Schacter et al., 1998). Importantly, this engram can vary in its future potential; it may be sufficient to support some types of retrieval goals but may be inadequate for others (Davachi & Dobbins, 2008).

Results from human neuroimaging studies have generally shown that encoding activity in the ventrolateral PFC, hippocampus, and the posterior parahippocampal cortex is enhanced for recollected items relative to forgotten items (e.

g. Uncapher et al., 2006). In contrast, robust correlates of familiarity-based recognition at encoding have not been identified that often (Kensinger & Schacter, 2006; Uncapher & Rugg, 2005).

Using ERPs to delineate the cerebral processes occurring when information is encoded into episodic memory, Mangels et al. (2001) selectively averaged ERPs on the basis of later retrieval during a recognition test. Items later retrieved on the basis of familiarity (known) were distinguished at encoding from later missed items by an enhanced left fronto-temporal negative wave around 400 ms similar to the N400, but did not demonstrate a negative posterior sustained potential and a positive frontal sustained potential like items retrieved with conscious recollection (remembered) did. They suggested that item-specific conceptual processing is sufficient to produce familiarity-based recognition, but additional processing is necessary for conscious recollection.

Davachi et al. (2003) used event-related fMRI to examine the relation between activation in distinct medial temporal lobe subregions during memory formation and the ability to later recognize an item as previously encountered (item recognition) and to later recollect specific contextual details about the prior encounter (source recollection). Encoding activation in hippocampus and in posterior parahippocampal cortex predicted later source recollection, but was uncorrelated with item recognition. In contrast, encoding activation in AMTL predicted later item recognition or stimulus familiarity, but not subsequent source recollection. These outcomes suggest that the subregions within the medial temporal lobe code for distinct properties of an episodic event and thereby subserve distinct, but complementary, learning mechanisms.

Ranganth et al. (2003) used event-related fMRI to examine the degree to which recollection and familiarity were supported by different MTL subregions. Their results showed that encoding activity in the AMTL selectively predicted familiarity-based recognition and was directly related to familiarity-based recognition confidence ratings, whereas activity in the hippocampus and posterior parahippocampal cortex selectively predicted recollection. Collectively, these results support the view that different subregions within the MTL memory system implement distinctive encoding processes that differentially sustain familiarity and recollection. In the AMTL, activation during encoding has been shown to be higher for items that were subsequently rated as highly familiar, whereas during retrieval, activation is lower for items that were highly familiar than for items that were forgotten.

Referring to these studies the "binding of item and context" (BIC) -Model by Diana et al. (2007) argues that during encoding the AMTL must be more active for items that are subsequently judged as more familiar because increased processing at study leads to strengthened item representations, allowing deactivation of the medial temporal lobe cortex during retrieval to the extent that the item is familiar. A more familiar item will lead to a larger deactivation because better encoding leads to a more efficient and sharper item representation. Thus, AMTL regions seem to sustain familiarity-based recognition not only by retrieving item-specific information but also by coding for the specific aspects of an event that can support later familiarity. These neuroimaging findings suggest that different forms of recognition-memory outcome can be predicted based on the success of qualitatively distinct encoding processes.

Previous ERP and fMRI studies investigating the correlation between MTL activity and later familiarity-based versus recollection-based recognition compared brain activity at encoding on the basis of subsequent success or failure during different types of later memory tests (Mangels et al., 2001; Davachi et al., 2003; Ranganath et al., 2003) without directly manipulating encoding processes per se. However, it might be useful to search for encoding operations which can enhance the probability of familiarity-based recognition already during learning. Consistently with the previously mentioned hypothesised representational resolution of the AMTL, past cognitive research suggests that, for example, processing the meaning of a stimulus (e.g., is the word concrete or abstract?) compared to processing perceptual aspects of a stimulus (e.g., is the word in upper or lower case?) at the time of study leads to a consistent increase in familiarity (e.g. Gardiner et al., 1996). Fittingly, in psycholinguistic research, it has been shown that semantic processing can induce activity modulations in the AMTL (see below). This has been observed for the presentation of semantically incongruent sentence endings like "I ordered a ham and cheese *scissors*." as well as for novel semantic relationships. Thus, we investigated whether the role of AMTL in declarative memory indeed results from its involvement in processing semantic aspects of an event in an event-related fMRI study (Meyer et al., 2010). For this purpose, a sentence comprehension task was employed which varied the demands of syntactic and semantic processing of the sentence-final word. By presenting those sentence-final words together with new words in a following incidental recognition memory test, we were able to determine the mnemonic consequences of presenting words in diverse sentential contexts. Greater semantic processing during comprehension activated regions in AMTL and led to response suppression in partly overlapping regions when the word was successfully retrieved. Data from a behavioural follow-up study as well as from a previous ERP study supported the view that enhanced semantic processing at study enhances familiarity based remembering in a subsequent test phase (Meyer et al., 2007; Meyer et al., 2010).

Neuropsychological case studies also support the importance of the AMTL region for familiarity-based recognition and of the hippocampus for recollection. Brain lesions including both the hippocampus and the surrounding MTL cortices disrupt both familiarity and recollection, whereas selective hippocampal damage disrupts recollection while leaving familiarity unaffected (Yonelinas et al., 2002; Mayes et al., 2002; Holdstock et al., 2005).

Investigating subjects with semantic dementia, Davies et al. (2004) found a significant contribution of the perirhinal cortex to semantic memory function as performance on a range of semantic tests correlated with perirhinal volume. Moreover, atrophy of the human perirhinal cortex, and of directly connected areas, was associated with semantic memory impairment but not episodic memory impairment. Using an implicit lexical-decision priming task to examine the integrity of the underlying semantic network, Rogers and Friedman (2008) also observed a substantial degradation of semantic memory in patients with semantic dementia. To clarify which neural structures, when atrophic, alter lexical–semantic function in patients with very mild Alzheimer's disease, Venneri et al. (2008) correlated the lexical attributes of words produced in a semantic fluency task with grey matter density values from MRI scans of mild Alzheimer's disease patients. The voxel-based morphometry (VBM) analyses showed a significant positive correlation between the lexical attributes characterising residual linguistic production in early Alzheimer's disease (AD) patients and the integrity of the perirhinal and parahippocampal cortex. Interestingly, there were no correlations within these structures with scores on neuropsychological tests not involving semantic memory. In a similar vein, we investigated 25 patients with single-domain amnestic mild cognitive impairment (aMCI) (Meyer et al., 2013). This syndrome is discussed as a potential AD prodrome. All participants underwent extensive neuropsychological testing and anatomical scanning with structural magnetic resonance imaging. Using VBM to identify brain regions that show a significant correlation between regional brain volume and behavioural measures of memory, we found that performance in a variety of mnemonic tests was directly related to the integrity of the AMTL. In a second study we tested 24 participants with single-domain aMCI in a yes/no recognition memory task using ERPs and VBM (Hoppstädter et al., 2013). The early frontal ERP old/new effect, the neural correlate of familiarity-based memory, was absent in aMCI, whereas the control group showed a significant early old/new effect at frontal electrodes. This effect was positively correlated with behavioural episodic memory performance. Analyses of brain morphology revealed a focused grey matter loss in the inferior and medial temporal lobes in aMCI versus healthy controls. Moreover, the positive correlation between gray matter volume in the AMTL and the familiarity-related early frontal old/new effect supports the notion that this effect relies upon the integrity of the AMTL.

Bowles et al. (2007) examined recognition memory in a patient who underwent surgical resection of left anterior temporal lobe structures for treatment of intractable epilepsy. This resection included a large portion of perirhinal and entorhinal cortex but spared the hippocampus. The results of four experiments based on three different experimental procedures (remember-know paradigm, receiver operating characteristics, and response-deadline procedure) indicated that the patient exhibited impaired familiarity with preserved recollection.

In a further study we investigated structure–function relationships between the hippocampus and declarative memory performance in healthy subjects

(Pohlack, Meyer et al., 2014). For this purpose, 50 healthy young male participants performed the California Verbal Learning Test. Hippocampal volume was assessed by manual segmentation of high-resolution 3D magnetic resonance images. We found a significant positive correlation between hippocampus-dependent memory measures like short-delay retention, long-delay retention and discriminability and percent hippocampal volume. No significant correlation with measures related to executive processes was found. In addition, percent amygdala volume was not related to any of these measures. This study showed a direct association between hippocampal volume and declarative memory performance in healthy young adults using standard neuropsychological testing procedures. These findings illustrate that individual differences in episodic memory function are partly driven by differences in hippocampal volume. They extend previous functional studies that provided support for a crucial role of the hippocampus in episodic memory by linking structural instead of functional, correlates to episodic memory performance.

Numerous models have been proposed to provide a conceptual or neuroanatomical framework for MTL-based recognition memory processes. Many current models of recognition memory assume two distinct underlying processes such as recollection and familiarity (or item versus source, or item versus associative retrieval). However, various competing dual process models exist ranging from simple 2-parameter measurement models to more complex neurocomputational models of the MTL and surrounding cortex like the model by Aggleton and Brown (2006) or the Complementary Learning Systems Model by Norman & O'Reilly (2003). For instance, Fernandez and Tendolkar (2006) referred to the perirhinal cortex as the 'gatekeeper' of declarative memory, arguing that its role is to direct encoding resources towards less familiar items. This same familiarity signal is then relevant at retrieval for making item memory judgments. This model predicts the decreasing activation that is seen with repetition of items in the perirhinal cortex; however, it does not make specific predictions for the hippocampus and the parahippocampal cortex. Mayes et al. (2007) have proposed the domain dichotomy model, which also argues that the hippocampus is essential for recollection, whereas the perirhinal cortex is important for familiarity (no role for the parahippocampal cortex is specified). In addition, they suggest that hippocampally-dependent recollection is necessary to support memory for new associations between items from different processing domains (e.g. faces and words), but familiarity could support learning of new associations between items within processing domains (e.g. an association between two faces). In a neurocomputational model of recognition memory derived from converging biological, psychological and computational constraints (Norman and O´Reilly, 2003) familiarity is assumed to arise from a sharpening mechanism in the perirhinal cortex. This process causes stimulus representations to become sharper over repeated exposures resulting in a smaller amount of neurons which are distinctively tuned to represent a particular item while other neurons are inhibited. As a consequence, the total activity of the MTL cortices in response to a familiar relative to a novel item is decreased. Additionally, by assigning overlapping representations to similar stimuli, the binding characteristics of the MTL cortices allow to represent the shared structure of events and therefore make it possible to generalize to novel stimuli as a function of their similarity to previously encountered items. From this view it follows that the MTL cortex cannot support recall of details from specific events owing to its inability to sufficiently differentiate the representations of different events. This can be achieved by hippocampal processes using separated representations to encode the details of specific events while minimizing interference ("pattern separation").

The sharpening model is supported by a number of recent findings. Intracranial recordings in monkeys performing visual recognition tasks indicated that up to 25% of neurones in the perirhinal cortex react strongly to items that are new but only weakly when the items have been seen before. Moreover, these neurons show single-exposure learning, i.e. the responses are already attenuated on the second appearance of stimuli. Such response reductions are found even after extended delays involving the presentation of many other stimuli (Brown & Aggleton, 2001; Aggleton & Brown, 2006). A study with intracranial recordings in humans also demonstrated a dramatic decrease in the number of cells in the anterior parahippocampal region responding to repeated stimuli as compared with novel stimuli (Viskontas et al., 2006).

Norman and O'Reilly's model highlights the perirhinal and parahippocampal cortex as an intermediary between the hippocampus and the neocortex. However, the roles of the perirhinal and the parahippocampal cortex are not differentiated, and thus this model provides little insight into the observed differences in activation across these regions.

Although the "binding of item and context" (BIC) model (Diana et al., 2007) is similar to other recent models of MTL organization, it differs in some important aspects. The key innovation of this model is that recollection and familiarity are not thought to have a simple one-to-one mapping to regions of the MTL. Rather, MTL subregions are important for processing different types of information (items, contexts, and bindings). The demands of the encoding and retrieval tasks in a given experiment are supposed to determine which subregions will be recruited during recollection-based processing and familiarity-based processing. In contrast to most accounts of the role of the MTL which focus on possible delineations between the functions of its various regions in their service of declarative long-term memory, such an informational account of MTL function stipulates that the engagement of different areas within this region is better characterised by what type of information is being processed (e.g. items, contexts, item/context associations) and the cues that are presented than the processes themselves.

Both the item-context (Davachi, 2006) and binding-in-context (BIC; Ranganath, 2010) theories of MTL function conceptualize the role of the AMTL as encoding and later retrieving information about items, while the hippocampus binds this item-specific information with contextual information stored in the parahippocampal cortex as relational associations. Because of these roles, the distinct areas can be differentially related to familiarity and recollection, but this relationship is secondary to the stimulus-dependent engagement of the area. This fits well to a growing body of evidence suggesting that the MTL is crucial for solving problems that do not strictly depend on long-term memory, such as some types of perception, working memory or contextual conditioning. That signifies that the aforementioned mnemonic accounts of MTL function either insufficiently account for this evidence, or that they require unparsimonious additions. Novel theoretical viewpoints are necessary, therefore, to provide a framework in which both mnemonic and non-mnemonic data can be interpreted. One such viewpoint is a representational account of MTL function. Like informational accounts, representational theories propose that the recruitment of a given MTL structure is stimulus-dependent. They diverge, however, in that informational accounts emphasize mnemonic processing of these stimuli, whereas representational theories assert this stimulus-dependent engagement will occur regardless of the cognitive process involved (Saksida & Bussey, 2010), thereby also shifting the theoretical focus away from the MTL as an exclusive LTM system. A representational account proposes that, instead of being specialized for declarative memory per se, some structures in the MTL process representations of high-level stimuli (e.g. objects, scenes) and context, which can be called upon for mnemonic but also for other purposes (e.g. language, conditioning, perception, working memory). This view is in line with Fanselow's (2010) view that there are nor hard-wired memory circuits but that mnemonic processing is allocated to specific circuits through a dynamic process.

Recent evidence indeed indicates that the hippocampus mediates rapid context associations with and without consciousness in humans and animals for long-term and short-term retention (see Henke, 2010). For instance, studies on contextual fear conditioning in animals and humans found an involvement of the hippocampus during fear learning. According to configural or relational learning theories it is assumed that the hippocampus plays a major role in the formation of the representation of context by integrating multiple cues into a unified or configural representation (e. g. Eichenbaum, 2004). Hippocampal lesions can spare configural discriminations only when item-location binding is not integral to the problem (Bussey et al., 1998). Amnesic patients compared to matched controls show deficits in reconstructing the spatial locations of a small array of objects even after a short delay (Watson et al., 2013). They were particularly impaired when two objects swapped places during the delay phase, which demanded object identity-to-relative-location bindings. To create an experimental conditioning scenario that requires configural processing we constructed a cue-array context paradigm that is comprised of two feature-identical picture stimuli, which are only differing in the arrangement of their context components (Baeuchl, Meyer et al., in press). This paradigm should ensure that focusing on single elements is not a sufficient strategy to distinguish between the two context pictures and thus to predict the CS-US association. For contextual fear acquisition, we paired one context (CS+) with an aversive electrical stimulus, whereas the other (CS-) was never followed by aversive stimulation. Blood oxygen level dependent activation to the CS+ was present in the insula, inferior frontal gyrus, inferior parietal lobule, superior medial gyrus and caudate nucleus. Furthermore, the amygdala and hippocampus were involved in a time-dependent manner (Fig. 1). Psychophysiological interaction analyses revealed functional connectivity of a more posterior hippocampal seed region with the anterior hippocampus, posterior cingulate cortex and superior parietal lobule. The anterior hippocampus was functionally coupled with the amygdala and postcentral gyrus.

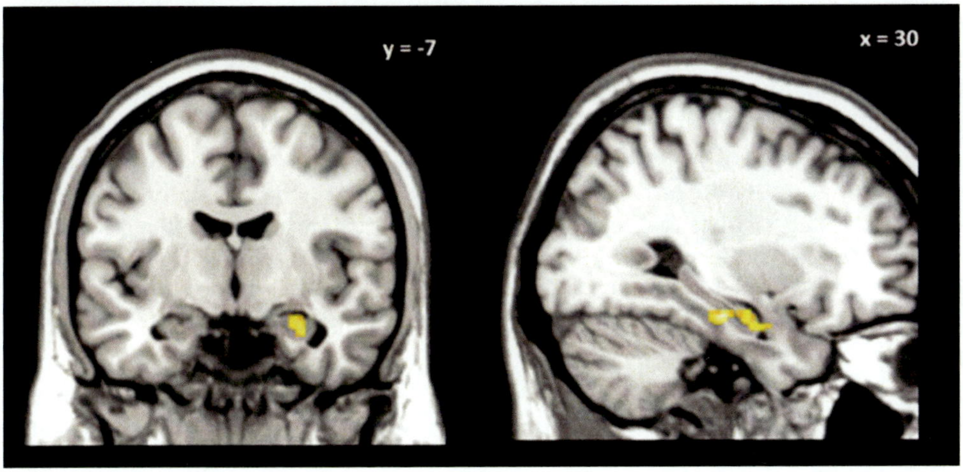

Figure 1: *Transient brain activity (linearly decaying over time) for the contrast CS+unpaired > CS- at a cluster-level threshold of $p < 0.05$ (family-wise error corrected), cluster-size $k = 200$. Plane coordinates are in MNI (Montreal Neurological Institute) space.*

The involvement of the MTL in particular processes of language comprehension, however, is less well understood. For example, testing of language functions in patient H.M. revealed a mixed pattern of results (MacKay et al., 1998): Although his general language abilities appear to be intact (Kensinger et al., 2001), he exhibits a distinct performance deficit, especially appearing in the detection and understanding of ambiguities. We recorded event-related potentials (ERPs) directly from the AMTL and the hippocampus, while epilepsy patients listened to sentences that either were correct or contained semantic or syntactic violations (Meyer et al., 2005). Semantic violations elicited a large negative ERP response peaking at 400 ms in the AMTL. In contrast, syntactically incorrect sentences elicited a negative deflection of 500–800 ms in the hippocampus. The results suggest that functionally distinct aspects of integration in language comprehension are supported by different MTL structures: The AMTL is involved in semantic integration, whereas the hippocampus proper subserves processes of syntactic integration. An analysis of phase synchronisation within the gamma band between AMTL and hippocampal recording sites showed that both of the above-mentioned ERP components were preceded by an increase of phase synchronization. In contrast to these short phasic increases of phase synchronization in both violation conditions, correct sentences were associated with a long-lasting synchronization in a late time window, possibly reflecting the integration of semantic and syntactic information as required for normal comprehension. In the case of a phrase structure violation, a new and unfamiliar linguistic input requires a new relational moment. Sentences with a syntactic violation cannot be represented with the acquired rules, with the consequence that known words have to be bound in a novel, grammatically unknown manner. They may thus give rise to increased binding demands and by this activate the hippocampus.

N400-like effects in the AMTL have not only been recorded using semantic violations (McCarthy et al., 1995; Meyer et al., 2005) but also during semantic priming (Nobre & McCarthy, 1995). Results from Nobre and McCarthy (1995) show that the so-called AMTL-N400 responds similarly to identical experimental manipulations as the scalp-recorded N400. Also the intracranially observed peak latencies around 350-450 ms were similar to the peak latencies for the negative ERP deflections recorded from the scalp. These data suggest that the N400 is at least in part a volume-conducted representation of activity in the AMTL structures. In order to investigate the neural basis of the N400 component directly, we simultaneously assessed ERPs and event-related fMRI during semantic priming in young healthy subjects. In addition, ERPs and structural brain data were obtained in older healthy adults and patients with aMCI, a population with neurodegenerative changes in the AMTL, as already mentioned above. In the fMRI results, the loci of the global maxima were found bilaterally in the AMTL. EEG-informed fMRI analysis addressing trial-to-trial fluctuations in semantic processing by relating single-trial N400 amplitudes to the BOLD signal provided a direct link between the scalp-recorded N400 and the corresponding BOLD signal in the AMTL. Patients with aMCI showed a smaller N400 effect when compared to healthy older adults. In addition, VBM showed that the magnitude of the N400 effect was related to AMTL integrity.

Taken together, our data and those of others clearly demonstrate MTL functions beyond declarative long-term memory. Instead of being specialised for episodic memory, some structures in the MTL process representations of high-level stimuli (e.g. objects, scenes) and context, which can be called upon for memory but also for other cognitions. The MTL can be conceived as a hierarchically organised representational scale where different areas within the hierarchy contain different representations. In this model the AMTL can be seen as a module for the integration of information across sensory modalities to form multimodal representations for conjunctions of a large number of features (see Suzuki, 1996, for review). Many neurons there signal the novelty, recency or familiarity of individual items. Previously encountered items typically evoke reduced neural responses. In addition, studies of long-term stimulus memory (e.g., stimulus–stimulus associations) suggest that the AMTL is critical for learning about and storing the co-occurrence of stimulus features across presentations. For these and other reasons it has been suggested that the AMTL operates as the kernel of a system for semantic memory (Eacott et al., 1994; Murray, 1996; Murray et al., 1998). The hippocampus instead contains representations at a higher level. In the hippocampus only few neurons signal the prior occurrence of individual items. However, many neurons signal information about spatial position or associations between items (see Brown & Aggleton, 2001 for a comprehensive review).

In sum, it might be better to understand the functions of the AMTL and the hippocampus in terms of the computations they perform and the representations they contain and to assume a dynamic and flexible allocation of specific circuits depending on task demands and anatomical constraints.

4 On the Neuroanatomical Parcellation and Multiple Functions of the Inferior Parietal Lobule

Juliane Klann, Ferdinand Christoph Binkofski and Svenja Caspers

Key words:
IPL, angular gyrus, supramarginal gyrus, anatomical parcellation, multimodal processing, spatial neglect, tool use, verbal working memory, language functions, apraxia

1. Anatomy of the Inferior Parietal Lobule (IPL)

The inferior parietal lobule (IPL) is situated within the ventral part of the posterior parietal cortex of the parietal lobe. It abuts the postcentral sulcus rostrally and the intraparietal sulcus dorsally. Ventrally, the Sylvian fissure demarcates the transition from the lateral aspect of the IPL to the caudal part of the parietal operculum. The caudal and ventro-caudal borders of the IPL are less well defined, since there is no sulcus as delineation. The IPL rather continues into the posterior superior and middle temporal gyri and the occipital gyri. Two major gyri can be differentiated within the IPL, namely the supramarginal gyrus rostrally and the angular gyrus caudally. These are typically separated by the primary intermediate sulcus of Jenssen, although the form and presence of this sulcus is highly variable (Ono et al., 1990).

1.1. Microstructural Parcellation of the IPL

In his famous map, Brodmann (1909) subdivided the IPL into a rostral area 40 and a caudal area 39, based on differences in cytoarchitecture and corresponding to the two major gyri. This largely corresponds to the description by Smith (1907) with a rostral area pariB and a caudal area pariA. The rostral area was a bit smaller, though, since a third area at the transition to the parietal operculum was identified as area pariC. This idea of a predominant bipartition was also adopted by von Economo and Koskinas (1925), who identified a rostral area PF and a caudal area PG. In addition, they found further local variations of the general pattern of area PF, such as the opercular part of PF (area PFop), the part of PF with a thin cortical ribbon (area PFt), the magnocellular part of PF (area

PFm), and the magnocellular and columnar part of PF (area PFcm). Similarly, Sarkissov et al. (1949) introduced local variations within Brodmann's areas 40 and 39, namely areas 40op, 40p, 40i, and 39p.

Another influential subdivision was proposed by Vogt (1911), and Vogt and Vogt (1919) based on myeloarchitecture, delineating four areas 74, 88, 89, and 90. This parcellation was corroborated by Gerhard (1940) and Batsch (1956), who introduced further subdivisions of the major four areas. This myeloarchitectonic heterogeneity within IPL was also established by Hopf and Vitzthum (1957) and Hopf (1969).

More recent parcellations resembled those found in macaques (Pandya & Seltzer, 1982). Eidelberg and Galaburda (1984) found four areas within the IPL, arranged in a rostro-caudal sequence: areas PF, PFG, PG, OPG. Based on a sample of ten human postmortem brains, Caspers et al. (2006, 2008) could identify seven cytoarchitectonically distinct areas by means of an observer-independent, quantitative statistical mapping approach: a dorsal rostro-caudal sequence of five areas on the lateral surface, i.e. areas PFt, PF, PFm, PGa, and PGp, which have borders with intraparietal areas; and two ventral areas in the caudal part of the parietal operculum, i.e. areas PFop and PFcm, which follow caudally to the secondary somatosensory cortex. The rostral areas on the supramarginal gyrus (PFt, PFop, PF, PFcm, PFm) are cytoarchitectonically all characterized by a largely homogeneous distribution of pyramidal cells in layers III and V, with a pronounced superficial-to-deep increase in cell size in layer III. Layer IV is generally sparsely developed, while often being interrupted by strands of pyramidal cells from lower layer III and upper layer V. The caudal areas on the angular gyrus, areas PGa and PGp, are characterized by large pyramidal cells in middle to deep layer III and by a pronounced and well-developed layer IV. Additional features are attributable to the individual areas (Caspers et al., 2006).

The seven IPL areas are furthermore characterized by differences in receptor distribution (Caspers et al., 2013). While rostral IPL areas showed comparably higher concentrations of cholinergic nicotinic, GABAergic $GABA_A$, and glutamatergic AMPA receptors, caudal IPL areas had relatively higher concentrations of serotoninergic $5\text{-}HT_{1A}$ and $5\text{-}HT_2$ receptors. Similarity analyses revealed a rostral, middle, and caudal part of IPL, in which the receptor distribution within the areas was more similar to each other as compared to the surround.

1.2. Connectional Architecture

Similar to the parcellations based on microstructural criteria, connectivity information was used to parcellate the IPL into distinct regions with a characteristic connectional pattern. Mars et al. (2011) and Wang et al. (2012) found five connectionally distinct regions, mainly ordered in a rostro-caudal sequence and thus largely resembling the cytoarchitectonic parcellation of Caspers et al. (2006, 2008). These differences in connectivity encompassed a distinct structural connectivity as measured by using diffusion tensor imaging as well as a distinct functional connectivity of each region as revealed by correlations of resting-state time-series. Ruschel et al. (2014) found a tri-partition based on differences in structural connectivity, resulting in a rostral, middle and caudal IPL cluster, which resembled the parcellation of the IPL based on its receptor architecture (Caspers et al., 2013). A similar parcellation was found based on functional connectivity patterns, with seven distinct IPL clusters, which were grouped into a rostral, middle and caudal group based on similarities in functional connectivity (Zhang & Li, 2014).

Connectivity of the IPL is mainly provided via the arcuate and the superior longitudinal fasciculus. Strong connections can be found to various frontal, superior parietal and posterior temporal areas. The more caudal the IPL, the stronger and more extensive is the connectivity with temporal as well as rostral and medial prefrontal areas (Caspers et al., 2011). Within the frontal lobe, the inferior frontal gyrus and adjacent aspects of the precentral and middle frontal gyrus are strongly connected with the IPL, particularly its rostral aspect (Caspers et al., 2011; Catani et al., 2005; Mars et al., 2011; Parker et al., 2005; Powell et al., 2006). The more rostral parts of the inferior frontal gyrus, particularly area 45, is more heavily connected to middle and caudal IPL, predominantly via the extreme capsule (Saur et al., 2008; Weiller et al., 2011). Additional connections with varying intensity exist with different prefrontal and frontal polar areas (Caspers et al., 2011; Rushworth et al., 2006). While the ventral, language-related pathways involving the arcuate fasciculus seem to be more lateralized to the left (Catani et al., 2005), the more dorsal paths, amongst other involved in visuospatial attention, was found to be right-lateralized (Thiebaut de Schotten et al., 2011). Similar connection patterns can be identified using resting-state functional connectivity (Mars et al., 2011; Yeo et al., 2011).

Overall, these connectivity patterns measured in humans using in-vivo diffusion and resting-state imaging are largely similar to the patterns found in macaque monkeys using invasive tracer techniques (Andersen et al., 1990; Cavada, 2001; Cavada & Goldman-Rakic, 1989a,b; Mesulam et al., 1977; Neal et al., 1990a,b; Gregoriou et al., 2006; Rozzi et al., 2006; Seltzer & Pandya, 1984). Considering the fiber tract reconstruction on diffusion imaging data to be indirect and thus prone to false positives and negatives, this overall similarity in the connectivity of the IPL between the species is striking. The differences, though, might be of even more interest. The connectivity to the prefrontal cortex is much more pronounced in humans as compared to macaques, structurally as well as functionally. This provides further evidence for the evolution of particularly the frontal cortex from monkeys to humans, also including novel connections to evolve which seemingly to a considerable degree engage the IPL.

2. Functions of the inferior parietal lobule (IPL)

The anatomical fragmentation of the IPL into seven different areas induces the consideration of a parallel functional parcellation. In line, the IPL is engaged in a widespread range of functions, starting with sensory-motor control, motor skills, object and tool use, reaching to spatial reception as well as language, speech, verbal working memory and number processing. Within this context it is important to notice that the IPL is surrounded by the primary somatosensory, visual and acoustic areas. This location can explain why the IPL is engaged in so many synthetic functions. In many aspects, it can be regarded as an important computational buffer for processing of multisensory information (e.g. Seghier et al., 2013, p. 43).

2.1. Motor Functions and Object Use

The IPL's rostral part (areas PFop, PFt and PF) is involved in motor and action related functions like simple motor behavior, tactile reception, motor control of spatially/timely complex movements, and tool use. The last two functions additionally involve the middle part of the IPL (areas PF and PFm). Beside the partition along cytoarchitectonically different brain areas, lateralization also cues distinctive functions: While tactile perception is guaranteed through left rostral IPL, e.g. its damage impairs the tactile recognition of an object (astereognosis), the right rostral and middle IPL are involved in spatial coding and spatial attention during motor learning and motor acts (Mesulam, 1999). Moreover, motor learning recruits a bilateral fronto-parietal network complemented by intraparietal sulcus, hippocampal, cerebellar and subcortical regions (King et al., 2013; Seitz, 2001). Herein, the rostral IPL seems to specifically serve the processing of spatially/timely complex motor sequences. Thus, lesions affecting the supramarginal gyrus are reported to lead to impaired control of complex movements (Goldenberg et al., 2007; Goldenberg & Karnath, 2006). The lesion data is convergent with results of functional brain imaging studies, which uncovered the right rostral and middle IPL to be involved in the control of spatial characteristics of complex motor behavior or attention (Halsband & Lange, 2006; Rauch et al., 1995). In line with the idea of the IPL being a multisensory computational buffer, lesion data demonstrated that the right IPL serves for the integration of sensory information as well as verbal auditory and nonverbal visual feedback processing (Halsband & Lange, 2006).

Furthermore, the IPL is part of a bilaterally arranged action system, hosted in the parietal cortex (Rizzolatti & Matelli, 2003; Binkofski & Buxbaum, 2013). The system is anatomically and functionally split into two subsystems: One subpart is associated with the dorso-dorsal stream, including the intraparietal sulcus (IPS) and superior parietal lobe (SPL). It warrants the processing of actions directed to currently visible stimuli on the basis of their structure (size, shape, and orientation). The other subpart involves mainly the IPL (ventro-dorsal stream) and is specialized on abilities of skilled object-related actions (Buxbaum, 2001; Fridman et al., 2006; Buxbaum & Kalénine, 2010; Johnson-Frey, 2004; Pisella et al., 2006; Randerath et al., 2010; Vingerhoets et al., 2009). More precisely, the two streams were deduced from monkey data, and further subdivide the dorsal stream of visual perception as it was defined formerly by Mishkin and colleagues (Mishkin et al., 1983; Mishkin & Ungerleider, 1982). In humans, recent evidence shows the ventro-dorsal stream to mastermind the processing of sensorimotor information based upon longer-term object use. In line, lesion data reports on disordered pantomimic and/or real object use after damage within the ventro-dorsal stream/IPL, mirroring an impaired conceptual knowledge about the skilled handling of objects. The disorder related to these deficits is called limb apraxia (LA). In contrast to LA, optic ataxia (OA), a disorder characterised by misreaching in visually guided movements, typically arises from damage within the dorso-dorsal stream. In accordance with the idea of a preserved dorso-dorsal stream in LA, numerous studies prove intact online reaching and grasping actions in LA patients. The performance of visually guided actions usually deteriorates only when they have to be performed ''offline'', e.g. when persons are blindfolded before they have to execute the action or movement (Buxbaum, Johnson & Bartlett-Williams, 2005; Haaland, Harrington, & Knight, 1999; Jax, Buxbaum, & Moll, 2006; Laimgruber, Goldenberg, & Hermsdörfer, 2005). This may be interpreted in terms of an underlying deficit in the anticipatory planning. Moreover, apraxia is linked to a comprehension deficit. Some patients are reported to show up with problems in the understanding of motor acts. This disorder was found to be more related to dissociation between conceptual and production components than to comprehension of symbolic or representational content of the motor act itself (Halsband et al., 2001).

The so far described capabilities of object use, targeting the ventro-dorsal stream, also cover the more specific ability of tool use. Tool use is associated with area PFt in the rostral part of the IPL (Peeters et al., 2009). In general, tool use seems to involve both hemispheres in naturalistic multistep tasks like preparing coffee, fixing a cassette recorder etc., meanwhile only patients with left brain damage show up with deficits in the use of single familiar tools or tool/object pairs (Hartmann et al., 2005; Schwartz et al., 1998). Moreover, only left lesions have been demonstrated to be associated with errors in (a) matching objects to pantomime actions (mainly caudal IPL; Buxbaum, Kyle & Menon, 2005; Kalénine, Buxbaum & Coslett, 2010; Vaina, Goodglass & Daltroy, 1995; Varney, 1978; Vignolo, 1990), (b) pantomiming an action stimulated by an object stimulus (mainly rostral IPL; Barbieri & De Renzi, 1988; Goldenberg, Hartmann & Schlott, 2003; Goodglass & Kaplan, 1963) or (c) matching objects subserving the same purpose (Caspers et al., 2010; De Renzi, Scotti & Spinnler, 1969; Rumiati et al., 2001; Vignolo, 1990). Left hemisphere damage also leads to impaired inference of functions from structure, when novel tools linked to their complementary objects by transparent mechanical relationships have to be applied (Goldenberg & Hagmann, 1998; Heilman et al., 1997), or when alternative uses of familiar tools are to be detected (e.g. a coin for screwing, Heilman et al., 1997; Roy & Square, 1985). In line with the lesion data, it was stated that the rostral IPL warrants the ability to correctly infer the function of an object from its structure (Barbieri & De Renzi, 1988).

2.2. Spatial Functions

In contrast to the bilaterally hosted motor and action related functions, spatial skills seem to predominantly focus on the right parietal cortex. More specifically, the right IPL and especially its middle and caudal parts (areas PF, PFm, PGa, and PGp) subserve visuo-spatial and visuo-motor functions like the estimation of directions, processing of extra- and peri-personal space as well as the localization of objects. Nevertheless, the left caudal IPL together with the IPS is involved whenever language or calculation are engaged, e.g. the processing of visuo-spatial components in reading and spatial imagery of magnitudes (Seghier, 2013; Simon et al., 2002).

Lesions within the right caudal IPL lead to spatial hemineglect (Gainotti et al., 1972; Colombo et al., 1976; Bisiach et al., 1979; Driver et al., 1992). The hallmark of hemineglect is the ignorance of the visual items in the contralesional side of space irrespective of completely intact vision, and therefore is interpreted as an awareness disorder. It manifests itself symptomatically in shaving only the right side of one's face, sparing those parts of a meal on the left side of a plate/eating food placed on the right side only etc. Additionally, constructive skills like drawing a clock and therein positioning the numbers within the right half of a given circle are evident. Under the many explanations of the causes of hemineglect, the most common hypothesis is an underlying attention deficit (e.g. Mesulam, 1999, 1981). Another popular assumption suggests disturbed mental representations of sensory stimuli (Rizzolatti & Berti, 1990; Bisiach et al., 1981) or a transformation disorder of (multimodal) sensory input into egocentric coordinates (Vallar, 1997; Karnath, 1994, 1997).

The cortical network subserving visuo-spatial functions seems not to be limited to the right IPL, as was shown by a lesion study where hemineglect was related to right temporal cortices (Karnath et al., 2001). This may be interpreted as proof for a temporal node playing a crucial role within the well-known right fronto-temporo-parietal attention network (Corbetta & Shulman, 2011, 2002). Convergent with this view, functional connectivity analyses identified interconnections between these parts of the brain. Within this network, the IPL seems to guarantee control of spatial attention rather than spatial attention itself (e.g. arousal, reorienting, detection of behaviorally important novel input; Corbetta & Shulman, 2011; Halsband, Gruhn & Ettlinger, 1985).

2.3. Verbal and Speech Functions

The left perisylvian network is well-known as serving speech- and language functions, these abilities are also related to left supramarginal (rostral IPL – PFop, PFt and PFcm) and angular gyri (caudal IPL – PGa and PGp), which are amongst others anatomically interconnected with frontal and temporal parts of the perisylvian language network (Caspers et al., 2011; Seghier, 2013). Once again and in line with the idea of a functional segregation parallelizing cytoarchitectonical parcellation, individual studies report the IPL to be engaged in several speech and language functions and processes, reaching from the selection of articulatory gestures (Tremblay & Gracco, 2010) to verbal integration within complex comprehensive contexts like sentences (Lerner, Honey, Silbert & Hasson, 2011).

As was shown for visual perception, auditory perception was also assumed to be processed within a system consisting of two major pathways, connecting temporal auditory and frontal regions. Recent brain imaging and electrophysiological data suggest a 'ventral' and a 'dorsal' auditory stream, both connecting the primary auditory cortex with prefrontal regions along the superior temporal gyrus via the uncinate fasciculus. In contrast to the ventral, the dorsal pathway projects along the left IPL. With the help of diffusion MRI tractography (Parker et al., 2005), white matter connections were detected along the dorsal stream connecting classical speech areas and the IPL in the left hemisphere, stressing the crucial role of the IPL in speech and language processing. Remarkably, the arcuate fasciculus, which interconnects BA 44 and 45 with IPL and, farther on with posterior superior and middle temporal cortex, displays the anatomical representation of the dorsal stream (Parker et al., 2005; Saur et al., 2008; Weiller et al., 2011). It is noteworthy that these anatomical findings are convergent with the predictions of the DIVA (Directions Into Velocities of Articulators) model of speech production (Guenther et al., 2006). DIVA supposes a feedback process for motor speech planning, which relies on Broca's area and involves a somatosensory error map located within the rostral part of the IPL.

Furthermore, the caudal parts of the IPL (angular gyrus: areas PGa and PGp) are documented to be involved in reading, writing, naming, and verbal repetition (Henseler, Regenbrecht & Obrig, 2014; Seghier, 2013; Zukic et al., 2012; Dronkers et al., 2004). This is in line with lesion data demonstrating that damage to the left angular gyrus leads to dysgraphia/agraphia, dyslexia/alexia and anomia. Moreover, dysgraphia as part of Gerstmann's syndrome as well as isolated repetition problems and conduction aphasia are additionally related to damage of the supramarginal gyrus (rostral part of the IPL) (Fridriksson et al., 2010; Zukic et al., 2012; Damasio & Damasio, 1980). Since a proportionally heavy deficit in verbal repetition is seen as the hallmark of conduction aphasia, the rostral IPL is interpreted to play a crucial role in verbal working memory. More specifically, this seems to be associated with phonological problems in short term memory (Baldo et al., 2008; Dell et al., 2007). Convergent imaging data, revealing the left supramarginal gyrus to foster phonological short-term memory functions, confirms the role of the IPL in language processes (e.g. Ravizza et al., 2004). This is very much in line with further evidence which demonstrated activation within the supramarginal gyrus, when the input language was switched from one to another language, a task in which cognitive control of language is focussed (Price et al., 1999).

In contrast, another finding reports both, the angular and supramarginal gyri, to be involved in the retrieval of foreign words with high imagery content (Halsband, 2006; Halsband and Lange, 2006). In convergence with the view of the angular gyrus being part of a more conceptual-semantical network, semantic content and lexical meaning are more connected to activity within the angular gyrus (caudal part of IPL) (Binder et al., 2009; Borovsky et al., 2007; De Leon et al., 2007; Vigneau et al., 2006; Price, 2000). This may be due to the formerly suggested grounding of language functions in somatosensory experiences ("action-perception theory"; Pulvermüller, 1999). According to this view, both, linguistic semantics and action perception, rely on action related networks, including the angular gyrus. This hypothesis is supported by lesion data as well as functional brain imaging studies. Both types of evidence prove the fronto-parietal junction to underlie action knowledge as well as the comprehension of action words (Higuchi et al., 2009; Pulvermüller, Shtyrov & Ilmoniemi, 2005; Perani et al., 1999).

In addition, the IPL is associated with sequential processing. More precisely, the caudal IPL (corresponding to PGa and PGp; BA39) together with anterior speech regions was reported to increase neural activity as syllable sequence complexity accelerated (Bohland & Guenther, 2006). The rostral parts of the IPL (BA40) are linked to the handling of the temporal order of speech syllables (Moser et al., 2009). Furthermore, it seems to play a role for processing more complex constructions, as demonstrated by an fMRI study on sentence production (Haller et al., 2005). More complex stimuli than discourse are less frequently studied. There is some data on the relationship between expressive and receptive skills in spoken language (Awad et al., 2007), sign language communication (Braun et al., 2001) and reading (Brownsett & Wise, 2010). They all underpin the important role of the left angular gyrus (caudal IPL) for expressive language, irrespective of its output modality (spoken, sign or written language). This was recently supported by a brain imaging study demonstrating the involvement of the left IPL in spoken discourse rather than non-speech related repetitive tongue movements (Geranmayeh et al., 2012). The important role of the angular gyrus in complex language production was confirmed by a lesion study using voxel-based lesion–symptom mapping (VLSM) on 50 aphasic patients (Borovsky et al., 2007). Whenever expressive discourse behavior and language production in terms of semantic context were impaired, damages of frontal and/or temporal regions combined with a strong focus on the left angular gyrus (caudal IPL) were found.

Altogether it can be summarized, that the IPL seems to be part of the language network, for it is engaged in different speech and language processes on multiple linguistic levels reaching from phonology to discourse. In line with the anatomical connection (arcuate fasciculus) of PFop, PFt and PFcm to BA 44, an area of the language network functionally more dedicated to modality specific oral speech and articulation processes (Horwitz et al., 2003), the rostral IPL is related to temporal ordering of sound and articulation (speech functions). In contrast, the caudal IPL is associated with modality independent conceptual and semantic processes including the connection between language and action networks that may be explained by the assumption of language being grounded in action and sensual experiences. Here, the anatomical connection (the arcuate fasciculus) links PGa and PGp with BA 45 (Caspers et al., 2011), a language area associated with modality independent language processes (Horwitz et al., 2003). Therefore, the angular gyrus recently was entitled a "cross-modal hub where converging multisensory information is combined and integrated to comprehend and give sense to events, manipulate mental representations, solve familiar problems, and reorient attention to relevant information" (Seghier, 2013, p. 43).

3. Summary

As the cytoarchitectonic parcellation of the IPL into seven distinct areas suggests, this part of the parietal cortex displays a multifunctional area engaged into several different processes and functional networks. Functional segregation of the IPL already has been demonstrated to partly reflect anatomical fragmentation: While its rostral parts (areas PFop, PFt and PFcm; supramarginal gyrus) are associated with processes of speech and articulation, phonological short-term memory, simple motor behavior, tactile reception and general higher somatosensory functions, its middle part (areas PF and PFm) is linked to motor attention, motor control and motor planning, especially in the left hemisphere. The IPL's caudal part (PGa and PGp) is dedicated to spatial attention, spatial perception, spatial memory, mathematical cognition, modality-independent language functions as well as conceptual and discourse related processes, and visuomotor integration. Considering this high degree of variable functions involving caudal IPL, it was interpreted to play a more general role as a cross-modal hub, which warrants comprehension, manipulation and orientation based on processes of multisensory combination and integration.

Based on the fact that the three parts of the IPL are somehow present in the monkey, future work will also have to explore evolutionary aspects of the relationship between cytoarchitectonic and functional parcellation. So far, it is already evident that the human IPL cytoarchtectonically parallels that of the non-human primate in respect to PF (human: PFt and PF), PFG (human: PFm), PG (human: PGa) and Opt (human: PGp). Furthermore, hints towards a similar functional role in action processing and tool use are apparent for monkey areas PF and PFG and human areas PFt and PF. Another important aspect that needs further investigation as of now concerns the correlation between each part of the IPL and its function within different cortical networks, using the evolving knowledge over the last years about the relation between structure and function of the IPL in both species.

5 Role of the First and Second Person Perspective for Control of Behaviour: Understanding Other People's Facial Expressions

Denise Potthoff and Rüdiger J. Seitz

Key Words: Empathy, Theory of Mind, Perspective Taking, Medial Frontal Cortex, Perception, Action, Emotion, Valuation, Social Interaction, Neuroimaging

Abstract

Humans typically make probabilistic inferences about another person's affective state based on her/his bodily movements when viewing body language like emotional facial expressions, emblematic gestures and whole body movements. Furthermore, they deduce tentative predictions about the other person's intentions. Such interpretations reflect the valuating first person perspective of humans which allows the subject to adopt a second person perspective as in theory of mind and in empathy. Neuroimaging investigations have shown that the medial frontal cortex is a critical node in the circuits underlying theory of mind, empathy, and intention of action. It is suggested that personal perspective taking in social interactions is paradigmatic for the capability of humans to generate personally discriminable accounts of the complex world and to control behaviour.

1. Introduction

The mechanistic model of the action-perception cycle describes the spatio-temporal contingencies of behaviour as highly interwoven processes of sensory perception and action production (Fuster, 1990; Guillery et al., 2005). Physical activity, however, includes the impact of cognition at all levels of processing. Specifically, action has been linked to perception by motor intention (Navchev et al., 2008; Passingham et al., 2010). Conversely, perception is linked to action by comprehension which allows the subject to recognize an object by dedicated movements (Binkofski et al., 1998). Moreover, humans perceive the physical nature of their complex environment with their different senses including audition and vision. While much of this information will remain below the level of explicit awareness, humans can turn their window of attention to certain objects or events in their environment to explore their physical properties. This processing of information involves a number of important computations. First of all, there are different processing streams that mediate the analysis of the physical properties of objects, their use, and their spatial configuration concerning the objects themselves, their relation to adjacent objects as well as the temporal order of events (Tsuchiya et al., 2008; Ungerleider & Haxby, 1994). Thereby, the subject becomes aware of the formal characteristics of the event or object and generates a simplified probabilistic representation of the information sampled (Mesulam, 2008).

In this contribution we will show that mental activity related to the first and second person perspective has largely been neglected concerning the generation of probabilistic representations of the information sampled but is important to understand the processes underlying control of human behaviour. Specifically, we will summarize experimental findings addressing the following questions:

1. Which brain areas are engaged in processing subconsciously affective information as presented by emotional facial expressions?
2. Which brain areas are engaged in classification of emotional facial expressions?
3. Which brain areas are engaged in discriminating emotional facial expressions?
4. What do these findings mean with respect to personal control of behaviour?

2. The First Person Perspective

Simultaneously and independently from perception of the physical features of objects and events in the outside world, their personal meaning is evaluated by mental processes summarized as valuation (Seitz et al., 2009). This judgement is fast and typically below awareness underlying the default first personal perspective: "What does it mean to me?" Importantly, the complexity of the outside world is put into simplified accounts reflecting the subjective perspective inherent in the individual (Fuchs, 2009). Concerning the interactions of people, humans are capable of estimating the warmth and competence of other people and to adjust their own behaviour accordingly (Fiske et al., 2007).

As illustrated in Figure 1, the mental act of valuation is linked to perception by attention which directs the subject to a given sensation in the outer or inner world. The personal value of an object or event is coded in terms of immediate key motivations such as desire or appetite as well as ultimate goals like success or survival (Rolls, 2006). Conversely, perception is linked to valuation by the process of attribution, as the subject classifies the perceived information in emotional categories (Damasio et al., 1998; Eccles & Wigfield, 2002). This includes the internal sensations of pleasure, attractiveness or social esteem as well as threat, aversion or avoidance (Rolls, 2006; Eisenberger & Cole, 2012). It should be noted that the subject's conclusion about the physical properties of objects and events is generally assumed to be virtually identical among different subjects, while in contrast it is well known that the personal relevance of the same object or event can be profoundly different among subjects. Evidence from electrophysiology in nonhuman primates and from functional imaging in man shows that physical properties and subjective assumptions about objects are represented in different brain circuits including dopamine neurons in basal ganglia (d'Acremont et al., 2013; Prevost et al., 2010; Schultz 2013). Notably, explicit verbal labelling of objects or events by top-down semantic processing modulates the visual word form area (Song et al., 2012). On the executive side, the process of valuation is linked also to action. Importantly, the link between valuation and action is asymmetric such that valuation can set the subject into the position to act in a certain way. The mental processes linking action to valuation is the process of implicit and explicit strategic motor planning which involves the dorsal medial prefrontal cortex (DMPFC) including the supplementary motor area (SMA; Farrow & Frith, 2002; Jackson et al., 2006; Passingham et al., 2010; Sumner et al., 2007; Tusche et al., 2010; Vogeley et al., 2001). There is a tight link of the sense of agency to the bodily self mediated by a large scale networtk encompassing both the pre-SMA and SMA (Ferri et al., 2012; Haggard et al., 2002; Moore et al., 2010). Both structures are targets of the basal ganglia and cerebellar output (Akkal et al., 2007; Qin & Northoff, 2011). In addition, the first person perspective will optimize subsequent actions of the subject by estimating predicted reward and expected costs (Friston, 2010; He et al., 2013; Vlaev et al., 2011; Walton et al., 2004). However, the result of the selected actions and the reactions of the other people will become apparent to the acting subject only by perception. From animal experiments we have learnt that neurons in the DMPFC (Kennerley & Wallis, 2009; Kennerley et al., 2011) and striatum (Kim et al., 2009) code values of chosen actions. Furthermore, gamma-band activity signifies the number of relevant items maintained in working memory in left Brodmann area 9 and right infraparietal lobule (Roux et al., 2012).

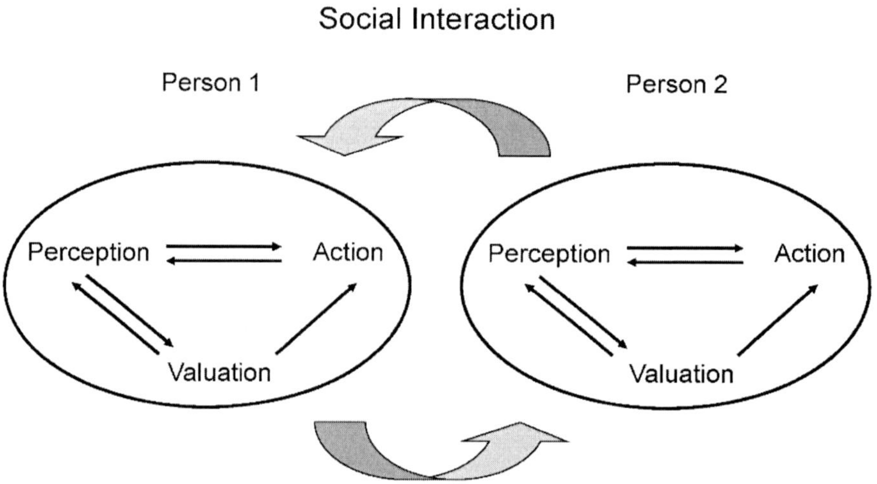

Figure 1: *Schematic flow of information affording control of human behavior in each of two interacting subjects. Note the reciprocity of the processes and the flexibility of the personal perspective (after Seitz et al. 2009).*

3. The Second Person Perspective

In social interactions persons need to adapt the second person perspective to decode the other persons' affect and intentions. In fact, humans have an innate and highly developed capability to infer the meaning of body movements (Meltzoff & Decety, 2003). Likewise, humans are capable of rapidly identifying the emotional state of the counterpart behind her/his facial expressions, gestures and whole body movements (Conty et al., 2012; Lindenberg et al., 2012; de Lussanet et al., 2008). This allows the acting person in a social encounter to behave appropriately with respect to the given contextual situation and the persons around her/him. In case the acting person behaves selfishly, she/he does not care about other people. However, people are educated to behave such that the rights of the contemporary people are not compromised. This implies that another person is acknowledged as a creature akin to oneself (Collange et al., 2009). The appropriate behaviour, therefore, ought to be selected on the basis of how the emotions and intentions of other people are interpreted. For this purpose two mental activities have been described: theory of mind and empathy (Singer, 2006). Theory of mind implies understanding the other person`s point of view and intention (Gallagher et al., 2000; Frith & Frith, 2003). Empathy implies the understanding of the other's emotion that accompanies sensory signals (Ruby & Decety, 2001; Shamay-Tsoory et al., 2009; Singer et al., 2004). Both concepts are considered to have some degree of conceptual overlap when it comes to 'warm' (emotionally driven) and 'cold' (cognitively driven) empathy or theory of mind (Bush et al., 2000; Cox et al., 2011; Fan et al., 2011). Specifically, the subject asks the question: "What does it mean to her or him?". In other words, the subject is concerned with the emotional state the other subject is in. Thus, the acting person needs to recognize the state of emotion as expressed by body movements including facial expressions of emotions. Importantly, this process needs to be done rapidly to allow the acting subject to behave appropriately. When humans make inferences about the affective state of the person they interact with, they make predictions about her/his future acts (Behrens et al., 2009). Evidence for this role of the DMPFC was obtained from virtual lesions induced by transcranial magnetic stimulation and transcranial current stimulation (Reinhart & Woodman, 2014). Furthermore, the making of an emotional facial expression by a person comprises also the inference of the cause for her/his emotional state and behaviour. Thus, subjects attempt to grasp likely explanations why the other subject may be in this or that affective state (Figure 1).

In essence, bodily expressions of emotion are paradigmatic for the predisposition of humans to reason about the meaning behind other people`s behaviour. In fact, humans guide their behaviour according to the meaning they read from the body movements of the persons they interact with. In the following we will report about experiments addressing by which networks in the brain this is being accomplished. Again, it is important to realize that both, theory of mind and empathy, reflect probabilistic representations of personal perceptions such that internal mental states represent external states, events or objects in a probabilistic manner (Friston et al., 2014).

4. Subliminal Processing of Emotional Facial Expressions

Due to its high sending capacity of various different stimulus patterns, the human face is a powerful communicator of socially relevant messages (Ekman, 1969). Recently, more than 20 composed facial expressions of emotions have been identified (Du et al., 2014). Although emotional signals are rapidly extracted as evident from electrophysiology (Eger et al., 2003), many of them are overwritten in succession so rapidly that they cannot be perceived consciously. However, according to Dehaene and colleagues (2006), beneath the threshold of consciousness, stimuli can still be processed subliminally and preconsciously. Although subliminally perceived facial expressions were found to bypass selective attention (Harry et al., 2012), Rohr and colleagues (2012) have demonstrated that their processing is nevertheless specific in terms of their degree of self-relevance. The affective primacy hypothesis provides an explanation why even subtle emotional cues are suited to affect people's behaviour and interpretation of events. According to the theory and subsequent research, an affective response does not need a strong elicitor or extensive cognitive processing to be generated, instead very shortly occurring but strongly meaningful emotional ones suffice to determine how a person emotionally reacts (Murphy & Zajonc, 1993; Zajonc, 1980). This particular effect can be measured on the behavioural, as well as the physiological level through brain activation patterns and gamma-band activity (Duan et al., 2010; Nomura et al., 2003; Ruys & Aarts, 2011; Smith, 2011; Yamada & Decety, 2009; Winkielman et al., 2005).

There is broad consensus that the brain processes emotion including facial expressions with emotional content in a holistic manner (Adolphs, 2002; Fusar-Poli et al., 2009; Kilts et al., 2003; Seitz et al., 2008; Schulte-Rüther et al., 2007; Vuilleumier & Pourtois, 2007). Interestingly, the activation patterns found under conditions of limited awareness did not appear to differ strongly from those observed during conscious processing (Brooks et al., 2012; Killgore et al., 2004; Phillips et al., 2004; Sabatini et al., 2009). As social subjects, healthy people continuously try to attribute meaning to an emotional expression they are confronted with. This recognition process typically activates parts of the DMPFC and inferior frontal cortex (IFG, LaBar et al., 2003; Prochnow et al., 2013a; Seitz et al., 2008). Simultaneously, facial expressions tend to be matched to an observed expression (Sato et al., 2013) which has been interpreted as emotional contagion by some authors (Moody et al., 2007). Empathizing emotionally with another person consistently leads to activation of the IFG and adjacent anterior insula which consequently have been suggested to play a key role in this process (Carr et al., 2003; Fan et al., 2011; Lamm et al., 2007; Prochnow et al., 2013a; Seitz et al., 2008; Shamay-Tsoory et al., 2009). More medially located regions of the frontal cortex located in the anterior cingulate (ACC), paracingulate cortex or the pre-SMA become engaged when people empathize in a more cognitive-evaluative manner – which is also referred to as forming an affective theory of mind (Frith & Frith, 2003; Hooker et al., 2008; Prochnow et al., 2013b; Schulte-Rüther et al., 2007; Völlm et al., 2006). In a meta-analysis, the dorsal mid-cingulate cortex was identified as the key substrate of higher order empathy (Fan et al., 2011).

In our study (Prochnow et al., 2013b) we were interested in whether emotional facial expressions below the level of subjective awareness (40 ms) were processed similarly to facial expressions that are consciously perceived (400 ms presentation). In both conditions people were instructed to attribute mood to an emotional facial expression while in the subliminal condition it was masked with a neutral expression. We hypothesized that unconsciously perceived emotional facial expressions alter the perception and empathic judgments of the neutral expression by distorting judgments towards the subliminally presented emotional facial expression. In line with the affective primacy hypothesis (Murphy & Zajonc, 1993; Zajonc, 1980) and based on multiple reports of mirror neuron recruitment in basic empathy (Leslie et al., 2004; Schulte-Rüther et al., 2007), we expected IFG activation during the subliminal presentation of emotional facial expressions owing to their important role as empathic cues in face-to-face situations. In addition, we hypothesized that consciously accessible and subliminal facial expressions of emotion share important nodes within the empathy and face processing network, especially in the DMPFC and the temporo-parietal junction.

The behavioural part of our study showed that compared to consciously accessible facial expressions of emotion which were correctly classified to almost 100%, neutral masking impaired the recognition of the preceding subliminal emotion. This is in congruence with observations of Murphy and Zajonc (1993). However, a more detailed analysis revealed that the subliminally presented affective states had an effect on the judgments of the neutral facial expressions and, thus, were suited to act as affective cues. For example, the neutral expression was classified more often as angry when it was preceded by subliminal anger as compared to subliminal happiness and sadness. In addition, our results provided evidence for a positive–negative valence discrimination of facial expression below the level of awareness. Nevertheless, we found only a trend for the discrimination of two affective states of the same valence as shown by Rohr and colleagues (2012).

The behavioural study was corroborated by our fMRI data revealing that facial expressions engage occipital, posterior temporal, parietal, inferior frontal and dorsolateral prefrontal brain areas regardless whether they were presented above or below the threshold of awareness (Figure 2). In the light of a stage concept of empathy with pure emotional contagion as the basis of emotional empathy and cognitive-evaluative forms of empathy (Decety & Lamm, 2006; Fan et al., 2011; Moody et al., 2007; Shamay-Tsoory et al., 2009), our fMRI data support the notion that emotional facial expressions do not require conscious processing to make an essential contribution to empathy. As hypothesized, the IFG was recruited not only when people were confronted with supraliminal expressions but also in response to the 40 ms masked subliminal affective states. Responsiveness to very subte emotional stimuli was also observed in the amygdala showing an early automatic response after approximately 40 ms and later attention modulation response at 400 ms (Luo et al., 2010). Consciously accessible subliminal faces also shared activity along the posterior portion of the right superior temporal sulcus and the DMPFC, regions which are considered crucial in cognitive-evaluative forms of empathy and theory of mind (Döhnel et al., 2012; Frith & Frith,

2003; Grosbras & Paus, 2006; Kampe et al., 2003; Prochnow et al., 2013a; Saxe & Wexler, 2005; Seitz et al., 2006; Seitz et al., 2008). The strength of activation in the pre-SMA which has been linked to valuation of thought (Seitz et al., 2006; Seitz et al., 2008) was similar in both conditions, as shown by regional data analyses. Other regions which were not specific to subliminal or supraliminal expressions were the caudal part of the intraparietal sulcus which is likely to reflect visual attention to the supraliminal emotional and neutral facial expressions (Corbetta et al., 2005; Nickel et al., 2005), as well as the fusiform face area (FFA, Grill-Spector et al., 2004), an area responding selectively to human faces. Strikingly, activation of the left face-sensitive region was more intense under conditions of awareness. This accorded with the notion of the critical role of feedback processing for conscious visual perception (Koivisto et al., 2012; Rees, 2007). However, the lacking effect in the right FFA can be explained by the accumulated activation by the subliminal face and the subsequent face mask which prevented the subliminally-generated activation to die out (Dehaene et al., 2006).

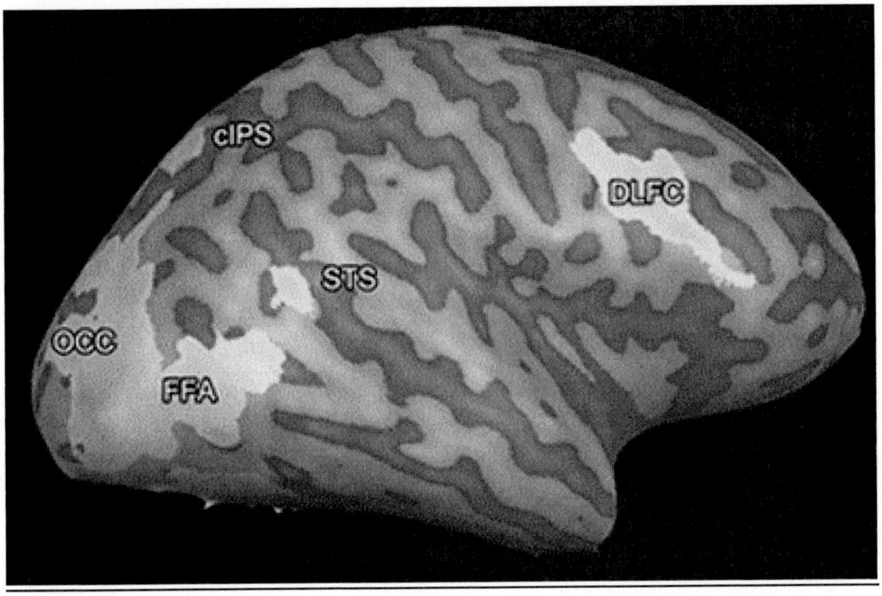

Figure 2: *Attribution of mood to subliminally presented facial expressions. a) Cortical activation areas in occipital, inferior parietal, inferior and superior temporal and mid-frontal cortical areas. b) Significant difference as compared to supraliminally presented facial expressions in the left fusiform face area (FFA). From Prochnow et al. (2013b).*

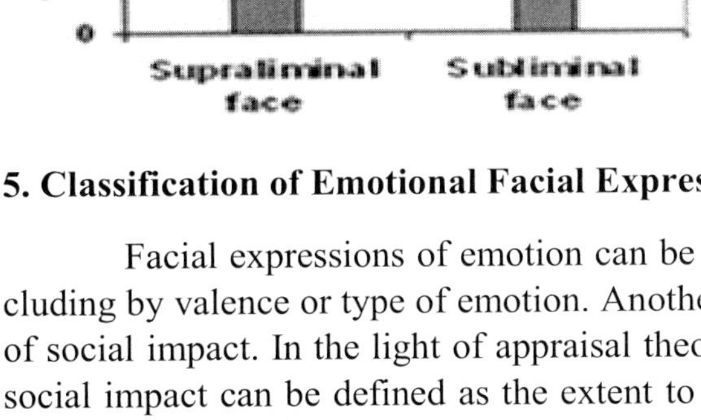

5. Classification of Emotional Facial Expressions

Facial expressions of emotion can be classified in a variety of ways including by valence or type of emotion. Another possible criterion is their degree of social impact. In the light of appraisal theories (Ellsworth & Scherer, 2003), social impact can be defined as the extent to which a specific affective state is associated with behavioural consequences to the observer (cf. Rohr et al., 2012). For example, an angry expression signalling possible threat is highly relevant for the well-being of the observing person who might instinctively engage in allying the other's anger. For efficient social functioning, identification of a specific affective state alone does not meet the requirements of everyday social interactions.

A successful recognition should immediately lead to the decision whether the affective state is of high or low social impact for oneself. This consequently leads the individual to reason about the origin of the observed affective state and the counterpart's associated intentions. As mentioned earlier, theory of mind and empathy are closely related concepts (Shamay-Tsoory et al., 2009). While empathizing with another person facilitates the recognition of affective states, employing cognitive-evaluative forms of empathy can offer valuable clues why someone is looking so angrily at us.

The complex process of recognizing a specific affective state and its associated social impact draws on a number of probably interacting brain regions. Emotional contagion and emotional empathy can activate brain areas which are discussed to accommodate the putative human mirror neuron system (Rizzolatti & Craighero, 2004) in order to create a representation of the observed state in the observer's brain. In accordance with this assumption many research studies report activation of areas such as the IFG or intraparietal lobule in basic empathic processing (Carr et al., 2003; Lamm et al., 2007; Schulte-Rüther et al., 2007; Seitz et al., 2008; Shamay-Tsoory et al., 2009; et al., 2013a; Prochnow et al., 2013b). When cognitive-evaluative forms of empathy are employed and a theory of mind is formed on the information retrieved during empathizing, current neuroscientific research points again to the involvement of the DMPFC (Fan et al., 2011; Gallagher & Frith, 2003; Hooker et al., 2008; Hynes et al., 2006; Krämer et al., 2010; Vogeley et al., 2001)

To investigate the areas involved in reasoning about another person's affective state, we required 26 healthy subjects to select a phrase that described best the putative reason of an emotional facial expression (Prochnow et al., 2014a). Specifically, participants were presented with depersonalized photographs from male and female actors displaying happiness, sadness, anger or fear in difficulty-adjusted degrees. Angry and happy affective states were considered to represent a high degree of social impact due to the related behavioural consequences for the observer, while sad and fearful expressions were considered to have low social impact (cf. Rohr et al., 2012). By pressing one out of four response buttons, they had to indicate which out of four sentences represented the possible cause for the facial expressions, e.g. "He was threatened by someone" or "He got a parking ticket". In the control condition scrambled images were shown and a button press in response to unrelated sentences was used to control for visual, reading and motor related brain activity.

The study aimed at mapping the brain regions involved in empathic reasoning. Due to their self-relevance for the observer, we hypothesized that affective states of high social impact are processed in a fast, preferential, and accurate manner compared to those of low social impact. We expected not only faster reaction times and more accurate choices but also less pronounced brain activation in emotion-related areas as a result of the less cognitive resources consuming preferential processing. On the contrary, we predicted that affectives states of low social impact lead to more profound processing because people lack routine to process these less self-relevant expressions in everyday life. In addition, we expected empathic reasoning to go along with activation in brain regions associated with cognitive-evaluative forms of empathy and theory of mind in the DMPFC and anterior prefrontal cortex.

Data analysis revealed that participant's performance on reasoning about the origin of a specific affective state was more accurate for expressions of high social impact. Contrary to our hypothesis, response times were longer when the affective state had high social impact compared to low social impact. However, longer response times were related to lower accuracy for expressions of high social impact while the contrary effect was observed for expressions of low social impact. This observation pointed towards an advantage effect of intuitive reasoning when the degree of social impact is considered high. Even though more mistakes were made when the subjects took more time to respond to expressions of high social impact, they were still more accurate compared to expressions of low social impact.

Independently of social impact, facial expressions evoked brain activation in typical regions such as the occipital cortices, the right FFA (Grill-Spector et al., 2004), the premotor cortices, and the inferior parietal lobule. The latter areas have been repeatedly associated with the putative human mirror neuron system (Rizzolatti & Craighero, 2004), as well as basic emotional empathy (Lawrence et al., 2006; Lamm et al., 2007). In addition, we observed activation in the left superior DMPFC and the anterior prefrontal cortex (Figure 3). The DMPFC has been identified as a core region of cognitive-evaluative empathy (Fan et al, 2011) due to its involvement in theory of mind (Gallagher et al., 2000; Hooker et al., 2008; Moore et al., 2010; Ullsperger et al., 2007). The left anterior prefrontal cortex has been repeatedly implicated in cognitive perspective-taking (Hynes et al., 2006; Völlm et al., 2006). The early recruitement of brain areas associated with cognitive aspects of empathy or even cognitive theory of mind may at a first glance appear surprising. It may reflect, however, goal-directed behaviour in order to perform the task correctly. The activation increase observed in the DLPFC is in accordance with decision-making in an ambiguous social-affective context (Baumgartner et al., 2011; Hall et al., 2010; Heekeren et al., 2006; Krain et al., 2006; Prochnow et al., 2013a).

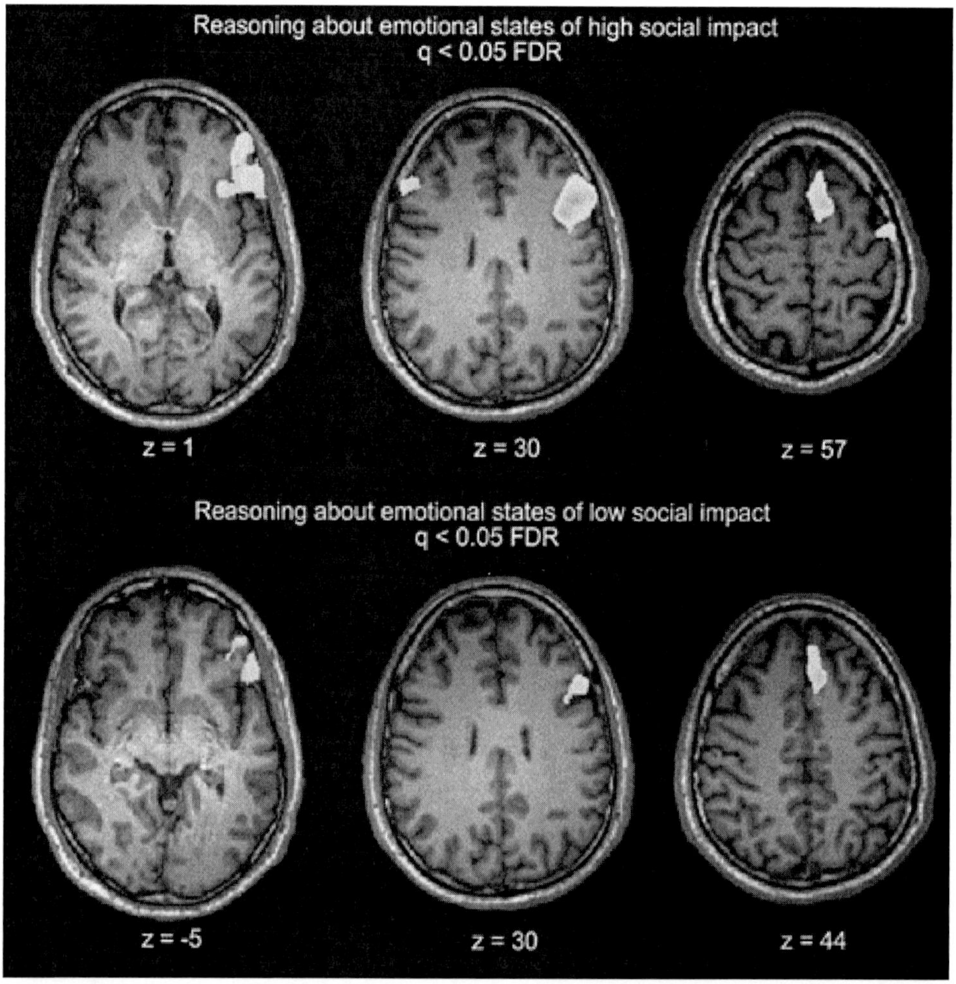

Figure 3: *Reasoning about affective facial expressions with high social impact (top row) and low social impact (bottom row). Note the stronger activation pattern involving the left inferior frontal gyrus and the dorsal medial prefrontal cortex in facial expressions with high social impact. From Prochnow et al. (2014a).*

6. Discrimination of Affective Body Movements

People are equipped with a wide range of patterns of behavior to communicate nonverbally. Whether these are facial expressions, gestures, variants of prosody, posture or other body movements, they all offer an observer the possibility to get important information about the sender's current affective state. According to Ekman and Friesen (1976), some classes of affective states are considered universal in their performance and perception. These are happiness, sadness, anger, disgust, surprise and fear. In real life, these so called basic emotions can occur purely but also in combination with each other, e.g. anger and disgust combined might signal contempt. Facial expressions are often combined with gestures. Different from the basic facial expressions of emotion, emotional or emblematic gestures are sequences of body movements which are culture-specific (Kendon, 1997; Lindenberg et al., 2012). Together, facial expressions and gestures constitute two main pillars of body language (Duncan, 1969). A high degree of routine allows us to decode even very subtle affective cues which are only visible for fractures of seconds (Bar et al., 2006; Jiang et al., 2009; van den Stock et al., 2011). However, the dynamic character of both, facial expressions and gestures, makes social interactions challenging.

We used fMRI to map the brain activation patterns related to different stages within the processes of observing and discriminating facial expressions and gestures conveying an emotionally relevant message (Prochnow et al., 2013a). We created an fMRI paradigm in which we presented block-wise sequences of short video-clips displaying either a male or female face showing a specific affective state, or the upper part of a male's body presenting a specific emblematic gesture. The video-clips started with a neutral expression and neutral posture, respectively, and dynamically evolved into a meaningful expression. Brain activity was captured at two events of interest: On the one hand, during an early stage of observation when the expressions were still ambiguous in valence, and on the other hand at the time point when our subjects were able to discriminate the gestures as positive or negative or the facial expressions as angry or not angry. Subjects responded with pressing one of two response buttons. We contrasted facial expressions and gestures against scrambled images to control for visual effects and additionally included a motor control condition in which the subjects watched the video-clips and had to respond in an alternating fashion.

We hypothesized that observing the evolving but still ambiguous expressions would trigger low level empathy as reflected by activation of empathy-relevant brain areas such as the IFG and DMPFC (Carr et al., 2003; Fan et al., 2011; Lindenberg et al., 2012; Lotze et al., 2006; Schulte-Rüther et al., 2007; Seitz et al., 2008). Also, we predicted the subsequent discrimination to result in activation of decision-relevant brain areas such as the dorsolateral prefrontal cortex (DLPFC) which has been shown critical for information manipulation (Rowe et al., 2000) and stimulus discrimination (Krain et al., 2006; Stoeckel et al., 2003).

Data analysis revealed that during the observation of the evolving and still ambiguous facial expressions and gestures led to activation increases in the frontal, temporal, and parietal lobes (Figure 4). Within the temporal cortex, a portion of the inferior temporal gyrus became active which can be associated with the visual processing via the ventral visual path, also refered to as the 'what-stream' relevant for recognition and form representation (Borowsky et al., 2005).

We also observed activation in the IFG and the closely adjacent anterior insula which are considered as putative parts of the human mirror neuron system affording empathy (Carr et al., 2003; Schulte-Rüther et al., 2007; Shamay-Tsoory et al., 2009). Viewing dynamically changing body language also yielded an increase of brain activation in the DMPFC which has been previously implicated in integrating an observed affective state in a personal frame of reference (Carr et al., 2003; Lindenberg et al., 2012; Schulte-Rüther et al., 2007; Seitz et al., 2008). At the moment of discrimination, the right DLPFC became engaged. The degree of activation within the DLPFC correlated with activation in parts of the right DMPFC and the left premotor cortex, among others. Due to the involvement of the DLPFC in tasks involving different types of decisions (Hall et al., 2010; Hosseini et al., 2010; Krain et al., 2006; Stoeckel et al., 2003), our results argue for a specific role of this region in social-affective discriminative decisions complementing earlier results by Mériau et al. (2006).

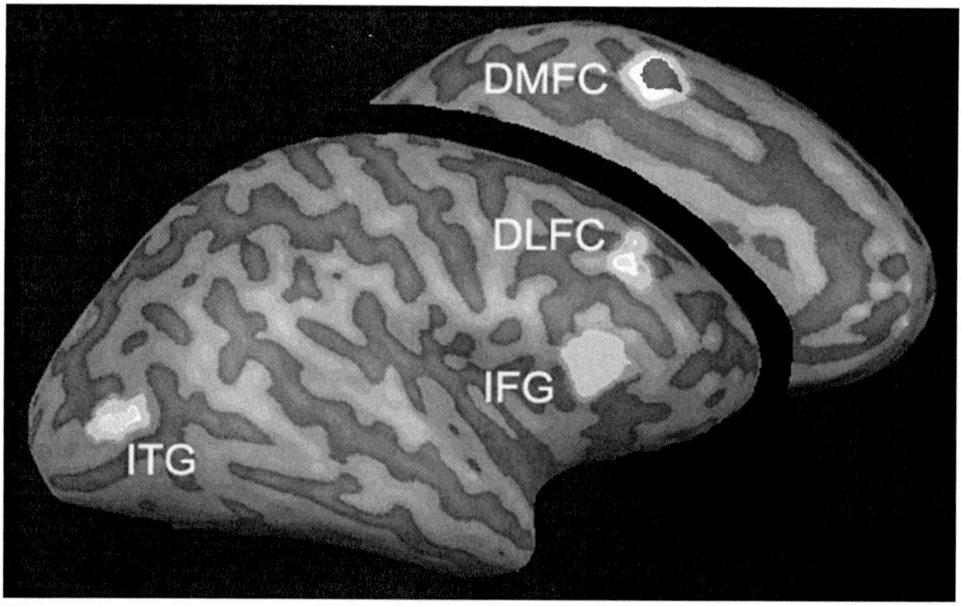

Figure 4: *Common activations in perception and discrimination of emotional face expressions and emblematic gestures. Involved for perception and discrimination were the inferior temporal (ITG) and inferior frontal gyrus (IFG), for perception the dorsal medial frontal cortex (DMFC), and for discrimination the dorsolateral prefrontal cortex (DLFC). From Prochnow et al. (2013a).*

Svenson (1996) offered a theory explaining the different steps people need to take when making a decision. Accordingly, the moment of the decision is preceded by a predecision period during which choice alternatives are generated and compared until one reaches an acceptable degree of acceptance. The DLPFC has been implicated in the computation of these decision values (Camus et al., 2009). Often, the decision is followed by a consolidation period in order to evaluate the decision and its possible consequences (Svenson, 1996). In the current study, we instructed our subjects to observe the evolving expressions and to indicate their decision by a button-press as soon as they felt confident enough to discriminate them. Thus, the event of interest we studied here is likely to reflect the actual decision. Possible post-decision consolidation effects can be neglected, since our subjects did not receive any feedback. Thus, unlike other observations (Grabenhorst & Rolls, 2011), the DLPFC activation we observed here might reflect reward-independent decision-making in a social-affective context.

7. Probabilistic Perspective Taking

The discussion so far is open to further, possibly speculative hypotheses. First, when people set out for initiating and maintaining certain behaviour, they have to identify the appropriate social situation, adapt to restrictions in their social or cultural environment, and determine how to reach their goal. Typically, subjects will make formal classifications and subsequent decisions intuitively in a probabilistic manner, since information is available only for a short period of time, distorted by noise, or due to elusive competing computations. Behavioural decisions in social context involve, in addition, the discrimination of right and wrong, good and bad, pleasant or unpleasant. Such discriminations lead to the selection of an appropriate action and the suppression of inappropriate actions. There is good evidence in the literature that the DLPFC is specifically involved in the discriminative decision process (e.g. Stoeckel et al., 2003; Prochnow et al., 2013a, b, c). Specifically, spatial, sensory, emotional and abstract discriminations involve the right DLPFC (Eickhoff et al., 2011; Hall et al., 2010; Hosseini et al., 2010; Stoeckel et al., 2003) with more demanding tasks resulting in higher activation (Duncan et al., 2008; Niendam et al., 2012). The DMPFC is relevant for unexpected stimuli, not the valence of the stimuli as evident from recordings of feedback related negativity (Ferdinand et al., 2012). The difference between the symbolic discriminations performed on literal or numerical data and spatial, sensory and emotional data is that the former can be ascribed to correct or faulty solutions, while in the latter domain the discriminations are intuitive and reached by high subjective estimates of certainty. The DLPFC is a critical node with more intense connections in subjects with high intelligence (Cole et al., 2012). This network involves the inferior frontal cortex, the medial frontal cortex, and the parahippocampal area.

Second, in a more general sense, people interpret the signals of the complex outside world in simplified personal terms. These accounts are manageable for the given subject affording a basis for self-control of behaviour. Accordingly, behavioural decisions involve different degrees of ambiguity which is heavily influence by the credibility of the subjective assumption. Ultimately, subjects take a positive stance to their decisions, as much as they believe to have taken the right decision. Usually, a given subject can be certain of how to classify the object or event in the outside world, which will make her/him say: "I know this is so and so". The statement "I know" refers to an objectivity which can be probed by others in reality. In case the subject is less certain, she or he may say: "I think this is so and so". In case the subject is certain about his appraisal but cannot prove it, she/he will say: "I believe this is so and so". In fact, in this broad sense, believing is a mental activity that leads to the first person perspective that something is real or true, although this cannot be proven. Thus, the proposition "I believe" provides a deep sense of certainty or personal trust and is a cognitive-emotional evaluation process which has been labeled credition (Seitz & Angel, 2012). The process characterizing the statement "I believe" also has a second-person perspective (Churchill, 2012). For example, we usually use "I believe" to express respect for the belief of the listener even despite 100% confidence on our own belief. Above that, the use of "I" may assume that my belief may turn out to be wrong, while simultaneously there is some reason for me that nevertheless "I" want to hold that belief. The reason is usually a desire for being released from distress or an impending demand of decision making. This is object of reinforcement learning, such that a personal belief about the probability of a representation involves an implicit judgement of certainty which is updated by subsequent experience (Chang et al., 2012). In support of such a model repetitively occurring stimuli induce an illusion of truth (Chang et al., 2010; Henkel & Mattson, 2011). Neuroimaging data have shown that the DMPFC is critical for attributing a meaning to a certain event in the complex environment (Azari et al., 2001; Sugiura et al., 2009). Conversely, the ventromedial prefrontal cortex influences sensory processing by belief (Goel & Dolan, 2003). Further, anxiously attached adults are automatically more responsive to positive facial expressions in brain areas involved in perception of facial emotions (Donges et al., 2012).

Third, probabilistic estimates of external uncertainties ultimately may become transcendental or religious beliefs (Döhnel et al., 2012; Harris et al., 2008). The cognitive processes underlying a religious belief may vary depending on the situational and cultural context and have been proposed to represent interpretations of one's own mental states, perceptions, and motivations (Boyer, 2003; Eccles & Wigfield, 2002; Krüger et al., 2009; Seitz & Angel, 2014; Vogeley & Roepsdorf, 2009; Vandenbergh et al., 1999). But observations in delusional belief have suggested that there are three mental processes of normal belief generation (Bell et al., 2006). These include (1) attentional monitoring systems of ambiguous perceptions leading to first-person experience, (2) the bias of individual attributions to perceptions for causal explanations, and (3) belief evaluation processes giving priority to indirect sources of information (Langdon & Coltheart, 2000). Another possibility which is not mutually exclusive to this hypothesis is the possibility that sensory and likewise mental information is processed in parallel channels. According to Morewedge and Kahneman (2010) there is a type 1 process which is intuitive and implicit and overrules the abstract and rational type 2 process. In fact, it was hypothesized that type 1 processes represent a faulty intuition system that gives major biases of intuitive judgment controlling the rational operations. Religiousness has been proposed to include dual implicit/intuitive and abstract/rational cognitive processing (Watts, 2007). Such a dual pathway was shown to engage different brain areas (Kuo et al., 2009). Notably, religious beliefs involve the DMPFC (Azari et al., 2001; Han et al.. 2008). In the end, deities have been described as intentional agents with mental states (Norensayan et al., 2012) suggesting that the belief in a person-like God is a special form of mentalizing and is known to be of great relevance for control of behaviour.

Part 2:

Clinical Neuropsychology, Brain Dysfunction and Neurorehabilitation

6 Neurophysiological Assessment and Brain Communication in Non-Responsiveness and Paralysis

Boris Kotchoubey, Ujwal Chaudhary, Francesco Piccione and Niels Birbaumer

Key Words:
brain-computer interface (BCI), classical conditioning, consciousness, event-related potentials (ERP), functional magnetic resonance imaging (fMRI), locked-in syndrome (LIS, also complete LIS: CLIS), minimally conscious state (MCS), near-infrared spectroscopy (NIRS), outcome prediction, vegetative state (VS, synonym unresponsive wakefulness syndrome, UWS)

Abstract

Problems of assessment and communication with non- and low-responsive patients (particularly those in locked-in state, LIS, or in complete locked-in state, CLIS) are discussed. First of all, the extant literature routinely draws a strong borderline between the patients with severe disorders of consciousness and those who are "only" severely paralyzed but assumed to be in full awareness. We show that this strong distinction does not hold because there are numerous mixed cases and even transition states between the two groups of disorders. Methods of the preliminary assessment of non-responsive patients are described, and the most important results obtained by using these methods are listed. While LIS patients can use the already existing Brain-Computer Interface (BCI) systems for communication, all attempts to teach a CLIS patients in using a BCI have failed. The possible reasons of this failure and potential ways of solution of the specific CLIS problems are discussed.

1. Varieties of Non-Responsiveness

Many neurological patients are highly restricted in their behavioral responses ("low-responsive"), or even do not have any overt behavior at all ("non-responsive"). Most textbooks strictly distinguish between two categories of non- and low-responsive patients: those with severe motor deficits and those with deficits in the domain of cognitive functions including consciousness. First of all, therefore, these categories of patients should be briefly depicted. After this we will show that the usual distinction between motor and cognitive impairments might be useful in theory but does not hold in real life.

Examples of the former category (i.e., severe motor disorders) are locked-in syndrome (LIS), severe aphasias, high-level spinal cord injury, or some paralyzing degenerative diseases (e.g., amyotrophic lateral sclerosis, ALS). LIS (Bauer et al., 1979) is usually a result of a lesion in the anterior pons, the part of the middle brain where all motor pathways from the primary motor cortex to the spinal cord and the brain stem come together in a very narrow space. Most frequently, the damage to this area results from a thrombosis or embolism of the basilar artery with subsequent infarct in the tegmentum pontis. Such a sudden catastrophe leads to the immediate loss of almost all movements. As a rule, i.e., in the "classical" LIS, vertical eye movements remain intact because the third cranial nerve innervating these movements leaves the brain just above the level of the lesion (Kotchoubey & Lotze, 2013).

In contrast to such catastrophic events as the stroke of the middle brain (i.e., LIS), or a traumatic spinal cord injury leading to a complete paralysis below the level of the lesion, degenerative diseases such as ALS are chronic, slowly developing conditions. ALS is characterized by degeneration of motor neurons at the levels of both motor cortex and spinal cord. Also these diseases can result in a profound paralysis of the entire musculature quite similar to the classical LIS, and eye movements (or, sometimes, movements of face or fingers) can remain as the last communication channel relating the patient to his or her caregivers (Kübler & Birbaumer, 2008). Therefore, it may be useful to speak about a locked-in *state* independently of its etiology (contrary to the term locked-in *syndrome* which is specifically attributed to the pontine lesions). Also inflammatory processes in the nervous system (peripheral polyradiculoneuropathy in form of a Guillain-Barré Syndrome) can similarly lead to a locked-in state. If ocular paralysis is also present and no motor action is available any longer, a complete locked-in state (CLIS) is diagnosed.

Looking now at the presumably alternative category of low- and non-responsive patients, the typical representative is coma. Coma is defined as the complete loss of consciousness and behavioral responses, mainly due to a direct lesion or indirect impairment of brain stem. As an acute condition coma is usually related to deadly peril due to dysfunction of the respiratory and circulatory systems. Therefore coma patients need intensive medical care. Coma can last from a few seconds to maximal four weeks. After this time, most coma patients regain consciousness. Of the rest, some die and others evolve into a vegetative state (VS), also referred to as Unresponsive Wakefulness Syndrome (UWS) (Kotchoubey, 2009; Laureys et al., 2010). This condition can be described as "wakefulness without awareness". VS/UWS patients appear to be awake for some time, and their reflexes are preserved or even enhanced, but, by definition, these patients do not have any kind of subjective experience or sensation and do not demonstrate any voluntary activity or attempt to communicate with other people. If minimal and instable signs of subjective awareness can be observed, the diagnosis is not a VS/UWS, but a minimally conscious state (MCS: Giacino et al., 2002). MCS patients can sometimes follow simple instructions, e.g. to look right or left, or pronounce understandable words or other vocalizations appropriate to the situation (Bruno et al., 2011). They can grasp an object, show in its direction, keep, and adjust the position of their hand or arm in accordance to the object's shape, but they cannot use it.

A patient is *not in MCS* any longer, but has regained consciousness, as soon as at least one of the two criteria is fulfilled: consistent communication at least at the simplest level, or functional use of two different objects. To establish consistent communication, it should be shown that the patient can correctly answer six simple alternative questions such as "Do I show to the ceiling?" or "Are we now in a hospital?" in a row. Answers can be non-verbal (e.g., close eyes = yes, open eyes widely = no), but unambiguous. To establish functional use of objects, even a rudimentary use is sufficient. For example, a patient does not merely grasp a comb (which can be done also in MCS), but brings it to her hair; it is not necessary that she is able to make a nice hairstyle.

Thus far, we have two different categories of low- and non-responsive patients, the one with severe motor impairments, and the other with severely impaired consciousness. In fact, however, the border between the two groups is unclear. Let us start with the former category. Patients with **classical LIS** have presently much better chances than before to restore to normal life, and many of them have later reported their experiences of an acute locked-in condition. All of them remember at least partial disorders of consciousness (e.g., Bauby, 1997; Pantke, 1999; Tavalaro, 1998), which is in a strong contrast to the doctrine that LIS and disorders of consciousness are completely different conditions that have only superficial, behavioral similarity. Even lesions restricted to the typical area in the anterior pons can result in cognitive deficits in addition to motor deficits (Pistoia et al., 2008); wider lesions, which extend in the rostral or posterior direction, are consistently accompanied with disorders of perception and attention. Further, the pontine infarct resulting in a classical LIS can be combined with other infarcts in other brain regions, whose neuropsychological effects are masked by the severe paralysis and cannot be diagnosed in time (Chia, 1991). Finally, a subarachnoidal hemorrhage (which leads to coma and VS/UWS) can result in a vasospasm in the basilar artery, resulting in a secondary LIS (Lacroix et al., 2011).

Concerning **ALS**, the situation is not much different. Since the pioneering study of Ludolph et al. (1992) we know that in many ALS patients degenerative processes are not restricted to motor regions only, but can be observed in various areas of the frontal and temporal cortex. These morphological changes are further related to the corresponding changes in cognitive and emotional functions (e.g., Abrahams et al., 1996). Although more than a half of ALS patients remain cognitively intact even at the late stage of the disease, others have various degrees of cognitive disorders. **Guillain-Barré Syndrome**, as a disease of the peripheral nervous system, is not expected to be related to problems of cognition and consciousness. However, it can combine with encephalitis (Fisher Syndrome), and particularly in chronic forms of the disease it is still unknown how higher brain function can respond to the blackout of motor functions. To sum up, *all conditions, in which a "pure" paralysis is frequently assumed, can involve different degrees of impairment of cognitive functions including disorders of consciousness*, beyond the motor impairment.

On the other hand, the rate of misdiagnosis in **VS/UWS** is about 40% and, what is worse, it has remained at this level of imprecision for at least for 15 years notwithstanding huge efforts to improve clinical diagnostics (Andrews et al., 1996; Schnakers et al., 2009). Even if most misdiagnosed patients are probably in MCS, indirect estimations indicate that about 5 to 10% patients with the diagnose VS/UWS can have levels of consciousness higher than the MCS, and some of them are probably in LIS (Kotchoubey et al., 2013). Moreover, Formisano et al. (2011) have recently shown that "functional LIS" (in fact, CLIS, as such patients do not have even a minimal behavioral response) can be a transition phase from VS/UWS (or MCS) to normal condition. The rate of misdiagnosis of MCS is not known, but since MCS patients are characterized by strong fluctuations of their state, and since such fluctuations are even a part of the definition of the MCS, this diagnosis may be expected to be at least as difficult as (or even more difficult than) VS/UWS. In sum, *a considerable portion of the patients diagnosed as severe disorders of consciousness may be (partially) conscious but unable to express their thoughts, wishes and feelings in their behavior.*

This means that from a pragmatic point of view, it is not necessary to strictly subdivide low- and nonresponsive patients into two opposite categories. Rather, we can ask a practical question of whether a patient can communicate. The answer to this question is not dichotomous (yes/no), but depends on the patient's actual state, availability of appropriate communication means, and other, e.g., social factors.

2. Assessment of Communicative Abilities

By definition, behavioral responses of the target patient group are either minimal, or unreliable or virtually absent. Neumann and Kotchoubey (2004) showed that even in patients with minimal but quite reliable responses, neuropsychological tests for assessment of cognitive functions cannot be applied in their standard form but need to be adjusted according to the patient's facilities. The authors demonstrated how this adjustment can be done for such well known cognitive tests as the Standard Progressive Matrices, the Wisconsin Card Sorting Test, the Verbal and Nonverbal Learning test, the Rivermead Face Memory Test, and the Aachener Aphasia Test. In most non- and low-responsive patients, behavior is unreliable, if present, and the analysis should be based on neurophysiological responses. Two well-known neurophysiological methods used, event-related brain potentials (ERP) and functional magnetic resonance imaging (fMRI), have recently been supplemented with Near Infrared Spectroscopy (NIRS).

2.1. EEG and Event-Related Potentials

Several large studies used ERP (EEG components, strongly related in time and phase with particular events, e.g., stimuli; see Figure 1) in non-responsive patients. In the earliest study (Schoenle & Witzke, 2004) sentences with semantically congruent and incongruent endings were acoustically presented to 66 patients with definite or "suspected" VS/UWS. A component N400, which is typical for brain responses to semantic incongruence, was found in 22 patients. Among 54 severely brain damaged but conscious patients, the N400 was obtained in 49 cases.

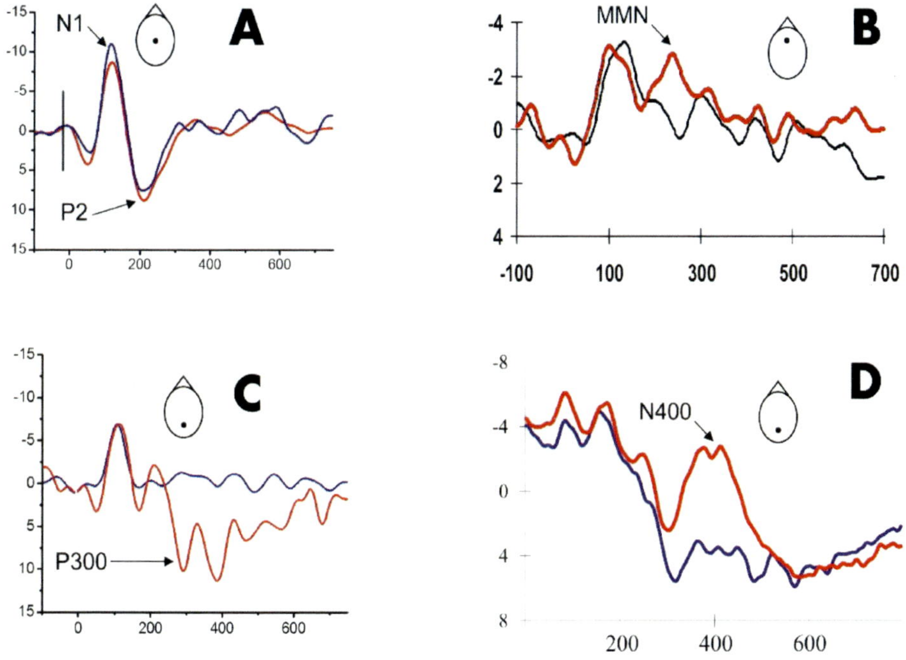

Figure 1. *Examples of ERP components used in the assessment of non- and low-responsive patients. Red lines: "odd" stimuli (i.e., rare deviant stimuli in panels A, B, and C; semantically incongruent stimuli in panel D). A: the primary cortical N1-P2 complex that does not differentiate between stimulus categories. B: mismatch negativity (MMN) as a sign of simple (attention-independent) auditory discrimination. C: the parietal P300 (or P3b) as a target response. D: the N400 as a response to semantically inappropriate stimuli. X-axes are in msec, please not different time scales for different ERP components. Y-*

axes are in μV, negativity is plotted upwards. The schematic head sign indicates the appropriate site of recording of a given component.

In contrast to this study, in which ERP components were visually evaluated by an expert, Kotchoubey et al. (2005) applied a quantitative assessment of ERP. Compared to the results in Schoenle and Witzke (2004), they reported even higher rates of N400 in both VS/UWS and MCS patients. Also the P3 component was found in about 25% of the patients. These finding have recently been confirmed by Cavinato et al. (2009), Fischer et al. (2010), Steppacher et al. (2013), and others.

A specific kind of ERP paradigm consists of active instruction tasks. If a brain response of a patient demonstrates that he or she attempts to follow an instruction (e.g., to move the right or left hand), this is a direct indication of the presence of consciousness and thus the ability to use a communication device. To date, such proof has been provided in patients with CLIS (Kotchoubey et al., 2003; Schnakers et al., 2009), but not with VS/UWS or MCS. Schnakers et al. (2008) asked eight VS/UWS and 14 MCS patients to count their own name and found a significantly larger P3 amplitude to this stimulus than to other (passively listened to) stimuli in the MCS group. No ERP response in any condition was recorded in the VS/UWS group. The characteristic P3 increase with the active instruction was also found when the target stimulus was a name unfamiliar to the patient. Similar results were obtained by Faugeras et al. (2011), Chennu et al. (2013), and Risetti et al. (2013). Obviously, at least some MCS patients are able to intentionally follow instructions. To summarize, *a large portion of non-responsive patients diagnosed as severe disorders of consciousness* (VS/UWS, MCS) *exhibit cortical responses to stimuli of different levels of complexity.*

As a common result of most studies, ERP do not differentiate between VS/UWS and MCS (Faugeras et al., 2011, 2012; Fischer et al., 2010; Kotchoubey et al., 2009; Perrin et al., 2006; Wijnen et al., 2007). Two notable exceptions are Schoenle and Witzke (2004) and Schnakers et al. (2008). In the former, however, the presence of ERP components was subjectively evaluated by a non-blinded rater. The latter included probably a particularly severe VS/UWS group because even N1 was totally absent, although this component is typically recorded in most VS/UWS patients.

The data from Kotchoubey et al. (2005) shed light on this issue. Most MCS patients have moderate (4-7 Hz) slowing of the background EEG oscillations (e.g., Leon-Carrion et al., 2008). If they are compared to VS/UWS patients with a similar EEG pattern, no difference in any ERP component can be found; however, much more negative results are found in VS/UWS patients with a severe slowing of the EEG rhythmic activity (< 3 Hz). Therefore, the results of other studies comparing VS/UWS and MCS may critically depend on the exact "mixture" of VS/UWS patients with moderate versus severe background EEG disturbance in a particular sample.

The problem of diagnosis in DoC is closely related with that of prognosis of the outcome. Even taking into account important clinical variables such as etiology and time since the accident leaves a high degree of uncertainty. Therefore, a search for neurophysiological *predictors* remains an important task.

Kotchoubey et al. (2005) retrospectively collected 6-month follow-up data in 43 patients with severe disorders of consciousness. Clinical improvement was observed in 9 VS/UWS patients (4 MCS, communicative) and 10 MCS patients (all communicative). Patients who showed an MMN later improved significantly more frequently than patients without an MMN, and the same tendency approached significance for the N400. The importance of the MMN was confirmed by Wijnen et al. (2007). Although they examined only ten VS/UWS patients, all of whom recovered, the study had several important advantages: it was prospective (rather than retrospective as in Kotchoubey et al., 2005), the sample was homogenous, and each patient was examined every two weeks for a period of 3.5 months.

The MMN finding is noteworthy for two reasons. First, the MMN reliably predicts the outcome of acute coma (meta-analysis of Daltrozzo et al., 2007). The acute pathological process in the brain and the chronic conditions such as VS/UWS differ substantially in their morphology and pathophysiology, and thus factors determining their temporal course are generally different. Nevertheless, the same ERP component may be an important index of brain function in both coma and chronic disorders of consciousness. Second, the fact that the MMN predicts recovery of consciousness may appear strange given that the component is largely independent of the actual state of consciousness. The presence of an MMN does not indicate that the patient is able to consciously perceive stimuli at the moment of examination, but that this ability is not detected by clinical methods. Rather, the MMN may manifest the yet silent reserves of the brain that will later be realized in form of conscious awareness.

The predictive trend for the N400 observed by Kotchoubey et al. (2005) was replicated in a recent study, the largest and most careful study to date (Steppacher et al., 2013). It involved a total of 175 low- and non-responsive patients, of which fifty-three VS/UWS and 39 MCS patients were followed up from two to 15 years (mean 8.3) after the accident. The target ERP components were determined using both blind expert assessment and a careful mathematical analysis. Both methods yielded the same result: The presence of the N400 was strongly associated with clinical improvement during the following years. The predictive value of the N400 depended neither on the diagnosis nor the etiology (traumatic, hypoxic, others). In contrast, the presence of oddball P3 was unrelated to the outcome in any diagnostic group.

Contrary to the other reports, a significant predictive effect for P3 was found in a study with 34 traumatic VS/UWS patients (Cavinato et al., 2009), and for middle-latency auditory EP components in a study with 39 MCS patients (Luauté et al., 2010). In the latter study ERP were recorded in the acute period, and the patients were followed up to five years. All of them were in MCS after one year (additionally, 12 VS patients were investigated, but none of them changed the diagnosis after one year).

The lack of consistency in these data should not be surprising, as it has at least two reasons. First, the patient samples differ among studies in terms of the diagnosis (VS/UWS, MCS, coma), etiology (purely traumatic versus mixed groups) and time post ictum (from days in Faugeras et al., 2011, to years in Luauté et al., 2010). Second, the result of a prediction study critically depends on the initial set of independent variables which the search for predictors starts with. This set was rather small in all studies mentioned above. Including additional variables might radically change the final results. Reliable information on the predictive role of ERP and other neurophysiological variables (e.g., sleep EEG and fMRI) can only be obtained in a large multi-center longitudinal study involving a broad set of potential clinical, neurophysiological and demographic predictors.

Only a few studies applied non phase locked EEG components in addition to the ERP. Cruse et al. (2011) reported that their EEG analysis revealed the ability to consistently follow verbal instructions in three of 17 patients with the diagnosis VS/UWS, indicating a rather high level of consciousness in these presumably unconscious individuals. However, the methods used in this study have been strongly criticized (Goldfine et al., 2013). Further research in this direction is necessary.

2.2. fMRI

For a long time low- and non-responsive patients were regarded as inappropriate for fMRI examinations, largely for two reasons: uncontrolled movements leading to uncorrectable artifacts, and components (e.g., magnetic pumps or devices for artificial ventilation) incompatible with strong magnetic fields. However, these restrictions concern only a portion of the population of non-responsive patients. Ethical rules dictate that patients who can be examined should be selected carefully in advance, so that only those are fMRI-examined whose data can really be analyzed. Such careful advance selection can minimize a loss of patients' data.

Because fMRI examinations cannot be performed at a patient's bedside but need a special environment, and because fMRI facilities are not available at any site, patients have to be transported, resulting in substantial stress and additional costs. On the other hand, the fMRI approach possesses two important advantages. First, the activity of deep brain structures can be recorded. Questions of great political and ethical importance, e.g., whether a patient can feel pain, experience pleasure and non-pleasure, cannot be answered using EEG because the brain areas responsible for pain and emotional experience are not accessible by means of EEG/ERP. fMRI, however, can record the activity of the amygdala (negative emotions), nucleus accumbens (positive emotions), and other affective brain structures. Thus Yu et al. (2013) demonstrated that many patients diagnosed as VS/UWS, whose neocortical structures were actually non-responsive to any complex stimulation, nevertheless adequately responded to other people's cries of pain and suffering; these responses concentrated, like in healthy controls, around the anterior and posterior insular regions and the anterior cingulate cortex (ACC).

The second advantage of fMRI is its ability to reveal whole networks of appropriate brain activations, rather than merely increase of some activity. We know that, e.g., pain stimuli are processed with a complex network called "pain matrix", which includes structures related to both sensory (thalamus, somatosensory cortex, posterior insula) and affective (cerebellum, anterior insula, ACC) aspects of pain. In ERP, we could only expect an increased response to pain as compared with non-pain stimulus, while fMRI data deliver much more detailed information about the ability of a patient's brain to process sensory and affective stimulus qualities, as shown by Markl et al. (2013) who recorded brain responses to pain in the above described regions of interests (ROI) in a large sample of behaviorally nonresponsive patients.

In addition to the studies of pain and emotions, two important fMRI-based approaches have been related to language comprehension and instruction following. Coleman et al. (2007) examined twelve non-responsive patients, five of whom demonstrated significant responses to comprehensible speech versus meaningless sounds ("mid-level speech perception"). Moreover, three of the five patients also exhibited significant brain responses to semantically ambiguous versus unambiguous sentences ("high-level speech perception"). Both groups of mid- and high-level responders included VS/UWS and MCS patients, thus there was no association between speech responsiveness and the diagnosis. Later on, these authors reported indications of high-level brain responses to speech sounds in four non-responsive patients (i.e., two of 22 VS/UWS, and two of 19 MCS; Coleman et al., 2009). Likewise, Fernandez-Espejo et al. (2008) found one (out of three) VS/UWS and one (out of 4) MCS patient with significant BOLD responses to intelligible speech. Kotchoubey et al. (2014) recorded BOLD responses to factually correct or incorrect sentences (e.g., March follows April vs. May follows April) in 55 non-responsive patients. Significant responses in the pre-defined ROI (Broca and Wernicke areas and the homologous areas of the right hemisphere) were obtained in 16 patients, indicating high level of language processing. Like in the other studies, there were no differences as a function of diagnosis, severity of morphological brain lesion or etiology.

The first active instruction task based on fMRI data was developed by Boly et al. (2007) who demonstrated that mental imagery of playing tennis and navigation in the own apartment elicit two significantly distinct patterns of brain activity in each and every healthy individual, with the maximum activity in the supplementary motor area (SMA) in the motor imagery condition and in the parahippocampal place area (PPA) in the spatial imagery condition. These two instructions were applied in a young female VS/UWS patient[1] whose results also did not differ from those of healthy controls. Obviously, the patient was able to understand and consistently follow the instructions, i.e., she was conscious (Owen et al., 2006). This single observation was the basis for two later larger studies. The first one examined 54 non-responsive patients (Monti et al., 2010). Five of them showed similar activation patterns. An attempt to communicate with these patients was undertaken, such that they were instructed to think of playing tennis when they wanted to answer a question with "yes", and to think of navigation in their home when they wanted to answer "no". Communication was established for a short time with one patient. The other study (Vogel et al., 2013), with 22 non-responsive patients, showed that the results are related to the outcome within the three months following the examination. Specifically, a significant clinical improvement (change of the diagnosis) was observed in 11 of 14 patients with significant responses in at least one of the two ROIs, and in only one of the eight patients without such activations. The difference between the two studies in terms of the general activation percentages (i.e., five of 54 versus 14 of 22) is explained by very different composition of the samples and different response criteria.

To conclude, there are presently no exact ERP or fMRI indicators of whether a patient will or will not be able to communicate using an assistive device or a brain-computer interface (BCI). It is further possible that such indicators cannot be established in general, i.e., they should depend on the properties of the device or BCI. While in the past, only single indices of brain activity were explored, presently there are attempts to delineate a general schema of looking for potential predictors of successful communication (Kotchoubey et al., 2013). According to the most far-developed schema, EEG/ERP should be regarded as the method of choice because of their rapidity, flexibility, availability at every site and high temporal resolution. First of all, patients with extremely severe EEG pathology (diffuse delta waves, flat EEG, or burst-suppression pattern) are mostly unable to communicate at least with our present methodologies. All other patients should be tested using a battery that includes at least four passive stimulation procedures and at least two active instruction tasks. If the results of all six paradigms are negative, communication chances are very low. If active paradigms yield positive results, communication should be attempted. If the results of the passive paradigms are positive, but those of the active paradigms are negative, other active paradigms should be applied using a technique with a better spatial resolution (fMRI or, possibly, functional near-infrared spectroscopy: fNIRS);

---

[1] VS/UWS criteria in the UK are less stringent than in the US and the continental Europe. Thus in the US or in Germany this patient might have been classified as MCS.

also passive emotional fMRIor fNIRS-based paradigms should be applied to the patient's affective awareness. If the result of any active imaging test is positive, an attempt to establish communication should be done.

3. Brain-Computer-Interfaces (BCI) in the Paralyzed: A Possible Tool for Differential Diagnosis

In many unresponsive patients (particularly last-stage ALS) brain-computer interfaces (BCI: Kübler et al., 2001) have been applied during the last two decades. The BCIs use a voluntarily controlled brain signal to replace lacking motor and speech motor signals. Most BCIs use non-invasive signals such as the EEG, fMRI and NIRS. In patients with functioning vision and eye control BCIs based on the sensorimotor rhythm (SMR-BCI: Pfurtscheller et al., 1996) and event-related potentials (oddball-BCI: Farwell & Donchin, 1988) show the results superior to other kinds of BCI (Birbaumer, 2006). It has been suggested that cognitive impairment and EEG changes in late stage ALS may contribute to the lack of success using EEG-BCI technology (Munte et al., 1998). Kübler and Birbaumer (2008) showed that ALS patients in LIS can use BCI at the same level as healthy individuals. The most successful application for communication has occurred in people at the early stages of the disease (Birbaumer et. al, 1999; Birbaumer, 2006; Kübler et al., 2001). However, patients in CLIS do not reach sufficient BCI control for communication. Hence there is a need to find an alternative learning paradigm and probably another neuroimaging technique to design a more effective BCI to help ALS patient in CLIS with communication.

3.1 Complete Paralysis and CLIS Require Alternative BCI-Paradigms

While in LIS with intact eye-control and other states of incomplete paralysis, circadian rhythm is irregular, sleep polysomnographic recordings over several nights in one CLIS patient with implanted ECoGelectrodes showed chaotic sleep patterns with unpredictable slow wave sleep (SWS) episodes during the day (Ramos Murguialday et al., 2011). Thus changes in circadian rhythm, sleep pattern and arousal with alterations of attentional performance may at least partially be responsible for BCI communication failures in CLIS. BCI sessions are usually scheduled during day-hours, without polysomnographic recordings and without on-line detection of sleep. Fading vigilance during learning of BCI-based communication methods may be a consequence, because sleep cannot be detected behaviorally in a motionless, eyes-closed, artificially-respirated CLIS patient (Birbaumer et al., 2014).

The lack of reliable brain communication in CLIS patients with an invasive BCI (Ramos Murguialday et al., 2011) is mirrored by the complete failure of noninvasive EEG-BCIs in complete paralysis. A meta15 analysis of all reported

ALS patients by Kübler and Birbaumer (2008) and a longitudinal study by Silvoni et al. (2013) indicate that non-invasive BCIs based on imagery or instrumental-operant learning (Birbaumer et al., 1999) failed to meet a 70%-correct threshold for sufficient on-line classification of ''yes'' or ''no'' responses. Birbaumer et al. (2012) hypothesized that ''loss of the contingency between a voluntary response and its feedback'' in individuals who are completely paralyzed would prevent learning even if auditory afferent input and cognitive processing (attention, memory, imagery) remained intact. If the voluntary response is cognitive, such as in covert goal-orientated imagery in the LIS, the feedback or reward does not follow a reliable environmental or internal change and the response consequently extinguishes. Psychophysical studies (Haggard et al., 2002) demonstrate that, if the behavioral response is elicited independently of a conscious decision and intention, the conscious awareness of the contingency and the conscious experience of the decision vanish. In CLIS, contingencies between goal-directed thinking and intentions are lost because there is no environmental response to the particular intention. This process was termed as the 'extinction of goal directed thinking' or 'extinction of thought'. A single case of a completely locked-in patient able to communicate with a BCI based on instrumental (voluntary) learning and training after entering that state without a history of BCI control would disprove this speculation. However, in the BCI literature and in extensive studies of operant physiological regulation in the curarized rat (Dworkin & Miller, 1986) no such case has been reported yet.

A possible way to address the 'extinction of thought' problem and prevent extinction may consist in the creation of artificial contingencies. For example, it would be possible to utilize transcranial magnetic stimulation (TMS) pulses or peripheral nerve stimulation applied to a specific body part or to different frontal or motor brain areas contingent on the elicited brain response or contingent on peripheral nerve responses of the BCI. Also extensive successful BCI training should prevent cessation of brain communication if the BCI response can be maintained in the CLIS. We believe that the absence of extensive contingent stimulation and reward during waking hours may lead to the loss of associative connections between intention to communicate and response or consequence. A particularly original and Hebbian solution to this problem in the monkey was recently proposed by Jackson et al. (2006). Transmission of external currents and magnetic fields into the brain to induce or accelerate learning of BCI control may also represent an interesting future extension of existing BCI systems (see Karim, Kammer, Cohen & Birbaumer, 2004 for a first attempt).

3.2 Classical "Reflexive" Conditioning of BCI Communication

After failure to replicate operant physiological regulation in the curarized rat, Dworkin (1993) proved successful classical conditioning of various physiological responses, i.e. firing rate of facial nerves, in this preparation. Stimulus–

Stimulus (S–S) conditioning does not rely on goal-directed voluntary-operant motor preparation and response execution. Based on these animal experiments (Birbaumer et al., 2008; Birbaumer & Cohen, 2007) classical semantic conditioning was attempted in a series of experiments involving healthy participants and ALS-patients at various stages of their disease, all of them in LIS or CLIS (Furdea et al., 2012; Ruf et al., 2013; De Massari et al., 2013).

Classical semantic conditioning in humans was extensively demonstrated by Pavlov's students and summarized by Razran (1961). Patients suffering from ALS in the advanced stage were artificially fed and artificially respirated. The complete paralysis was verified through repetitive recordings of eye movements and electromyographic (EMG) recordings from various muscles over a period of several weeks (Ramos Murguialday et al., 2011). No control of external sphincter or eye control was present. Because paralysis of eye movements is frequently accompanied by loss of clear vision due to drying of cornea and eye ball only the auditory and tactile modality remains for interactive purposes: Extended bed rest and skin deformations may also compromise tactile and somatosensory input channels. Lack of any type of communication with the patients was verified by relatives and nursing personnel and documented in repeated video recordings. Words or sentences belonging to different semantic categories were presented as CS (conditioned stimuli). One specific semantic category (i.e. the thought "no") was followed by an unconditioned stimulus (US), usually a non-painful electric shock. Obviously, classical semantic conditioning of autonomic responses or brain responses does not depend on goal-directed motor systems and involves only minimal attentional resources and effort. Thus, classical semantic conditioning may circumvent extinction of volition, goal-directed thinking, effortful selective attention and cognitive control, imagery and working memory functions during operant learning and, thus, represent a principle to maintain communication in complete paralysis. On-line classification of different components of EEG oscillations, ERP signals associated with "yes" or "no"-responses was performed (see Figure 2). De Massari et al. (2013), for example, reported 37 sessions of classical semantic conditioning of one CLIS patient and eight sessions of two LIS patients using wavelet classification and non-linear support vector machines of fronto-central slow cortical potentials (SCP) to "yes" and "no" questions resulting in correct classification above 70% in some sessions. After training of the classifier based on several hundred questions with well-known answers (e.g. "Rome is the capital of Germany"), personal and open questions (e.g. "you want to be turned to...") were presented. While useful communication needs at least 70% correct classification of brain signals over an extended period of sessions (Perelmouter & Birbaumer, 2000), in the reported CLIS patient only 7 out of 37 sessions resulted in sufficient classification (De Massari et al., 2013). Thus although the classical conditioning paradigm showed potential, the EEG could not be used reliably for successful communication.

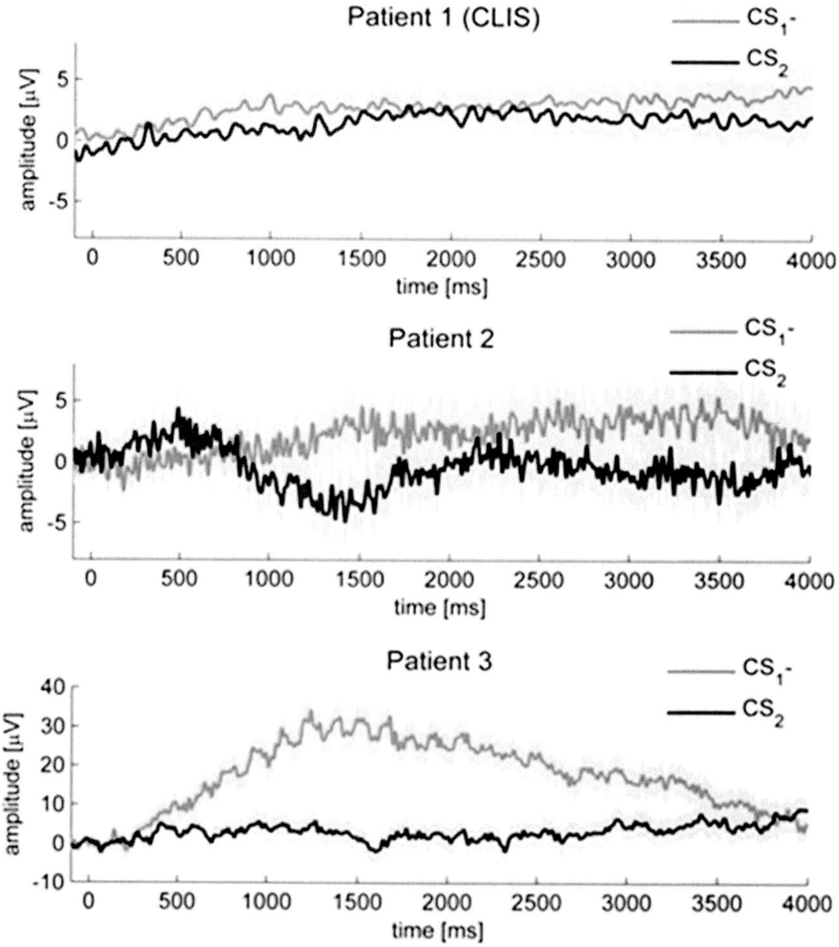

Figure 2. *Time courses of the averaged (195 trials acquired in the first four sessions) EEG signal recorded at channel CP3 in one CLIS patient (Patient 1) and two LIS patients (Patients 2 and 3). The time point 0 corresponds to the end of the sentence. Grey line: CS1, true sentences; black line: CS2, false sentences. Grey area shows the standard error of the average curve. From: Brain, doi: 10.1093/brain/awt102, with courteous permission of the Oxford University Press.*

4. Metabolic BCI

Another possibility to address these problems may include metabolic BCIs using fMRI or fNIRS (see Sitaram et al., 2007a, b). Metabolic changes and vascular variations are sensed by arterial receptors and may be utilized to control contingent reafferent perceptual responses (Adam, 1998).

4.1 fMRI-Based BCI for ALS Patients

fMRI measures increases and decreases of paramagnetic load of blood flow to activated pools of neurons, particularly to apical dendrites (Logothetis et al., 2001). Paramagnetic charge is determined by blood oxygenation level dependent (BOLD) flow, which reflects local metabolic deficiencies of the vascular bed supplying the neurons. Logothetis et al., 2001, have shown that the correlation of local blood flow change and the BOLD signal is particularly high for the neuronal inflow to the apical dendrites reflecting primarily intracortical activity. The fMRI-based BCI is difficult to apply on ALS patients because it is expensive, bulky and impossible to move to a patient's home. Moreover, the patient enclosed in the scanner does not experience a satisfying environment for communication. Still instrumental learning of BOLD control has turned out to be successful in neuropsychiatric disorders (Birbaumer et al., 2013).

4.2 fNIRS-Based BCI for ALS Patients

NIRS is an emerging neuro-imaging modality which employs near-infrared light to non-invasively or invasively investigate cerebral oxygenation changes in healthy and neurologically challenged adults and children (Strangman et al., 2002). It has reasonable spatial and good temporal resolution and is relatively robust to motion artifact, thereby enabling it to be suitable for investigating everyday tasks. Thus in contrast to functional MRI, a NIRS-based BCI can easily be applied at the bedside of these highly impaired and difficult to move patients in desperate need for communication.

Sitaram et al. (2007) published the first controlled evaluation of a NIRS-based BCI. Using motor imagery with a 20 channels NIRS system over sensorimotor cortex they reported 89% correct classification of right and left hand imagery without any training and the use of a hidden Markov model as a classifier. Recently, we demonstrated stable brain communication with NIRS using the classical conditioning procedure in a CLIS patient (Gallegos-Ayala et al., 2014), who was previously trained with an EEG-BCI (De Massari et al., 2013). While EEG-BCI application resulted in significant (above 70%) classification of ''yes'' and ''no'' responses in only seven of 37 sessions and no discriminatory response in brain oscillations at frequencies between three and 30 Hz, NIRS-BCI communication resulted in an overall stability of 72% up to 100% correct answers across 14 consecutive sessions (Figure 3). Blood oxygenation from frontal to central sensors increased during 25 s of ''yes''-thinking and decreased during ''no''-thinking. This clinical experiment is the first demonstration of stable BCI based communication using semantic classical conditioning in a CLIS patient which holds promise and raises the hope for communication in CLIS.

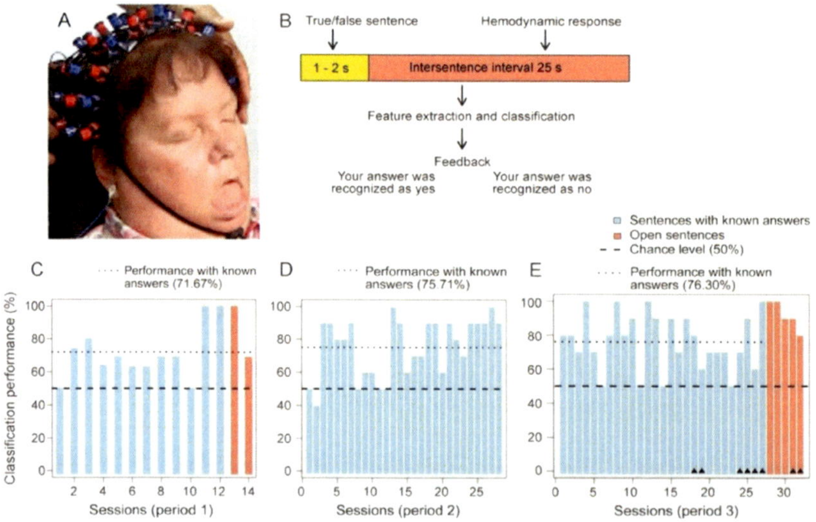

Figure 3. *A: Functional NIRS recording brain oxygenation/deoxygenation changes in a CLIS patient, using an ETG-4000 Optical Topography System (Hitachi Medical Co., Tokyo, Japan). B: The structure of a trial, as presented by the brain-computer interface (BCI) system. C: Classification performance (percentage of correct responses) during period 1, which consisted of 12 sessions with known answers (e.g., "Were you born in Munich?") and two final sessions with open answers (e.g., "Do you want to be moved now?"). Blue: sessions with known answers; orange: sessions with open answers. D. Classification performance during period 2, including 28 sessions with known answers. E: Classification performance during period 3, which included 27 sessions with known answers and five sessions with open answers. Sentences were presented auditorily by the patient's husband, except the sessions marked by a black triangle, in which stimuli were presented by an unfamiliar voice. Performance data in trials with open answers are estimates based on the answers the husband gave before the session. From: Neurology, DOI 10.1212/WNL.0000000000000449, with courteous permission of the American Academy of Neurology.*

Hence, to further validate these preliminary findings of our lab and refine the technology of fNIRSbased BCI for communication in CLIS-patients, extensive studies are presently being carried out on several CLIS patients using combined fNIRS and EEG based BCIs (Chaudhary et al., submitted). A particular challenge is the validation of answers to open questions, as validation often depends on family members and long-term nursing personnel introducing biases towards their own expectations. Frequent repetition of semantically differently phrased questions over days and weeks (i.e. ''you are not in constant pain'', instead of ''you are in constant pain'') might help to control for this problem.

5. Ethical Considerations of BCI in Complete Paralysis

Current legal systems in most industrialized countries provide the possibility to declare a ''patient will'' or ''advanced directive'' in case of medical emergencies. The patients' will declarations may include the patient's wish that ''artificial'' life preserving medical interventions such as artificial respiration and feeding and similar intensive care measures should be avoided. In most cases, however, these patients' wills are signed long before such medical emergency occurs. The underlying assumption of the signing persons (and these documents) is very often that the circumstances requiring life preserving measures are associated with a poor quality of life. In contrast to this widespread assumption, well-controlled studies in patients with LIS, ALS, chronic stroke and other chronic and untreatable neurological diseases show average and sometimes above average quality of life (Lulé et al., 2009; Kübler et al., 2005, 2006, 2008), despite paralysis and artificial respiration and feeding. Still, about 95% of all ALS-patients in most industrialized countries ''choose'' to die before tracheostromy and artificial respiration. Widespread hidden euthanasia is the rule and not the exception for these patients. In places with ''liberalization'' of assisted suicide and euthanasia such as The Netherlands, Belgium, or Oregon, more patients choose death before emergency measures are taken than in countries with less ''liberal'' euthanasia laws such as Germany and Israel. This indicates that ''patients' will'' declarations are affected by the social conditions and may be invalid at the decisive time points. They may serve as an excuse for the medical professions, insurance systems or family members to shorten anticipated long periods of care for these patients and avoid the financial and social burdens. Patients themselves may follow the social pressure, accept the poor quality-of-life prognosis, and ask for hastened death. If quality of life is measured objectively in the absence of doctors and family members, paralyzed and respirated ALS-patients judge their quality of life significantly better, and their level of depression significantly lower, than their caregivers (Kübler et al., 2005; Lulé et al., 2008, 2012; Matuz et al., 2010; Pantke & Birbaumer, 2012). The CLIS patient mentioned in Gallegos-Ayala et al. (2014) was completely paralyzed for 20 months, without any ability to communicate good mood and good quality of life. While single case reports do not provide scientific proof, a more extreme case than this is difficult to imagine in modern medicine. This example suggests that it is worthwhile to further investigate semantic classical conditioning for BCI communication in CLIS.

While there is no evidence that invasive BCIs had any advantage over non-invasive systems when using the established BCI paradigms (Ramos Murguialday et al., 2011), it is conceivable that novel paradigms might change this assessment. However, various ethical considerations must be taken into account when implanting invasive BCIs in patients who are unable to give informed consent. Most legal systems, e.g. in Germany, require that the relatives or legal guardians permits implantation, while consent by an ethics committee is not necessary. This regulation acts on the assumption that relatives or legal guardians are able to reconstruct the patient's will based on their acquaintance with the person. It also assumes that the relatives or legal guardians decide in the interest of the patient. The availability of BCI technology yielding the study results described may force us to deny hastened death requests formulated in ''patient wills'' or ''advanced directives'' signed long before the present state of a disease. We, however, do not generally deny the right of a person in a particular state of an intractable and often painful disease such as terminal cancer to ask for and receive death in dignity and without pain. The unsolved ethical problems associated with the advancements in neurotechnology and BCI research urge a broad and open-minded societal discourse (Vlek et al., 2012; Clausen 2008, 2009).

Acknowledgements:

We acknowledge the participation of all our patients, particularly of Joachim Faehnrich. The studies were carried out with funding from the Deutsche Forschungsgemeinschaft (DFG, Koselleck to Niels Birbaumer), the Bundesministerium für Bildung und Forschung (BMBF, EMOIO FKZ 16SV7196; BMBF MOTOR-BIC, FKZ 13GW0053), the Stiftung Volkswagenwerk (VW), the Eva und Horst Köhler Stiftung, the Baden-Württemberg Stiftung (GRUENS), the Indian-European collaborative research and technological development projects (INDIGO-DTB2-051), EU COST action TD1006.

7 Correlation Between Aging, Mild Cognitive Impairment and Alzheimer´s Disease Studied with MRI, FDG-PET and PIB-PET

Juha O. Rinne

Key Words:
Aging, cognitive impairment (CI), Alzheimer's disease (AD), MRI, PET, FDG, diagnostic work-up, memory complaint, longitudinal amyloid imaging, brain cognitive reserve

1. Introduction

Normal ageing is associated with some cognitive impairment, especially slowing of the information processing speed. However, significant memory impairment during ageing suggests the presence of a progressive memory disease or some other conditions (unsuitable medication, psychological or psychiatric causes etc.). Mild cognitive impairment (MCI) is a heterogenous syndrome that may progress to dementia, remain stable or even revert to normal. In amnestic MCI the patients have impairment of episodic memory in isolation or with impairment of some other cognitive domains. This impairment must be objectively verified and the activities of daily living must be unimpaired and the patient has no dementia (Petersen et al., 2001). Alzheimer´s disease (AD) typically affects episodic memory which progressively worsens with time. Eventually AD leads to widespread cognitive decline that impairs the activities of daily living. The ultimate cause of AD is still unknown. The typical pathological hallmarks of the disease are beta-amyloid plagues and intraneuronal neurofibrillary tangles that contain hyperfosforylated tau-protein. These changes have a typical temporal and anatomical order of progression (Braak & Braak, 1991; Braak & Braak, 1997; Thal et al., 2002). There are also several other pathophysiological processes occurring in the brain in AD including inflammation, astrocytosis, microgliosis, apoosis and necrosis leading to neuronal and synaptic dysfunction and death. The temporal relationship and interplay between these processes is not well known today. Brain amyloid accumulation has been suggested to be an early pathological sign of the AD process and the earliest changes in the amyloid biomarkers are found even years before the symptoms (Jack et al., 2013; Choi et al., 2014). Most probably soluble forms of beta-amyloid (oligomers and protofibrils) are the toxic species of amyloid. However, alternative hypotheses regarding the role of beta-amyloid in the pathophysiology of AD have also been suggested (Drachmann, 2014).

The diagnostic work-up of a person with memory complaint include clinical investigation, cognitive testing, laboratory examinations and structural brain imaging (computerized tomography (CT) or magnetic resonance imaging (MRI). In special situations cerebrospinal fluid (CSF) investigation or functional brain imaging (single photon emission tomography (SPET) or positron emission tomography (PET)) may be used.

2. Brain Magnetic Resonance Imaging (MRI)

In AD the typical changes in brain MRI include atrophy of the medial temporal lobe structures (including the entorhinal cortex and hippocampus), cortical atrophy and widening of the ventricles (Jack et al., 1992; Scheltens et al., 1992; Frisoni et al., 2010). There is a huge number of studies investigating brain MRI to separate normal aging, MCI and AD. It seems, at least at present, that in spite of development of new MRI techniques and analysis tools, medial temporal lobe atrophy, especially hippocampal atrophy, is the best MRI marker to predict further conversion to AD in patients with MCI (Risacher et al., 1992; Jack et al., 1999; DeCarli et al., 2007; for a review see Jack, 2011; Clerx et al., 2013). However hippocampal atrophy is not specific for AD and can be seen for example in old age or in dementing conditions such as Lewy-body related pathologies (Dementia with Lewy bodies and Parkinson´s disease), in frontotemporal dementia and in hippocampal sclerosis. Repeated MRI with volumetric evaluation of hippocampal volume is a reliable marker of progression, since volume reduction in AD is two to four time faster than in age matched controls (Fox et al., 1996). In the new suggested research criteria (see below) MRI imaging is considered either as a "progression marker" or as a marker of neuronal injury.

3. Metabolic and Amloid Imaging

In functional brain imaging patients with AD typically show symmetrical temporo-parietal hypometabolism that can be detected by fluorodeoxyglucose (FDG) PET (Minoshima et al., 1997; deSanti et al., 2001; Nestor et al., 2003; Mosconi et al., 2008). Figure 1 shows a typical pattern of hypometabolism in a patient with AD and a milder reduction in cerebral metabolism in a subject with MCI. A similar kind of change has been detected also in healthy individuals carrying apolipoprotein E epsilon 4 (ApoE4) allele, especially in those being homozygous for ApoE4 (Reiman et al., 1996; Small et al., 2000) and in healthy elderly individuals with familial (especially maternal) history for AD (Mosconi et al., 2013). This hypometabolism in typically AD-affected areas in healthy elderly has been shown to predict future global cognitive decline (de Leon et al., 2001; Jagust et al., 2006).

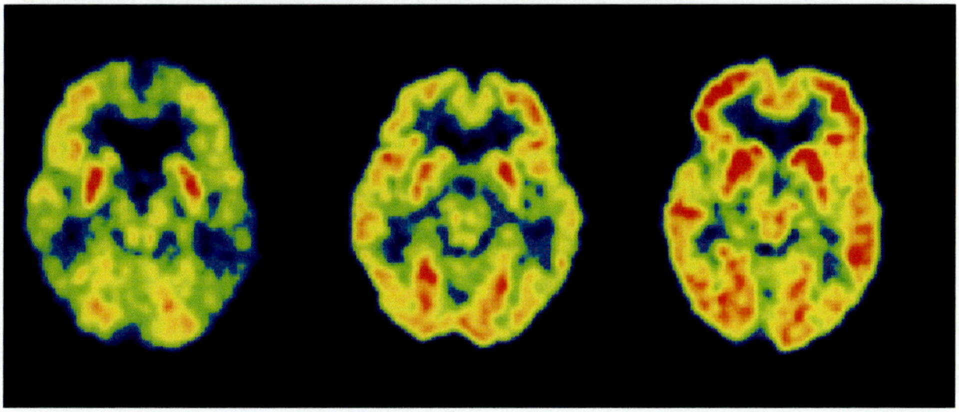

Figure 1. *Examples of axial [18F]FDG images in a patient with Alzheimer's disease (left panel), in a patient with mild cognitive impairment (MCI, middle panel) who converted to AD during follow-up and in a healthy control (right panel). Note the temporo-parietal (and to some extent frontal) hypometabolism in the AD patient, moderate temporo-parietal hypometabolism in the MCI patient and a normal pattern of glucose metabolism in a healthy age matched volunteer.*

In addition, patients with AD show widespread increase of cortical amyloid burden that can be detected with positron emission tomography (PET). [11C]PIB was the first in vivo amyloid imaging PET ligand (Klunk et al., 2004). Since then several new ligands have been developed, some with 18F label. Labelling the PET tracer with 18F has some advantages, since the half-life of 18F (around 109 min) is considerably longer than for 11C (around 20 min). This allows manufacturing in one site and shipment of the tracer to several, even remote imaging sites. Moreover the longer half-life allows investigation of several subjects using one synthesis batch which may lead to cost savings. Recently three [18F] labelled amyloid imaging tracers, [18F]florbetapir (Joshi et al., 2012), [18F]florbetaben (Rowe et al., 2008), [18F]flutemetamol (Vandenberghe et al., 2012) were accepted by FDA and EMA for the diagnostics of AD. It is good to remember that the current beta-amyloid imaging PET tracers bind preferentially or solely to the fibrillar beta-amyloid. However, as mentioned earlier, oligomeric or profibrillar forms of beta-amyloid are probably the important species of amyloid in the pathophysiology of AD.

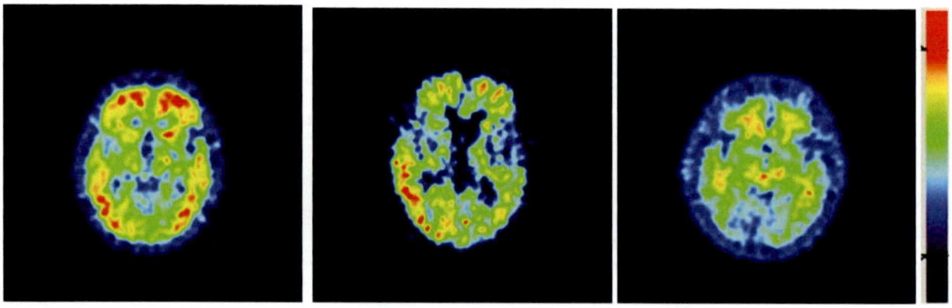

Figure 2. *Examples of axial [11C]PIB images in a patient with Alzheimer's disease (left panel), in a patient with mild cognitive impairment (MCI, middle panel) who converted to AD during follow-up and in a healthy control (right panel). Note the widespread cortical [11C]PIB accumulation in the AD patient (red colour), moderate accumulation in the MCI patient and virtual absence of cortical uptake in a healthy age matched volunteer.*

Comparative studies suggest that both amyloid imaging and MRI and amyloid imaging and [18F[FDG provide complementary information in detecting MCI or AD (Jack et al., 2008; Li et al., 2008; Trzepacz PT et al., 2014). In a study comparing amyloid imaging (with [18F]florbetaben, hippocampal volume and episodic memory found that positive [18F]florbetaben scan predicted conversion to AD during the next two years better than hippocampal volume (Ong et al., 2015). However while the association between [18F]florbetaben uptake and episodic memory decline over 2 years, the association between memory impairment and hippocampal volume became stronger.

Studies with amyloid imaging tracers have revealed that with advancing age increasing number of elderly individuals without cognitive impairment show increased cortical uptake (Pike et al., 2007; Mintun et al., 2006; Villain et al., 2012; Rowe et al., 2010; Scheinin et al., 2014). Positive amyloid imaging in an elderly individual indicates the presence of brain amyloidosis, but does not necessarily predict cognitive decline. On the other hand, already at the time of first clinical symptoms of MCI a considerable number of the patients have a widespread Alzheimer-type brain amyloid burden and decreased brain metabolism especially in the parietal and temporal lobes, which can detected as an increased [^{11}C]PIB uptake and a decreased [^{18}F]FDG uptake in PET imaging (Drzezga et al., 2003; Mosconi, 2005; Forsberg et al., 2008; Kemppainen et al., 2008). Increased amyloid imaging (Okello et al., 2009; Nordberg et al., 2013) or reduction in [^{18}F]FDG uptake (Drzezga et al., 2003) predict future conversion to AD in patients with MCI .

4. Longitudinal Studies

Longitudinal amyloid imaging studies in healthy controls and in patients with MCI and AD have revealed variable results the annual increase in amyloid ligand uptake varying from 0% to 3,8% in healthy controls, 1,3 % to 5,1 % in MCI and from 0 % to 3,4 % in AD (Engler et al., 2006; Koivunen et al., 2011; Jack et al., 2009; Scheinin et al., 2009; Grimmer et al., 2010; Sojkova et al., 2011; Villemagne et al., 2011). In these studies the patient populations, the number of subjects and the follow-up period (from 1 year to 3 years) varied contributing to the variation results (Table 1). Moreover, it was noted that the progression of beta-amyloid accumulation in patients with AD was influenced by ApoE4 allele, the progression being highest in ApoE4 homotzygotes (Table 1, Grimmer et al., 2010).

Patient group	N	Age	MMSE	Follow-up (yrs)	Change (% / yr)	Reference
Control	21	73[1] (63-90)	28[1] (24-30)	~1 yr	3.8 %	Jack et al. 2009
MCI	32	76[1] (61-88)	27[1] (24-30)	~1 yr	1.7 %	
AD	8	69[1] (54-80)	23[1] (17-26)	~1 yr	3.0 %	
AD	16	66 (51-81)	24.3 ± 3.7	2 yrs	No change[2]	Engler et al. 2006
Control	13	68 (59-79)	28 (25-30)	2 yrs	1.1 %	Scheinin et al. 2009
AD	14	72 (55-84)	24 (17-29)	2 yrs	1.0 %	
MCI-C	17	71.6 ± 7.2	26.2 ± 1.5	2 yrs	1.0 %	Koivunen et al. 2011
MCI-NC	12	70.8 ± 4.9	27.9 ± 1.3	2 yrs	2.5 %	
Control	106	73.1 ± 7.5	29.2 ± 1.0	~1.5 yrs / 3 yrs	0.9 %[3] / 1.7 %	Villemagne et al. 2011
MCI	65	73.4 ± 8.5	26.5 ± 2.9	~1.5 yrs / 3 yrs	1.3 %[3] / 1.8 %	
AD	35	71.7 ± 8.9	22.5 ± 3.7	~1.5 yrs / 3 yrs	3.4 % / 1.5 %	
AD	24	66 (52–77)	24 (15-30)	2 yrs	1.5 %, 5 %, 11% 0 1 2	Grimmer et al. 2010 (No of e4 alleles)
Control	11	66 ± 7	29 ± 1	2.5	No change	Ossenkoppele et al. 2012
MCI	12	67 ± 7	27 ± 3	2.5	5.1 %	
AD	8	62 ± 6	25 ± 2	2.5	No change	
Control	24	79.2 ± 8.1	29 ± 1.0	~1.5 years	0.9 %	Sojkova et al. 2011

[1] Median, others mean, [2] No absolute values given, [3] subjects with initially high PIB uptake
Note that some of the change %:s are estimates based on the numbers given in the articles

Table 1. *Some longitudinal amyloid imaging studies in healthy controls and in patients with MCI and AD.*

The largest longitudinal follow-up cohort is from the Australian Imaging, Biomarkers and Lifestyle (AIBL) study AIBL (Villemagne et al., 2013) which included 145 healthy controls, 36 individuals with MCI and 19 patients with AD. They investigated rate of beta-amyloid deposition ([11C]PIB PET), cerebral atrophy (MRI) and cognitive decline. The main findings were that it was estimated to take 19.2 years from the threshold of "PIB-.positivity" to the levels typically seen in AD. Moreover it was estimated to take 12 years from the low beta-amyloid levels seen in healthy controls to reach "PIB-positivity). Interestingly according to their data [11C]PIB PET became abnormal 17 years, hippocampal atrophy 4.3 years and memory 3.3 years before the onset of dementia (defined as Clinical Dementia Rating score of 1).

In spite of several studies investigating FDG and amyloid imaging changes in patients with MCI, only a few studies using the same tracers in the same individuals in a longitudinal setting has been published. Follow-up studies including both amyloid imaging and FDG indicate an increasing [^{11}C]PIB uptake and a decreasing [^{18}F]FDG uptake during the MCI phase (Kadir et al., 2012; Kemppainen et al., 2014), but the long-term interrelationship between these biomarkers, i.e. between the distribution and temporal development of the brain amyloid accumulation and metabolic changes, is not very well known. In a 3-year follow-up study in MCI no regional PIB-FDG correlations at baseline were seen, but negative association between [^{11}C]PIB and [^{18}F]FDG uptake in frontal cortex and posterior cingulate at follow-up scan was seen (Kadir et al., 2012). Another 2.5-year follow-up study found no significant correlation between the changes in global [^{11}C]PIB and [^{18}F]FDG uptake over the study period in MCI (Ossenkoppele et al., 2012). In our own study (Kemppainen et al., 2015) we evaluated the associations between brain metabolism ([^{18}F]FDG uptake) and amyloid accumulation ([^{11}C]PIB uptake) in patients with MCI and the long-term changes in these biomarkers and their relationship during the 5-year follow-up. Clinically, all patients converted from MCI to AD during the follow-up period, and thus the results reflect brain pathology both in MCI and mild AD phases, and the pathological changes during the conversion phase. [11C]PIB uptake was clearly higher in MCI patients at baseline compared to controls. This increase spread to encompass most of the cerebral cortex during the conversion to AD. [18F]FDG uptake was reduced especially in the temporal-parietal regions in MCI compared to controls at baseline, and showed wide reduction over the cortex at 5-year scan. The reduction in metabolism during the follow-up was significant in the posterior brain regions. In addition, brain amyloid load was positively associated with metabolism in posterior brain regions in MCI, but not anymore at AD. The results suggest that there are interactions between brain amyloid accumulation and metabolism during the AD process, including a possible compensatory up-regulation of posterior brain metabolism in the early phase.

These findings are in agreement and extend the results from an earlier cross-sectional study showing both local and distant positive correlations between [11C]PIB and [18F]FDG in MCI especially between precuneus metabolism and posterior and frontal [11C]PIB uptake (Cohen et al., 2009). Also, a follow-up study in AD showed widespread positive associations between baseline [18F]FDG uptake at mild AD and [11C]PIB uptake at moderate AD at 2-year time point (Forster et al., 2102). In addition, a higher baseline [11C]PIB uptake was associated with more severe decline in brain metabolism during the 2-year follow-up (Forster et al., 2012). Similar findings were also found out in a 2.5-year follow-up study in MCI (Ossenkoppele et al., 2012).

In earlier studies, first changes in the metabolic activity reflecting neuronal dysfunction are seen in the entorhinal cortex already at pre-symptomatic phase in subjects who later convert to MCI, when hypometabolism is found to be present also in the hippocampus and lateral temporal cortex (De et al., 2001; DeLeon et al., 2001). This somewhat different distribution of hypometabolism in these and other studies can be partially employing automated anatomical masking technique to sample the hippocampus on PET (HipMask) (Mosconi et al., 2005; Li et al., 2008). Individuals converting from MCI to AD have been found to have wider regional distribution of brain hypometabolism extending to several cortical regions, compared to non-converters (Mosconi et al., 2004; Brück et al., 2013).

The existing data suggest that there could be an up-regulation or relative preservation of posterior metabolism in MCI. One possible explanation is that posterior brain regions show metabolic compensation or are less susceptible to the early amyloid pathology compared to other cortical regions. This metabolic preservation is lost later during the progression towards clinical AD.

5. Cognitive Reserve

Brain cognitive reserve is a factor that can have an effect on amyloid and metabolic PET findings in MCI and AD. Therefore, subjects' educational background might also modulate the PIB-FDG association in different clinical stages of the disease i.e. high-educated patients with MCI could have higher [11C]PIB uptake and either higher or lower [18F]FDG uptake depending on brain region compared to low-educated patients. In earlier studies, MCI patients and patients with mild AD with higher educational level have showed more severe hypometabolism (especially in the temporal, parietal and occipital cortices), and higher amyloid load compared to lower educated patients at similar level of cognitive performance (Garibotto et al., 2008; Kemppainen et al., 2008; Morbelli et al., 2013). On the other hand, greater frontal metabolism in high-educated individuals with MCI compared to low-educated ones has been reported, which is thought to represent a compensatory mechanism during the AD process (Morbelli et al., 2013). Moreover, highly educated healthy subjects show an increased metabolism in the anterior cingulate area that corresponds to better connectivity between brain areas (Arenaza-Urquijo et al., 2013). Thus, in addition to age and apoE4 status, education can also affect brain amyloid load and brain metabolism and their relationship and influence the degree and extent of brain pathology required to lead to certain degree of cognitive impairment.

6. New Research Criteria for AD

The new suggested clinical criteria for AD have evolved from the increasing knowledge of cognitive and biomarker changes in the continuum from normal ageing to MCI and to AD. According to the model suggested by Jack et al., the earliest changes in AD process are abnormalities in beta-amyloid and tau (Jack et al., 2013). These changes begin several years, if not decades, before first clinical symptoms as suggested for instance by the AIBL study cohort (Villemagne et al., 2013).

There are also suggestions to include biomarker information at earlier stages. It has been suggested that there is a continuum from normal ageing with evidence of beta-amyloidosis (evidenced by PET or CSF beta-amyloid) to a stage where there is also evidence for neurodegeneration (evidenced by FDG PET, MRI, CSF tau). Some individuals may progress further, starting to express subtle cognitive decline and MCI due to AD pathophysiological process (Sperling et al., 2011; Albert et al., 2011). Thus the recommendation separates AD as an underlying pathophysiological disease process and the clinical stage. Thus an individual may have evidence of AD pathophysiological process without any evidence of cognitive impairment (preclinical stage of AD) or may have MCI due to AD.

The two main suggested new clinical research criteria for AD are the International Working Group (IWG-2) criteria (Dubois et al., 2014) and the National Institute on Aging – Alzheimer´s Association (NIA-AA) workgroup diagnostic guidelines (McKhann et al., 2011). These criteria separate AD pathophysiological process (that can be detected earlier) from clinical AD dementia. Both the criteria emphasize that these are currently meant for research purposes only. There are some differences between these criteria regarding terminology and required biomarker abnormalities and their application, but detailed comparison between these criteria is beyond the scope of this manuscript. Briefly, according to IWG-2 criteria AD could be diagnosed when clinical AD phenotype (typical or atypical) is associated with biomarkers consistent with the presence of AD pathology (positive amyloid PET or decreased beta amyloid level in CSF together with increased tau or phosphor tau). Volumetric changes in brain MRI or FDG PET are considered as "progression markers" and better serve to evaluate clinical severity and the progression of the disease. The NIA-AA criteria refer "AD" as a pathological process, whether symptomatic or asymptomatic, whereas IWG-2 criteria refer "AD" to the symptomatic stage. The NIA-AA criteria retain the term "MCI" whereas IWG-2 criteria use term "prodromal AD". According to the NIA-AA criteria, biomarker abnormalities can be used to support the diagnosis, but they are not required. On the other hand the NIA-AA criteria divide the biomarkers to reflect either beta-amyloid pathology (PET or CSF beta-amyloid) or to reflect neuronal injury (CSF tau, FDG PET, structural MRI). Individuals can be characterized into three stages based on biomarker information and cognition. At stage 1 individuals have only abnormal beta-amyloid marker. At stage 2 both beta-amyloid and neuronal injury markers are positive and at stage 3 individuals show positive beta-amyloid and neuronal injury marker accompanied with cognitive impairment. There have also been attempts to harmonize between the different new criteria suggested (Morris et al., 2014).

Recently the prognostic value of these criteria has been investigated. In a study including 73 individuals with MCI had evaluation of amyloidosis (CSF beta-amyloid) or neurodegeneration (hippocampal atrophy in MRI, FDG PET, CSF tau). The best predictor of conversion to AD was combined abnormality in amyloid and neurodegeneration biomarkers (Prestia et al., 2015), whereas of the individual biomarkers FDG PET showed best performance. In another study a considerable number (n = 1607) of individuals with MCI from several centers were identified and followed through up to three years (Vos et al., 2015). They found that using both beta-amyloid and neuronal injury markers as proposed by the NIA-AA criteria showed the most accurate prognosis. However more studies with longer follow-up are needed to determine the relative predictive value of these criteria (for instance it may take a longer time for an individual with MCI with only abnormal beta-amyloid biomarker at baseline to convert to AD than for an individual with abnormal beta-amyloid and neuronal injury biomarker).

Conclusions

Recent increase in the knowledge of the clinical course of AD and the biomarkers to detect AD process in vivo have indicated that there is a long pre-symptomatic period when an aged individual may have biomarker evidence of AD pathophysiological process but still be cognitively intact. It is yet unclear which factors will ultimately determine which of these individuals will progress to stages of mild cognitive impairment and eventually to AD dementia stage. Based on available literature it is obvious that an extensive brain amyloid accumulation is an early event in the Alzheimer process, and the amyloid load is still increasing during the MCI phase starting to plateau at AD stage, whereas [18F]FDG and brain MRI are more closely linked with the clinical progression of the disease. Which combination of these biomarkers will eventually turn out to be the most sensitive and best predictors of future AD remains to be seen. However these biomarkers can help to identify individuals at increased risk to progress into clinical stages with cognitive impairment and give the possibility for early intervention either by drugs (Miller, 2012) or by life-style intervention (Ngandu et al., 2015). This is probably the most efficient way to slow down or even halt the pathophysiological process, since it may be that already at early clinical stages the pathophysiological changes are so widespread and complex that the effect of drug treatment and interventions may be limited.

8 Voluntary Movement Deficits of Eyes and Limbs: Neuroanatomy and Diagnosis

Styrmir Saevarsson and Árni Kristjánsson

Key words:
voluntary movement disorders, limbs, eyes, neuroanatomy, assessment

Abstract

We present a systematic overview of voluntary eye and limb movement deficits that are caused by brain injury. The frontal lobes along with many other brain areas are believed to play a critical role in the voluntary movement of eyes and limbs. In particular, we explore the approximate locations of brain injury as well as the associated diagnostic procedures. The main findings of the review are that frontal regions are involved in saccades, smooth pursuit, grasping, unilateral action neglect, directional action neglect, anarchic hand disorder, utilization behavior, imitation behavior, motor perseverations, limb apraxia, imitation of meaningless gestures, limb apraxia (imitation of meaningful and meaningless gestures, tool and object use), but to a lesser extent in optic and kinaesthetic ataxia. Further, limb apraxia and anarchic hand disorder are the only voluntary movement deficits mainly associated with the left hemisphere of the brain. More fine-grained analysis may prove difficult due to limitations of findings and methods in lesion-symptom mapping. The overlapping networks for voluntary eye and limb action are evidence for a partially common module for eye-limb system control even if eye and limb movements are controlled by different brain regions.

1. Introduction

The motor system involves a functional division within the central nervous system. Voluntary movement deficit is a broad term that refers to many distinct disruptions in the voluntary motor system (also called pyramidal motor system) that are associated with various disorders such as reaching in optic ataxia and eye movements in visual search. Voluntary (endogenous, internally driven/evoked; endo-evoked) responses are made, for example, in response to arrows in the central visual field indicating likely target locations. Conversely, involuntary movement deficits, e.g. tremor, dystonia, and tics, are caused by injury in the involuntary movement system (also called extrapyramydal and cerebral systems) and are associated with movement disorders such as Parkinson´s dementia. Involuntary (exogenous, externally driven/evoked, exo-evoked, automatic) responses are characterized by a reflexive response to salient stimuli, such as abrupt movement in the peripheral visual field (e.g. Posner, 1980, 1989; Ebadi, 2005; Birian et al., 2006; see Blakemore et al., 2002 regarding awareness of the motor system). Voluntary control of the eyes and limbs involves a highly complex operation requiring coordinated interaction between various brain regions. For instance, simple flexing and extending of the fingers while the eyes are closed, evokes large brain activation in frontal and other areas in addition to primary motor and sensory areas (e.g. Filimon, 2010). Advanced neuroanatomical understanding of these mechanisms' function may help enhance the treatment and diagnosis of various neuropsychological deficits.

Neuropsychology concerns mainly higher order deficits, not primary deficits, with a few exceptions such as blindsight (Beaumont, 2008). Higher order functions refer to cortical operations such as organization, planning, decision-making, attention, etc. Areas such as the inferior parietal cortex are believed to operate as a sensorimotor interface (Mattingley et al., 1998). Conversely, primary order functions are characterized by lower brain functions such as color perception and movement execution. For example, the primary visual cortex, which the retinas of both eyes project elementary visual information to, is an area where this kind of primary function takes place. However, no clear-cut definition exists for the higher vs. lower order distinctions although our rough understanding is useful in the categorization of different disorders. Higher order deficits are especially interesting with respect to limbs and eyes since both are crucial for voluntary interaction with our environment. Many situations require the coordination of both involuntary and voluntary components of limb and eye movements, e.g. when using a wheelchair, where goals such as maintaining direction and remembering the route to the desired endpoint compete with various external sources of relevant information such as suddenly appearing-objects or pedestrians (e.g. Arai & Mardiyanto, 2011).

The main aim of this review is to describe and compare most voluntary motor deficits of eyes and limbs with respect to neuroanatomy as revealed by lesion-symptom mapping following various stroke-related neural injury and to outline neuropsychological assessment methods. The general neural mechanisms of voluntary movement are still not well understood for various reasons. For instance, some voluntary movement deficits are rare and can be difficult to diagnose (Birian et al., 2006). We aim to discuss and compare the neuroanatomical and diagnostic bases of different voluntary limb (i.e. action neglect, grasping, optic and kinaesthetic ataxia, anarchic hand disorder, utilization behavior, imitation behavior, motor preseverations, and limb aparaxia) and saccadic and smooth pursuit eye movement deficits. Precise understanding of diagnoses and neuroanatomy is important for the development of successful interventions. In particular, we explore how different brain areas are specialized for voluntary hand/limb and eye movements. This has not been addressed in previous reviews and studies on voluntary movement deficits following mainly stroke-related brain injury (see however a review by Filimon, 2010 on fMRI evidence). However, our aim is not to evaluate the quality of the various neuroanatomical analyses, which vary considerably (e.g. Karnath & Perenin, 2005), but rather to provide an overview of voluntary movement deficits following brain injury. Most importantly, we hope to be able to pinpoint research fields where further research is urgently needed.

Our review consists of four main parts. First, we introduce the neuropsychology of voluntary limb and eye movement deficits; second, the neuroanatomy and diagnosis of voluntary eye movement deficits; third, the neuroanatomy and assessment of voluntary limb movement disorders; and lastly we discuss and summarize the main findings.

2. Saccadic and Smooth Pursuit Eye Movements

A relatively simple model of motor function in general can be provided by eye movements. Relative to other motor movements, eye movements are typically more easily measured and the movements have less degrees of freedom and are easier to analyze than other types of motor movement, since the number of muscles involved in eye movement generation is typically an order of magnitude lower than for other movement types. Saccades (see below) are probably the simplest motor actions made by organisms that are capable of moving their eyes independently of the trunk or the head in the first place, making them ideally suited to investigations of motor control. Many have therefore argued for the importance of understanding oculomotion, arguing that understanding eye movements may then inform the study of other motor movements in general. In fact the ease with which simple eye movement tests can be administered means that they can be the first indicators of degenerative motor disease while limb movement deficits are more likely to be addressed in a clinical assessment (Amador et al., 2006).

But a problem with research into specific motor disorders in the eye movement domain is that patients with sufficiently small and focal lesions to disrupt specific aspects of eye movement functioning are rare. Lesions are typically larger than this would require, and are, by their nature, indiscriminate in the damage they cause. Many insights have therefore been gained by investigating experimental lesions in non-human primates (see Tehovnik et al., 2000; Pierrot-Deiselligny, Rivaud et al., 1991; Pierrot-Deiselligny, Rosa et al., 1991, for review). In addition, low prevalence rates of lesions to particular regions of human cortex may prevent a clear taxonomy of distinct eye movement disorders. It is therefore important to keep in mind that not many deficits following neural damage are specific to eye movements. Overlap with other conditions contaminates precise diagnoses of eye movement disorders.

In what follows in this section, we describe the basic characteristics of the most studied eye (saccades, smooth pursuit) movement types and describe the paradigms typically used to study them before going on to describe the effects of neural damage upon eye movements (e.g. directional action neglect). Generally speaking, in the field of eye movement research, more insights come from selective lesioning of the non-human primate brain than for voluntary limb movement deficits.

2.1. Saccades

Saccades are ballistic movements of the eye. Their vectors (or direction) and landing points are computed before they are executed, and once the command for the saccade has been made, relatively little changes can be made to the direction and landing point of the saccade (Leigh & Zee, 1999; Goldberg, 2000; Sparks, 2002). Saccades may be made either voluntarily or involuntarily (Kristjánsson, 2007). We can, in other words, plan to move our gaze to an item of interest in the field of vision. Such saccades are in that sense stimulus driven. Saccades can also occur involuntary in response to something that captures our attention. This is sometimes referred to as the visuo-motor grasp reflex (see e.g. Munoz & Everling, 2004; Fischer & Weber, 1993; see following discussion on the grasping reflex in section 3.1. as well in this context).

Furthermore, we can make saccades to locations in the visual field that have no stimulus. Such saccades are by their very nature internally generated. This difference between stimulus-driven and internally generated saccades is captured in a very popular paradigm for testing saccadic eye movements, the prosaccade/antisaccade paradigm (Antoniades et al., 2013; Kristjánsson, 2011; Munoz & Everling, 2004; Ross & Ross, 1980). This simple, yet surprisingly rich paradigm in terms of the information it yields, involves initial fixation on a central fixation point, and when the fixation point disappears, the task is either to make a saccade towards a stimulus that appears in the periphery on one side (prosaccade), or a saccade towards a mirror symmetric empty location on the other side of the fixation point (antisaccade). Hutton (2008) sums up what is probably the consensus in the literature, arguing that the paradigm involves a trade-off between bottom-up information such as target salience on the one hand and saccadic goals on the other. Observers may, in this way, often find their gaze drawn towards a location even if this goes against their intentions. Kristjánsson (2007) laid emphasis on *competition* between top-down and bottom-up influences in the generation of antisaccades, a view that accords well with the available data on the process (see below). The effects of neural damage upon antisaccade performance may therefore be very informative about neural control of saccadic eye movements, and by analogy, movement function. Large individual differences in antisaccade performance have been observed (Hutton, 2008) and many psychiatric and neurological disorders affect antisaccades in interesting ways (see below). One problem with antisaccade research is the lack of standardized methodology. This may be the reason for contradictory results in the literature (Antoniades et al., 2013). Antoniades et al. argue that standardized protocols are needed for research using antisaccades and have proposed such a protocol, which many authors have started to use.

2.2. Neuroanatomy of Saccades

As mentioned before, voluntary saccadic eye movements are among the simplest movements that humans make. However, it would be an overstatement to say that the simplicity in execution is matched in some way by simplicity in brain circuitry guiding this motor function in humans, but at the same time the neuroanatomy of eye movements is rather well studied (for an overview see Leigh & Zee, 2011).

The key centers for control of saccade generation are the superior colliculi (SC) of the midbrain, the frontal (FEF) and supplementary (SEF) eye fields in the frontal lobes and the parietal eye fields (PEF) in the parietal cortex (situated on the horizontal portion of the intraparietal sulcus, in regions adjacent to the superior part of the angular gyrus and to the supramarginal gyrus). All these regions have strong connections with eye movement control centers in the brain stem.

The SC can locate a saccade target and generate a movement towards it on their own (Moschovakis, 1996), such as through the retinotectal pathway (Jóhannesson, Ásgeirsson & Kristjánsson, 2012; Jóhannesson & Kristjánsson, 2013; Williams, Azzopardi & Cowey, 1995) a phylogenetically old pathway that links the retina and SC directly without going through the cerebral cortex. The superior colliculi convey signals to movement generation centers in the brain stem (Cullen & Van Horn, 2011). However, input from saccade centers in the cerebral cortex complicate this picture. The frontal eye fields and the supplementary eye fields in the frontal lobes have direct input to the SC influencing its activity. The FEF are in turn fed information from V1, and the SC also interacts with the PEF.

The dorsolateral prefrontal cortex (dlPFC) also influences saccadic execution and interacts with the SC. Parietal areas also influence the process (in particular the parietal eye fields) strongly influencing saccade execution. This means that the SC does not handle saccade control in isolation. Additionally, regions in the Cerebellum are believed to play an important role in fine-tuning saccadic eye movements (Leigh & Zee, 2011). Roughly, the consensus in the literature appears to be that the FEF are involved in the control of voluntary saccades (Gaymard et al., 1998; Pierrot-Deseilligny et a., 2002). Even though saccades are generated by the brain stem, without cortical input (from the FEF or SC) saccades or not generated (Schiller, True & Conway, 1979, 1980). In non-human primates, the FEF and/or SC therefore appear to be necessary for eye movements. The FEF and SC contain neurons that provide a command signal for saccade generation if they reach threshold for saccade generation. Note importantly, that the thresholds are flexible depending on task demands (Jantz, Watanabe, Everling & Munoz, 2013).

The PEF are thought to be particularly involved in generating stimulus driven saccades. The SEF are involved in initiating motor programs comprising multiple saccades or more complex motor programs, while the dorso-lateral prefrontal cortex (dlPFC) handles inhibition of reflexive saccades to external stimuli when they go against instruction and memory guided saccades – saccades that are to be made to remember locations rather than to visible stimuli. In addition Pierrot-Deisilligny et al. (2002) also propose that the dlPFC plays a critical role in the inhibition of reflexive saccades with the FEF subsequently generating the correct saccade in an antisaccade task. The dlPFC therefore plays an important role in tasks that have a memory component, in particular regarding tasks that involve memorizing instructions for saccades for later execution. Moreover, the cingulate eye field (in the anterior cingulate) is thought to manage motivation and the preparation of intentional saccades.

Evidence from functional magnetic resonance imaging supports this picture. Voluntary saccades cause greater FEF and parietal activity than reflexive saccades (Mort et al., 2003). The results of Bender et al. (2013) support the view that the FEF play a large role in the execution of internally generated saccades (see also, Reuter et al., 2010) while the parietal eye field is more involved with reflexive saccades.

One potentially important consideration arising from the results of Bender et al. (2013) is that since they used multivoxel pattern analysis, they argue that the *pattern* of activity is crucial for understanding neural control of eye movements, rather than control by specific regions. If this is true, lesion studies may be not nuanced enough to catch the critical neural patterns sufficiently well. It is important to keep this caveat in mind when the distribution of function is considered.

Eye movement related activity also occurs in the Cerebellum (Fukushima, Fukushima, Warabi & Barnes, 2013; Lekwuva & Barnes, 1996). The cerebellar dorsal vermis seems to be related to working memory functions during saccades (Fukushima et al., 2013).

2.3. Smooth Pursuit

To follow a moving visual stimulus with our eyes, or when we need to track a stationary stimulus while we ourselves move, we use smooth pursuit (SP) eye movements. SP eye movements have the curious characteristic that without a stimulus to be tracked, they cannot be made. Without a smoothly moving stimulus the movement would instead be a collection of jerky saccades (see e.g. Leigh & Zee, 1999; Chen et al., 1999; Krauzlis, 2004; Rashbass, 1961). Readers can easily try this for themselves by tracking their moving finger, and then trying to move their eyes in a similarly smooth manner across a stationary scene containing no moving stimulus. The latter task will be impossible to perform in a smooth way, and the movement profile will contain a number of saccades.

The generation of SP eye movement requires correction for retinal slip (movement of stimuli across the retina) and also requires prediction of future locations of the stimulus to be tracked, because of inherent processing delays in the visual system. Smooth Pursuit has an onset latency of ~100-130 ms (Carl & Gellman, 1987). Typically the gain is 0.9-1.0 degrees, while corrective saccades are often seen for targets that move faster than 20°/sec (Leigh & Zee, 2011). Recent reviews of the neural control of saccades and pursuit indicate that there is a lot of overlap in the neural control systems for saccades and pursuit (Fukushima et al., 2013).

2.4. Neural Control of Smooth Pursuit

Perhaps the most important aspect that distinguishes neural control of smooth pursuit from saccades, is the involvement of regions related to motion processing in extrastriate cortex, not surprisingly, perhaps, since motion analysis is obviously necessary for SP. The MST area is critical in monkeys and an area roughly corresponding to V5 in humans. SP is also thought to be mediated by pathways connecting visual areas (for example involved in motion processing) to motor control areas in the Cerebellum (Krauzlis, 2004).

Smooth pursuit eye movements are controlled by a network of frontal and parietal regions (Heide, Kurzidim & Kömpf, 1996), which means that there is nevertheless considerable overlap in neural control between saccades and SP (Leigh & Zee, 2011; Krauzlis, 2004).

2.5. Disorders of Voluntary Oculomotor Function Following Lesions

2.5.1. Superior Colliculi

The superior colliculi (SC) of the midbrain connect strongly with brainstem reticular saccade generators and therefore play a critical role in saccade generation. The SC contains neurons whose activity peaks right before saccades are executed. Neurons in the deep layers of the SC, and the intermediate layers fire before eye movements, and the superficial layers have cells that give responses to stimuli that are the targets of upcoming eye movements (Mohler & Wurtz, 1976).

The functional neuroanatomy of the human SC is predominantly contralateral during saccade generation (Krebs et al., 2010; Sylvester, Josephs, Driver & Rees, 2007). Chemical deactivation or induced lesions of SC lead to impairment in the ability to voluntary move the eyes into the contralesional field (Hikosaka & Wurtz, 1986; Heilman et al. 1987). Pierrot-Deseilligny et al. (1991b) studied a patient with damage to only the right SC, revealing that the SC play an important role in saccade initiation to contralateral items as well as saccade inhibition.

2.5.2. Frontal areas

The frontal eye field (FEF) connects strongly with brainstem saccade generation motor areas in the reticular formation (Leigh & Zee, 2011). It is well known how frontal areas serve an inhibitory function, which is useful for antisaccade generation. In a seminal study, Guitton et al. (1985) studied patients with FEF injury, reporting that such patients had great difficulty in suppressing reflexive saccades towards a stimulus during antisaccade task. They made erroneous saccades towards salient targets even though they were supposed to suppress these reflexive movements, and generate a saccade in the other direction. Note that these symptoms resemble limb apraxia (see section 3.9).

Rivaud et al. (1994) studied three patients with FEF brain injury. Their eye movement patterns indicated that the FEF plays a role in disengagement from fixation, the control of contralateral saccades and smooth pursuit. Additionally, damage to the FEF can have repercussions in effects upon other areas. Machado and Rafal (2004) argued that chronic damage to the FEF disrupts interactions between the colliculi and cortical control centers. This, in turn, causes hypoactivity in the contralesional SC and loss of strategic collicular control over central fixation. Henik, Rafal and Rhodes (1994) then reported that patients with prefrontal lesions show increased saccade latencies for the initiation of voluntary saccades (to blank locations) to the contralateral visual field during an antisaccade task. These symptoms resemble directional hand movement preservations (Heilman et al., 2008; see section 3.2 for further discussion).

The supplementary eye fields (SEF) are located slightly anterior and inferior to the frontal eye fields. The most notable deficit following damage to the SEF involves a difficulty in making preplanned sequences of saccades (Gaymard et al, 1993, 2003). These symptoms resemble optic ataxia (see section 3.3). Husain et al. (2003) studied a patient with a highly selective lesion of the SEF (with other regions intact). They found that the patient had difficulty with changing saccade direction from a previously learned instruction to meet newer task demands. They suggested that the SEF play a critical role in oculomotor control when there is response conflict. They also reported that the patient quickly corrected the mistakes made, suggesting that the SEF are not critical for error monitoring. Importantly, Husain et al. (2003) found that similar mistakes were not made on a comparable motor task indicating that the deficit was indeed eye movement specific. This result is consistent with neurophysiological studies on monkeys, which indicate that the SEF can flexibly map stimulus response relations (Chen & Wise, 1995).

Note that the potential role of the SEF may be of specific interest in the current review, since the SEF are part of the supplementary motor complex

(Krainik et al., *2001;* Nachev, Husin & Kennard, 2008) which has often been connected with action neglect (see section 3.2) of the current chapter.

In addition, lesions of the frontal eye fields cause impaired smooth pursuit (Leigh & Zee, 2011; Heide et al. 1996; Lekwuwa & Barnes, 1996) in particular a difficulty in generating pursuit into the ipsilateral visual field (Heide et al., 1996; Morrow & Sharpe, 1995; Krauzlis, 2004; see also MacAvoy et al., 1991 for converging evidence from lesioning studies of monkeys).

2.5.3. Dorso-Lateral Prefrontal Cortex (dlPFC)

According to Gaymard et al. (1998), the dlPFC is involved in the inhibition of reflexive saccades during an antisaccade task. Consistent with this, lesions of the dlPFC, cause impaired suppression of reflexive antisaccades (Condy et al., 2004). This accords well with the general claim that the dlPFC plays an important role in working memory function (Levy & Goldman-Rakic, 2000). The available evidence suggests that the dlPFC are involved in maintaining the required task in memory.

2.5.4. Parietal lobe

Unilateral neglect, or neglect for short, is a multimodal neuropsychological syndrome that can be described as a failure to respond and attend to objects on or to the contralesional side. It cannot be explained with primary motor and sensory impairments (Heilman et al., 1987; Saevarsson, Halsband & Kristjánsson, 2011). Neglect can be divided into output (i.e. action neglect) and input (i.e. perception) neglect. The disorder often follows parietal damage, commonly having a dramatic impact on eye movements to one side. Many different terms have been used to refer to this deficit such as directional action neglect (also called premotor neglect; Saevarsson, 2013a, b). The tight relationship between saccades and attention (Deubel & Schneider, 1996; Kowler et al., 1995; Kristjánsson et al., 2001), clearly suggests that the attentional problems that follow right parietal lesions should impact saccades and vice versa.

Eye movement latency increases both for saccades in ipsi- and contralateral space following right hemisphere damage, but typically there is a latency increase only into the contralateral field from left parietal damage (Pierrot-Deseilligny et al., 1991a). This asymmetry of symptoms is reminiscent of the well-known asymmetry in neglect (see e.g. Saevarsson, Halsband & Kristjánsson, 2011), reflected in the fact that neglect primarily occurs following right parietal lesions, but not following left parietal lesions.

Walker and Findlay (1996) studied saccadic performance in neglect patients, finding that the deficits in their saccade performance correlated overall rather well with their attentional dysfunction. For example, saccadic latency did not increase with simultaneously presented bilateral targets as compared to unilateral targets, as is typically seen with normal observers, indicating that the contralesional stimulus did not capture attention as such stimuli will do for normal observers. Walker and Findlay suggest that this reflects that the ipsilesional SC is over-inhibited. Some of their patients also showed visual extinction in that they did not make saccades to the contralesional target when bilateral targets were presented. Note that the patients exhibited normal speed-ups in saccade latency with a temporal gap between fixation offset and target onset (a normal "gap-effect" in other words, Kristjánsson, 2011).

Sharpe, Cheng and Eizenmann (2011) argued that parietal lobe lesions caused impaired suppression of reflexive saccades and impaired generation of antisaccades through a disconnection between parietal lobe and frontal lobe oculomotor areas (such as the FEF).

Parietal eye movement areas connect with the superior coliculli. Gaymard et al. (2003) showed how the lateral intraparietal area (LIP) contributes to saccade generation through its role in spatial attentional capture. Parieteo-tectal nerve fibers are involved in an online signal for triggering reflexive saccades to salient stimuli (Rafal, 1991; see discussion in Jóhannesson, Ásgeirsson & Kristjánsson, 2012). Damage to parieto-tectal neural pathways severely affects performance accuracy in an unpredictable landing point paradigm driven by unpredictable salient stimuli. Note importantly, that lesions in parietal areas have a larger effect on saccadic eye movements if they occur in the right than the left hemisphere (Lekwuva & Barnes, 1996). Again, this accords well with findings on neglect. Heide, et al. (1995) studied patients with parietal lesions using a double-step saccade stimulus. They found that if the stimulus first jumped into the contralesional hemifield and then into the ipsilesional one, observers could not make an accurate saccade to the target even though it was in their *non*-affected hemifield. This result suggests that parietal areas are involved in calculating saccade amplitude in a dynamic way.

Parietal lesions can have a devastating effect on smooth pursuit. This is, in particular, likely for lesions that have some overlap with extrastriate motion processing areas that are nearby in the cortex (Heide et al., 1996). Some evidence also suggests that area V5 (the analogue of MT/MST in monkeys) is critical for SP, which is perhaps not surprising given the role of these mechanisms in motion perception (Krauzlis, 2004).

2.6. Cerebellum

Evidence from Monkeys

The cerebellum has direct neural projections onto brainstem generation centers (Bötzel, Rottach & Büttner, 1993; Robinson & Fuchs, 2001). The cerebellar dorsal vermis is involved in working memory related activity (Fukushima et al., 2013) whereas the FEF and cerebellar areas are involved in movement preparation (Fukushima et al., 2013; Lekwuva & Barnes, 1996).

Importantly, the cerebellum also makes connections to cerebral saccade centers (Filippoulos, Eggert & Straube, 2013). The results of Barash et al. (1999) indicate that the cerebellum is involved in moment to moment recalibration such as in saccadic adaptation tasks (He & Kowler, 1989). Monkeys with damage to the posterior vermi (or oculomotor vermis) of the cerebellum showed hypometria and a permanent lack of short-term adaptation (Yamada & Noda, 1987). In fact the literature strongly indicates that lesions to the posterior vermis cause dysmetria (i.e. saccades that are shorter than the task requires).

2.6.1. Other results from cerebellar lesions in humans

Filippopulos et al. (2013) studied the role of the cerebellum in eye movements in 24 patients with cerebellar lesions. These patients showed saccades that were hypometric, had longer latencies, and exhibited errors of suppression in a memory guided saccade task. Lesions at various sites of the cerebellum (e.g. dorsal vermis or the Floccules) cause disorders of SP mainly of pursuit of targets moving in the ipsilesional direction of the hemifield.

Rambold et al. (2002) reported that the ventral paraflocculus of the cerebellum is critical for control of SP. The cerebellar vermis also plays an important role in SP; damage to the vermis harms the accuracy of pursuit initiation (Takagi, Zee & Tamargo, 2000). Damage to the cerebellar vermis may affect the trajectories of SP and saccades through impaired acceleration and deceleration. These findings are consistent with the proposal that the cerebellum may fine-tune the commands for SP, based on feedback (Krauzlis, 2004).

3. The Neuroanatomy and Assessment of Voluntary Limb Deficits

3.1. Grasping

Grasping reflex disorders are found in less than 10% of brain-injured patients in response to tactile stimulation of their affected hands and visual presentation of stimuli. Such disorders involve catching hold of a stimulus object without any explicit intention to use it. Some patients are able to suppress the grasp reaction voluntarily. However, most patients use their healthy hand to loosen the grasp of the other hand. Improper grasping can be diagnosed by stroking a patient´s palm in a gentle and repetitive way with an object such as a pen. The patient is instructed not to grasp the pen. De Renzi and Barbieri (1992) found grasping in 70% of patients with bilateral and unilateral anterior cingulate gyrus injury, but this was less prevalent following damage to the supplementary motor cortex. Grasping also occurred in 26% of patients with lesions of other frontal areas (the lateral motor and premotor areas). Hemispheric asymmetry of grasping has not been observed, however. Foot grasping has also been described as the flexion of toes in response to touching the sole, without movement of the stimulus. Moreover, five subvarieties of grasping (i.e. closing reaction, final grip, trap reaction, magnet reaction, and instinctive grouping) have been differentiated. Their neuroanatomical substrates have been specified neither for foot grasping nor for the subforms of grasping (De Renzi & Barbieri, 1992).

3.2. Action neglect

Action neglect is one form of unilateral neglect (see discussion in section 2.5.4) and can be explained by the lack of correct behavior or responses (e.g. in contrast to apraxia). Action neglect can be divided roughly into two main forms: motor and premotor neglect. Unilateral action neglect (also known as motor neglect, intentional motor disorder, intentional neglect, etc.; e.g. Mark, 1996) has been described as an underutilization of one side of the body without significant loss of strength, sensibility, or reflexes (Laplane & Degos, 1983). Common behavioral symptoms are, for instance, use of the ipsilesional hand when use of the other hand would be more convenient and appropriate, and difficulties using the affected limb in bimanual tasks such as clapping or opening a bottle. A subform of motor neglect called motor extinction has also been described. In short, it is detected when unimanual and bimanual limb movements are compared, and the contralesional limb shows significiantly poorer performance than the ipsilesional limb in bimanual tasks as opposed to unimanual tasks (Saevarsson, 2013a). Diagnosis is based on observing situations where the use of the contralesional hand would be more appropriate and on requesting patients to perform tasks that are normally performed with both hands, such as opening a bottle. The neuroanatomical injury most commonly believed to cause motor neglect is right unilateral damage to the frontal and/or parietal lobes, but subcortical brain injury is also connected to unilateral action neglect. Similar injury to the left side of the brain has also been reported to cause the affliction. The large inconsistencies across various studies are a considerable problem, however (Saevarsson, 2013a).

Directional action neglect (also known under other terms such as premotor neglect) refers to the voluntary response bias in or to the contralesional space of a non-affected ipsilesional body part that can occur on both sides. Hand movements are most often studied (Saevarsson, 2013a) although other movements, such as eye movements (see section 2.5.4), have been explored (e.g. Butter et al., 1988). Several different subtypes of directional action neglect have been described. For instance: directional hypokinesia refers to when initiation of a movement to one side is markedly slowed; directional akinesia refers to an inability to generate voluntary movements to one side; directional bradykinesia involves abnormally slow movements to one side; and directional hypometria refers to abnormally small amplitudes of a movement to one side. The neuroanatomy of directional action neglect is a controversial issue. Lesions in almost all subparts of the brain have been suspected to cause the deficit. Saevarsson (2013a) argues that right unilateral frontal and parietal lobe injury combined with subcortical brain injury is the most common cause of directional action neglect. Similar injuries on the left side of the brain have also been reported to cause this form of action neglect. It is unclear which brain injury causes subtypes of directional action neglect (e.g. Simon et al., 1995). Many different methods have been developed to assess directional action neglect. Best known is the verbal-manual landmark task approach. Patients are requested to estimate pre-bisected lines by indicating orally if they are bisected in the middle or not. The patients are then requested to bisect the same or a similar line manually. If patients perform markedly worse on the manual landmark task than the verbal landmark task they are categorized as suffering from directional action neglect as well as visual neglect. Furthermore, various reaching and pointing tasks have been developed where visual conditions are controlled (e.g. Saevarsson, 2013a, b; Saevarssson & Kristjánsson, 2013; Saevarsson et al., 2014; Mattingley & Driver, 1997).

3.3. Optic ataxia

Optic ataxia (also called visuomotor ataxia or visuomotor apraxia, Freund, 2001) refers to the condition in which patients are unable to use visual input to guide goal-directed hand movements precisely (Balint, 1909). Symptoms may include inexact and halting reaching movements to visual objects such as a pen held in front of the patient, in contrast to rapid and exact reaching to non-visual objects such as the tip of their nose or the center of their glabella. Optic ataxia tends to be less pronounced in central vision than in the periphery. Optic ataxia affects reaching movements of both hands although it can in some cases be stronger for the contralesional hand. Optic ataxia can be diagnosed by asking patients to touch their nose top with their index finger, and to watch and move a small object such as a pen, in front of them (Rossetti et al., 2005). The neuroanatomical injury that is believed to cause optic ataxia is believed to be in the parieto-occipital junction (bilaterally) and/or superior parietal lobe (Karnath & Perenin, 2005), as well as the posterior parietal cortex in both hemispheres (Freund, 2001; Rossetti et al., 2005).

3.4. Kinaesthetic ataxia

Kinaesthetic ataxia (also known as parietal hand syndrome) refers to a neuropsychological deficit characterizezed by involuntary changes in hand position. Additionally, patients do not perform voluntary movements when the limbs are out of their visual guidance. The disorder is believed to be caused by insufficient processing of afferent kinaesthetic signals. When movements are guided visually, patients´ grasping and hand coordination are still clumsy and their gait is staggering. Kinaesthetic ataxia can be diagnosed by observation of involuntary hand displacement when the patient´s visual attention is distracted or when a patient is simply blindfolded while imitating a certain hand movement. Neuroanatomical injuries found to cause kinaesthetic ataxia involve contralateral lesions to the affected hand of the anterior parietal lobe (Freund, 1987), lateral thalamus, or fiber tracts connecting these nodes (Goldenberg, 2010).

3.5. Anarchic hand

Anarchic hand disorder refers to a hand that can perform complicated movements that are clearly goal-directed, but, importantly, unintended (Della Sala et al., 1994; Brion & Jedynak, 1972). The movements are not under voluntary control and may interfere with voluntary actions of the non-affected hand. Patients may claim that the affected hand is disobedient or has a will of its own. For example, patients frequently refer to the affected limb in the third person (Marchetti & Della Sala, 1998). Normally, the action symptoms can be characterized by pulling and seizing various objects (Goldenberg, 2010). For instance, the alien hand may seize a phone from the other hand or undo shirt buttons. Patients may even be woken up by the anarchic limb as it tries to choke them (Banks et al., 1989). Some studies indicate that voluntary movements of an anarchic hand are impaired, especially in the presence of distractors, whereas involuntary hand movements are relatively intact (Cantagallo et al., 2010). Controversially, Tanaka et al. (1996) claimed that anarchic hand syndrome is a form of complex grasping or groping. Currently, the term "alien hand" is often used synonymously with "anarchic hand" (e.g. Biran et al., 2006) and several other abnormal types of hand behavior (Tanaka et al., 1996), although it was originally used to refer to the feeling of non-belonging of one´s own hand when it was held behind the patient´s back (Brion & Jedynak, 1972; Marchetti & Salla, 1998). Anarchic hand disorder is diagnosed by clinical observation, bimanual tasks (e.g. eating with a fork and knife), and the patient´s subjective complaints of their own limbs as alien to themselves (e.g. Bakheit et al., 2013; Brainin et al., 2008). The neuroanatomical injury that typically causes anarchic hand syndrome in its most dramatic form is normally found in the corpus callosum, contralateral left superior, and medial frontal lobe (in particular the supplementary motor area; Birian et al., 2006; Cantagallo et al., 2010; Coulthard et al., 2007; Marchetti & Della Sala, 1998). Injury to the parietal lobe and thalamic nuclei accompanied by sensory loss has been found to cause a variant of the affliction (see Birian et al., 2006 for an overview).

3.6. Utilization behavior

Utilization behavior is characterized by a tendency to grasp with both hands and apply objects that are present within reaching distance in a way that is inappropriate for the situation but not the object (Lhermitte, 1983; Lhermitte et al., 1986). For instance, when sitting in front of a plate, holding a knife and fork, patients may imitate gestures of eating. Clinical diagnosis of utilization behavior can be affected by enhanced suggestibility of brain-injured patients and it is therefore important that the patients are not aware of the purpose of the testing. Interesting objects (e.g. hourglass, newspaper, game pieces, pen and paper, mobile phone, parts of a brain model, comb, etc.) are placed on the side of a table where a patient is sitting while engaged in unrelated testing or conversation. Their spontaneous actions are then observed. If the patients use the objects, the examiner may ask why and the patient may claim that the examiner handed the objects to them and they therefore felt they should use them. The examiner may ask the patient not to use them and then observe their behavior further (Shallice et al., 1989). The behavior is not inhibited by verbal commands when it is related to the grasping reflex and a result of injury in large diffuse bilateral or unilateral medial frontal lesions, and perhaps the head of the caudate nucleus (Archibald et al., 2001; Lhermitte, 1983; Mori & Yamadori, 1982; Motomura, 1990; see also De Rensi & Barbieri, 1992). Shallice et al. (1989) suggested a differentiation between two forms of utilization behavior: an incidental and induced form. Incidental utilization behavior occurs when the examiner does not make any special attempt to draw the patient´s attention to objects placed on two ends of a desk. Induced utilization behavior takes place when the behavior is elicited by putting the objects in the patient's hands.

3.7. Imitation Behavior

Imitation behavior in patients is described as the imitation of actions such as gestures of the examiner or other people when patients are not instructed to do so. Imitation behavior is a subform of utilization behavior (Lhermitte et al., 1986). For instance, patients may repeat instructions or imitate the finger pointing of the examiner. A clear-cut command to stop the imitation can indeed stop it, but it will typically reoccur shortly. When patients are asked why they imitate others, they may claim that the examiner indirectly requested them to imitate him, or they may be surprised and say nothing (De Renzi et al., 1996). Clinical diagnosis is based on gestures, brief instructions, and clinical observation of spontaneous imitation behavior. The gestures are typically initiated without any explanation. The examiner performs various gestures in front of the patient such as hair stroking, yawning, and clapping. If the patient imitates the behavior, he or she is asked to stop. The examiner then performs other behaviors such as humming a tone, sighing, and saying "that is enough," to reconfirm the diagnosis (De Renzi et al., 1996). Neuroanatomical injury associated with imitation behavior normally occurs in bilateral medial and lateral frontal lobes as well as structures of the basal ganglia such as the caudate nucleus (De Renzi et al., 1996). This is at odds with the findings of Lhermitte et al. (1986) who pinpoint the bilateral and unilateral frontal lobe as well as lower mediobasal injury (i.e. thalamus, caudate nucleus, and internal capsule areas) for this affliction.

3.8. Motor Perseverations

Motor perseveration occurs when a patient continues to perform certain acts even if their intended purpose has been fulfilled. For instance, they may press a response button repetitively on their left hand with their right hand although only one press is required (directional perseverations; Heilman et al., 2008) or patients may spend a long time washing their hands although they are already clean. When patients are asked about their motor perseverations they describe them as compulsive and unintentional, or they may rationalize them with plausible motivations, such as difficulties in seeing items when crossing out letters or other items on a neglect task. Motor perseverations are often confirmed with clinical observation in various settings. For instance, the deficit can be diagnosed by requesting a patient to cross out objects (e.g. in standard neglect task) with a pencil where they are observed for perseverate cancelations of the same items. Neuroanatomical injury related to motor perseveration has been found to be in uni- and bilateral areas of superior mesial frontal lobe, bilateral frontal lesions, basal ganglia, and additional diffuse brain injury (Goldberg, et al., 1981; Goldenberg, 2010; Sandson & Alberg, 1984). Consistent with this, Annoni et al. (1998) claim that any cerebral lesion at any location can lead to some form of perseverative behavior.

3.9. Limb Apraxia

Limb apraxia occurs when brain-injured patients fail to perform skilled and purposeful movements even when the ipsilesional hand shows completely intact skills (Steinthal, 1871; Liepmann, 1920). The affliction is commonly associated with aphasia although the severity of either disorder may differ within individuals. The deficit cannot be explained by ataxia, athetosis, ballismus, chorea, dystonia, muscular weakness, myoclonus, tremor, seizures, non-motor cognitive disorders (e.g. language comprehension, agnosia, and attention deficits), nor sensory deficits (e.g. hemianopia; Heilman & Rothi, 2012). Apraxia is a heterogeneous disorder characterized by a wide variety of movement errors. Different forms of apraxia have been proposed based on different kinds of errors (e.g. eye opening, speech, visuospatial functions, and facial movements). This section will only cover three forms of limb apraxia. Limb apraxia has been explained by three domains of actions (Goldenberg, 2010): (1) imitation of gestures, (2) performance of meaningful gestures, and (3) tool and object use.

Patients rarely complain that they are suffering from an apraxia of gesture (Rothi et al., 1990), and neither they nor their families are typically aware of it before formal clinical testing. Imitations of meaningful gestures are sometimes partially preserved since patients are able to understand the meaning of a gesture such as the "two-finger military salute" without being able to mimic the position of the gesture itself. Patients are requested to imitate a demonstrated gesture with both their hands but their limb position for at least one hand is incorrect. If the patients do not understand the request, apraxia cannot be diagnosed. For instance, Heilman and Rothi (2012) and Goldenberg (1996, 2010) suggested various meaningful and meaningless finger and hand positions to evaluate imitation of gestures. For instance, patients were asked to mimic flipping a coin, using a toothbrush, waving goodbye, or putting their thumbs in their ears. Use of various tools and objects may fail because knowledge about the use of a tool or object may have disappeared (degraded semantic memory) or they may understand the use of the tool but are unable to perform the action (intentional motor deficit). For instance, a patient may try to cut bread by turning a knife upside down. Furthermore, problems can also start to appear when more complicated sequences of actions with objects and tools are evaluated, such as when patients are asked to prepare a meal (Hodges et al., 2000).

Neuroanatomy of limb apraxia: Impaired imitation of meaningless hand postures or gestures is associated with damage to the inferior parietal cortex in the left hemisphere, while disturbed imitation of meaningless finger stance is linked to inferior frontal (including the opercular portion) and precentral brain injury (i.e. motor cortex; Halsband et al., 2001; Goldenberg & Karnath, 2006) in the left hemisphere. Apraxia of meaningful gestures is associated with left hemisphere neural damage, particularly the inferior frontal cortex and underlying white matter (Goldenberg et al., 2007). Simple and multi-step tool and object use has been associated with injury to the parietal lobe of the left hemisphere. Studies have revealed no differences in neuroanatomical lesions between simple and multi-step tool and object apraxia (Goldenberg & Hagmann, 1998). The loss of knowledge about the use of tools or objects in association with a preserved ability to figure out possible functions has been related to bilateral temporal lobe brain injury (Hodges et al., 2000).

4. Discussion

Voluntary eye and limb movement defects are often associated with bilateral injury to frontal areas (e.g. Butter et al., 1988). However, voluntary movement deficits of eyes and limbs are related to various other brain injuries. Frontal brain injury is most commonly identified for voluntary limb and eye deficits, although the overlap is far from complete. The disorders are also associated with injury to parietal cortex, subcortical areas or white matter. This finding corroborates fMRI evidence that activation in the frontal and parietal cortex such as in the precuneus and frontal eye fields are part of the network for reaching and saccades (e.g. Filimon, 2010; Filimon et al., 2009). Apraxia and anarchic hand are the only voluntary motor deficits that were mainly associated with the left side of the brain, but not with right nor bilateral injury. Table 1 shows the main finding of the review – how different brain regions are associated with voluntary movement disorders. More fine-grained comparison analyses of the neuroanatomy of the disorders than is presented in table 1 is not feasible since the diagnostic and lesion-symptom approaches as well as the number of studies on voluntary movement deficits vary greatly.

Deficits	Frontal lobe	Temporal lobe	Parietal lobe	Occipital lobe	Cerebellum	Subcortical areas / white matter	Limbic lobe
Saccades	LR		LR		LR	LR	
Smooth Pursuit	LR		LR	LR			
Grasping	LR						LR
Unilateral action neglect	LR		LR			LR	
Directional action neglect	LR		LR			LR	
Optic ataxia			LR	LR			
Kinaesthetic ataxia			LR			LR	
Anarchic hand	L						
Utilization behavior	LR					LR	
Imitation behavior	LR					LR	
Motor perseverations	LR					LR	
Limb apraxia: imitation of meaningless gestures	L						

Limb apraxia: imitation meaningful gestures	L			L
Limb apraxia: tool and object use		LR	L	

Table 1. *Comparison of different voluntary movement deficits of limbs and eyes with respect to different areas of the brain. L refers to left side and R to right side of the brain.*

The underlying neuroanatomical causes of deficits of voluntary eye and limb movement remain in many ways controversial. It is not possible to identify specific voluntary movement deficits based on the location of brain injury for various methodological reasons. For instance, lesion-symptom mapping procedures addressed in this review vary greatly in quality and sample size and it may be questionable to compare studies within and between certain neuropsychological deficits (e.g. Saevarsson et al., 2014). For example, the findings of De Renzi et al. (1996) and Lhermitte et al. (1986) reveal differences in the incidence of imitation and utilization behavior in frontal injured patients – probably because of different selection criteria. Furthermore, diagnoses of voluntary movement deficits can be challenging. Symptoms of different voluntary movement disorders may be confused with one another. For example, abnormal actions in neglect and optic ataxia as well as utilization behavior may look very similar because of shared clinical features and differing diagnostic methods (e.g. Saevarsson, 2013a, b; De Renzi et al., 1996). Neuroanatomical methods such as simple descriptions of brain injury, Damasio and Damasio (1989) lesion template method, or more advanced voxel-by-voxel lesion-symptom mapping methods (Rorden & Bett, 2000) vary greatly in terms of quality and approach. For instance, exact drawings of certain injuries is more informative than descriptions and may therefore be less prone to error.

Future studies will need to address voluntary motor disorders with more detailed assessment and neuroanatomy, and comparing them precisely with other voluntary movement deficits. Eye and limb deficits are similar in many respects. For instance, symptoms of erroneous eye saccades can resemble limb apraxia. Results indicating a common frontal involvement in most voluntary movement deficits call for a more systematic study of various voluntary movement defects with respect to neuroanatomy and therapy.

9 Functional Connectivity Changes in BPD

Arun D'Souza

Key Words: *affective neuroscience, fMRI, functional connectivity, Theory of Mind, borderline personality disorder, emotion regulation, default mode network, biological markers, precuneus, ACC*

Abstract
The analysis of functional coupling of neuronal activity in patients with Borderline Personality Disorder (BPD) vs. healthy controls revealed increased connectivity of the default mode network (DMN) with other parts of the brain (such as the inferior frontal lobe) in patients, suggesting that BPD patients are dysfunctional in down-regulating the DMN during resting state. Decreased functional connectivity was found for patients compared to controls between the ACC and three brain areas involved in Theory-of-Mind (ToM) processes; the left superior temporal, right mid cingulate cortex, and right supramarginal/inferior parietal lobes. Increased functional connectivity was found in patients compared to controls between the precuneus and the left inferior frontal lobe, left precentral/mid-frontal, and left middle occipital/superior parietal lobes. Conclusion: Reduced functional coupling between the emotional and the *ToM* network showed a dysfunctional or even lack of modulation of the *ToM* network from regions involved in emotion processing in line with emotion regulation dysfunctions in BPD.

1. Introduction

Borderline personality disorder (BPD) is a severe psychiatric disorder with high mortality. Data suggest that BPD affects from 1.2% to almost 6% of the general population, approximately 10% of those who seek outpatient services, and as many as 20% of those who undergo inpatient treatment (Grant et al., 2008). Earlier studies reported that BPD affects 1–2% (Skodol et al., 2002; Torgersen, Kringlen & Cramer, 2001) of the general population and the prevalence rises as high as 15–20% in psychiatric settings (Lieb, Zanarini, Schmahl, Linehan & Bohus, 2004).

Up to 10% of those who meet criteria for BPD eventually commit suicide, this rate is 50 times that observed in the broader population (American Psychiatric Association Practice, 2001). Thus, BPD is associated with tremendous emotional and financial burdens to individuals, families, and society. In light of these costs, identifying precursors to the disorder must be a priority.

While in the population-based studies men and women are affected in equal proportion (Grant et al., 2008), the clinical population mainly consists of young women (Zanarini, Frankenburg, Hennen, Reich & Silk, 2006). Skodol and Bender (2003) stated that BPD is diagnosed three times more often in females than in males but that the reasons for this distribution remain unclear. The ratio of 3:1 may be an artefact of selecting samples (Skodol & Bender, 2003).

The significance of the disorder can indirectly be inferred from studies on making use of available therapies. Bender et al. (2001) showed that compared to depressive patients people suffering from BPD make significantly more use of both in-patient as well as out-patient psychiatric services. Some authors have estimated that, for example in the case of Germany, 15% of the total budget spent on treating psychiatric disorders is accounted for by BPD (Sanderson, Swenson & Bohus, 2002).

1.1 BPD and Emotional Dysregulation

Emotional dysregulation is hypothesised to be a core feature of BPD (Lieb et al., 2004). It has been shown to be of prognostic relevance for the development of a BPD, and criterion six (affective instability) of DSM-IV is strongly related to it (Tragesser & Robinson, 2009). Emotional dysregulation is usually characterised by strong emotional reactivity. According to the prominent model of Linehan (1993), emotions are said to be easily triggered in BPD patients, to rise quickly to an abnormally high level and to last longer than in healthy individuals. While emotional dysregulation is related to negative emotions in general, anger and rage are seen as prominent emotions in BPD (criterion eight in DSM-IV).

Some studies show higher reactivity of negative emotions in BPD. Herpertz et al. (1998) showed higher self-rated scores over a broad range of emotions in response to an emotional short story in BPD patients compared with patients with avoidant personality disorder. Levine et al. (1997) found a more intense experience of negative emotions in BPD subjects than in non-BPD controls. Koenigsberg et al. (2002) reported increased self-reported affective lability for anger, anxiety, and oscillation between depression and anxiety in BPD subjects compared with other personality disordered patients, while self-rated affective intensity was not associated with BPD in this study. Arntz et al. (2005) found stronger increases in fear as a reaction to an emotional film in BPD patients as compared with healthy and Cluster C personality disordered controls. Different fMRI-studies have shown significantly increased amygdala activation in response to facial expressions of different emotions (Donegan et al., 2003) and to emotionally aversive pictures taken from the International Affective Picture System (IAPS) (S. C. Herpertz et al., 2001). In a field study with frequent measurement points, Stiglmayr et al. (2005) reported stronger self-rated aversive tension in BPD subjects and a stronger fluctuation of tension over time as compared with healthy controls. In a similar design, Stein (1996) found greater negative affect and more fluctuations in negative affect over time in BPD as compared with healthy controls and patients with anorexia nervosa.

Other studies report basically higher negative emotionality in BPD over all types of negative emotions, independently of the presence of actual emotional stimuli. BPD groups typically indicate high levels of trait anger (Linehan, Tutek, Heard & Armstrong, 1994) and anxiety sensitivity (Gratz, Tull & Gunderson, 2008). Rusch et al. (2007) found elevated state and trait shame and other negative emotions in BPD subjects as compared with healthy participants and to women with social phobia. In an experimental study on the evaluation of non-interpersonal emotional situations by Sieswerda et al. (2005), patients with BPD appeared to be characterised best by a generally negative evaluative style.

1.2. Functional Imaging

Recently, O'Neill and Frodl (2012) reviewed the literature on brain structure and function in BPD. The most common finding amongst functional MRI studies is that of exaggerated activity in the amygdala of patients with BPD compared to controls during procedures that involve the processing of emotionally aversive stimuli (Donegan et al., 2003; S. C. Herpertz et al., 2001; Minzenberg, Fan, New, Tang & Siever, 2007). Of particular interest is an emotional linguistic study by Silbersweig et al. (2007) which examined the brain function of BPD patients compared to controls under conditions associated with the interaction between behavioural inhibition and negative emotion. In the study, a significant reduction in activity was seen in the ventromedial prefrontal cortex (including the medial OFC and subgenual ACC) in the BPD patients compared to controls.

A strong correlation was found between decreasing ventromedial prefrontal activity and decreasing constraint (impulsivity), whilst a strong correlation was also found for increased amygdala ventral striatal activity and increased negative emotions in the patients (Silbersweig et al., 2007); impulsivity and the experience of exaggerated negative emotions being diagnostic features of the disorder.

The majority of past BPD research has explored the psychological aspects of the disorder from characteristic behaviours to psychosocial triggers and risk factors, with high levels of childhood trauma found to be strongly correlated with occurrences of BPD (Cohen et al., 2006). Current theories propose that the experience of early life trauma (e.g. childhood abuse or maternal separation), genetics, neurobiological alterations, or a combination of the above may play crucial roles in the development of the disorder (Goodman, New & Siever, 2004; Steele & Siever, 2010).

In recent years, the spotlight has increasingly been focused on neurobiological abnormalities associated with dimensions of personality dysfunction, with a number of studies providing strong evidence for the existence of functional neurobiological disturbances in BPD (Foti et al., 2010; Goodman et al., 2004).

Due to its levels of location accuracy and non-invasiveness, functional magnetic resonance imaging (fMRI) has largely replaced positron emission tomography (PET) and other brain imaging methods in the study of brain activation patterns. By using magnetic fields and radio frequencies to measure changes in blood oxygenation, fMRI can be used as an indirect measure of neural activity, blood flow, or volume (O'Neill & Frodl, 2012). Using the symptomology of the disorder as a guideline, the majority of previous fMRI studies in BPD have looked at activation abnormalities in regions understood to be involved in the regulation of stress responses, emotion, and affect, amongst others. The most common finding amongst these studies is that of hypermetabolism in the amygdala of BPD patients compared to controls during tasks that involved the processing of emotionally aversive stimuli (Donegan et al., 2003; Sabine C. Herpertz et al., 2001; Minzenberg et al., 2007; O'Neill & Frodl, 2012).

Less common in the BPD literature is work considering "functional connectivity" amongst neural networks. As we use the term here, functional connectivity describes the relationship between different brain regions and within particular networks by assessing the correlation of their neuronal activity (Nierhaus, 2012). This can be done utilizing several different methods, including assessing resting state (on-going brain activity) fMRI data, and assessing task based (evoked brain activity) fMRI data, both of which we shall use in the present study.

Regions within one particular neural network, the default mode network (DMN), have been found to display their greatest levels of activity when at rest, and decreased activity during task based stimulation (Sheline, Price, Yan & Mintun, 2010). During these periods of "active rest", the DMN is thought to be involved in internal processes such as self-referential processing, inner speech, emotional control, episodic memory, and theory of mind processes (Spreng, Mar & Kim, 2009; Wolf et al., 2011). Research has shown the constituent regions of the DMN to include the medial temporal lobe, the medial prefrontal cortex, the posterior cingulate cortex, the precuneus, and the medial, lateral, and inferior parietal cortex (Broyd et al., 2009; Spreng et al., 2009; Wolf et al., 2011). Surprisingly, though interest in the DMN is on the rise generally, and, given the similarities between the DMN functional roles and the dysfunction observed in BPD making it likely that there exists some relationship between the two, there remains a dearth of research investigating abnormalities in DMN functioning in BPD. Of the research that exists, one study explored alterations in the functional connectivity of the DMN in patients with BPD during pain processing. Abnormalities in pain processing (self-harming as a means of regulating affect, decreasing dissociative symptoms, etc.) are another well documented characteristic of BPD (Ludascher et al., 2007). This particular study observed less integration of the left retrosplenial cortex and left superior frontal gyrus into the DMN in the BPD group than in the controls during pain appraisal (Kluetsch et al., 2012). The researchers suggest that for BPD patients not only may this result in difficulties interpreting painful stimuli as self-relevant, but that there is also an observable positive correlation between this signal strength in the posterior DMN and clinical measures of symptom severity and trait dissociation during pain appraisal (Kluetsch et al., 2012). An earlier study explored prefrontal and limbic resting state networks in BPD patients without any external stimulus. To our knowledge, it is the only study thus far to explicitly examine DMN connectivity in BPD, yielding results that showed an increase in functional connectivity in the left fronto-polar cortex (FPC) and the left insula, and decreased connectivity in the left cuneus in the BPD group (Wolf et al., 2011). The researchers opine that, with regard to the increased connectivity observed in the FPC, these findings may have implications in terms of processing of internal thoughts, self-referential information, and interpersonal interactions, and may in the future be found to be a potential biological marker for the disorder (Wolf et al., 2011). Regarding the increased activation in the insula, the researchers suggest that abnormal activation may be related to both dissociative symptoms and decreased pain sensitivity observed in BPD patients (Wolf et al., 2011).

As part of the present research's focus, we shall also attempt to address the gap in DMN BPD research by mapping the functional connectivity corresponding to a selected seed region of interest (ROI; precuneus) within the DMN in a sample of BPD patients compared to healthy controls. The precuneus was chosen as a region of interest as previous research has suggested it to play a crucial role in the DMN, with involvement in reflective, self-related processing, empathy, awareness and conscious information processing, and episodic memory, amongst other things (Fransson & Marrelec, 2008; Vollm et al., 2006; Zhang & Li, 2012). Additionally, abnormal functional connectivity of the precuneus during default mode has been documented in a range of psychiatric disorders with features also common to BPD (Broyd et al., 2009; Sheline et al., 2010; Whitfield-Gabrieli et al., 2009), providing a basis for similar research in BPD.

For the task based portion of this study, again a selected seed region of interest from which to map functional connectivity was used, in this case the seed region being the anterior cingulate cortex (ACC). The ACC is known to be involved in emotion processing, empathy, and cognition (Bush, Luu & Posner, 2000; Ruocco, Amirthavasagam, Choi-Kain & McMain, 2013; Vollm et al., 2006, see also 1.2.5), with previous studies observing divergent neural dynamics in the ACC of BPD patients compared to healthy controls (Dziobek et al., 2011). However, despite this knowledge there also remains a lack of research examining functional connectivity of the ACC in BPD samples. In the present study we will investigate functional connectivity between the "emotion network" and the theory of mind processing regions of BPD patients by analysing responses to Theory-of-Mind (*ToM*) stimuli, using ACC as the seed region. The overall aims of the study were twofold; to examine functional connectivity within the DMN, and to examine the functional connectivity between the emotion network and the *ToM* regions, as research investigating both is as yet still lacking. For the DMN investigation, the brain activity of the BPD patients during resting state was observed for any abnormalities (where precuneus was the ROI).

1.3. Hypotheses

There is an increased functional connectivity in the DMN during resting state in BPD patients compared to healthy controls.

There is decreased functional connectivity between the emotion network and the *ToM* network in BPD patients compared to healthy controls.

2. Methods

2.1. Design

Data acquisition consisted of two separate sessions that were covered in one day per participant and took place at the Trinity College Institute of Neuroscience, Dublin, Ireland. In the first session all participants were asked to undergo a comprehensive psychological assessment that included filling in questionnaires and a structured interview conducted by a licensed psychiatrist. The average time spent on the first session was 90 minutes. Subsequently, participants underwent MR imaging for 50 minutes during the first and last 15 minutes of which anatomical images were acquired. Most session days were conducted on a Tuesday afternoon. Participants spent roughly three hours at the institute. Prior to the study, participants were informed about all its aspects and signed a written consent form.

All participants were screened for their suitability of undergoing MRI (i.e. no internal metal parts, non-claustrophobic) and gave their informed consent according to the guidelines of the St. James's and Ethics Committee of the Adelaide and Meath Hospital incorporating the National's Children's Hospital (AMNCH) in Dublin, by which the study had been approved.

2.2. Participants

As BPD is much less frequently found in men (75% of those with the disorder are women: Oldham, 2004), it was decided to have the participant groups consist solely of women to avoid potential gender based differences. The BPD patient group was receiving continuous treatment from the South-West mental health services in Dublin. The BPD participants were all attending outpatient clinics for years. Thus, patients were well known to the service and mainly were treated in outpatient and home care, when necessary with crisis admission. Only when the continuous care consultant indicated these inclusion criteria did we further interview them for suitability to the study. Diagnosis according to DSM-IV was thus confirmed by a second psychiatrist. SCID-II was used to diagnose BPD and SCID-I was used to exclude comorbid axis-I disorders other than MDD. A cohort of 21 healthy female volunteers with ages between 20 and 47, and a mean age of 30.1 years (*SD*=8.0), was recruited from the local community. An effort was made to match both samples with respect to gender and age in so far as similar age ranges were chosen and the distributions regarding age and education levels did not significantly differ from each other.

Healthy volunteers did not undergo conventional SCID-I/II interviews; however, they completed the same battery of psychometric assessment on the day of testing and immediately before MRI scans were obtained. This battery importantly included scales of Depression (BDI and HRSD) on the basis of which one healthy volunteer had to be excluded from the control subjects' sample.

The volunteers and patients were carefully screened for medical conditions to ensure that none had a personal history of neurological disorder, severe medical illness, head injury or substance dependency. Healthy participants were excluded if they had a personal history of any psychiatric disorder (axis I or axis II: APA, 1994) and the BPD participants were excluded if they had any additional psychiatric disorder other than comorbid major depression (MDD) at present or in the past. Demographic variables and inclusion and exclusion criteria were assessed using a standardised questionnaire and through structured interview based on SCID-I by registered psychiatrists.

One patient had not completed the first session and another patient had not completed the second session. Three patients had to be excluded from functional MRI analysis due to excessive movement at some point during the scanning session. The cut-off point chosen for this purpose was a head movement of >3.5mm in any direction which relates to the size of one voxel used in the functional analysis.

Exclusion criteria for all patients and controls were severe medical illnesses, drug or alcohol dependency, other psychiatric axis one diagnosis other than depression. The details on the samples sizes used for each study please are given in each chapter. The samples used in this study were made up of seventeen BPD-patients (Pat) and the nineteen participants (HC) they were compared to.

2.3. Methods

fMRI Task

The stimulus material consisted of two types of cartoons, puns (PUN) and jokes requiring mentalizing (TOM) as well as a control condition that consisted of unfunny pictures containing an incongruity that could not be resolved meaningfully (INC). All pictures were low in aggressive, violent, and sexual content and were used in previous studies (Samson, Hempelmann, Huber & Zysset, 2009; Samson, Zysset & Huber, 2008). In order to investigate brain activity during resting state rest trials (NULL) were interleaved during which participants observed a blank screen. All participants processed a total of 120 trials (30 INC + 30 PUN + 30 TOM + 30 NULL). Stimuli were presented every 10 s on average and with variable stimulus onset delays (0, 400, 800, 1200 or 1600 ms). Each stimulus was onset for 6000 ms during which participants were instructed to make a response. Below each picture (cartoon) the word "understood" was printed on the left side and the words "not understood" were printed on the right side. Participants were asked to press the corresponding button (left/right) with their index or middle finger, respectively, depending on whether they understood the joke. The functional neuroimaging part started after 15 minutes of the scanning session (during which the structural image was acquired) and took about 18 minutes.

Being not relevant to the research question of the present study, the PUN and INC trials were excluded from the analysis and only TOM and NULL trials were further considered for contrasts.

MRI Data Acquisition

Magnetic resonance images were obtained with a Philips Achieva MRI scanner (Philips Medical System, Netherland BV, Veenphuis 4–6, 5684 PC Best, The Netherlands) operating at 3 Tesla. For the cognitive paradigm run, 26 axial slices (3.5 mm× 3.5 mm× 3.5 mm resolution, 0.75 mm spacing), parallel to the AC-PC plane and covering the whole brain were acquired using a single shot, gradient recalled EPI sequence (TR 2000 ms, TE 30 ms, 90° flip angle). One functional run with 620 time points was acquired, with each time point sampling over the 26 slices. Prior to the functional run, 180 anatomical slices T_1-weighted 3D-MPRAGE sequence (repetition time, 11.0 ms; echo time, 4.4 ms; total acquisition time, 7 min 30 sec; number of acquisitions, 1; field of view, 250 mm× 256 mm × 160 mm; matrix: 256 mm × 256 mm; resolution: 0.9 mm × 0.9 mm × 0.9 mm) with the same spatial orientation as the functional data were acquired.

Data Analysis

SPM8 Pre-Processing

A standard Statistical Parametric Mapping (SPM8, Functional Imaging Laboratory, University College London, UK) analysis was conducted on fMRI data of all subjects in order to obtain the regions with the strongest activation for the contrast [TOM>NULL] in the tasks. The CONN Toolbox was then be used to extract the mean voxel time series ROI for a 10 mm radius regions around the maximum of activation within the precuneus (for the default mode network) and ACC (for the emotion network) for each subject separately.

CONN Toolbox

The CONN resting state software (http://www.nitrc.org/projects/conn/) performs seeded voxel correlations by estimating maps showing temporal correlations between the BOLD signal from given seed and that at every brain voxel. The toolbox implements a *CompCor* strategy for physiological noise source reduction, first-level General Linear Model for correlation and regression connectivity estimation, and second-level random-effect analyses.

Using CONN resting state software the data were temporally band-pass filtered ($0.009 < f < 0.08$). Several sources of spurious variance along with their temporal derivatives then were removed from the data by linear regression, such as signal from regions centred in the white matter, cerebrospinal fluid, movement and effects of rest. This regression procedure removes fluctuations unlikely to be involved in specific regional correlations.

First level analysis: A method previously introduced by Bokde et al. (2006). For whole brain mapping of ROI coupling, the time series representing right and left ROI was separately regressed on all fMRI time series in each individual's dataset (without prior convolution by a model of the hemodynamic response function). This results in maps of the regression coefficients for the effect of (right and left) ROI activity on all other brain regions for each participant in the study.

Second level analysis: In order to identify locations of significant group, side and group-by-side effects on ROI coupling a 2x2 mixed effects ANCOVA was performed using the ROI coupling as the dependent variables as well as age and individual BDI-depression scores as covariates. This model was specified to include a main effect of group (with 2 levels, BPD patients, and healthy volunteers) and a main effect of side (with 2 levels, left, and right). Statistical significance was based on a threshold of $p<0.05$ (*FWE*, voxel level corrected). The anatomic localisation of significant clusters was identified using the AAL toolbox (Tzourio-Mazoyer et al., 2002, see 2.9).

Further, structural equation modelling (SEM) was applied to the data in order to test the functional connectivity within the default mode and affect/emotion regulation network.

Functional Coupling Analysis

To compute functional connectivity maps corresponding to a selected seed region of interest (ROI), the regional time course was correlated against all other voxels within the brain. Based on data from a previous resting state study by Sheline et al. (2010), the connectivity within the affective network was explored. Correlation maps were produced by extracting the BOLD time course from a seed region, then computing the correlation coefficient between that time course and the time course from all other brain voxels. The anterior cingulate cortex (ACC; +/- x=10, y=-35, z=2) was extracted as the seed regions of interest in the affective network that was modulated between TOM trials and NULL events, and the precuneus (+/- x=7, y=-60, z=21) as the seed ROI in the resting state network during NULL events. The principal techniques used were computation of whole brain, voxel-wise intrinsic functional connectivity maps.

Statistical Analysis

We analysed resting-state functional MRI data to determine significant differences in functional connectivity between BPD and control participants using a family wise error (FWE) whole brain corrected threshold of $p<0.01$. The threshold was reduced to $p<0.025$ from $p<0.05$ because the connectivity was analysed within the two different networks. Moreover, mean connectivity data were extracted from areas that showed significant differences between patients and healthy controls.

3. Results

Default Mode Network

After visual inspection of the resting state network the differences between patients and controls were calculated. The resting-state network for all participants ($N=36$, Figure 1) with right precuneus used as the seeding region showed a standard DMN pattern, as described in detail by previous resting-state network studies (Buckner, Andrews-Hanna, & Schacter, 2008).

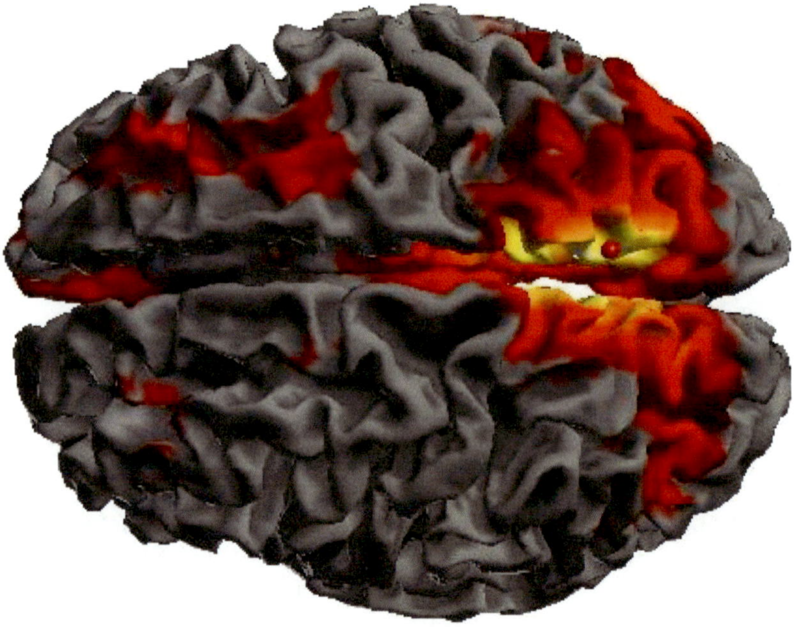

Figure 1: *Resting state network, (Pat+HC), seed region: Precuneus. Functional connectivity superimposed on a 3D standardised template, dorsal view.*

Increased functional connectivity was found in patients, compared to controls, between the precuneus (seed region) and three brain areas which were located left inferior frontal lobe, left precentral/middle frontal, and left middle occipital/superior parietal (Table 1, Figure 2).

Table 1: *Default mode network: Pat > HC, seed region: Precuneus.*

K	$FWE_{cluster}$	Region	FWE_{voxel}	t	Coordinates [mm]		
					x	y	z
259	0.067	L Inf. Frontal Operculum	0.025	5.98	-42	14	16
		L Inf. Frontal Triangularis	0.350	4.72	-48	18	20
		L Inf. Frontal Triangularis	0.535	4.36	-38	22	16
401	0.014	L Precentral	0.137	5.17	-42	10	48
		L Mid. Frontal	0.335	4.72	-48	6	52
		L Precentral	0.915	3.95	-42	2	44
384	0.016	L Mid. Occipital	0.674	4.31	-24	-64	40
		L Sup. Parietal	0.888	4.01	-22	-74	54
		L Precuneus	0.913	3.95	-8	-74	54

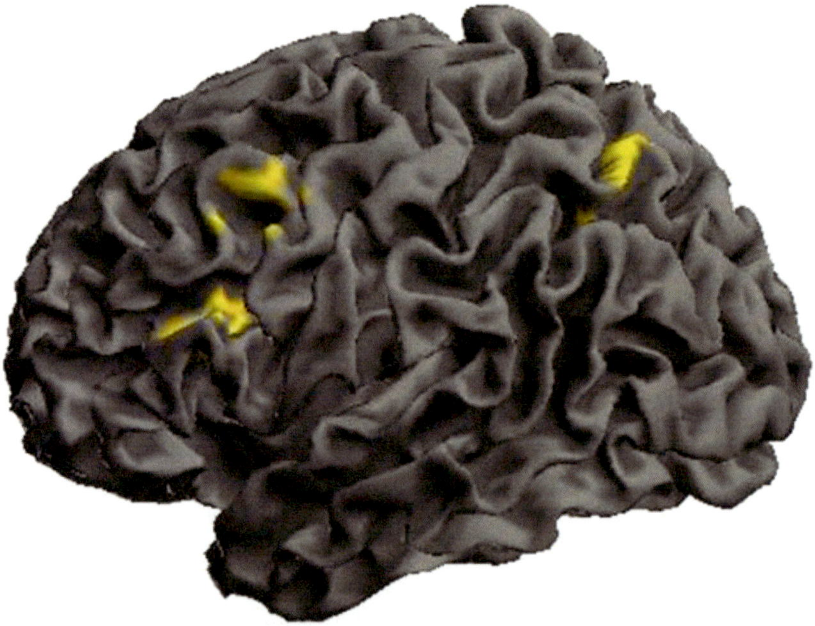

Figure 2: *Resting state network: Pat > HC. Increased functional connectivity between precuneus (seed) and left IFG (visible), L precentral, L midfrontal, L midoccipital, L sup. Parietal, superimposed on a 3D standardised template, lateral view.*

Affective Network

During trials where brain activity was modulated between TOM and NULL conditions, decreased functional connectivity was found for patients compared to controls between the ACC (seed) and three brain areas left superior temporal, right mid-cingulum, and right supramarginal/inferior parietal (corresponding to the cognitive neuroscience term "temporo-parietal junction", RTPJ).

Table 2: *Connectivity changes PAT<HC for [TOM-NULL]; seed region: ACC*

K	$FWE_{cluster}$	Region	FWE_{voxel}	t	Coordinates [mm]		
					x	y	z
603	0.001	L Sup. Temporal	0.016	6.09	-60	-4	-2
		L Sup. Temporal	0.192	5.05	-60	4	-5
		L Sup. Temporal	0.486	4.57	-42	-35	22
1507	<0.001	R Mid. Cingulum	0.070	5.49	14	-26	40
		R Mid. Cingulum	0.203	5.03	10	-20	35
		R Mid. Cingulum	0.241	4.95	10	-40	50
844	<0.001	R Supramarginal	0.072	5.48	66	-32	36
		R Supramarginal	0.134	5.21	58	-32	40
		R Inf. Parietal	0.326	4.79	52	-35	45

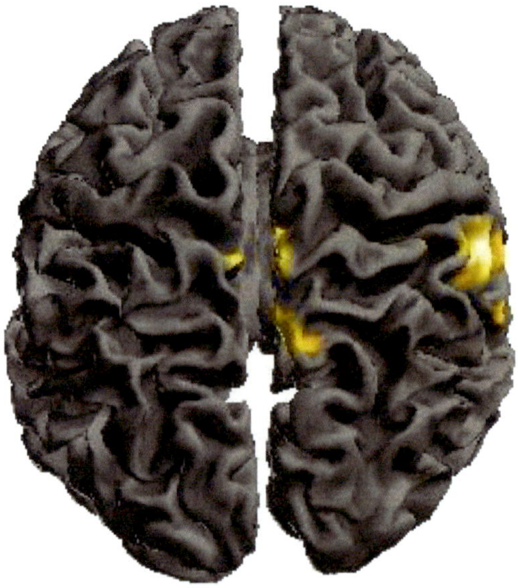

Figure 3: *Connectivity changes PAT<HC for [TOM-NULL]. Decreased functional connectivity between ACC (seed) and RTPJ and right MCC, superimposed on a 3D standardised template, caudal view.*

4. Discussion

The objectives for the present BPD functional connectivity study were, firstly, to test for abnormalities in brain activity during resting state (specifically monitoring the precuneus), and, secondly, to test for differences in connectivity between the ACC (the core region of affective network) and all other parts of the brain during mental processing of Theory-of-Mind stimuli vs. resting state.

The main finding of the present study was decreased functional connectivity of ACC with MCC, left STS, and right TPJ during processing of *ToM* stimuli (or mentalizing) in BPD patients. ACC has an important role in integration of neuronal circuitry for affect regulation and can be identified as a distinctive region in understanding psychopathology (Stevens, Hurley & Taber, 2011). It was for this reason that we selected ACC as the seed region for the affective network. While the MCC was shown to be involved in both self-and other-perspective (Vogt, 2005), bilateral STS and TPJ belong to the core neural network of mentalizing (Dodell-Feder, Koster-Hale, Bedny & Saxe, 2011; R. Saxe & Wexler, 2005). Especially the right TPJ includes areas that are recruited exclusively by mentalizing (Scholz, Triantafyllou, Whitfield-Gabrieli, Brown & Saxe, 2009) and seems to be the only brain region for which this is true (R. R. Saxe & Pelphrey, 2009). Our data suggest dysconnectivity between the emotion (regulation) network and the *ToM* network in BPD compared to healthy controls supporting the theory of BPD as an emotional regulation disorder (Linehan, 1993). An important testable prediction from this finding might be that BPD individuals have altered *ToM* processing compared to healthy controls when placed under emotional stress.

As extensive comorbidity has been documented for BPD with both Axis I disorders and other Axis II disorders of the DSM-IV (usually mood disorders, anxiety disorders, or substance disorders), comorbidities are a potential limitation in this study, although MDD was the only comorbidity that was clinically diagnosed in our BPD sample.

In order to identify the above mentioned dysconnectivity as a biological marker for BPD, future studies should also carry out functional connectivity analyses in the most commonly documented comorbidities of BPD which are major depressive disorder (MDD), attention deficit hyperactivity disorder (ADHD), and post-traumatic stress disorder (PTSD) which is of particular interest given that both disorders are highly related to experiences of trauma (Pagura et al., 2010; Philipsen et al., 2010; D. J. Stein et al., 2010; Zetzsche et al., 2006).

The second network investigated in the recent study was the default mode network. The approach of measuring BOLD signal independent of any task makes the method independent of any differences of performance between sessions and/or subjects. Therefore, resting-state fMRI can be easily employed in patients with potentially limited ability for participation in task paradigms. However, the rapid employment of these techniques by the imaging community over the past decade is due, in part, to both the ease of data acquisition and the similarity of results to previous finding using task-induced approaches (Nierhaus, 2012).

The comparison of functional connectivity during rest revealed higher activity in BPD patients in areas that are not commonly found in the DMN. A first conclusion that may be drawn from this finding is that the DMN is altered in BPD. While there was no decrease in connectivity from the precuneus to any brain area, patients activated left IFG (comprising BA 44 and 45 which together are known as Broca's area), left mid-frontal, left precentral, and left mid-occipital/superior parietal in addition to the standard DMN regions and thus exhibited significantly higher activity in these regions compared to healthy controls. To further conclude that any processes of speech processing were at work during resting state would probably be too premature at this stage. This hypothesis however could be tested by investigating true "task-negative" resting state connectivity by contrasting it to the connectivity during a cognitive task that involves processing of language.

Recent neuroimaging studies also show involvement of BA44 together with, precentral/pre supplementary motor area (pre-SMA), mid-frontal, and mid-occipital in selective response suppression in go/no-go tasks and has therefore been interpreted as core neural substrates of error processing (van Gaal &

Lamme, 2012). Our data suggest that error processing could be active in BPD even in absence of external stimuli and hence of external errors. This does not necessarily mean that subjects are aware of this process as van Gaal, de Lange and Cohen (2012) were able to show that the "inhibition network", and in particular the left inferior frontal gyrus, is active during unconscious error processing.

Particularly in resting state connectivity studies caution must be made with regard to gender differences, which did not apply to our all-female sample. Healthy men and women differed in connectivity patterns across precuneus subregions (Zhang & Li, 2012).

In the past, other distinct neural networks have been identified in healthy subjects during resting-state conditions, including lateral fronto-parietal and medial–frontal networks (Damoiseaux et al., 2006; Smith et al., 2009). These resting-state networks (RSNs) have been suggested to reflect a dynamic functional organisation of the brain (Fox et al., 2005), a notion supported by the finding of a close correspondence between RSNs and activation patterns underlying a wide range of cognitive processes, such as attention, memory, behavioural inhibition and executive control (Smith et al., 2009). Thus, the investigation of multiple RSNs may provide a rich source of information with regard to the functional architecture of altered brain states in patients with mental disorders, as previously shown in patients with schizophrenia (Calhoun, Maciejewski, Pearlson & Kiehl, 2008), affective disorders (Calhoun et al., 2008), and also BPD (Wolf et al., 2011). Investigating other RSNs in BPD and its comorbidities may hold future research potential. The only study that has attempted this is recent work by Wolf et al. (2011) – who likewise found increased connectivity in BPD between precuneus and left inferior frontal lobe using a similar method.

In terms of the practical limitations of the methodology, we must look to past studies. The majority of past PET functional studies examined patients only during resting state, with results producing very little consistency (O'Neill & Frodl, 2012). One reason for the lack of consistency amongst these PET studies could be that at resting state the patients' emotional state is not known, thus the range of neural activity could be vast, especially with a patient sample typified by emotional fluctuations. Whereas in the past studies, mostly involving specific tasks or images, the patients' emotional states could be more accurately predicted and the resulting images compared with more reliability (O'Neill & Frodl, 2012). This would suggest that when investigating neurobiological functioning in BPD patients, studies which employ specific emotion related stimuli provide a more reliable measure than resting state studies (O'Neill & Frodl, 2012). This may hold true for DMN functional connectivity studies in BPD as well, and is worth noting for future studies.

Given the similarity in symptomology observed between the two disorders, research methodologies in BPD have often followed those of PTSD. It has been suggested that DMN connectivity may have potential as a predictor of posttraumatic stress disorder symptom severity in acutely traumatised subjects (Lanius et al., 2010). Considering this and the more recent findings of Kluetsch et al. (2012) (who related signal strength in the posterior DMN to symptom severity), it may be of interest to future researchers to further explore this avenue.

Apart from that it will be necessary to study the sub-regions of the precuneus and their role in DMN function, specifically within BPD, as Zang and Li recently (2012) provided evidence for different roles in eight sub-regions of the precuneus. Thus, examining the precuneus as a whole may lead to distorted data as a number of studies have observed positive connectivity with the default network for ventral but not dorsal precuneus (Buckner et al., 2008; Zhang & Li, 2012).

Finally, co-occurrent Axis I-disorders and medication use in this sample of patients with BPD have to be considered as potential limitations. However, the question of whether patients with BPD with psychiatric comorbidities should be excluded to homogenise clinical sample characteristics remains controversial (Lis, Greenfield, Henry, Guile & Dougherty, 2007).

The sample size in the present study was modest, though comparable to that of most functional imaging studies of psychiatric populations. Nevertheless a failure to detect possible differences at a behavioural level might be explained by a lack of statistical power. Also, because the samples consisted of only female patients with relatively typical clinical presentation, conclusive inferences for male BPD patients who make up a smaller proportion of all BPD patients and often exhibit atypical clinical features cannot be made.

A strength of the study is that the samples did not include any patients with a comorbid generalised anxiety disorder or with co-morbid panic disorder. Both the BPD and the healthy sample were clinically assessed and one healthy participant was excluded for scoring outside the normal range on depression/impulsiveness scales.

For conclusion, a promising finding is the reduced functional coupling between ACC as seed region for the emotional network and the theory of mind (mentalizing) network indicating dysregulation between these two networks in line with emotion regulation dysfunctions in BPD. Moreover, higher resting state functional connectivity is also of interest since it may be linked to higher arousal in BPD which needs to be investigated further in future studies.

In summary, patients with BPD display a specific pattern of disturbance in cognitive and emotional empathy and expression of social signals. Given the importance of social cognition (on the part of both the sender and the recipient (Roepke, Vater, Preissler, Heekeren & Dziobek, 2012) for maintaining stable interpersonal relationships and establishing therapeutic alliance, these deficits should be further explored in future studies.

Acknowledgements

I thank my TCIN colleagues Thomas Frodl, Angela Carballedo, and Aisling O'Neill for their assistance with the study and the Irish Research Council for Science, Engineering, and Technology (IRCSET) for supporting me and funding my research.

10 Borderzones of Neurorehabilitation - A Personal Statement

Arto Laihinen

> **Motto**: "The important thing is not to stop questioning. Curiosity has its own reason for existing. One cannot help but be in awe when contemplating the mysteries of eternity, of life, of the marvellous structures of reality."
>
> **Albert Einstein**

Key Words: restoratio ad integrum, salutogenese, plasticity, palliative treatment, nursing care, neurobiology, synapse, positron emission tomography (PET), Barthel Index, Phase of Rehabilitation, CNS, neurorehabilitation

1. Introduction: Concept and Domain of Neurorehabilitation

Neurorehabilitation means restoration of function after the acute phase of neurological illnes, e. g. stroke or a brain trauma. The aim of rehabilitation is either (1) to reach full health (restitutio ad integrum) or at least an improvement of the condition to variable extent, or alternatively (2) to prevent deterioration of the condition.

In this part of m text, I deal with neurorehabilitation, which has characteristics of its own among the different areas of general rehabilitation. Most often, neurosurgical rehabilitation is included within neurorehabilitation. The difference between neurorehabilitation and geriatric rehabilitation is somewhat gliding, but it could be stated – if we are not focussing on the age of the patients – that patients on a geriatric rehabilitation ward are usually multimorbid and a neurological disease - if there is any - is only part of the disease panorama.

In section five I deal with the borderzone between rehabilitation and palliative care and discuss the role rehabilitation in patients whose condition cannot be stabilized, but is continuously deteriorating, e.g. in cases of amyotrophic lateral sclerosis or in certain malignant brain tumours like glioblastoma multiforme.

Rehabilitation can be vocational, where the aim is the restoration of the working capability or medical rehabilitation, which aims at a normalization of the patient's condition without reference to his working capacity. Rehabilitation is carried out either on a ward in a clinic or on an out-patient basis – in this latter modality the patients stay overnight at home and spend their days in the rehabilitation institution. Some out-patient rehabilitation units have a transport service of their own.

Rehabilitation is carried out by highly skilled staff consisting of medical doctors (the role of specialists of neurology is important) and therapists including physiotherapists, occupational therapists, experts of physical treatment (e. g. massage, functional electrical stimulation, etc.), psychologists (note the special role of neuropsychologists), speech therapists and social case workers and dietitians. This interdisciplinary team has to be well coordinated so that it can deal also with demanding and multimorbid patients.

2. Borderzone: Neurobiology and Rehabilitation

Even though rehabilitation is part of clinical medicine, it is based on information about pathobiology. The concept of plasticity (Hara, 2015) is the main topic of basic science dealing with rehabilitation. Plasticity in the Hebbian sense means that there are compensatory mechanisms in the Central Nervous System (CNS), which allow – more or less – the restitution of the nervous function. It is assumed that the basis of plasticity is the modification of synapses – in this way, adjacent areas to the destroyed regions are able to carry on the functions which were either lost or reduced. On the other hand, nonsynaptic plasticity, e.g. modifications of the membrane permeability may also play a role in plasticity.

The traditional way of thinking was that neurons in the CNS are post-mitotic, meaning that they do not divide any more after the embryonic period. Recently, there has been evidence based on, e.g., electron microscopy and isotope techniques, that neurogenesis actually does take place in the mature CNS of mammals (Gould et al., 1999; Ernst et al., 2014; Seib & Martin-Villalba, 2014; Winner et al., 2011). New neurons are formed, e.g., in the hippocampus dealing with mechanisms of memory or forgetting ("new-born neurons may not have the engrams of the past"), and also elsewhere in the brain such as the olfactory bulb. In the living brain, this can be studied only indirectly: It is assumed that neurogenesis is correlated to angiogenesis (Sierra et al., 2011; Small et al., 2004) and perfusion can be measured with different techniques including PET and SPECT.

Furthermore, functional imaging studies of the human brain such as fMRI and PET have provided new insights into this topic – it is now possible to study brain function not only during the acute phase of the neurological disorder (e.g. stroke) but also successively in the time-course of gradual recovery (Mountz, 2007; Weiller, 1998; Calautti et al., 2001; van Meer et al., 2012). Both intrahemispheric and interhemispheric mechanisms of adaptation can be studied. Enhanced cortical excitability and reduced laterality correlate with spontaneus functional recovery after stroke (Cramer, 2008). These processes are time-dependent, increasing in the early weeks after stroke and decreasing over months thereafter, and a reduction is greater among stroke patients with stronger functional recovery while the persistent increased activity over both the hemispheres is greatest in those patients with the poorest outcome (Cramer & Crafton, 2006; Ward et al., 2003).

A concrete example of the studies concerning motor recovery which has led to a new therapeutic approach is the so-called therapy of Taub, where the affected limb is under constraint and cannot be used, which leads to the activation of the affected hemisphere (Laible et al., 2012; Liepert et al., 2000; Rijntjes et al., 2011). These results can be analyzed quantitatively with PET. Motor recovery and aphasia as well can be studied using serial PET or fMRI studies (Abel et al., 2015).

3. Borderzone: Acute Neurology and Rehabilitation

It is sometimes stated that rehabilitation begins already in the ER (emergency room). This may be an overexaggeration, but actually there is a bridge between acute medicine and rehabilitation; this link is called early rehabilitation. This is carried out on special wards which allow intense treatment including artificial respiration. There is also much more staff on these wards than on normal rehabilitation wards.

3.1. Phases of ehabilitation:

The criterion of these phases is the so-called Barthel-Index (BI) which records need of help in everyday life. The rehabilitation phases are defined according to the BI in the following way:

A: Acute medine
B: Early rehabilitation BI 0-30
C: Intermediate state BI 35-65
D: Advanced rehabilitation BI 70-100
E: Aftercare

There has been, however, considerable discussion about the Barthel-Index because it is supposed to overemphasize motor performace, while cognitive and linguistic functions are not given proper value. Still, the BI has kept its position as a criterion when the phases of rehab are classified.

Rehabilitation on the ward	B+C
Out-patient rehabilitation	(partly C +) D.

4. Borderzone: Nursing Care and Rehabilitation

In early rehabilitation (Phase B) no rehabilitation is possible without extensive nursing care. In intermediate rehabilitation (phase C), as BI increases, less and less nursing care is needed. Finally in the rehabilitation phase D, most patients do not need nursing care any more but mostly they are independent.

The concept of an active or activating nursing care, denotes the care given when the nurse is participating in rehabilitation trying to support the patient to be as independent as possible In reality therapy (frequently begun with: "Good morning - today its this and that day"), through the daily routines there is an attempt to activate the patient and to point out that good orientation in time and space is crucially important.

5. Borderzone: Palliative Care and Rehabilitation

In rehabilitation, we have the starting point that the condition will get better or will at least be stabilized (see the Introduction). In palliative care with patients who have a terminal disease, we have to accept the situation that the health condition is getting worse and finally eventually leads to death. In spite of this unfortunate development, rehabilitation may at least partly and particularly at early phases of these disorders improve the quality of life of the patients. Usually, it is, however, very difficult to integrate the rehabilitation treatment of this kind in everyday routines and the working set-up of a normal rehabilitation clinic. The strategy preferred is to give rehabilitative treatment in the palliative unit itself. The rehabilitation program ought to be gentle and individialized to the specific needs of the patients.

Psychological care and support are of utmost importance with these patients. What should be avoided, is a situation where patients have unwarranted wishes of full recovery via the rehabilitation measures. Finally, when the malignant disease does progress, the patients are extremely upset and have difficulties coping with the situation.

Certain patients, e.g. with early ALS (Degenhardt, 2002; Weisser et al., 2015) or patients suffering from cancer (Salakari et al., 2015) including malignant brain tumours (e.g. glioblastoma multiforme) may profit to some limited extent from rehabilitation imroving the quality of life, still the disease will progress and the time window for efforts in the area of rehabilitation is inevitably of short duration. Often, it is very difficult for the patients to accept this transition from rehabilitation to palliative treatment. Actually, this process ought to be seen as a continuum, where at the beginning the rehabilitative approach is more important and toward the end the role of palliation becomes more relevant.

What helps at least to some extent, is that the patients are well informed and that there is an adequate doctor-patient relationship, in which the prognosis can be discussed openly with the patient and his family and where the patient can get the necessary support, preferrably in a good setting of Hospice Care.

6. Conclusion

Above, I discussed rehabilitation mainly from the point of biological determinants. Rehabilitation can also be approached from other points of view. The proposal of Antonowsky (1978) is in this sense interesting. The core message is that health can be dealt with basically in the same way as disease, analyzing the different "risk factors" or "determinants" of health (e.g. good nutrition, sufficient sleep, enough exercise, good genes etc.). Antonowsky coined the term "salutogenesis". The term describes an approach focusing on factors that support human health and well-being, rather than on factors that cause disease. What is relevant is the relationship between health, stress and coping in the actual situation of the patient.

Consequently, the aim of rehabilitation would be to support all these positive factors enabling the patient to overcome his handicap. The role of team work in rehabilitation is very important because this kind of support needs collaboration between all the different professional groups, which participate in the rehabilitation.

Rehabilitation ought to be scheduled according to the rules of evidence-based medicine, which means that different ways of rehabilitation are compared with each other in large series, this would allow solid statistical evaluation. Multicenter international studies are needed to have samples, which are inclusive enough. Thus the most efficient ways of rehabilitation (which would hopefully be also the most cost-effective) would be found.

In the future, rehabilitation ought to be available to everybody who is making a recovery from a difficult acute neurological disease. Access to rehabilitation should be straight-forward, without a complicated process of repeated bureaucratic correspondence with the health authorities (health insurance provider or "Krankenkasse") – or perhaps, this procedure could be made immediately after the commencement of the acute illness (stroke, brain trauma, etc.) has taken place, thus creating a registry of "would-be" rehabilitation cases. In the final analysis, these patients would be followed-up in order to obtain statistical data for the detailed evaluation concerning efficacy of the different forms of evidence-based rehabilitation.

Part 3:

Neuropsychology: A Bridge to the Sciences, Arts and Education

11 Neuropsychology and Dentistry. Is there any Connection?

Tibor Károly Fábián, Anita Beck, Wolf-Rainer Krause, Pál Fejérdy, Péter Hermann and Gábor Fábián

Key Words: dental fear, orofacial pain, cranial nerves, oral immunity, salivary gland, autonomic innervation , prevention, communication, mind-body therapies, brainstem

1. Introduction

Although dentistry is a profession dedicated to treating somatic disorders of the oral/orofacial region primarily, there is also a collection of various psychological and pathopsychological conditions dentists should deal with (Fábián et al., 2007/b; Fábián et al., 2012/a; Fábián et al., in press). The most common and widely known phenomena are dental fear and several related manifestations like odonto/dental phobic reactions, needle phobia or panic attack (Carlsson et al., 1980; Berggren & Carlsson, 1984; Berggren et al., 1997/b, 2000; Botto, 2006). However, the oral region is an area that appears to be particularly predisposed also for a large number of different functional and somatoform psychosomatic disorders (Kreyer, 2000; Fábián & Fejérdy, 2010; Beck et al., 2012; Fábián et al., 2012/b; Fábián & Hidalgo Wulff, 2014; Fábián et al., in press). Therefore, another large group of psychogenic manifestations in dentistry is formed by several oral psychosomatic manifestations (Fabian et al., 2007/a; Fábián et al., in press). The reason behind this may be that there are rich psychological and neuroanatomical couplings of the mouth, teeth and other oral structures based on their highly important and rather unique psychological and physiological functions (Fábián et al., 2007/a; Fábián et al., in press).

The orofacial region is affected by psychogenic manifestations much more frequently, compared to most other parts of the body (Fábián et al., 2007/a, Fábián et al., 2012/a; Fábián et al., in press). In general, roughly 10 percent of the dental patients may be counted as *risk patient* for any psychogenic manifestations (Doering & Wolowski, 2007, Fábián & Fejérdy, 2010) which is a significant proportion, and the incidence may increase (Sugawara et al., 1998, Fábián & Fejérdy, 2010). Thus, the importance of psychogenic manifestations should not be underestimated, but considered as a rather important and difficult problem of dentistry (Fábián & Fejérdy, 2010; Fábián et al., in press). The most important *primary consequences/risks* of oral psychogenic manifestations are: moderate or excessive loss of teeth and other oral tissues; chronification and/or aggravation of the oral (orofacial) symptoms and/or the psychiatric condition behind the symptoms; long-run disturbances of a patient's relationship to dentists; highly increased expenses because of the repeated dental treatments; legal procedures because of unsuccessful and/or expensive treatments; consequences of all premised elements on the general health and quality of life of the patient (Fábián & Fejérdy, 2010; Fábián et al., in press). It should also be considered that, even two or three of such patients may unbalance a dentist's entire schedule and can occupy a large percentage of the dentist's time; which should also be considered as a rather difficult problem (Fábián & Fejérdy, 2010; Fábián et al., in press).

Problems relating to dental fear primarily occur in the childhood, adolescence or early adulthood (before the age of 20) (Hällström & Halling, 1984) and most patients suffering from dental fear experience at least partial remission at times (Hällström & Halling, 1984). The most common reasons of dental fear are bad (painful or fearful) dental experiences, lack of control over the social situation in the dental chair, lack of control over personal emotional reactions, feeling of powerlessness during treatment and social learning processes with a negative image of dentists (Moore & Birn, 1990; Fábián et al., in press). A large proportion of these patients are aware of having been exposed to fear-provoking dental treatment in the past (Berggren & Meynert, 1984; Moore et al., 1993; Berggren et al., 1997/a; Skaret et al., 1998). In some cases, an unconscious psychological trauma may also be a cause of dental fear reactions (Fábián et al., in press).

There are also various oral psychosomatic manifestations (Fábián et al., 2007/a; Fábián et al., in press) caused by either acute psychological stress conditions (existential trauma, workplace problems, relationship problems with the sexual partner, etc.) or by chronic conditions like depression, neuroses, chronic anxiety, death anxiety, schizophrenic or paranoid reactions (etc.). These manifestations more frequently appear in women, usually in the second half of life, although they can appear in children or in young adults as well (Fábián et al., 2007/a; Fábián et al., in press). The most frequent symptoms are atypical facial pain, burning mouth syndrome, myofascial pain, temporomandibular dysfunction, bruxism and other parafunctions, gagging, psychogenic denture intolerance, psychogenic taste disorders, certain recurrent oral ulcerations or inflammations, some oral allergic reactions, psychogenic occlusal problems, tic, psychogenic salivation problems, and oral discomfort, but any other symptoms mimicking somatic symptoms of jaws, mouth and teeth may appear. The symptoms may appear singly or in combination (Fábián et al., 2007/a; Fábián et al., in press). Since the appearing psychogenic symptoms may mimic a great variety of (most) somatic symptoms of jaws, mouth and teeth, a clear-cut diagnosis and proper differential diagnosis could be rather difficult (Pomp, 1974; Fábián & Fejérdy, 2010; Fábián et al., 2012/a; Fábián & Hidalgo Wulff, 2014), even if a history of symptoms that are inconsistent with the physical findings and a history of a precipitating life event after which the symptom first appeared are hallmarks of such psychogenic manifestations (Marxkors & Muller-Fahlbusch, 1981; Laskin & Block, 1986; Muller-Fahlbusch & Sone, 1982; Green & Laskin, 2000; Dworkin & Sherman, 2006)

2. Psychological Couplings of the Oral Region

Tooth loss (or other oral damage) may profoundly affect the psychosocial well-being of patients, even those who are apparently coping well with the dental treatment and dentures (Fiske et al., 1998; Allen & McMillan, 2003), and complete edentulousness can be a serious life event (Bergendal, 1989; Trulsson et al., 2002; Fábián & Fejérdy, 2010; Fábián et al., 2012/a, Fábián & Hidalgo Wulff, 2014). The rich psychological couplings of mouth, teeth and other oral structures are rooted in their widespread and psycho-emotionally highly important functions (Fábián et al., 2007/a; Fábián et al., in press). They are important aspects of an individual's facial aesthetics and sexual characteristics (Fábián et al., 2007/a; Fábián et al., in press); they play an important role in speech and nonverbal-communication; serve as a primary zone of interaction with the environment (Ament & Ament, 1970); take part in sexual contact; and act as organs of various senses (Fábián et al., 2007/a; Fábián et al., in press).

The oral region is tremendously important already in a baby's life (Ament & Ament, 1970; Fábián et al., 2007/a; Fábián et al., in press) as an organ of pleasure, as an organ of contact with the mother as well as an organ of testing, learning, understanding, and social signaling (Ament & Ament, 1970), especially (but not exclusively) in the highly important oral stage of personality development in which breast-feeding plays a prominent role in the communication between the mother and the infant (Fábián et al. 2007/a; Fábián et al., in press). Also of great importance is the symbolic value of the mouth, teeth and other oral structures (Fábián et al. 2007/a, Fábián et al. 2012/a; Fábián et al., in press).

Because of the multiple psychological couplings and importance of the mouth and teeth, it is no wonder that many of the psychopathological mechanisms related to sexuality, aggressiveness, auto-aggressiveness, or death anxiety can lead to orofacial manifestations. Especially if the above mentioned important psychological and symbolic functions are damaged by tooth or mouth disorders (Fábián et al. 2007/a; Fábián et al., in press).

3. Neuroanatomical Couplings of the Oral Region

Neuroanatomical couplings of the oral region are rather peculiar compared to other parts of the body. In general, those tissues, which are of mesodermic origin in most parts of the body, are of *ecto*dermic (ectomesodermic) origin in the orofacial region indicating a strong coupling of the orofacial and the nervous structures. In good accordance with this consideration, there is an interesting recent finding that stem cells present in the human dental pulp have a tendency to differentiate into functionally active neurons under certain experimental circumstances (Király et al., 2009) which may be another indication of the above mentioned relatively strong coupling of certain oral tissues and nervous tissues. Further, innervation of the orofacial region is originated from the brain stem (instead of the spinal cord); which may also form a base of the strong influence of the psycho-emotional functions on the orofacial tissues and their function. It is also obvious that there is an exceptionally rich representation of the oral region in a large number of various brain structures.

The neuroanatomical structures that are of particular importance in the complex neuropsychological processes of oral and orofacial pain are (according to Gebhardt et al., 1984; Fields & Basbaum, 1994; Peyron et al., 2000; Strasbaugh & Levine, 2000; Zimmermann, 2004; Baldry, 2005; Fábián & Fejérdy 2010): (1) pain related *sensory receptors* and their *associated afferent trigeminal nerve* fibers; (2) the *brainstem* including the *nuclei of the trigeminal nerve*, and their connecting nervous paths (*interneurons*) towards the ascending and descending pain tracts and the reticular formation; (3) the *ascending pain tracts* which could be either those which conduct pain signals of the spinal cord, or other not yet characterized ascending nervous paths conducting pain stimuli of the trigeminal nerve; (4) *descending inhibitory tracts*, and the *local* ("segmental") *inhibitory interneurons*; (5) the *reticular formation* which is responsible primarily for pain related changes of arousal level, attention as well as for pain related autonomic changes and mediation of descending inhibition of pain; (6) the *thalamus* which is responsible for pain related affective, autonomic and hormonal changes as well as for determination of quality and localization of pain; (7) *other subcortical structures* including the periaqueductal grey, the locus ceruleus, and nuclei of the raphe which modulate pain impulses and mediate descending inhibition; (8) the *somatosensory cortex* responsible for the integration of pain related sensory stimuli with other sensory inputs; (9) the *frontal cortex and limbic system* which are responsible for the highest integration resulting in pain experience, pain-related cognitive and emotional activities, changes of mood, as well as initiation of pain related behavioral, autonomic and hormonal responses (Gebhardt et al., 1984;

Fields & Basbaum, 1994; Peyron et al., 2000; Strasbaugh & Levine, 2000; Zimmermann, 2004; Baldry, 2005; Fábián & Fejérdy, 2010).

Considering neuroanatomical specificities of the orofacial muscles it may be mentioned first that the masticatory and facial muscles are highly sensitive muscles having rather small motor units (Silverman, 1961; Graber, 1995) and a rather extended representation in the motor cortices compared to other muscles (Sergl, 1996). Motor nervous supplies of the orofacial muscles are conducted by several cranial nerves including the mandibular nerve (which is a branch of the trigeminal nerve), the facial nerve, the hypoglossal nerve and the accessory nerve (Griffin & Harris, 1975). Thus, (in contrast to most other muscles, which are supplied via the spinal cord) motor nervous supplies of masticatory and facial muscles are maintained *directly* from the brainstem via several cranial nerves. The brainstem is a structure mediating numerous important psychoemotional processes such as pain, arousal, attention, mood (i.e. depression) and anxiety as well as defensive and reproductive behaviors (Clark et al., 2006). Therefore, the brainstem seems to be an ideal structure to regulate muscles having unique functions strongly interrelated with emotions including speech (chewing muscles, tongue, lipthe, and facial muscles), expressing emotions nonverbally (facial muscles), fighting and aggressiveness (chewing muscle) or sexuality (lips, tongue).

The functioning of the orofacial muscles is influenced not only by the brainstem, but also by the motor cortices and other brain centers including the limbic system, thalamus, cerebellum, as well as the basal ganglia and brainstem reticular formation (Harris & Griffin, 1975). Therefore, psychoemotional and psychosocial stress factors also significantly influence muscle tone and contraction through these higher brain centers. Taking all these data together, it is no wonder that the facial and masticatory muscles are highly sensitive to psychoemotional processes (Heggendorn et al., 1979; Graber, 1995; Fuhr & Reiber, 1995), increase of their tone (muscle tension) occurs rather frequently (Heggendorn et al., 1979, Graber, 1995, Fuhr & Reiber, 1995), and their reaction (increase of tension) to stress is stronger and longer lasting compared to other muscles of the body (Heggendorn et al., 1979). It is also likely that increased activity of the facial and masticatory muscles has an extraordinary role in the attenuation (elimination due to motor activity) of psychoemotional stress (Sato et al., 2010).

Neuroanatomical aspects of the control of oral immunity should also be considered. Highest central components, which significantly influence immunity, are located in *higher cortical*, *limbic* and *neurosensory systems* receiving and integrating a great diversity of signals arising from inside and outside the body (Chrousos, 1998; Ligier & Sternberg, 2000). The influence of personality, cognitions and certain psychoemotional states on immune responses are also related to this structures. The *lateralized cortical control of immunity* (resulting in upregulation during left hemispheric and downregulation during right hemispheric activity) is likely to occur also due to certain cortical areas (Gruzelier et al., 1998; Clow et al., 2003). Other highly important central components influencing immune response significantly are located in the *hypothalamus*. Especially important are the parvonuclear neurons of the *paraventricular nuclei*, which release corticotrophin-releasing hormone (CRH) leading to the production of adrenocorticotrop hormone (ACTH) in the *anterior pituitary gland* and the consequent release of glucocorticoids in the *adrenal cortex* (referred to as *hypothalamic-pituitary adrenocortical axis*, HPA axis) (Chrousos, 1998; Ligier & Sternberg, 2000; Krahwinkel et al., 2004). Other key elements are located in the *brain stem*, including the *locus ceruleus* and other mostly noradrenergic cell groups of the pons and medulla as well as the *paragigantocellular* and *parabrachial nuclei* of the medulla (Chrousos, 1998; Ligier & Sternberg, 2000), elements which influence the immune reactions primarily due to the activation of the *sympathetic nervous system*. (Besides HPA axis, this latter system of the sympathetic autonomic response is certainly also under the control of hypothalamus (Weinberg, 1977).

Activation of the HPA axis has profound effects on the immune and inflammatory response, because liberated glucocorticoids alter leukocyte trafficking and function, decrease production of various pro-inflammatory mediators and inhibit their effect on numerous target tissues (Breivik et al., 1996; Chrousos, 1998; Szabó, 1998; Ligier & Sternberg, 2000). Glucocorticoids also suppress the expression of inducible nitric oxide synthase (iNOS) (Szabó, 1998; McCann, 2000; Fábián et al., 2009/a). Glucocorticoids also appear to cause a shift from a Th1-type $CD4^{+}$cell response (favoring cellular over humoral immune response) to a Th2-type $CD4^{+}$cell response, favoring humoral over cellular immune response (Chrousos, 1998; Ligier & Sternberg, 2000). The efferent *sympathetic nervous system* modulates the immune- and inflammatory response via regional innervations of immune organs, including bone marrow, spleen, thymus, lymph nodes, Peyer's patches, tonsils, adenoids and appendix (Breivik et al., 1996; Chrousos, 1998; Ligier & Sternberg, 2000). The sympathetic nervous system also reaches all sites of inflammation via the postganglionic sympathetic neurons (Chrousos, 1998; Ligier & Sternberg 2000). The sympathetic nervous system also reaches the salivary glands and likely influence the level of salivary immunoglobulin A (sIgA) (Gruzelier et al., 1998) and other salivary defense proteins like salivary alpha-amylase, HSP70/HSPAs, and others (Fábián et al., 2003, 2004, 2007/b, 2008/a,b, 2009/b, 2012/b). The sympathetic *activation of adrenal medulla* leads to the release of catecholemines (i.e. epinephrine, norepinephrine and dopamine) into the blood which leads to release of certain immune activator/modulator cytokines into the blood and the alteration of immune cells and immune accessory cells containing receptors for cathecolamines.

In relation to the neuroanatomy of regulation of the salivary glands it should be noted that salivary fluid secretion (flow rate) and protein secretion are primarily mediated by the parasympathetic and sympathetic autonomic innervation (Ishikawa et al., 2006; Ferreira & Hoffman, 2013). Parasympathetic innervations arise from the medulla (inferior salivary nucleus, ISN) and pons (superior salivary nucleus, SSN) regions of the brainstem (Ferreira & Hoffman, 2013). Preganglionic fibers synapse either in the otic ganglion (ISN) or in the submandibular ganglion (SSN) and postganglionic fibers target salivary glands via either the auriculotemporal nerve (ISN) or via the lingual nerve (SSN) both of which are branches of the submandibular division of the trigeminal nerve (Ferreira & Hoffman, 2013). The primary sympathetic salivary centers are located in the thoracic ganglion of the upper thoracic segments of the spinal cord (Ferreira & Hoffman, 2013). Preganglionic fibers from the thoracic ganglion synapse at the superior cervical ganglion and postganglionic sympathetic fibers target the salivary glands through the external carotid artery plexus and its branches (Ferreira & Hoffman, 2013). Recently, an extraordinary role in the attenuation of psychoemotional stress due to autonomic activity (i.e. similar to that of shedding tears) was hypothesized in relation to the psychoemotional stress induced alterations of saliva secretion (Fábián & Fejérdy, 2010; Fábián et al., 2012/a; Fábián et al., in press).

There are also rather complex neuroanatomical couplings of the *various oral sensory functions* like taste, the oral thermal and tactile sense, and the oral propriocetive/sensorimotor function. The *sense of taste* is maintained by the gustatory apparatus. The peripheral parts of this apparatus include the chemoreceptors of taste buds located in the epithelium covering the tongue, the inferior surface of the soft palate, the palatoglossal arches, the posterior surface of the epiglottis and the posterior wall of the oral part of the pharynx (Williams & Warwick, 1980; Fábián & Fejérdy, 2010) as well as the peripheral processes of unipolar nerve cells in the genicular ganglion of the facial nerve (entering the tongue via chorda tympani and n. lingualis), the inferior ganglion of the glossopharyngeal nerve and the inferior ganglion of the vagus nerve (Williams & Warwick, 1980). The central parts of the gustatory apparatus include the tractus solitarius, the nucleus of the tractus solitarius and its ascendent connections including the nucleus ventralis posterior medialis of the thalamus, the antero-inferior part of the sensorimotor cortex and the insula (Williams & Warwick, 1980) as well as several other connections to numerous hypothalamic nuclei and the limbic system (Williams & Warwick, 1980). Relayed fibers also reach the frontal cortex.

In relation to taste it should be mentioned that *psychological factors can lead to significant alteration of taste sensation*. There are numerous central nervous mechanisms that can be viewed as being behind psychological alterations in taste sensation including conditioned learning processes (Chang & Scott, 1984) and modulation of glutamate-, GABA- or substance-P related orosensory (taste related) synaptic transmission of the rostral nucleus of the solitary tract (rNST) in the brainstem (Smith et al., 1998; Grabauskas & Bradley, 1998). The latter may occur by means of local changes in the brainstem, or by means of descending regulatory cortical connections of rNST from the insula (Shipley 1982; Smith et al., 1998) and the amygdala (Halsell, 1998). Recent findings also indicate that psychological stress induces release of HSP70/HSPA proteins into the extracellular space in the brain (Guzhova et al., 2001; Lancaster et al., 2004; Mokrushin & Pavlinova, 2008) which may alter central nervous mechanisms of flavor discrimination via modulation of glutamatergic synaptic transmission in the olfactory cortex (Mokrushin & Pavlinova, 2008), and consequent modulation of retronasal olfaction (involved in taste sensation coupled flavor discrimination). Since glutamatergic synaptic transmission is also strongly involved in taste pathways (Bradley & Grabauskas, 1998; Smeraski et al., 1998; Smith et al., 1998), the premised stress induced release of HSP70/HSPA in the brain is likely to modulate taste sensation also by direct means (Fábián & Fejérdy, 2010).

Thermal and tactile sensation is initiated by specific tactile and thermal receptors and their signal is transferred via the *associated afferent trigeminal nerve* fibers and processed in the trigeminal somatic afferent nuclei especially in the spinal nucleus and the principal sensory nucleus of the trigeminal nerve (Williams & Warwick, 1980). Although not all details are fully understood yet, data clearly indicate that the ascendent connections reach the thalamus, the reticular formation, several other cranial nerve nuclei, the cerebellum and various subcortical structures (Williams & Warwick, 1980). Relayed fibers also most certainly reach the somatosensory cortex as well as the frontal cortex and the limbic system. Both thermal and tactile sensations are highly important in the recognition of harmful substances or foreign bodies in the mouth. The tactile sensation of the oral mucosa, gingiva and periodontal tissues also serves as the basis of the *oral stereognosis* which is the ability to recognize and discriminate form or shape in the oral cavity (Jacobs et al., 1998).

The *oral proprioceptive/sensorimotor function* includes the mandibular and lingual position sense as well as the ability to recognize and properly manage morsels and foreign bodies (i.e. piece of bone or fishbone etc.) in the mouth. This complex function is based on the proprioceptive sense of the periodontal tissues and the fine proprioceptive sensory function of the muscle spindles as well as the consequent fine motor control of the masticatory and other orofacial muscles

(Fábián & Fejérdy, 2010). The proprioceptive impulses from the masticatory (and likely also other orofacial) muscles and the periodontal ligament travel to the *mesencephalic nucleus* of the trigeminal nerve. Although details have not been established yet, it is likely that efferent fibers originating from the mesencephalic nucleus directly influence motor function via muscle spindles of the masticatory (and maybe also other orofacial) muscles (Williams & Warwick, 1980), and ascendent connections of the nucleus reach the thalamus, the reticular formation, several other cranial nerve nuclei, the cerebellum and various subcortical structures (Williams & Warwick, 1980). It is also likely that relayed fibers reach the somatosensory cortex as well as the frontal cortex and the limbic system.

The proprioceptive sensation of the periodontal tissues serves as the basis of *occlusal perception*, which is responsible for the recognition of the consistence of a morsel between the occluding teeth while chewing. In relation to occlusal perception it should be mentioned that, *there is great variation in the occlusal sensory perceptive and discriminative abilities among patients*. This phenomenon is of considerable clinical importance because these abilities can be so highly sensitive in certain patients that it may lead to occlusal dysesthesia (Baba et al., 2005) especially if the occlusal relief was changed and the patient has to adapt to a new relief (because of tooth loss, new dentures, orthodontic treatment etc.). Erroneous integration and consequently increased perception of peripheral signals (due to the malfunction of serotonin and norepinephrine systems) were hypothesized as a possible (patho)-mechanism behind this phenomenon (Toyofuku & Kikuta, 2006). On the other hand variation of the neuroplasticity of the brain can also help to explain the great variation among individuals regarding occlusal sensory perceptive and discriminative abilities related adaptation capacity to tooth loss and/or occlusal changes (Carlsson & Johansson, 2014).

The fine propriceptive/sensorimotor function of masticatory and facial muscles is primarily regulated by the alpha and gamma motoneurons of the innervating cranial nerves (Griffin & Harris, 1975; Williams & Warwick, 1980; Fábián & Fejérdy, 2010). The *alpha motoneurons* are responsible for the maintenance of muscle tone as well as for volitional and/or reflex contraction of the muscles (Graber, 1995; Fuhr & Reiber, 1995). The *gamma motoneurons* (also referred to as *fusimotor fibers*) are responsible for the "fine tuning" of the muscle spindles which determine the muscle stretch related discharge of afferent fibers leaving the muscle spindles. Since the premised afferent fibers bring about monosynaptic facilitation of alpha motoneurons in the *mesencephalic nucleus* of the trigeminal nerve, in this way an alpha-gamma linkage control of muscle tone and muscular contraction develops (Harris & Griffin 1975); which serves as the most crucial mechanism behind sensorimotor function (Fábián & Fejérdy, 2010).

Besides these hypothesized basic mechanisms of the oral proprioceptive/sensorimotor function, there is also an *inhibitory control* of muscular contraction due to *Golgi tendon organs*. In this case afferents originating from the Golgi tendon organs bring about synaptic inhibition of the alpha motoneurons via a disynaptic (or possibly polysynaptic) nervous path (Harris & Griffin, 1975; Munro, 1975). Further, the function of both alpha and gamma motoneurons are also influenced by *afferent sensory fibers*, therefore a wide variety of peripheral stimuli including pain, touch or pressure (Hunt & Paintal, 1958; de Laat et al., 1985, van der Glas et al., 1985, 1988; Munakata & Kasai, 1992; Kossioni & Karkazis, 1995) can influence the fine proprioceptive/sensorimotor function of orofacial muscles through alteration of muscle tone and muscle contraction (Fábián & Fejérdy, 2010). The alpha and gamma motoneurons are also influenced by higher brain centers like the vestibular nuclei, brainstem reticular formation, limbic system, red nucleus, tectum and tegmentum of the midbrain, the cerebellum, the corpus striatum, the thalamus and hypothalamus and many parts of the cerebral cortex (Williams & Warwick, 1980). Thus, there is a considerable neuroanatomical basis for the phenomenon that *emotions* as well as *psychoemotional and psychosocial stress factors* can influence the oral proprioceptive/sensorimotor function significantly (Fábián & Fejérdy, 2010).

4. Management of the Psychogenic Manifestations in Dentistry

There are three major aspects of the management of psychogenic manifestations in dentistry, namely: prevention, diagnosis and treatment (Fábián & Fejérdy, 2010; Fábián et al., 2012/a). *Cornerstones of prevention* are screening of risk patients, proper treatment planning and proper communication with the patient (Fábián & Fejérdy, 2010; Fábián et al., 2012/a). *Screening of risk patients* is primarily based on the collection of a detailed patient's history as well as on careful evaluation of medical-psychosocial and orofacial status (Fábián & Fejérdy, 2010; Fábián et al. 2012/a). For *proper treatment planning* assessment of both mental (psychosocial) as well as physical (biomedical) conditions should be evaluated carefully (Bensing, 2000; Green & Laskin, 2000; Fábián & Fejérdy, 2010; Fábián et al. 2012/a). Accordingly, a patient's subjective need as well as the normatively determined need for dental treatment should also be evaluated carefully (Mazurat & Mazurat, 2003/a, b; Graham et al., 2006; Fábián & Fejérdy, 2010; Fábián et al., 2012/a); and it should always be considered that the success of a treatment strongly depends on the patients' perception of the value of such replacement (Mazurat & Mazurat, 2003/a, b). It should be also kept in mind that most patients are rather focused on social meaning and esthetics of the mouth than to physical (physiological) function of the teeth when defining subjective need for dental treatment (Graham et al., 2006; Fábián & Fejérdy, 2010; Fábián et al. 2012/a). In fact, there is a discrepancy between the normative need and the perceived need in many cases. Therefore, treatments without a subjective need in the patients may lead to overtreatment and discomfort (Mazurat & Mazurat, 2003/a, b; Fábián & Fejérdy, 2010; Fábián et al. 2012/a). It may also occur that the patient's wishes related to the dental treatment may not harmonize with the reality and the possibilities of a dental treatment. It is a matter of considerable significance that the clinician carefully weighs the option of nontreatment in such cases (Stein, 1983; Fábián et al., 2007/a; Fábián & Fejérdy, 2010; Fábián et al. 2012/a). The financial means and compliance of the patient as well as the amount of stress and possible complications of the planned treatment should also be taken into consideration during planning (Fábián & Fejérdy, 2010; Fábián et al. 2012/a). Further, planning of a time-schedule ensuring enough time to carry out a high quality, precise, "lege artis" dental treatment should also be considered as one of the most important points to prevent triggering psychogenic symptoms (Fábián & Fejérdy, 2010; Fábián et al. 2012/a). *Communication with the patient* is also a key factor of the prevention certainly. Further major aspects of the proper and efficient patient-dentist communication are good interpersonal relationship and mutual trust (Fábián & Fejérdy, 2010; Fábián et al. 2012/a), although basic techniques of communication such as verbal following (Deneen et al., 1973), verbal reflection (Deneen et al., 1973) as well as greeting the patient and using the patient's name should also not be forgotten (Fábián & Fejérdy, 2010; Fábián et al. 2012/a). A good interpersonal relationship and mutual trust can be created with friendliness, genuineness, congruence, readiness to help, empathy, respect, warmth, as well as eliciting feelings, paraphrasing and reflecting. Silence as well as humor may also be very useful in certain cases (Fábián & Fejérdy, 2010; Fábián et al. 2012/a).

The most important diagnostic tools for the diagnosis of psychogenic manifestations in dentistry are collecting detailed patient's history and careful evaluation of all relevant psychosocial, medical and dental anamnestic data including their understanding in the context of a biopsychosocial model of orofacial disorders (Ross et al., 1953; Engel, 1977; Green & Laskin, 2000; Dworkin & Sherman, 2006; Fábián & Fejérdy, 2010; Fábián et al. 2012/a). Careful clinical examination of the oral and orofacial region and general health status as well as X-ray, MRI and other specific examinations are certainly also cornerstones of a proper diagnostic process (Fábián & Fejérdy, 2010; Fábián et al. 2012/a). Since psychogenic symptoms may mimic a great variety of somatic symptoms, a clear-cut diagnosis and proper differential diagnosis of PDI could be rather difficult; therefore, it should be emphasized that the diagnosis of PDI is a presumptive one in many cases (Fábián & Fejérdy, 2010; Fábián et al., 2012/a). The diagnosis may change later in the course of the disease as the clinical findings change and/or stabilize; therefore, continuous monitoring and evaluation of the patient over time are also essential (Fábián & Fejérdy, 2010; Fábián et al. 2012/a). It should be also emphasized that the diagnosis of psychogenic symptoms is a diagnosis of exclusion in many cases (Fábián et al., 2007/a; Fábián & Fejérdy, 2010; Fábián et al. 2012/a); therefore, a detailed differential diagnosis considering possible disorders of the teeth, or oral- and maxillofacial tissues should also be carried out (Fábián & Fejérdy, 2010; Fábián et al. 2012/a) and any other possible somatic causes behind the symptoms should also be excluded (Fábián & Fejérdy, 2010; Fábián et al. 2012/a). Further, referral to other professionals such as maxillofacial surgeon, neurologist, psychiatrist, clinical psychologist, neuropsychologist, otorhinolaringologist, ophthalmologist, internist, rheumatologist, etc., may also be needed, and especially recommended in the case of (pseudo)neurological symptoms (Sarlani et al., 2005/a.b; Fábián & Fejérdy, 2010; Fábián et al. 2012/a).

In relation to treatment possibilities it should be considered that the majority of dental patients with psychogenic symptoms refuse to accept a psychological background of their symptoms (Ross et al., 1953; Schwichtenberg & Doering 2008; Fábián & Fejérdy, 2010; Fábián et al. 2012/a), and instead of psychiatrists or psychotherapists, they first visit a dentist and insist on the somatic origin of their symptoms (Ross et al., 1953; Fábián & Fejérdy, 2010; Fábián et al., 2012/a). Therefore, a simple referral to a psychiatrist and/or psychotherapist would not solve the problem in most cases. Consequently, an initial psychosomatic dental therapy is needed prior to definitive therapy, which is the scope of the dental profession's duty (Moulton et al., 1957; Pomp 1974; Fábián & Fejérdy, 2010; Fábián et al. 2012/a). The most important goals of an initial dental psychosomatic therapy are avoidance of further useless invasive dental treatment (Brodine & Hartshorn, 2004; Reewes 2nd & Merrill, 2007; Baad-Hansen, 2008; Fábián & Fejérdy, 2010; Fábián et al. 2012/a) as well as obtaining a decrease in symptoms and the motivation of patients to participate in a definitive psychosomatic therapy which is the highest level of care for patients with psychogenic oral/orofacial manifestations (Fábián & Fejérdy, 2010; Fábián et al., 2012/a). The gradual escalation of psychogenic aspects of therapy and the avoidance of the irreversible forms of treatment are "cornerstones" of the initial dental psychosomatic therapy (Laskin & Block, 1986; Fábián & Fejérdy, 2010; Fábián et al. 2012/a). The initial dental psychosomatic therapy utilizes several placebo and/or palliative methods (i.e. physiotherapies, medication, medicinal herb therapy, diet therapy, complementary and alternative medicine etc.) combined with certain psychotherapeutic approaches and administration of any mind-body therapies which are the "basic therapeutics" for psychosomatic disorders (Iversen, 1989; Binder & Binder, 1989; Krause, 1983, 1994, 2000; Fábián et al., 2006, 2009/c, 2012/a; Fábián &

Fejérdy, 2010; Fábián, 2012). If the initial dental psychosomatic therapy is not efficient enough a definitive psychosomatic therapy should be offered for the patients (Fábián & Fejérdy, 2010; Fábián et al. 2012/a). The definitive psychosomatic therapy is the highest level care for patients with oral/orofacial psychogenic symptoms that utilizes any available dental, medical and psychotherapeutical treatment possibilities in an evidence based manner (Fábián & Fejérdy, 2010; Fábián et al., 2012/a). In contrast to the initial dental psychosomatic therapy the definitive psychosomatic therapy is clearly *not* within the scope of *every* dentist's duties (Fábián & Fejérdy, 2010; Fábián et al. 2012/a). The definitive psychosomatic therapy should be carried out by *specialized dental professionals* (Dahlström et al., 1997; Hertrich & Joraschky, 1996; Dworkin et al., 2002; Fábián & Fejérdy, 2010; Fábián et al. 2012/a) as members of a specialized *psychosomatic team* including *experienced* dentists and other medical and psychological/psychotherapeutical professionals (Fábián & Fejérdy, 2010; Fábián et al. 2012/a). Although clinical experiences clearly indicate that there is also a major role for specialized dental professionals in the definitive psychosomatic therapy in most cases, close collaboration with medical professionals (especially with psychiatrists and neurologists) and with psychologists/psychotherapists is clearly needed (Dahlström et al. 1997; Hertrich & Joraschky, 1996; Von Korff et al., 2005; Turner et al., 2006; Schwichtenberg & Doering, 2008; Fábián & Fejérdy, 2010; Fábián et al., 2012/a).

5. Specific Considerations about the Management of Dental Fear

Dental fear is also considered a psychogenic manifestation appearing in relation to dental treatments. The basic principles of prevention, diagnosis and treatment of dental fear are the same as in the other psychogenic manifestations introduced above. However, the phenomenon of dental fear is different in many aspects from other oral/orofacial psychogenic manifestations which dentists should deal with. Therefore certain specific considerations relating to dental fear should be discussed in relation with the management of dental fear as follows.

Prevention of (or at least a reduction in) of dental fear should be integrated into dental treatment for all patients regularly (Kreyer, 1989; Hermes et al., 2006; Fábián & Fejérdy, 2010; Fábián et al. 2012/a), especially because traumatizing dental events (such as fearful and/or painful dental treatment) may trigger other psychogenic oral/orofacial symptoms (Müller-Fahlbusch & Sone, 1982; Fábián & Fejérdy, 2010; Fábián et al. 2012/a). The most common reasons for dental fear are bad (painful or fearful) dental experiences (Moore & Birn, 1990), lack of control over the social situation in the dental chair (Moore & Birn, 1990), lack of control over personal emotional reactions (Moore & Birn, 1990), feeling of powerlessness during treatment (Moore & Birn, 1990) and social learning processes with a negative image of dentists (Moore & Birn, 1990).

The most important method for both prevention and treatment of dental fear is *communication* (Fábián & Fejérdy, 2010; Fábián et al. 2012/a). Great care should be taken (1) to avoid fear by producing terms or phrases which describe dental treatment or dental instruments (Fábián & Fejérdy, 2010; Fábián et al. 2012/a) as well as (2) to make only those promises that can be fulfilled (Botto, 2006; Fábián & Fejérdy, 2010; Fábián et al., 2012/a). It is also important to give the patient the perception of being in control (Botto, 2006; Fábián & Fejérdy, 2010; Fábián et al. 2012/a). For such purposes, the "*tell-show-do*" technique (Addelston, 1959) may be used, which includes describing in simple terms what is about to occur ("*tell*"); than allowing the patient to see, feel, explore and manipulate the tools or instruments ("*show*"); and then starting the procedure ("*do*") (Addelston, 1959; Allen, 2006).

Methods for *distraction* to refocus the patient's attention away from the potentially painful/fearful stimulus or procedure may also be used advantageously (Allen, 2006; Botto, 2006; Fábián & Fejérdy, 2010; Fábián et al., 2012/a). Offering brief breaks during treatment is the simplest method for such purposes (Allen, 2006). Other simple forms of distraction include rubbing the patients' cheek or asking them to hold their legs up in the air during a critical procedure (i.e. administrating local anesthesia, or making a dental impression) (Botto, 2006). Music expressing positive emotions (Suda et al., 2008) may also be used for distraction during treatment (Vinard & Ravier-Rosenblaum, 1989; Botto, 2006). Audiovisual methods like video games (Allen, 2006), two-dimensional DVD-glasses and three-dimensional virtual reality technology (Askay et al., 2009) may also be used advantageously. Mind-body therapies including hypnosis, self-hypnosis, photoacoustic stimulation, relaxation and several biofeedback methods are also suitable for distraction during the dental treatment (Fábián et al., 2009/c, 2012/a; Fábián & Fejérdy, 2010; Fábián 2012).

In some cases certain *pharmacological methods* including premedication with anxiolytics relative analgesia (inhalation of nitrous oxide-oxygen mixture), conscious sedation (intravenously administered benzodiazepines) and occasionally general anaesthesia as well as several *psychotherapeutic approaches* may also be used to manage dental fear (Fábián & Fejérdy, 2010; Fábián et al. 2012/a)

6. Summary

Although dentistry is a profession dedicated to treating somatic disorders of the oral/orofacial region primarily, there is also a collection of various psychological and pathopsychological conditions dentists should deal with (Fábián et al., 2007/b; Fábián et al., 2012/a; Fábián et al., in press), especially because the orofacial region is affected by psychogenic manifestations much more frequently when compared to most other parts of the body (Fábián et al., 2007/a, Fábián et al., 2012/a; Fábián et al., in press). This is very likely because of the rich psychological couplings of the mouth, teeth and other oral structures (Fábián et al., 2007/a; Fábián et al., in press) and because of the rather unique and intimate neuroanatomical couplings of the oral region with the brain through an innervation originating from the brainstem and because of an exceptionally rich representation of the oral region in various brain structures.

Because of the above considerations it is no wonder that a patient can be dissatisfied with his or her dental treatment even though the treatment at issue was carried out conscientiously and properly from a somatic point of view (Mazurat & Mazurat, 2003/a,b; Fábián & Fejérdy, 2010; Fábián et al. 2012/a, Fábián & Hidalgo Wulff, 2014); thus normative evaluation by the dentist and subjective evaluation by the patient related to the dental treatment may be rather divergent (Lechner & Roessler, 2001; Fábián & Fejérdy, 2010; Fábián et al. 2012/a; Fábián & Hidalgo Wulff, 2014). When symptoms appear, both the potential somatic and psychogenic pathways of pathomechanism should be considered carefully. If psychogenic symptoms appear, factors not related to the somatic pathways become more important (Fábián & Fejérdy, 2010; Fábián et al., 2012/a; Fábián & Hidalgo Wulff, 2014), notwithstanding the possibility that there may also be certain somatic component of a psychogenic symptom. On the other hand there are complex neuropsychological processes behind any psychogenic symptoms, thus psychogenic processes are coupled with various somatic processes at the level of neuropsychological regulation. Because of the intimate contact of the orofacial region and the brain psychological and also somatic aspects of the dental treatments may influence certain neuropsychological processes. Thus, both psychogenic and somatic aspects of the dental treatment may release psychological manifestations via either psychological or neuropsychological pathways.

All the above considerations clearly indicate that there is a rather important connection between neuropsychology and dentistry, even if this connection is recognized more in theoretical rather than clinical aspects today. However, considering the rather intensive development of both dental and neuropsychological sciences it is well possible that this connection may reach significant impact on the clinical dental practice in the next future.

12 Neuropsychology of Asymmetrical Visual Aesthetic Preferences across European and Asian Cultures

Mohammadsaeid Marandi

Key Words: Aesthetic processing, cross-cultural variations, fMRI, beauty recognition, Western-Eastern, theory of mind, hemisphere specialization, symmetry-asymmetry

Abstract

This chapter aims to review both theoretically and experimentally the issue of visual asymmetric aesthetic preferences due to the directionality of scanning scripts across cultures. In this relation, results of three studies examining different cultures and subcultures in Europe and Iran on the phenomenon respectively revealed differential intracultural as well as cross-cultural aesthetic processing. However, surprisingly it was shown that intracultural differences were linked to biological factors such as behavioral laterality and age, whereas cross-cultural variations were more related to visuo-spatial features. Interpretations of the results are also discussed subsequently.

1. Introduction

Aesthetic processing in human beings has been considered to involve assessment of entities related to beauty, harmony, 'well-formedness' and the like which is sensationally dependent (Jacobsen, 2010). However, evidence reveals that aesthetic processing involves evaluating and producing *concepts* such as beauty, ugliness and harmony affected by determinants such as 'stimulus symmetry', 'complexity' familiarity and social status appeal (Jacobsen, 2010). Such processing can be viewed from various standpoints such as biology, evolution, cultural and subcultural ones etc. (Jacobsen 2006, 2013). In addition to the necessary and most efficient multidisciplinary awareness and method to this process, a requirement should be considered to link the mentioned methods to the brain underpinnings which govern all aspects of aesthetic appreciation (Jacobsen, 2010).

Numerous neural networks characterized by dynamic configuration are considered to govern the multidimensional aesthetic appreciation processing (Jacobsen, 2010). fMRI studies have demonstrated that brain distributed networks underlie visual aesthetic related tasks (Chatterjee et al., 2009; Cupchik et al., 2009; Fairhall & Ishai, 2007; Vartanian et al., 2013) including the motor cortical area as revealed in fMRI and MEG results respectively (Kawabata & Zeki, 2004; Cela-Conde et al., 2009). Studying neural activation patterns in response to aesthetic tasks using fMRI techniques research has demonstrated that the network not only possesses reward specific assessment capabilities variant in valence of emotions (Vartanian & Goel, 2004), but also shares aspects of social and moral evaluation; there are cultural differences and individual variations inside any culture in beauty recognition (Jacobsen, 2006, 2010).

A wide range of cognitive processing of the functions of the brain, as vast as vision and social cognition, has recently been shown to be affected by values, practices and beliefs of culture according to cultural neuroscience results. Awareness of the interaction between mind/brain and processes of reciprocal evolution of culture/gene is the requisite of research on the mind architecture of human beings (Chiao & Immordino-Yang, 2013).

Generally the dichotomous Western-Eastern styles of thinking and cognitive abilities, which in our study lead to convergence of brain laterality and aesthetic appreciation, have been debated for long. Typically the logical, analytical functions of the left hemisphere have been associated with the rational and technological thinking of the West (Ornstein, 1977; see Dr. Claus H. Bick's remarks reported in Harrington & Oepen, 1989), whereas the functions of the right hemisphere have been linked to the intuition and mysticism of the East (Ornstein, 1977). In this respect, criticisms have been made about the overemphasis of left brain functions in Western education and communities (Ornstein, 1977; see again Dr. Claus H. Bick's remarks reported in Harrington & Oepen, 1989).

Cross-cultural studies emphasize analytic/holistic perceptual contrast between Western and East Asian cultures in which western people reveal object relevant tendencies as well as properties and contexts considered independent, whereas East Asians demonstrated 'contextual relationship' and contexts considered interdependent respectively (Goh & Park, 2009; Ketay et al., 2009). Likewise, the N400 technique showed that Asian-Americans, connected to self-construal interdependency, proved to be *sensitive* to semantic incongruity as compared with European Americans who did not demonstrate such tendency (Goto et al., 2013). In general, the West reveals inclination toward objects, categorical relationship or self-relevance while the East Asia emphasizes details of contexts, 'similarities' and group-relevance (Gutchess & Indeck, 2009). Accordingly, there is substantial evidence which shows that culture affects neural circuitry as relevant in 'social perception', visual perception, 'long-term memory', attention, 'theory of mind' and 'context memory' respectively (Freeman et al., 2009; Goh & Park, 2009; Gutchess & Indeck, 2009; Ketay et al., 2009; Kobayashi Frank & Temple, 2009; Yang et al., 2013).

Although symmetry is a crucial concept in scientific fields, substantial evidence has revealed existence of asymmetry in the physical and biological world as well as in art development and exploitation (McManus, 2005). In this relation, research showed that asymmetrical style of presenting an entity in terms of directionality of main elements of artistic works and positioning a target people's interactions in advertisement affects their expressiveness and perception respectively (Bennett et al., 2010; Puccinelli et al., 2006).

In this relation, cross-cultural differences in asymmetrical aesthetic appreciation in terms of the order of drawing items or preferences of directionality of objects have been attributed to the subjects' reading and writing system of scanning across Indian nations as well as Arabic and American subjects respectively (Vaid & Singh, 1987, Heath et al., 2005). However, with similar aesthetic tasks across English speaking subjects who read and write left to right and Arabic speaking ones who read and write in the opposite direction, no significant differences were reported in terms of cultural effect on asymmetrical aesthetic positioning and preferences (Altmann et al., 2006, Treiman & Allaith, 2013).

In addition, biological factors relevant to the brain functional specialization indexed by age, sex, and handedness have been evident in lateral aesthetic preferences. In this respect, for instance, left handed male children's chronological switch from left-to-right preferences to the opposite direction preferred by adults accounts for the interference of age in this relation (De Agostini et al., 2010).

Also, localization of gender-specific handedness and perception of emotional valence of faces in the right-handed males' right hemisphere, recall of more information in the left hand side by males, and technical demonstration of the right hemisphere specialization for aesthetic preferences in males as compared to females respectively show the interaction of gender as a variable in this regard (Bourne, 2008; Puccinelli et al., 2006; Cela-Conde, 2009).

Concerning sensorimotor laterality, results showed more males within left-handed and left-legged subjects than females, whereas in perceptive measures this was reversed and there existed more left-eyed females than males (Chernigovskaya et al., 2005). In another study, using a dichotic task, it was found that significantly earedness corresponded to footedness as compared with handedness (Elias et al., 1998).

Notwithstanding efforts to define and enumerate asymmetric functions of the hemispheres of the brain, the core dichotomous asymmetries of the brain functions have been considered to be related to the language/visuo-spatial aspect. Concerning the visual specialization of both hemispheres for lower/higher-frequency spatial relations of visual outputs, the right hemisphere has been considered to be susceptible to higher-frequency discriminations more. Therefore, it has been suggested that narrower sub-process dependent phases of the viso-spatial ability should be considered rather than a broad one in this process (Hugdahl, 2000).

To this end, seeking aesthetic preference etiology, it has been concluded that despite clear cultural indefinite variations in such domains as music composition, dancing, and painting styles, studies are more and more disclosing outstanding neuropsychological results which are considered to be the underlying impetus for certain aesthetic preferences universally. Regarding the preferred aesthetic aspects, shape and spatial orientation are among the ones which are claimed to be neuropsychologically and physiologically relevant. Traditionally, these preferred aesthetic features were viewed as perfect cultural variations, whereas nowadays they are considered to pertain to physiological and neuropsychological realms such as hemisphere specialization, handedness and sex (Strachan, 2000). Other evaluation approaches of aesthetic judgment and response have also suggested cognitive neuroscience and scientific psychology as the basic method of investigation respectively (Jacobsen, 2010, 2013; Palmer et al., 2013).

The rest of this chapter aims to report and review the results of a series of experiments, in preparation, which pertain to differences in lateral aesthetic preferences across European and Iranian cultures as well as within Iranian subcultures as one of the intended reasons of experimentation. Since there is still an unclear relationship between lateral aesthetic preferences, hemisphere specialization and the effect of language scanning directionality, if any, three experiments were designed to disentangle cultural and linguistic effects through examining aesthetic preference directionality among subcultures in which native speakers read and write in distinct languages with the same scanning directionality in addition to the cultures with opposite scanning methods.

2. Methods

2.1. Subjects

Adult Iranians: A sample of 173 adult Iranians between 18 and 60 years of age was selected (M: 23.66; SD: 8.46), balanced for cultural differences, to participate in our study in the cities of Isfahan, Tehran, and the province of

Khouzestan (60 females). They were from different regions, cities and ethnicities in Iran with distinct mother languages which are normally read from right to left (87 Farses, 86 subcultures).

The major language in Iran is Farsi which is spoken among Fars ethnicity members who comprise the majority of the population. However, other languages are spoken in Iran most of which are represented by their native speakers in this study including Turkish, Kurdish, Lori, Gilaki and Arabic as the major ones and other subgroups such as Laki, Khalaji. Since in this study we had unequal numbers of speakers of each we classified them into three major groups according to the numbers of their representatives: Farsi, Turkish, others.

Adolescent Iranians: 115 Iranian adolescents aged 15-17 (M: 16.53; SD: 0.57) of different Iranian ethnicities (70 Farses, 43 subcultures) were selected to form our sample in this study (52 females). Their mother languages included the major ones: Farsi, Turkish, Kurdish, Lori, Gilaki, and Arabic.

European/Iranians: A sample of 120 Europeans and Iranians between 18 and 66 years old (M: 29.57; SD: 13.36), balanced for nationality (60 Europeans, 60 Iranians) and gender (44 females &16 males for each nationality group) was selected to participate in our study. European subjects consisted of 50 Germans and the rest were from eight other European countries all of whom read and write from left to right. In order to control for the direction of the script as a variable only Iranians whose mother tongue was Farsi were chosen for this study.

2.2. Procedure

In all our studies, having filled out a general information questionnaire (GIQ), the subjects took two tests: the Sensorimotor Laterality Inventory (SLI) (Coren et al., 1979) and the Visual Aesthetic Lateral Preference Inventory (VALPI) in the form of self-reports.

2.3. Materials

The GIQ included questions about subjects' age, gender, field of study, interests in arts and paintings etc. followed by checkboxes or completion formats.

The SLI is a reliable test which includes 13 behavioral self-assessment questions about the Ss' preferences which correspond to four different motor and perceptual modalities in performing routine and daily tasks: hand, foot, eye, and ear. Since from these laterality measures handedness played a crucial role, we replaced item 4 (dealing cards) which was not familiar to all of the subjects, with a question about the Ss' preferred hand for writing.

The VALPI was made in the form of a photo album and an answer sheet. The A4-size images of twenty asymmetrical realistic paintings together with their mirror reversed copies were set in a photo album. In order to avoid any artifacts due to side effects of positioning of the images, both vertical and horizontal paintings were chosen in this experiment. Therefore each image and its flipped version were arranged either side by side or in a vertical order so that the viewers could compare the picture pairs easily. The first six images were vertical and the rest were horizontal, and within each of these painting styles both the sequence of paintings and positioning of mirror images were randomized. For adult and adolescent Iranian studies, the images were arranged randomly in two different styles in the albums; one started from the right side of the album and the other started from the left side. Then, two photo albums of the same type with the same arrangement of pictures were provided for each style. The pictures were generally of four different themes: animals, landscapes, portraits and scenes. The answer sheet consisted of twenty numbered items of two small vertical boxes. The Ss were asked to circle the letters "a" or "b" in the boxes which they would think might correspond to the preferred picture.

2.4. Scoring

Concerning the SLI, in order to give the same weight to different modalities, we computed the laterality indices for each preference separately, and so the mean of the averages of the four modalities formed our laterality value. There were three questions for each modality except handedness which had four. For each question, +100 and -100 were allocated to the options “right” and “left” respectively and 0 to ‘both”, then the average for each preference was calculated by subtracting the value of the left choices from the right. The values ranged from -100 to +100.

The index for visual aesthetic lateral preference inventory (VALPI) was the difference between the number of the right choices and the left ones in percentages (Right - Left/ Right + Left X 100). The minimum value was -100 and the maximum +100.

Concerning the classification purposes, for both the directionality and laterality measures, for the VALPI, the scores between -40 and +40 were considered “mixed”, equal to or below -40 were categorized as “left”, and equal to or above +40 were classified “right”. However, due to unequal numbers of sensorimotor laterality across levels, for the SLI, scores between -100 and 40 were classified as ‘left and mixed’ and scores equal to and above 40 were considered as ‘right’.

3. Results

In order to determine the factors involved in variations of lateral aesthetic preferences (AP) as well as sensorimotor laterality (SL) across cultures, as mentioned in this chapter, the results of the three studies will be reviewed under five subsections:

a. Distributions of AP & SL levels
b. The effect of culture on AP & SL
c. The interaction of biological factors with culture on AP & SL
d. The interaction of environmental and psychological factors with culture on AP & SL
e. The effect of visuo-spatial factors on AP.

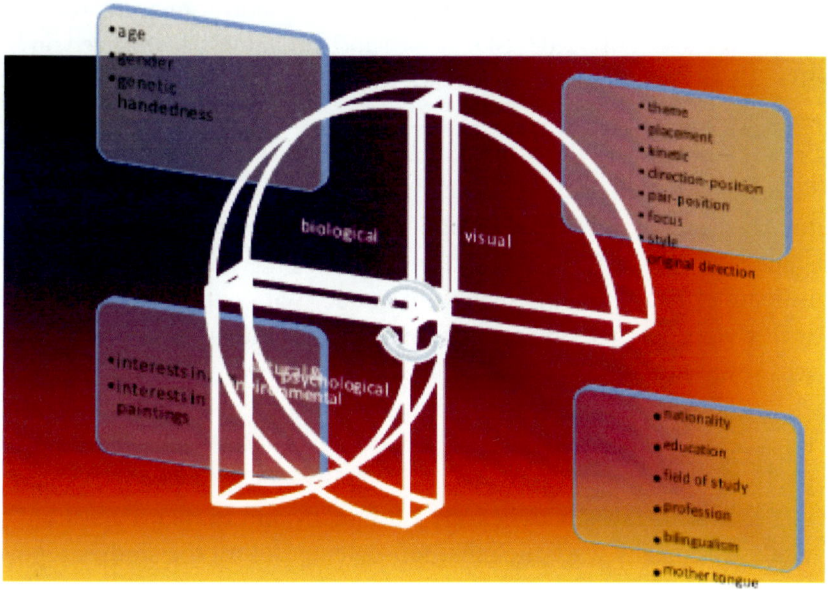

Figure 1. *Interaction schemata of biological, visual, psychological, cultural and environmental factors.*

3.1. Distributions of AP and SL levels

In the adult-Iranian study, as for AP, 12.7% were left oriented, 67.6% mixed and 19.7 right, but the effect of cultural distribution was not significant. However, the effect of culture was significant on SL distribution, *p< .o5*: of the adult Iranian subcultures18.6% were left and mixed and 81.4% were right, whereas of the adult Iranian Farses, 34.5% were left and mixed and 65.5% right. Similar significant results, regarding the effect of the cultural factor in handedness emerged in this study, *p< .05*. In neither measure was there any significant cultural effect regarding the adolescent-Iranian study. However, considering the results of the European/Iranian study, there was only a significant effect of the cross-cultural factor in the distribution of the AP levels, $p < .001$. According to the results, of the Europeans, 26.7% were left, 60% mixed and 13.3 right oriented, while of the Iranians, 6.7% were left, 53.3% mixed and 40%right oriented.

3.2. The Effect of Culture on AP & SL

As for the relationship between AP and SL, results showed a considerable correlation coefficient which is very close to significance in the adult Iranian subcultural group only, $p < .052$: in this respect, adult Iranian Ss were much less lateralized on AP (M: -2.03, SD: 32.48) and much more lateralized on SL (M: 57.89, SD: 32.88) as compared to the adult Iranian Farses respectively (M: 10.37, SD: 42.80; M: 44.63, SD: 50.68).

Therefore, the adult Iranians Farses and subcultures revealed the most significant differences on aesthetic and laterality measures respectively, $p < .05$, $p < .05$. Similar significant results were found on handedness and eyedness in the same study respectively, $p < .01$, $p < .05$. In the same study, also, there was a significant effect on the interaction of gender with culture on earedness, $p < .01$: females were less lateralized than males in the subcultural group, while this trend was reversed in the Fars group.

There was no such effect in the adolescent-Iranain study between subcultures and Farses on AP (M: 2.24, SD: 29.52; M: 10.23, SD: 33.42) and SL (M: 61.13 SD: 34.45; M: 56.57, SD: 45.13) respectively. But the greatest difference, in this section, was between the Europeans and Iranian Farses on AP, $p < .001$: while Europeans were the most left-oriented of all the studies reported here (M: -8.83, SD: 40.75), Iranian Farses were the most right-oriented (M: 23.87, SD: 35.47).

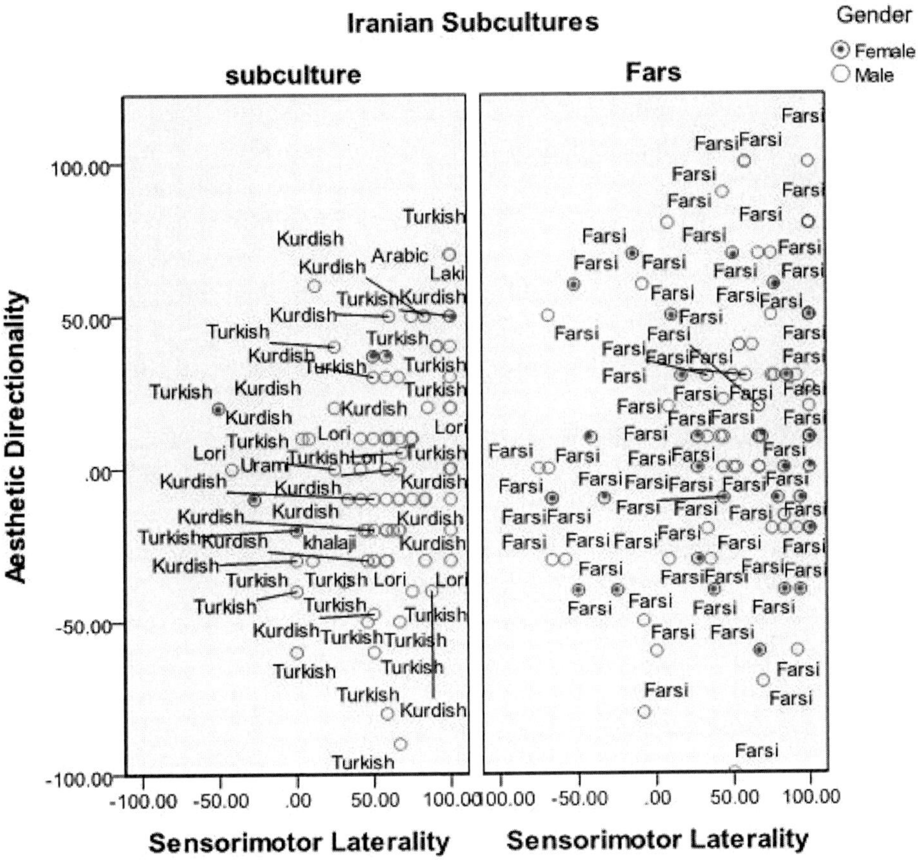

Figure 2. *Interaction between sensorimotor laterality and aesthetic preferences across adult Iranian subcultures.*

3.3. The Interaction of Biological Factors with Culture on AP & SL

As far as the interaction of the biological factors are concerned, there was only a significant positive correlation between age and AP in adult Fars Iranians as compared with subcultures, which means the older the Ss, the more right-oriented, $p < .01$.

3.4. The Interaction of Environmental and Psychological Factors with Culture on AP & SL

As for the environmental and psychological factors, education revealed significant interaction with culture in the adult-Iranian group on AP, $p < .05$: While subcultures with pre-university education scored positively (M; 0.49, SD: 27.90), the Ss in the same group with university education scored negatively (M: -2.70, SD: 33.74) on the same measure. This trend was reversed in Farses respectively (M: 0.01, SD: 39.27; M: 24.92, SD: 43.94). Also, adult-Iranian Ss showed a significant interaction between their interests in paintings and culture on the same measure, $p < .05$: Ss with no interests in paintings received positive scores in subcultures (M: 7.71, SD: 33.09), whereas Ss with their interests in paintings had negative scores in the same group (M: -5.81, SD: 37.70). Under the same conditions, Farses displayed the opposite trend respectively (M: -0.62 SD: 40.47 ; M: 17.36 SD: 43.68).

There was no effect for environmental and psychological interaction with culture in the adolescent-Iranian group. However, interestingly there was a significant interaction between profession and culture in the European-Iranian study on perceptual laterality, $p < .05$: European students were less lateralized (M: 35.98, SD: 50.05) than European non-students (M: 54.76, SD: 59.71), but the trend was reversed for Farses respectively (M:57.99, SD: 39.99; M: 33.92 SD: 44.32).

3.5. The Effect of Visuo-Spatial Factors on AP

Results revealed a significant interaction between culture and two visuo-spatial features in the European-Iranian study: kinetic element, $p < .001$ and theme, $p < .001$. Both Europeans and Iranians in this study were less lateralized on pictures with dynamic elements as compared with the static pictures respectively (M: 0.0006, SD: 22.15, M: 12.96, SD:27.45; M: -21.79, SD: 20.31, M: 34.48, SD: 24.09). Regarding the theme of the pictures, there were two points of the convergence for Europeans and Iranians on animals and scenes with parallel directions, and two points of divergence on portraits and landscapes with opposite directions for each cultural group.

Last but not least, the only interaction between picture set and culture belonged to the adolescent-Iranian study which was very close to significant level, $p = .055$: adolescent subcultures scored in opposite direction on the two picture sets (left-to-right, M: -6.36, SD: 25.39; right-to-left, M: 10.45, SD: 31.38). On the contrary, adolescent Farses scored in the same direction on the same feature (left-to-right, M: 13.47, SD: 34.12; right-to-left, M: 6.38, SD: 32.69).

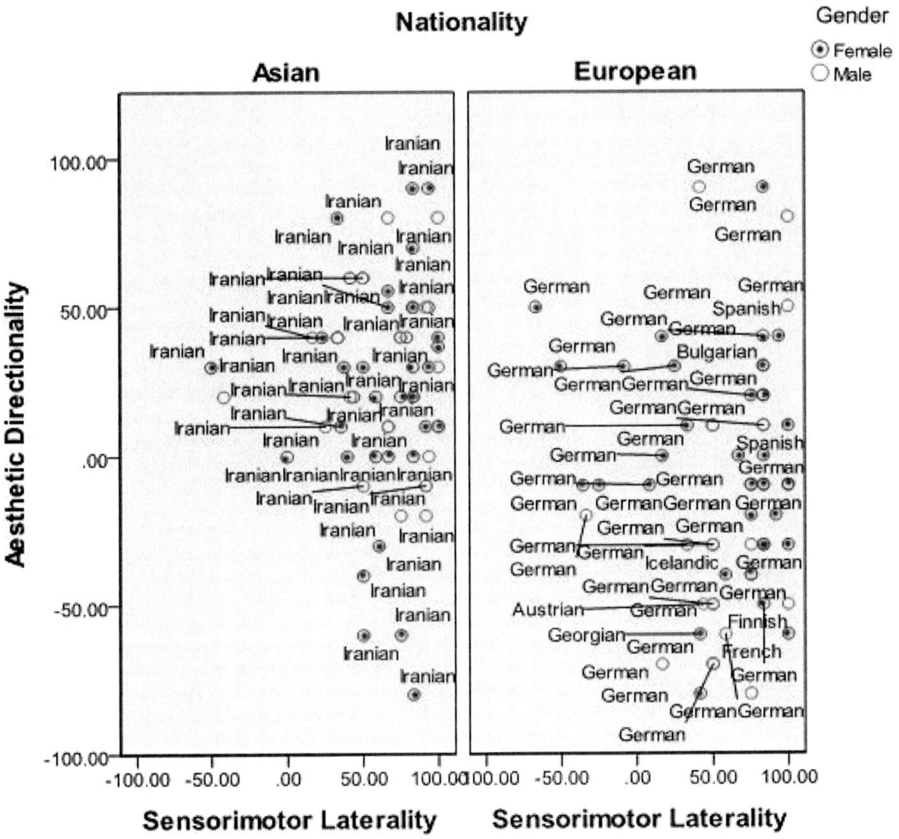

Figure 3. *Interaction between sensorimotor laterality and aesthetic prefences across European/Iranian cultures.*

4. Discussion

Examining both theoretical and experimental evidence on the hypothesis that differential visual asymmetric aesthetic preferences might pertain to the direction of the script, statistical analyses showed that the differences emerged not only across distinct cultures but also within territorially unified subcultures. Controlling for biological, environmental, psychological and visuo-spatial factors, however, it was revealed that intracultural variations on this issue were related to biological traits. On the contrary, results yielded significant differences in visuo-spatial features across cultures as related to aesthetic preferences.

As for the biological relationships between culture and aesthetic judgments within subcultures regardless of the directionality of the scanning process, inferences may follow in favor of the concept of bilateral compensatory processing of the brain hemispheres rather unilateral right hemisphere bias for visuo-spatial features.

Also, examining the second hypothesis (accounting for the right side bias which has been considered to conform to the Western style of scanning scripts) is further replaced, according to the results, by the directionality rather than mere placement of the main elements in a picture in European subjects.

13 What does Neuroscience Tell Us about How to Help Children with Mathematical Difficulties?

Ann Dowker

Key Words: Mathematical development, Dyscalculia, Educational interventions, Brain imaging, Brain development, Individual differences, Brain stimulation

Developmental arithmetical difficulties are an extremely common problem with a serious negative impact on both the individual and society. The prevalence of developmental dyscalculia has been estimated as approximately 6% (Butterworth, Varma & Laurillard, 2011), though there are many debates about the exact definition and nature of such a condition (Kaufmann, Mazzocco, Dowker et al., 2013). Certainly, a much higher proportion of people have severe numeracy difficulties that persist into adulthood. Parsons and Bynner (2005) reported that about 22% of a large adult British sample had numeracy difficulties severe enough to cause them serious practical and economic problems, as compared with about 5% who had comparably severe literacy difficulties. Therefore, interventions to treat, ameliorate or if possible prevent such numeracy difficulties are extremely important, and anything that helps to inform such interventions is of vital importance.

This chapter will describe ways in which neuroscience has informed the study of children's mathematical difficulties and the development of interventions to help them. I will concentrate on the main ways in which so far it has informed such interventions: by increasing our understanding of numerical cognition and of discrepancies and dissociations between different components of it. This chapter will also refer briefly to a few studies that look at more direct ways of applying neuroscience to intervention, for example by using brain stimulation; but these are still in a very early stage of development.

1. Methods of Studying the Neural Basis of Mathematical Abilities.

The oldest method of study involves studies of impairments (or sometimes selective preservation) of mathematical abilities in patients with brain damage. More recently there has been increasing use of functional and structural brain imaging studies of mathematics in typical and atypical individuals. Very recently, there have also been interference studies: both 'negative' interference, whereby techniques such as transcranial magnetic stimulation have been used to simulate brain lesions, and 'positive' interference, where brain stimulation has been used to enhance mathematical learning.

2. The Study of Acquired Mathematical Disabilities, and Selective Preservation of Mathematical Abilities, in Patients with Brain Damage.

Henschen (1920) was the first to study mathematical disability on its own rather than as a symptom of aphasia. He defined 'acalculia' as a primary impairment of arithmetical calculation, caused by focal brain injury. He considered this to be independent of other disorders such as language disorders.

More recently, several case studies have been carried out of patients with global and relatively pure mathematical disabilities resulting from brain damage, usually involving parietal areas. For example, "Signora Gaddi" was described by Cipolotti, Butterworth and Denes (1991). Following a stroke affecting the left parietal cortex, she had severe difficulties with all aspects of number. She could deal with numbers only up to fou, and only if she was permitted to count them. This was despite the fact that she had no lasting problems with language, spatial ability, memory, reasoning, or any other non-mathematical abilities which could explain such a deficit.

By contrast, some patients with widespread brain damage affecting many other cognitive functions have shown unimpaired arithmetical ability. It is notable that arithmetical ability is often one of the longer-preserved functions in Alzheimer's disease and other forms of dementia (e.g. Cappelletti, Butterworth & Kopelman, 2012) A particularly striking example of such a patient was 'Mr. Bell', described by Rossor, Warrington and Cipolotti (1995) "Mr. Bell" had Pick's disease and had profound deficits in language and memory. However, he could still add, subtract, and compare the sizes of 2- and 3-digit numbers. In contrast to "Signora Gaddi", the left parietal lobe was one of the few areas in his left hemisphere that was *un*damaged.

While some patients show global impairment or global preservation of numerical ability, many show much more selective impairments, and this is one of the findings that has had a strong and positive impact on our interventions for children with mathematical difficulties.. For example, patients with acquired dyscalculia demonstrate single and double dissociations between different arithmetical operations: addition, subtraction, multiplication and division (Cipolotti & Delacycostello, 1995; Dagenbach & McCloskey, 1992; McNeil & Warrington, 1994; Van Harskamp & Cipolotti, 2001). They demonstrate double dissociations between oral and written presentation modes (Campbell, 1990; McNeil & Warrington, 1993); between transcoding (reading and writing numbers) and calculation (Caramazza & McCloskey, 1987; Cipolotti & Butterworth, 1995); and between subitizing and counting (Demeyere, Lestou, & Humphreys, 2010; Demeyere, Rotshtein, & Humphreys, 2012).

The study of patients with brain damage also provides evidence for the broad distinction that the developmental psychologists Greeno, Riley and Gelman (1983) proposed between three major components of mathematical knowledge: factual (knowing facts such as addition bonds and multiplication tables), procedural (knowing *how* to carry out numerical tasks, ranging from basic counting to such arithmetical operations as long multiplication and long division) and conceptual (understanding the properties of numbers and the relationships between numbers and between arithmetical operations).

In this context, double dissociations have been reported between factual and procedural knowledge (McCloskey, 1992; Warrington, 1982). They are also found between factual/ procedural and conceptual knowledge (Delazer, 2003; Delazer & Benke, 1997; Girelli & Delazer, 1996; Hittmair-Delazer, Sailer and Benke, 1995; Rosca, 2010; Warrington, 1982). For example, Puvanendran, Dowker and Demeyere (2015, submitted) report a patient with Broca's aphasia resulting in poor verbal working memory, who demonstrated very poor fact retrieval, but excellent derived fact strategy use.

Double dissociations between exact calculation and estimation in patients have inspired many theories about the nature and neurological substrates of estimation; and in particular have indicated that the two can be relatively functionally indepeendent. For example, Warrington (1982) studied a patient who suffered a stroke affecting the left posterior parieto-occipital region of the brain. This patient was selectively impaired in the retrieval of number facts, and as a result was inefficient and inaccurate at calculation. Arithmetical reasoning was essentially unaffected. In particular, *he was unimpaired – indeed superior to most people- in tasks involving arithmetical estimation*.

Some patients have shown some preservation of approximation and estimation in the face of even more severe mathematical difficulties.. For example, Dehaene and Cohen (1991) studied a patient "Mr. N" with a left subcortical lesion. He could not perform any exact calculations reliably, even adding 2 + 2, but could still carry out approximations. He could locate numbers approximately on a number line; could usually say which was the larger of a pair of 2-digit numbers; and could reject wildly wrong answers to addition sums. For example, he was prepared to accept the sum '5 + 7 = 11', but rejected '5 + 7 = 19'. By contrast, another patient, with a left inferior parietal lesion, had difficulty with such approximation tasks but was still able to carry out some exact calculations through preserved rote knowledge of some addition and multiplication facts.

Most studies of patients have dealt with patients who have experienced strokes, trauma, or other forms of selective injury to particular areas of the bran. Similar results have also been found for people who develop Alzheimer's disease and other degenerative brain disorders. For example, Kaufmann, Montanes, Jacquier, Matallana, Eibl, and Delazer (2002) found that people in the early stages of Alzheimer's disease showed a variety of dissociations between arithmetic facts, arithmetic procedures, and the ability to understand, and compare numbers. No component appeared to be a necessary prerequisite for other components.

One of the largest-scale studies of dissociations between components of numerical abilities was carried out by Cappelletti, Butterworth and Kopelman (2012). They investigated numeracy skills in 76 participants. Forty were healthy controls and 36 were patients with either neurodegenerative disorders or focal brain lesions. The participants were given a comprehensive battery of numerical and calculation tasks. In addition, patients with degenerative disorders and herpes simplex encephalitis patients also performed non-numerical semantic tasks. Results showed that all patients, including those with parietal lesions, had intact processing of number quantity. Patients with impaired semantic knowledge had much better preserved numerical than semantic knowledge. Most patients with selective brain damage showed impaired calculation skills, even when they did not have parietal lesions; but most with dementia did not. Patients also showed dissociations between different aspects of arithmetical ability.

It must be emphasized that neither typically developing children nor those with mathematical difficulties are equivalent to patients with brain damage. Children's mathematical difficulties involve problems in learning, not damage to a previously fully developed system; and they very rarely involve any clear-cut brain damage or abnormality. However, the studies of patients still provide us with hypotheses about the componential nature of numerical ability, which have received much support from other sources.

3. Brain Imaging Studies of Mathematical Abilities

Recently, with the development of increasingly sophisticated techniques of functional brain imaging, the evidence from patients has received increasing support from imaging studies of people without brain damage. Different aspects of arithmetic do seem to make different demands on different parts of the brain; though it must always be remembered that most arithmetical processes, like many other cognitive functions, involve networks between multiple areas. For example, some of the studies by Dehaene and his colleagues (e.g. Dehaene, Tzourio, Frank et al., 1996; Dehaene, Spelke, Pinel et al., 1999) have found that the left parietal cortex is particularly involved in exact calculation, while approximation and estimation may depend more on the right hemisphere. For example, Castelli, Glaser and Butterworth (2006) found that continuous and discontinuous quantity tasks resulted in different patterns of brain activation. Chochon, Cohen, Van de Moortele and Dehaene (1999) found that multiplication activated predominantly the left parietal lobe, number comparison mainly the right parietal lobe, and subtraction activated both equally.

Thus, different studies disagree as regards the details of brain organization for arithmetic. But most suggest that the parietal cortex is involved bilaterally. There may be a bias toward the right hemisphere in magnitude comparison and approximation, and a left hemisphere bias for exact calculation. Some studies (e. g. Rickard, Romero, Basso et al., 2000) suggest bilateral and symmetrical involvement of the hemispheres, even though different regions are differentially activated by different numerical tasks. Others, e.g. Dehaene et al. (1996) and Chochon et al. (1999) suggest greater hemispheric specialization.

The results of some studies (e,g, Kazu, Hitagaki & Mori, 2000) suggest that the left parietal cortex is particularly important in the verbal retrieval of learned facts, while other parts of the brain play a greater role in tasks which require more arithmetical reasoning.

Gruber et al. (2001) used functional MRI to compare the areas of the brain that are active in calculation and in non-arithmetical tasks that make demands on language, visual-spatial processing, attention or memory. They concluded, on the basis of similarities between areas activated by arithmetical and non-arithmetical tasks, that most of the cortical areas that subserve arithmetic "do not exclusively represent modules for calculation but support more general cognitive operations that are instrumental but not specific to calculation". However, there were also brain areas that were more specifically activated by arithmetical tasks: the left dorsal angular gyrus and the medial parietal cortices.

Some recent studies have attempted to combine structural and functional brain imaging to provide converging evidence as to Van Eimeren, Grabner, R.H. Koschutnik, K. et al (2010). They found links between functional activation and structural integrity of grey and white matter regions in the left temporoparietal cortex, thereby contributing to our understanding of the role of both the function and structure of this brain region in calculation

4. Individual and Developmental Differences in Arithmetic: Are These Reflected in the Brain?

Until recently, it was very difficult to carry out neuroimaging studies with sufficiently large samples to enable the analysis of individual differences, because brain imaging techniques were so labour-intensive and expensive that only a few people could realistically be studied at any one time. It was even more difficult to study development, because most brain imaging techniques were unsuitable or untested for suitability for children. A partial exception to both these issues involved the use of EEG and its offshoots; but such techniques had their own problems, as they had very poor spatial resolution. In an earlier paper for the special issue of 'Journal of Physiology-Paris', edited by Ulrike Halsband, I mentioned that there were very few functional brain imaging studies of children, and that most of our knowledge of the relationships between brain and cognition in children had to be extrapolated from studies of adults (Dowker, 2006).

However, there are studies on such topics that go back remarkably early: well before the advent of modern brain imaging technology. Notably, an early

EEG study by Genkin (1960; reported by Krutetskii, 1976) indicated that electrophysiological responses of the inferior parietal lobes during a mathematical task were less strong in children with mathematical difficulties than in children who were performing normally in mathematics. Genkin suggested that the inferior parietal lobes are less well developed in children with pronounced mathematical difficulties.

This finding has received some support from later research using more advanced imaging techniques. For example, Isaacs et al. (2001) studied a group of children who had been born very prematurely and weighed less than three pounds two ounces at birth. A relatively high proportion of these children had specific arithmetical difficulties. Structural brain imaging showed that within this group, those who were experiencing difficulty in arithmetic, had smaller left parietal cortices than those who were not experiencing any such difficulty. This finding suggests that the size and functioning of the left parietal lobe could be a factor in individual differences in arithmetical development, though of course it must be noted that the developmental patterns of extremely premature babies may differ from those of full-term babies in a number of ways.

Menon, Rivera, White et al. (2000) carried out a fMRI study of 16 healthy young adults, and compared those who performed perfectly on a simple arithmetic test and those who occasionally made errors. The focus was on discovering whether there were differences either in the overall functioning of the left parietal lobe or in any of its subregions. The main difference was that perfect performers showed *less* activation of the left angular gyrus. This may be due to greater automatization resulting in less need for rehearsal.

Ansari, Grabner, Koschutnik et al. (2011) studied 24 adult participants with varying levels of mathematical competence were given problems of all four arithmetic operations. Researchers looked at the brain regions that responded more to erroneously versus correctly solved arithmetic problems. Overall accuracy was high. A robust main effect of accuracy (incorrect vs. correct) was observed in both medial and lateral regions of the prefrontal cortex. Furthermore, mathematical competence was found to modulate the activation of an area in the right dorsolateral prefrontal cortex. Specifically, the individuals with relatively higher mathematical competence activated this region more for incorrectly solved trials than did less mathematically competent individuals. This may indicate that more mathematically competent people not only make fewer errors, but monitor their performance better, and are more aware when they do make errors.

Price, Mazzocco and Ansari (2013) found that high school mathematics scores correlated positively with single digit calculation activation in the left supramarginal gyrus (associated with linking words to meanings) and bilateral anterior cingulate cortex (associated with cognitive monitoring). Surprisingly, mathematics scores were negatively related to greater activation in the right intraparietal sulcus during calculation. This may indicate that for high school pupils procedural calculation strategies for single-digit arithmetic, as opposed to automatic retrieval, are associated with better performance. This clashes somewhat with some other findings, but certainly indicates both that brain activation patterns are related to individual differences, and that these can vary with the exact nature of the tasks.

Research is just beginning to investigate developmental changes in brain activation during mathematical tasks. So far, studies suggest some change with age from predominant use of frontal regions to predominant use of parietal regions. This has been found both for magnitude comparisons (Ansari, Garcia, Lucas et al., 2005) and for mental arithmetic (Rivera, Reiss, Eckert & Menon, 2005). This may indicate greater automatization resulting in a reduced load of working memory as children grow older. It may also indicate that experience and/or maturation has a role to play in the increasing specialization of brain areas associated with mathematics. However, one study by Cantlon, Brannon, Carter and Pelphrey (2006) showed that 4-year-olds already do show increased activation of the intraparietal sulcus in magnitude comparison tasks.

DeSmedt et al. (2011) investigated brain activation during single-digit addition and subtraction in 28 children aged 10–12 years. Large problems and subtractions activated a fronto-parietal network, including the intraparietal sulci. The left hippocampus was active during the solution of small-number problems and addition (unlike in adults). Children with lower levels of arithmetical fluency showed higher activation in the right intraparietal sulcus during the solution of relatively small problems.

Thus, there is increasing evidence that different components of arithmetic and of number representation can involve different areas and networks of the brain (e.g. Cappelletti, Lee, Freeman, & Price, 2010; Castelli, Glaser, & Butterworth, 2006; Gruber, Indefrey, Steinmetz, & Kleinschmidt, 2001; Stanescu-Cosson, Pinel, Van de Moortele, Le Bihan, Cohen, & Dehaene, 2000).

However, we may conclude that there is still some uncertainty and disagreement about the extent and nature of the associations and dissociations between specific functions and specific brain areas, but that findings from brain imaging studies concur with the findings from patients in supporting the view that arithmetical ability is not a single entity.

Thus, dissociations between arithmetical abilities in patients have given rise to many of our hypotheses about the componential nature of arithmetic. These have been supported and extended by results of functional brain imaging; and by behavioural studies

5. Implications for Interventions

The evidence converges strongly on the conclusion that arithmetical ability is not unitary, but is made up of many different components. These may be grouped into several categories (e.g. procedural, factual and conceptual); but each of the categories has numerous subcomponents. Levels of performance in different subcomponents are influenced by a multitude of interacting factors: brain-based (both innate and acquired), social, cultural and educational. Thus, any statement that arithmetical ability is purely the product of a single factor – whichever this may be - is inevitably over-simplified.

Moreover, two children (or adults) with arithmetical difficulties are the same (Dowker, 2005; Dowker & Sigley, 2010). It is important to find out what specific strengths and weaknesses an individual child has, and to investigate particular misconceptions and incorrect strategies that they may have.

Admittedly, some educators were recognizing such issues long before most of the evidence that neuroscience has provided. Weaver (1954, pp. 300-301) wrote that "Arithmetic competence is not a unitary thing but a composite of several types of quantitative ability: e.g. computational ability, problem-solving ability, etc.... (T)hese abilities overlap to varying degrees, but most are sufficiently independent to warrant separate evaluations...Children exhibit considerable variation in their profiles or patterns of ability in the various patterns of arithmetic instruction... (E)xcept for extreme cases of disability, which demand the aid of clinicians and special services, remedial teaching is basically good teaching, differentiated to meet specific instructional needs".

However, Weaver's view was unusual in the mid-20th century, and was not at that time backed up by much concrete evidence. As indicated above, more recent evidence, including that provided by neuroscience has confirmed this view (Dowker, 2005, 2009). Partly for this reason, and partly due to greater public awareness of the importance of mathematical difficulties, the emphasis on the need for targeted interventions in numeracy has greatly increased in recent times. By the first decade of the 21st century, the need for interventions for children who were low-attaining in mathematics was receiving more emphasis from the British government (Gross, 2007) and was strongly emphasized by the Williams Review (DCSF 2008). Meanwhile, mathematics interventions and other approaches to supporting children who were low-attaining in mathematics were increasing in number (Dowker, 2009). Notable examples of targeted numeracy interventions are Mathematics Recovery (Wright, Martland & Stafford, 2006), Numeracy Recovery (Dowker, 2001), and the more recently-developed Numbers Count (Dunn, Matthews & Dowrick, 2010; Torgerson, Wiggins, Torgerson et al., 2011).

Some interventions are very intensive, such as Mathematics Recovery, or Numbers Count, typically involving half an hour per day of individualized intervention by qualified teachers.

Mathematics Recovery was originally developed in Australia and has been successfully extended to the UK and elsewhere (Wright et al., 2006; Willey, Holliday & Martland, 2007). It is delivered by teachers and advanced-level classroom assistants who have received 60 hours of training, and begins with an extensive video-recorded assessment interview of the child which is analysed to determine the most appropriate support. It is a highly intensive programme, requiring half an hour of individual intervention per day, which involves a variety of components of number and arithmetic but places particular emphasis on methods of counting and number representation and on the concept of broad developmental stages.

Numbers Count was developed in the UK in response to the Williams Review (DCSF 2008) and is delivered by specialist teachers who have received Masters level training (Dunn, Matthews & Dowrick, 2010). Like Mathematics Recovery, Numbers Count is a highly intensive programme, which comprises a dedicated assessment and diagnosis phase followed by half an hour of individualized intervention per day. It involves careful assessment of individual children's strengths and weaknesses, followed by the individualized intervention, which is targeted to addressing specific weaknesses, and emphasises the development of number concepts through multisensory teaching.

The effectiveness of the Numbers Count programme has already received some investigation (Torgerson, Wiggins, Torgerson et al., 2011). 2621 Year 2 children, across 27 English local authorities, took part in Numbers Count. They received an average of 40 half-hour individualized Numbers Count lessons in a term, delivered by teachers who had received Masters level training. The participating children were given the Sandwell Test of numeracy before and after entering the programme, and were retested 3 months and 6 months later.

Before entering the programme, their Number Age was on average 11 months below their chronological age. On average, they gained 14 months in Number Age in one term, a ratio gain of over four (months gained in Mathematical Age divided by mean duration of intervention in months). They were performing at Chronological Age level by the time they exited the programme. The gains were maintained over six-month follow-up. The children are now receiving long-term follow-up to investigate whether and to what extent the effects persist.

Both Mathematics Recovery and Numbers Count are targeted at children who have quite marked difficulties in mathematics, typically the lowest-attaining children in the class, and are highly intensive, they each involve half an hour of intervention per day delivered by specially trained teachers. However, there are many children who are not among the lowest-attaining in mathematics but who are nevertheless at risk for persistent numeracy difficulties, for whom such intensive intervention is unlikely to be an economic or practical possibility. Lighter-touch interventions are likely to be needed for such children (children who are low-attainers in mathematics but are not performing poorly enough to qualify for the most intensive interventions).

There are at least 15 to 20% of children who experience significant mathematical difficulties, but for whom very intensive intervention may not be a practical or cost-effective possibility. Less intensive, but still targeted, interventions are needed for this group.

6. Catch Up Numeracy

The Catch Up Numeracy intervention has been developed in collaboration with the CatchUp Trust (Dowker & Sigley, 2010; Holmes & Dowker, 2013). Catch Up® is a not-for-profit UK registered charity.

The programme is based on the 'Numeracy Recovery' scheme piloted in Oxford from 1998-2004 (Dowker, 2001, 2005). The target pupils for the intervention are pupils in Years 2 to 6 who have numeracy difficulties. Schools have selected whichever children they feel were likely to benefit; but the main target group are children with moderate mathematical weaknesses rather than the smaller number with extreme mathematical difficulties. Children in the project receive interventions from trained teachers or teaching assistants during two 15 minute sessions per week.

Initially, each child is assessed individually by a trained teacher/teaching assistant using 'Catch Up Numeracy formative assessments' which the member of staff then uses to complete the 'Catch Up Numeracy learner profile'. This personalised profile is used to determine the entry level for each of ten Catch Up Numeracy components and the appropriate focus for numeracy teaching. Children are provided with mathematical games and activities targeted to their specific levels in specific activities.

Children stay in the programme for one term, though teachers may adjust the length of intervention in the light of the pupils' progress.

The components addressed in the project are not regarded as an all-inclusive list of components of arithmetic, either from a mathematical or educational point of view. Rather, they were chosen because teachers regarded them as important to children's learning and relevant to topics in the British National Curriculum, and because earlier research (Dowker, 1998, 2005, 2007) had shown them to have considerable individual variation even among typically developing schoolchildren.

These components are:

(1) Counting verbally (subcomponents: counting verbally from 0 or 1; counting on from a given number; counting back from a given number).

(2) Counting objects (subcomponents: counting objects; order irrelevance; repeated addition of objects; repeated subtraction of objects)

(3) Reading and writing numbers (subcomponents: reading numerals; reading number words; writing numerals).

(4) Hundreds, tens and units (subcomponents: number comparison; adding tens and units; subtracting tens and units).

(5) Ordinal numbers. The ordinal task involves showing children pictures of bead strings and telling them that the bead with the dot in the middle is the first (or in some pictures tenth) bead. One bead in each picture is shaded, and the children are asked to say which bead it is (e.g. second; fourth; ninth; etc.).

(6) Word problems.

(7) Translation (subcomponents: translating from objects to numerals; translating from numerals to objects; translating from number words to numerals; translating from number words to objects).

(8) Derived fact strategies.

(9) Estimation.

(10) Remembered number facts.

An evaluation of outcomes involved 493 primary school children (mean age 104.49 months; s.d.14.63 months). 395 of these received the Catch Up intervention program. 50 were given the same amount of time for individualized mathematics work, which usually involved reviewing work done in the school lessons and was not specifically targeted to assessed individual strengths and weaknesses. 48 children received no intervention, except for the usual school instruction. They were all given Gillham and Hesse's (2008) Number Screening Test before and after the intervention.

At the beginning, the Catch Up intervention group had a mean age of 103.44 months (s.d. 13.25). Their mean mathematics age was 96.89 months (s.d. 16.65). The matched time group had a mean age of 107.83 months (s.d. 13.21). Their mean mathematics age was 95.98 months (s.d. 14.7). The no-intervention group had a mean age of 103.65 months (s.d. 13.88). Their mean mathematics age was 93.91 months (s.d.15.52).

ANOVAs with Group (Catch Up intervention vs. Matched Time controls vs No-Intervention controls) as the grouping factor revealed no significant group differences in chronological age, or mathematics age.

After approximately five months, the ratio gain (months gained in mathematics age divided by the number of months between initial and final testing) was investigated. The 395 children who received Catch Up intervention showed a mean ratio gain of 2.87 (s.d. 2.89); i.e. they made more than twice as much progress as would be expected from passage of time alone. The 50 children who received matched time intervention showed a mean ratio gain of 1.47 (s.d. 1.78). The 48 children who received no intervention showed a mean ratio gain of 0.86 (s.d. 3.17).

An ANOVA, with Group as the factor and Ratio Gain as the dependent variable, showed a highly significant effect of group ($F(2, 490) = 14.67$; $p < 0.001$. Tamhane 2 post-hoc tests showed that the Catch Up intervention group made significantly higher ratio gains than either of the other groups, who did not differ significantly from each other.

The findings suggest that individually targeted interventions are effective for children with mathematical difficulties, and may work better than similar amounts of individual attention in mathematics that are not targeted to a child's specific strengths and weakness. The matched-time control group made somewhat more than the expected gain over time; but those in the Catch Up Numeracy group made more than twice the expected gain.

One consideration is that improvements might be related to a 'regression to the mean' effect, whereby individuals who are scoring very low at the start seem to show improvement because of a general statistical tendency to score closer to the mean on subsequent occasions: In other words, they start out so poorly that they can only get better. Thus, regression to the mean can lead to an exaggeration of the effectiveness of an intervention. This risk was reduced in this study by the inclusion of control groups starting from a similarly low initial point. Regression to the mean would presumably lead to an overestimation of the level of improvement in all three groups, and could not readily account for the fact that the Catch Up group improved so much more than the other groups. Nevertheless, in order to control to some degree for the influence of the initial mathematics age, an additional ANOVA was carried out with group as the grouping factor, ratio gain as the dependent variable, and initial Mathematics Age as a covariate. There was indeed a significant effect of initial Mathematics Age ($F(1, 435) = 6.03$; $p = .014$), indicating greater change in those who started with lower scores, but the difference between the Catch Up group and the other groups continued to be highly significant, even after controlling for this factor ($F(2, 436) = 8.53$; $p = .000$). Thus, though this potential source of bias must be taken into account, it is unlikely that the greater effectiveness of the Catch Up intervention than the other non-targeted interventions can be attributed to a statistical artefact.

More systematic research is needed in order to compare different programmes. It is likely in fact that different programmes will be differentially appropriate for children with different levels of mathematical difficulty: The more severely impaired may need more intensive programmes than the less severely impaired. It is also desirable to carry out longitudinal studies and extend the intervention studies to investigate whether, despite the apparent lack of a simple hierarchy of components, interventions with certain important components also lead to improvement in other components.

More generally, this research strongly supports the view that children's arithmetical difficulties are highly susceptible to intervention. It is not the case that a large number of children are simply 'bad at maths', and that this cannot be ameliorated, although further research is still needed to establish the degree to which such improvements are maintained.

Further research is now needed (i) to refine further our understanding of the components, whether intervention for one component affects progress in other components and whether there are any components for which intervention has a particularly large impact on general mathematical performance, (ii) to investigate the possibilities and consequences of extending the intervention upwards and downwards in age, (iii) to compare the effectiveness of individual intervention with paired or small group intervention, and (iv) to compare the Catch Up Numeracy intervention against other interventions for children who have difficulties in numeracy: investigating the relative effectiveness of interventions for children with different characteristics (for example, age on entering interventions, gap between Chronological Age and Mathematics Age at start of intervention, level and type of arithmetical difficulties, and performance on other cognitive tests such as those measuring verbal and spatial ability), and considering their costs and benefits, financial and otherwise, for children, schools and beyond. But even when such research is done, it is likely that there will prove to be no single best intervention programme, and that different programmes would be suitable for different groups of children.

7. Other Ways in Which Neuroscience May Inform Interventions

So far, the main ways in which neuroscience has informed interventions have been indirect, involving increased understanding of the nature of numerical ability, and, in particular, of the fact that it consists of many components that can be selectively preserved and impaired.

There have recently been some studies that have used neuroscience in somewhat more direct ways in interventions. For example, some studies have used neuroimaging techniques to study the effects of interventions.

Kucian, Grond, Rotzer et al. (2011; see also Cohen Kadosh, Dowker, Heine et al., 2013) developed Calcularis, a set of computer games designed to improve number representations; and to strengthen links between numbers and spatial processes; after five weeks of training, both dyscalculic and typically developing children improved in both spatial number representation and arithmetical abilities. The dyscalculic children underwent fMRI scanning before and after training. They showed changes in brain activity, with more activation of parietal areas and less of frontal areas in arithmetic tasks. This suggested that the intervention was leading to changes in both brain and cognitive function, similar to those that occur in development (Ansari et al., 2005; Rosenberg-Lee, Barth & Menon, 2011).

By contrast, not all studies show such clear-cut relationships between parietal or frontal lobe activation and responses to intervention. Supekar, Swigert, Tenison et al. (2013) studied 8-year-olds' responsiveness to one-to-one tutoring in mathematics in relation to brain characteristics shown through pre-tuition structural and functional brain imaging. They found that the main predictive characteristics involved the hippocampus: its volume, and its functional connectivity with the dorsolateral and ventrolateral prefrontal cortices and the basal ganglia. Thus it appeared that the main predictors involved brain regions associated with learning and memory, rather than those specific to numerical processing. These results must be treated with caution, due to the many others that do show the importance of parietal and frontal activation in development, but is an indicator of the complexity of the topic and the need for further research.

Even more direct ways of involving neuroscience in mathematics interventions involve actual brain stimulation. Cohen Kadosh, Soskic, Iuculano et al. (2010) used transcranial direct current stimulation (TDCS), a method that can selectively inhibit or excitate neuronal populations by modulating GABAergic (anodal stimulation) and glutamatergic (cathodal stimulation) activity. They trained 15 participants for six days with artificial numerical symbols, while they applied concurrent TDCS – or sham stimulation - to the parietal lobes.

The polarity of the brain stimulation specifically enhanced or impaired the acquisition of automatic number processing and the mapping of number into space. Anodal stimulation to the right parietal lobe and cathodal stimulation to the left parietal lobe improved performance. By contrast anodal stimulation to the left parietal lobe and cathodal stimulation to the right parietal lobe reduced performance. The improvement in the first group was still present six months after the training. More recent studies (Iuculano & Cohen Kadosh, 2014) have given some preliminary evidence that transcranial direct current stimulation to the parietal lobes may improve response to numerical training in people with developmental dyscalculia.

It has to be noted that such studies are still in a preliminary stage, and that we do not as yet know how long the effects of such stimulation last, and whether they apply to all components of arithmetic or only some. Moreover, brain stimulation is a facilitator of learning, not a substitute for learning: Improvement occurs when brain stimulation is combined with cognitive training, not as a result of brain stimulation on its own. Also, we have to bear in mind the possibility that brain stimulation may have costs as well as benefits, especially perhaps if given to people who are already performing adequately (Sarkar, Dowker & Cohen Kadosh, 2014).

8. Conclusions

The study of neuroscience has already extensively informed the development of interventions for individuals with mathematical difficulties. Future studies integrating brain imaging studies with behavioural and educational studies are likely to give much more information, especially as brain imaging techniques undergo further development and refinement.

Acknowledgements

Some of this work was carried out in collaboration with Graham Sigley of the Catch Up Trust. I am grateful to Donna Clarke and Julie Lawes of the Catch Up Trust and Wayne Holmes of the Department of Education, Oxford for all their help. The Esmee Fairbairn Charitable Trust and the Caxton Trust provided financial support. Peter Morris and Chongying Wang helped collect data. Simon Yearley provided data on 55 children in Croydon schools receiving Catch Up Numeracy.

Part 4:

Animal Behaviour and Pet Ownership Relationships

14 Comparing Individuals within and across Situations, Groups and Species: Metatheoretical and Methodological Foundations Demonstrated in Primate Behaviour

Jana Uher

Key words:
Cross-species and cross-cultural comparative methodology, Scientific measurement and quantification, Configurational comparability/ structural or construct equivalence, Patterning and positioning effects,, Limitations of assessment methods, Weeper capuchin (*Cebus olivaceus*), mandrill (*Mandrillus sphinx*), toque macaque (*Macaca sinica*), Rhesus macaque (*Macaca mulatta*), Sex/ gender differences and species differences

Abstract
Individuals are explored in various kinds of phenomena and contexts. But how can scientists compare individual variations across phenomena with heterogeneous properties that require different methods for their exploration? How can measurements of individual variations be made directly comparable between different studies, groups of individuals or even species? This research applies the Transdisciplinary Philosophy-of-Science Paradigm for Research on Individuals (TPS-Paradigm) to elaborate metatheoretical concepts and analytical methodologies for quantitative comparisons of individual variations within and across situations, groups and species using behavioural phenomena as examples. Established concepts from personality psychology, differential psychology and cross-cultural and cross-species research are systematically integrated into coherent frameworks and extended by adding concepts for comparing individual-specific variations (i.e., "personality") between species. Basic principles for establishing the functional comparability of behavioural and situational categories are elaborated while considering that individuals from different groups and species often show different behaviours and encounter different situations and therefore cannot be studied with identical variables as is done in assessment-based research. Building on these principles, the chapter explores methodologies for the statistical analyses of the configurational comparability of constructs and of mean-level differences between groups and species. It highlights that situational properties are crucial for quantitative comparisons of individual variations. Fundamental differences between observational methods and assessment methods are explored, revealing serious limitations and fallacies inherent to comparisons of individuals on the basis of assessments. Implementations of the methodological principles

and concepts presented are illustrated with behavioural data from four primate species (weeper capuchins, mandrills, toque macaques and rhesus macaques).

Introduction

Comparisons between individuals are central to many fields of study, such as to neuropsychological, behavioural, social and "personality" research. In these fields, diverse kinds of phenomena (e.g., morphology, physiology, behaviour, the psyche) are explored in a multitude of contexts in which they are embedded. Individuals are compared with one another within and across different biosocial and sociocultural groups, such as groups of individuals of particular age, sex/gender, socio-economic status, nationality and language (Mischel, Shoda, & Ayduk, 2007).

Researching individuals of nonhuman species provides unique opportunities for comparing between-individual variations also across species that differ in their behavioural and social systems, ecological adaptations and phylogenies. Such comparisons are important for exploring the mechanisms and processes of the evolution of population differences within and between species (Capitanio, 2004; Hammock & Young, 2005; Uher, 2008a,b). Cross-species comparisons are also essential to unravel the ways in which humans are, in fact, unique (Tomasello, 1999; Uher, 2013).

The complexity of each of the various kinds of phenomena studied in individuals and the diversity of comparisons that can be made between individuals within and across different situations, cultural groups and species (e.g., cross-situational, cross-cultural and cross-species) entail particular challenges to research methodology. In many fields of psychological and social science research, assessments have become a primary source of information for the scientific exploration and comparison of individuals (Mischel et al., 2007). Judgements on individuals play important roles not only in research but also in everyday life (e.g., at work, schools).

But assessments are prone to various fallacies of the human mind (Uher, 2015a,b,c). Specifically, because individuals are members of the same species, they share basic organismal properties and are therefore substantially similar to one another (Uher 2011a,b). To judge individuals, people therefore abstract from properties that are common to all individuals and focus on the *minor variations* that are informative for differentiating highly similar individuals from one another, such as fine-grained differences in individuals' faces and behaviours. The particular kinds of minor variations that people use most frequently and in socially shared ways for differentiating individuals in their everyday lives are mentally represented in more pronounced ways. The corresponding individual variations are then considered to be *salient,* and they appear in people's minds to be much larger than can actually be observed (Lahlou, 1998; Uher, 2015b).

By contrast, to differentiate individuals of different biosocial and sociocultural groups, people tend to homogenise in their minds within-group differences and to exaggerate between-group differences, and they attribute salience to the particular properties on which these discriminations are based (Connolly, 1998; Gillespie, Howarth, & Cornish, 2012). This also influences people's perceptions of individuals because people may pay more attention to observable properties that match their implicit ideas and social beliefs but less attention to other properties that do not match, thus reinforcing stereotypical representations of individuals from different groups. Stereotypical beliefs about differences between individuals of different gender/sex, age group, ethnicity, nationality, language, amongst others, are found all around the globe (Schneider, 2005).

Salient individual and group differences form important parts of the everyday knowledge and social belief systems that human communities develop and maintain (Jovchelovitch, 2007; Uher, 2013). These socio-cognitive category systems enable humans to quickly form impressions of other individuals that are sufficiently viable for the purposes of first encounters. These category systems are lexically encoded in complex everyday vocabularies that enable people to efficiently communicate their impressions of individuals to others and to develop, maintain and propagate pertinent knowledge, attitudes and social beliefs (Dunbar, 1996; Goldberg, 1982; Lahlou, 1996, 2001; Uher, 2015d).

In fact, it was argued that these socio-cognitive and linguistic abilities first enabled our human ancestors to deal with unknown individuals of other communities in peaceful ways, thus enabling peaceful exchange, traffic and trade between different communities—abilities of fundamental importance for human evolution (the so-called *personality-constructs-promote-peaceful-anonymous-contacts-hypothesis*; Uher, 2013). These human abilities are also important for present-day humans' ability to live in large-scale societies in which they have to deal with many anonymous others in their everyday lives (Blaffer-Hrdy, 2009; Uher, Werner & Gosselt, 2013b).

These social beliefs, ideas and vocabularies inevitably influence the assessments that people make about individuals. For standardised assessments, questionnaire scales are widely applied. They require respondents to judge the assumed degree to which particular characteristics described in statements are applicable to a target individual and to indicate their graded judgements using a set of predetermined category units. The data that can be generated by this procedure constitute much of today's empirical research in many fields of psychology and the social sciences (Baumeister et al., 2007; Schwarz, 1999). Assessment data are also used widely in economic, medical, educational and governmental research (Hammersley, 2013; Menon & Yorkston, 2000) and increasingly also in basic and applied animal behaviour research (Tetley & O'Hara, 2012; Uher & Asendorpf, 2008).

Assessment tools are popular because they are rather easy to implement, time and cost efficient and because they produce highly standardised sets of data. But the ways in which respondents use these tools and by which they generate their answers to standardised scales are still not well understood (Diriwächter, Valsiner & Sauck, 2004; Rosenbaum & Valsiner, 2011). In assessments, people are required to judge a target individual on the basis of their previous experiences with that individual—thus, in retrospect. Therefore, assessments are inherently based on the raters' memory and mental reconstruction of events that they have perceived in the past and of impressions that they have previously formed (Uher, 2015a,b,c).

But human memories are fallible; the accuracy of reconstructions of past experiences is well known to be constraint and biased by errors in memory and reasoning (Fahrenberg, Myrtek, Pawlik, & Perrez, 2007; Gigerenzer, Todd & the ABC Group, 1999; Schacter, 1999; Shweder & D'Andrade, 1980; Uher, 2013). Moreover, memories are never just recalled in identical ways but are always reconstructed anew in the context of the given situation (Bartlett, 1932; Schacter & Addis, 2007; Uher, 2015a,b,c,d). Memory recall and thus, also the construction of assessments therefore depend on the states of mind that individuals may have in particular situations (Omi, 2012; Uher, 2013).

The item statements and answer categories used in assessment tools are commonly worded in everyday terms so that the raters can understand them without detailed instruction or even training of how to use these tools to generate data (as is the case in observational methods; see below). Thus, scientists capitalise on the raters' commonsense knowledge for interpreting the meaning that the statements and category units provided in a particular assessment tool may have for these raters in view of the specific assessment task at hand. Given this, it may be inevitable that assessment methods activate all kinds of sociocultural and stereotypical beliefs, lay theories and implicit norms and values, such as those about gender/sex (Lloyd & Duveen, 1992), ethnicity (Howarth, 2009), age and social status (Schneider, 2005; Uher et al., 2013b) that are widespread in all human communities.

From the particular requirements of assessment methods it follows that assessment data reflect properties of the raters' personal and socially shared ideas, beliefs, knowledge and psychical representations about the phenomena to be assessed but they cannot reflect properties of these phenomena in and of themselves (Uher, 2015a,b,c). Knowledge and belief systems are always context-dependent (Jovchelovitch, 2007). Therefore, they can be used flexibly and in context-sensitive ways in everyday life—and thus, also for assessments (Hammersley, 2013). As a consequence, assessment-based findings depend on the particular contexts of the raters, such as their particular stages of development (Toomela, 2010), educational level (Vygotsky, 1934) and their abilities to reflect on themselves, their world (Omi, 2012) and their life histories (McAdams, 1985). Assessments also depend on the raters' particular situation (Bandura, 1986; Lazarus, 1981; Mischel, 1968; Rotter, 1954); therefore, numerous studies could demonstrate that (experimentally induced) motivations and goals significantly influence the outcomes of assessments (Biesanz & Human, 2010).

Information obtained with assessments also depend on the context of particular groups of individuals that raters may implicitly consider (Heine, Lehman, Peng, & Greenholtz, 2002). This accounts for numerous, apparently puzzling findings from comparative research on individuals such as repeated findings showing that the average scores of "personality" assessments of people from different nations did not correspond to national character stereotypes (e.g., McCrae, Terracciano & 79 Members of the Personality Profiles of Cultures Project, 2005; McCrae, Terracciano, Realo, & Allik, 2007a,b; Perugini & Richetin, 2007; Terracciano, Abdel-Khalak, Ádám, Adamovová et al., 2005).

Given the context-sensitivity of social beliefs, values and knowledge and the inherently memory-based generation of assessments, standardised assessment methods are not appropriate for valid comparisons between individuals and for exploring and explaining real world issues in the increasingly pluralistic societies we live in today (e.g., in occupational, clinical, educational and economic settings). Moreover, the standardised data formats produced with assessment methods obscure the fundamental metatheoretical and methodological challenges that are inherent in any comparative study. For how can scientists establish comparability between phenomena, events or properties that are heterogeneous and that require for their exploration different kinds of methods and different units of measurement? How can quantitative measurements be made directly comparable between specialised disciplines, as this is possible in the physical sciences? Establishing such comparability is important to enable the interdisciplinary collaboration that is necessary to comprehensively explore the complex phenomena researched in individuals, such as the complex interplay between genes, brain and behaviour.

This research applies the Transdisciplinary Philosophy-of-Science Paradigm for Research on Individuals (TPS-Paradigm, see below; Uher, 2015a,b,c) to elaborate the metatheoretical concepts and analytical methodologies that are required for systematic quantitative comparisons between individuals within and across different situations, groups and species. These elaborations are made and illustrated using the phenomena of behaviour as example. Behaviours are chosen because they can be directly perceived in all kinds of individuals including those who are not able to self-report (e.g., young children, nonhuman animals). But behaviours also feature some challenging properties, such as the momentariness and dynamic fluctuations of behavioural events, which hinder direct comparisons between individuals and considerably complicate scientific measurements (Uher,

2015a). Explorations of other physical phenomena of individuals (e.g., morphology, physiology) can directly build on these principles. They also apply to explorations of the phenomena of the psyche; but because psychical[2] phenomena cannot be directly perceived in others, additional methodological peculiarities must be considered (Uher, 2015b,c,d).

First, the chapter outlines the relevant foundations that the TPS-Paradigm provides for research on behavioural phenomena and for scientific measurement and quantification. Using these fundamentals, established concepts for exploring variations within and between individuals and groups are systematically integrated and extended to the level of species, highlighting three central viewpoints on which all kinds of comparative explorations are based. Building on these concepts, the chapter elaborates basic principles for establishing the comparability of behavioural categories between groups and species that show different behaviours and that therefore cannot be studied using exactly the same behavioural variables. These principles are used to scrutinise the widespread practice of using "identical" variables to establish comparability in assessment-based research. Then the chapter explores methodological approaches needed to statistically analyse the configurational comparability of constructs and mean-level differences between groups and species, showing that situational properties are essential for quantitative comparisons. Implementations of the principles and concepts presented are illustrated by behavioural data from four nonhuman primate species.

The Transdisciplinary Philosophy-of-Science Paradigm for Research on Individuals (TPS-Paradigm)

The TPS-Paradigm comprises interrelated philosophical, metatheoretical and methodological frameworks for exploring individuals. In these frameworks, concepts, approaches and methods from various scientific disciplines were systematically integrated, further developed and complemented by novel ones; therefore it is a *transdisciplinary* paradigm (Uher, 2008a,b, 2011a,b, 2013, Desideratum 1a). It is called a *philosophy-of-science* paradigm because it emphasises the importance of making explicit the philosophical presuppositions that are made in a given scientific system and the metatheories and methodologies that are derived from them, and it aims to make these explicit in the fields that it explores (Uher, 2015a). The TPS-Paradigm therefore provides the necessary foundations from which to scrutinise established theories and methods from various fields of research for their commonalities and differences and to refine and develop metatheories and methodologies that are applicable across disciplines.

---

[2] The TPS-Paradigm uses the term *psychical* rather than psycho*logical* because "events, processes and structures that are properly called psychical do not become psychological until they have been operated upon in some way by the science of psychology" (Adams & Zener in Lewin, 1935, p. vii).

The potentials of the TPS-Paradigm for enabling such explorations were already demonstrated, amongst others, in critical analyses of taxonomic "personality" research. In this field, the TPS-Paradigm revealed fundamental mismatches between the researchers' (implicit and explicit) concepts of "personality" and the methodological rationales underlying the selection approaches, methods of data generation and reduction principles that are used for developing comprehensive "personality" taxonomies (Uher, 2015b). Further mismatches were revealed between widely established interpretations of the taxonomic "personality" models, constructs and data thus-derived and their actual abilities to reflect individual-specificity in the targeted phenomena (Uher, 2015c). Basic concepts of the TPS-Paradigm were also used to explore the phenomena of the psyche, their microgenetic, ontogenetic and (potential) phylogenetic development and their roles in the emergence of language, social institutions and societies (Uher, 2015d).

At the heart of the TPS-Paradigm is the metatheoretical definition and differentiation of various kinds of phenomena that are explored in research on individuals (i.e., the phenomena of morphology, physiology, behaviour, the psyche, semiotic representations, artificially modified outer appearances and contexts). These differentiations are made on the basis of *three metatheoretical properties* that can be conceived in different forms for each given phenomenon: *1)* spatial location in relation to the studied individual's body, *2)* temporal extension and *3)* spatial extension, i.e., physicality versus "non-physicality"[3]. These three spatio-temporal properties are considered because they determine a phenomenon's perceptibility by individuals in everyday life and—thus, also its accessibility by researchers and the methodologies required for explorations (Uher, 2015a,b,c).

What is Behaviour? Metatheoretical Definition and Methodological Implications

Behaviours are defined in the TPS-Paradigm as the "external changes or activities of living organisms that are functionally mediated[4] by other external phenomena (Millikan, 1993) in the present moment" (Uher, 2013, 2015a,b,c). Thus, behaviours are not just movements[5] (e.g., freezing in prey animals). Vice

---

[3] In the TPS-Paradigm, the term "non-physical" is put in quotation marks as it denotes properties that are not simply contrasted against the physical but are complementary instead (see Uher, 2015a).

[4] In the TPS-Paradigm, the meaning of the term *mediation* refers to the Latin *mediare*, to be in the middle, not to the meaning established in statistics (where it is differentiated from moderation).

[5] Importantly, the TPS-Paradigm conceives neither of physiological responses nor of mental activities as behaviours, in contrast to behaviourist and cognitivist paradigms (Skinner, 1957; Koffka, 1935). Moreover, it makes no a priori assumptions about the potential causes of behaviours in other kinds of phenomena as is implied by concepts of behavioural "responses" or "goal-directed" actions, amongst others. Instead, the TPS-Paradigm considers that different metatheoretical properties can be conceived for other kinds of phenomena that therefore require different methodologies for their exploration and thus also for explorations of their interrelations with behaviours (Uher, 2015a,b,c).

versa, not all movements, external changes or activities are behaviours (e.g., mere chemical by-products such as heat); they are behaviours only if their functions have *reference to* other external phenomena or to connections with them (Millikan, 1993). Hence, the meaning and function of behaviours can be explored only by considering the particular contexts in which they occur (cf. the behavioural situation, below; Uher, Addessi, & Visalberghi, 2013a; Uher et al., 2013b).

The TPS-Paradigm conceives of *functions* as temporal interrelations that regularly occur between particular kinds of phenomena, events or properties—thus, as established effects (derived from the Latin *effectus* meaning "worked out, brought about, accomplished"). Importantly, functions thus-defined neither imply purpose nor intention because teleological properties presuppose that possible prospective outcomes are simulated and evaluated on the basis of retrospective analyses of experiences made in the past, which is possible only for psychical phenomena (Uher, 2015d). Moreover, functions denote not only causal connections of various kind (Kausal-Zusammenhänge) but also compositional connections (Gefüge-Zusammenhänge) in which the interacting elements co-occur in coordinated ways and match and cooperate with one another such that the entirety of their joint interactions results in complexes and functions of higher organisation (Rothschuh, 1963; Uher, 2015a,c).

Behavioural phenomena are located external to the body of the individual under study and can therefore be directly perceived by observers. But observations are complicated because behaviours are bound to the present moment. Moreover, behavioural events often have only low temporal extensions but unfold continuously and dynamically in time and are therefore often highly fluctuating. Hence, behaviours can be observed and thus be recorded only in the particular moments in which they occur. Methods allowing for the real-time recording of momentary events are referred to as *nunc-ipsum methods* (from the Latin *nunc ipsum* for at this very instant) in the TPS-Paradigm (Uher, 2015a).

Behaviours are immaterial physical phenomena in and of themselves (e.g., sound waves, movements); therefore, rather constant spatial and temporal units suggesting clear demarcations of single events are largely absent. But spatio-temporal units can be identified on the basis of the physical matter of individuals' bodies (e.g., arms, torso) and of their external physical surroundings (e.g., trees) to which behaviours are bound. This boundedness to matter allows for identifying behavioural events that are repeatable at least to some extent although the units that can be identified in this way vary in their spatio-temporal extensions (e.g., arm movements to pick apples from a tree). These peculiarities have important implications for scientific measurement and quantification as explored below.

The phenomena of contexts—Situations and behavioural situations

Contextual phenomena (derived from the Latin *contexere* to interweave, link together) can be identified and conceived only with regard to the particular individual under study. Specifically, individuals interact with only those external physical events that are relevant for them given their particular physical and psychical properties; hence, the same physical surroundings are not the same for all individuals (Bandura, 1986; Lewin, 1936; Rotter, 1954; von Uexküll, 1909). Dualistic conceptions, such as of "individual versus environment" or "nature versus nurture" are therefore misleading and inherently circular (Uher, 2015a,b,c).

Considering this, the TPS-Paradigm defines a *situation* as the particular constellation of events of all kinds of phenomena both external and internal to the body of the studied individual that are present in a given moment. Thus from the universe of all external physical events, an individual's situation comprises all those particular events that are present in a given moment and that are therefore directly perceptible by the individual, consciously or not. Because individuals' bodies are always present, a situation also comprises internal physical events (e.g., physical condition, food deprivation). It also comprises all psychical events that are ongoing, thus also all those memories and psychical representations that the individual retrieves and reconstructs in the given moment, such as representations of events that are absent in and of themselves (Uher, 2015a).

Behavioural situations are situations of special kind that denote the particular constellation of those external physical events that functionally mediate an individual's external changes or activities in a given moment—his or her behaviours. Thus, the events that constitute behavioural situations are external to the individual in and of themselves. But the criterion for demarcating these particular events from the universe of all external physical events present in a given moment is bound to the properties of that individual. This criterion is the events' effectiveness to make functional the individual's external changes or activities that thereby become behaviours. Importantly, this demarcation is based on individuals' *external* bodily events that can be directly observed (i.e., behaviours) rather than on internal ones (i.e., psychical events). This facilitates the identification of those particular external properties that may functionally mediate the behaviours of a particular individual in a particular situation, which may be neither directly apparent nor known a priori. To identify the functions that a given behavioural event may have for particular individuals in particular situations, behavioural scientists therefore explore proximate spatio-temporal interrelations in the empirical occurrences of different behavioural events with one another and with other events in the individuals' external surrounding (see below; e.g., Preuschoft, 1992; Preuschoft & van Hooff, 1995).

Exploring individuals' behaviours in different kinds of situations, as intersubjectively categorised on the basis of particular constellations of observable properties (see below), constitutes an important approach for researchers to explore the possible psychical relevance and meaning that particular situational properties may have for particular individuals even if these individuals cannot be interviewed about their personal views, such as young children (Shoda, Mischel, & Wright, 1994; Wright & Zakriski, 2003) and nonhuman animals (Hinde, 1974, 1982). Such analyses presuppose metatheoretical and analytical concepts that enable scientists to quantify their study phenomena appropriately.

Philosophy-of-science principles of scientific measurement and quantification

Using concepts of the science of measurement—metrology (JCGM, 2008), the TPS-Paradigm elaborated the philosophy-of-science foundations of scientific quantification, highlighting two central requirements. First, researchers must specify the sets of the elements to be quantified in the phenomena under study; this is called the *set-theoretic requirement*. Second, the elements thus-defined must be compared with designated fixed standards to express their ratio as a real number; this is called the *algebraic requirement* of scientific quantification (Uher, 2015a,b,c). The TPS-Paradigm refers to numerical data that fulfil the set-theoretic and algebraic requirements as *scientific* quantifications—as opposed to (subjective) quantifications in which these requirements are not fulfilled. It highlights that the opportunities for meeting these two requirements are unequivocally determined by the three spatio-temporal properties that it considers. Importantly, these requirements must be fulfilled *with regard to the phenomena under study* and not only with regard to the phenomena that are used as data (Uher, 2015a,b, submitted).

What are *data*? In many fields of research, scientists seldom directly explore the phenomena under study in and of themselves (e.g., behaviours) as is the case when, for example, in medical investigations body tissue is dissected and dyed, thus changed and destroyed. Research on individuals mostly relies on persons (e.g., researchers, observers) who convert information from their observations of single occurrences of the phenomena under study into information encoded in signs (Uher, 2015c). The TPS-Paradigm highlights that *signs* are composite kinds of phenomena that consist of physical phenomena that are external to individuals' bodies (e.g., vocalisations, ink on paper) and of psychical phenomena (e.g., meanings) that particular individuals attribute to these external physical phenomena and that first make them signs. Behavioural and material signs (e.g., spoken and written language) are developed and used to physically represent meanings and all kinds of phenomena that individuals can perceive and/or conceive of (e.g., behaviours, buildings, deities). This enables the transmission of meanings also in absence of the particular objects to which they refer and across time and space, making signs important means for communication and the development and transfer of knowledge (Uher, 2015d).

The signs used in science (e.g., numerals, lexically encoded variables) and to which scientists attribute particular meanings (e.g., mathematical properties, behavioural events observed) are commonly called data. Data can be stored and analysed, thus manipulated, decomposed and recomposed *in lieu of* the actual phenomena of interest and in ways that may not be enabled by these phenomena in and of themselves (Uher, submitted).

The essence of data generation

The pivotal point for generating data are the decisions that observers and researchers make on the ways in which particular information from the actual phenomena under study can be appropriately represented in signs (i.e., data). When information from one kind of phenomenon are represented in another kind of phenomenon, this is called *conversion* in the TPS-Paradigm. Human individuals explicitly and implicitly convert information between different kinds of phenomena all the time they are communicating (Uher, 2015d). To enable systematic conversions and standardised encodings of information that are considered to be relevant for a given investigation, researchers must therefore specify the particular operations and practices that are used to implement these decisions—hence, the *methods of data generation* (Uher, 2015a).

The choice of the particular method of data generation depends on the theoretical definition of the object of research and on its operational definition in a given study. Therefore, researchers must specify the particular intersubjective agreements that are made about which particular pieces of information about the properties and events of the phenomena under study as perceived and conceived by human individuals (e.g., observers) can be demarcated and categorised in what particular ways. These specifications are essential for meeting the two requirements of scientific quantification.

Fulfilling the set-theoretic requirement for scientific quantification

The set-theoretic criterion of scientific quantification requires researchers to specify all the elements to be quantified. Thus, to scientifically quantify individual behaviours, researchers must specify all studied elements of the set *B* of behavioural events, the set *S* of behavioural situations that (may) functionally mediate these behaviours, the set *I* of individuals in which they are explored and the set *T* of occasions and periods of time in which they are recorded in a given study (Uher et al. 2013a).

The fact that quantifications of individual differences always depend on the particular set *I* of individuals to which a given target individual is compared is known as *reference group effect* (Heine et al., 2002). It is also well known that differences in the studied elements of the set *T* can influence empirical results, such as the effects that aggregations have on the reliability of measurements (Epstein, 1979, 1980). But it is often not well considered that the same principle equally applies to the elements of the sets *B* of behaviours and *S* of behavioural situations because the functions and meanings that behaviours may have for individuals depend on the particular situation in which they occur. Moreover, in the same sample of individuals, different behavioural events generally occur with different average frequencies in both the same and different kinds of situations (Uher, 2011a,b). Thus, comparing behavioural occurrences between individuals without considering such behaviour-specific and situation-specific variations can bias quantitative measurements.

The methodological necessity to specify the studied elements in *all* sets considered tends to be overlooked likely because the different kinds of phenomena impose different demands on researchers and observers for meeting this requirement. Specifically, the elements of the sets *I* and *T* can be specified easily by conceiving of individuals (on the basis of their bodies) as discrete physical material entities and by using the standard instruments for measuring time that are widely used also in everyday life. But to specify which particular elements of the sets *B* and *S* are being explored in a given study requires researchers and observers to decide on how to demarcate distinct kinds of events in the heterogeneous properties that can be perceived in these complex phenomena and on how to categorise these events. This entails particular challenges.

Challenges and principles for developing category systems in behavioural research

Developing category systems that specify all the elements of the sets *B* and *S* that are explored in a given study is complicated because, in behavioural phenomena, clear-cut and mutually exclusive categories often cannot be easily defined as this may be possible, for example, for categorisations of chemical elements. Demarcating and categorising different kinds of events is complicated because the momentary and fluctuating occurrences of behaviours hinder direct comparisons of their observable properties across different occasions and across different situations and individuals.

Demarcating behavioural events in the flow of their occurrence is also complicated because the spatio-temporal units that can be identified in behavioural phenomena often vary considerably in their extensions and are therefore identically repeatable only to some extent. For example, human individuals can smile in very different ways. They can turn the corners of their mouths up in different ways, with open or closed mouth. In addition, individuals may also produce laughter lines around their eyes with different levels of intensity. Given this considerable variability that is perceptible in the spatial properties of these behaviours, what entity can be demarcated and categorised as *one* ($n = 1$) smile? Which particular entities can be considered to be of the same kind, thus as identically repeatable at least to some extent? Moreover, smiles also differ in their temporal extension. Can a quick smile and a long-lasting smile be conceived as events of the same kind?

Whereas demarcations of behavioural events are made on the basis of the similarity in their *perceptible spatio-temporal forms*, these properties cannot be used for categorising the events thus-specified. The TPS-Paradigm emphasises that in research and in everyday life categorisations of behaviours are based on their *known or theoretically assumed functions* (e.g., slapping someone on the shoulder to kill a midge versus to bully that other individual). In fact, functionally similar behaviours often differ from one another in their spatio-temporal forms. In school children, for example, slapping and verbally insulting others can be considered functionally similar in particular kinds of situations (e.g., to win over others), but their particular spatio-temporal forms differ considerably (cf. Murray-Close & Ostrov, 2009).

Likewise, empirical co-occurrences of different behavioural events across the individuals studied (as studied, e.g., with factor analysis) cannot be used to derive summary categories of behavioural events—contrary to widespread practices in "personality" research. Rather, empirical co-occurrences of functionally related behaviours can also be low (e.g., of contact and non-contact aggression; Uher, 2011b; Uher et al., 2013a). But no matter such empirical inconsistency, in their everyday lives, people commonly categorise behaviours of *similar function* as behaviours of *similar kind* (e.g., as "aggression") and they also do so in standardised assessments.

In behavioural research, hierarchical *category systems* in which more specific categories of behavioural events are summarised by more abstract categories are established on the basis of the functions and meanings that the behaviours may have for the individuals studied. Hence in category systems, researchers specify not only events to be studied but also the *theoretical* interrelations of the specified elements both within and between the sets *B, S, I* and *T*. This is prerequisite for exploring the empirical interrelations between the elements studied—thus, for their scientific quantification as explored below.

As functions denote temporal interrelations that regularly occur between particular kinds of phenomena, events or properties, functions can be identified by means of contextual pre-post analyses of behavioural sequences studied in observations and by experimentation (Hinde, 1974, 1982; Preuschoft, & van Hooff, 1995; Visalberghi, Valenzano, & Preuschoft, 2006). But the particular external situational properties that are, in fact, functionally mediating particular behaviours in particular individuals are not always known a priori or directly apparent and they may not even be consciously perceptible by human individuals (e.g., subliminal odours; Li, Moallem, Paller, & Gottfried, 2007). Therefore, it may be possible that observers and researchers specify properties that actually do not fulfil mediating functions for the particular behaviours of the particular individuals studied. This is ultimately a matter of research. A first step towards identifying functional interrelations is to specify the situational properties (i.e., the elements of the set *S*) that can be directly perceived and intersubjectively conceived by multiple human observers. Given this, initial specifications may refer only to properties that are salient to individuals of particular sociocultural communities or only to humans. But with accumulating evidence, these specifications allow for exploring which particular constellation of properties can legitimately be assumed to fulfil mediating functions for particular kinds of behaviours in particular kinds of individuals.

Behavioural events are sometimes also categorised with regard to their *degrees of functional intensity*. This presupposes that their known or theoretically assumed functions and meanings that they may have for particular individuals, groups or species are considered to be qualitatively comparable. In school children, for example, slapping and verbally insulting others may be considered functionally comparable because both behavioural events represent offences in particular situations. But because of their different perceptible properties, differences in their degrees of intensity—thus quantitative differences—cannot be readily specified. For example, one may assume that slaps constitute a more offensive behaviour than verbal insults. But how could this be quantified? Can five verbal insults be considered to be as equally harmful as one slap?

Moreover, the functional intensity of behaviours also depends on the particular behavioural situations in which they occur. Slapping another child for taking away a toy may be considered less aggressive, and thus less intense, than slapping others who offer to play together (cf. Wright & Zakriski, 2003), even though the perceptible properties of the slap, in and of themselves, may be exactly the same in both kinds of situations. Often there are no natural entities on which decisions can be made about intensity differences between functionally related behaviours. Such decisions are thus arbitrary to some extent; they depend on the current state of knowledge and, in particular, on the particular social values that are socioculturally attributed to behaviours.

Further challenges arise because the spatial, temporal and functional properties that can be identified in behaviours are sometimes interrelated. For example, play behaviours necessarily involve physical activity; an individual that does not move at all does not play. But a motionless position may still have a social function, such as when individuals rest next to others rather than alone. Therefore, functional properties of the same behavioural event can be encoded in different behavioural categories (e.g., locomotive, play and social behaviours) even in the same study (for an example, see Uher et al., 2013a). This multiple categorisation of functional properties of one and the same behavioural event corresponds to the intuitive categorisations of behaviours that people make in their everyday lives.

In sum, in category systems researchers specify the known or assumed *theoretical* interrelations of the studied elements both within and between the sets *B, S, I* and *T*. This specification is prerequisite for exploring the empirical interrelations between the elements studied—thus, for their scientific quantification as explored below.

Principles for developing encoding schemes

Once the category system is developed for an investigation, researchers must specify encoding schemes that enable observers to quickly recognise relevant properties in the phenomena under study and to categorise and encode occurrences of defined events systematically and in standardised ways into raw data. During live observations, these requirements must be fulfilled real-time—i.e., nunc-ipsum, while the behaviours occur. Video-based observations decelerate this task and facilitate perceptions of the relevant properties, such as by enabling repeated and slow-motion playback. To establish behavioural encoding schemes, researchers can capitalise on the broad range of methods developed in ethology (e.g., Martin & Bateson, 2007; Lehner, 1998).

Importantly, researchers must consider that behavioural observations are never free of implicit decisions made by the observers (Pelligrini, 2011). This is because categorising individual behaviour is an important ability that humans use frequently in their everyday social lives and for which they have developed comprehensive sets of socio-cognitive categories. To ensure that observers interpret and use the encoding schemes for generating data as specified for the purposes of a given study, observers are instructed and trained. Therefore, researchers must specify the observable properties that are used to demarcate and categorise the particular kinds of events studied. This is especially important for abstract behavioural categories (e.g., "aggression") that are sometimes used to encode a heterogeneous set of behavioural events that could also be encoded in several more specific coding categories (e.g., "verbal insult", "slap"). The defining properties must be explicitly and sufficiently described in intersubjective ways such that different observers demarcate and categorise behavioural events and encode their occurrences in very similar ways as statistically tested by inter-observer reliability.

The TPS-Paradigm emphasises that encoding schemes can rely *only* on those properties of the events and phenomena under study that are or can be (technically) made *directly perceptible* and intersubjectively conceivable by multiple human individuals. In their encoding schemes, researchers must therefore address the particular forms that can be conceived for the given study phenomenon with regard to each of the three spatio-temporal properties because these properties determine a phenomenon's general accessibility by human individuals. Therefore, these properties also determine the accessibility of further, more specific properties on which demarcations and categorisations of events may be based in a given study (e.g., sound) and that are therefore also specified in the encoding schemes (Uher, 2015a,b,c, submitted).

For enabling systematic encodings, behavioural categories are defined on the basis of properties that occur in comparable constellations in all kinds of events that are assigned to the same category and that differ from those of events that are assigned to other categories. Such definitions can be based, for example, on the different communication modes such as by specifying the particular constellations of verbal, vocal, facial, gestural or postural properties that occur in all behavioural assigned to a particular category.

As behaviours are functionally mediated by other external events and are thus always contextualised, behavioural encoding schemes must also specify properties of the particular behavioural situations studied (Uher, 2013, Desideratum 2c). In behavioural studies, these specifications are always contained at least implicitly because they are carried out and their category systems are set up for investigations in particular settings, such as school classes or experimental laboratories. As with behavioural categories, defining encoding schemes for behavioural situations can rely only on those properties that are or can be made consciously perceptible by human observers. Situational categories can be defined in various degrees of abstraction. For example, descriptions of the situations in which school children are observed could refer to social settings in general. More specific sub-categories could differentiate contacts to adults or peers, to familiar or unfamiliar peers, same or opposite sex peers in conflict, play or teaching situations, involving one other individual, a group or an anonymous mass, amongst others. The degree of specification of situational properties depends on the purpose of the given study.

In sum, specifying the perceptible properties on which the demarcations and categorisations of behavioural events are based makes painfully apparent that identifying similarity—thus, establishing comparability—between events other than those that can be conceived to be identically repeatable at least to some extent is always a matter of decision, theoretical interpretation, degree of abstraction and the particular aim and purpose of the given study. These decisions are seldom made explicit but they are always involved in every observation of individual behaviour in both research and everyday life.

Such decisions are also involved in assessments but the standardisations that are implemented in these methods obscure the complexity of these decision. Assessment instruments comprise standardised statements and answer categories that are often global and abstract and not further specified in terms of perceptible properties of events to which they may refer. In contrast to observers in a behavioural study, raters are neither instructed nor trained to use the fixed encoding schemes provided in systematic and standardised ways for generating data. As a consequence, the particular elements of the set *B, S, I* and *T* that raters may implicitly consider when generating assessments and the ways in which they encode the elements considered in the predefined scales remain unspecified. Therefore, assessment methods fail to fulfil the set-theoretical requirement of scientific quantification, in contrast to observational methods (Uher, submitted).

Fulfilling the algebraic requirement for scientific quantification

The algebraic requirement of scientific quantifications states that researchers must directly compare the elements specified with designated standards of measurement to express their ratio as a real number. Most widely used in science are spatial standard units of measurement, such as of distance (e.g., meter). But such comparisons are complicated in immaterial phenomena that are momentary and fluctuating and in which identifiable events vary in their spatio-temporal extension (e.g., behaviours, neuronal action potentials).

Specifically, in behavioural research, direct comparisons with standards of measurement are possible only for some kinds of properties and often only under experimental conditions (e.g., measuring physical force with a dynamometer). But in most observational settings in either research or everyday life, properties of behavioural events can seldom be directly compared with designated standards of measurement in the moments in which the events occur (e.g., for measuring spatial distances between individuals that are socially and physically interacting in a group).

Specifying observable quantitative properties of the events under study

The possibilities to *directly* quantify occurrences of behavioural events are rather limited because, in nunc-ipsum methods, observers must decide quickly on how to demarcate, categorise and encode events in the continuous and dynamic flow of behaviours. Mostly, observers record only the occurrences and non-occurrences of specified events, thus using binary scales. But in some behavioural events, quantitative properties can be directly identified, such as by defining spatial distances between individuals on the basis of their bodily properties (e.g., body contact, arm-length distance) or by counting the occurrences of distinct events. To enable observers to systematically identify quantitative properties and to encode them in standardised ways in the data, researchers must specify the particular properties that are considered to be quantitative in the particular phenomena under study.

Quantitative properties are divisible properties of events that are categorised as being of the same kind, thus of events that are considered to be qualitatively similar (Hartmann, 1964; Uher, submitted). The TPS-Paradigm emphasises that these properties must be directly perceptible and intersubjectively conceivable by multiple human observers. Researchers must also specify rules for the determinative assignment of these properties to numerals so that observers can encode their occurrences always in exactly the same way. For example in the great ape species, scratching usually occurs at a speed that enables human observers to perceive and count the single flexions of their fingers while they occur (Uher, Asendorpf & Call, 2008). In capuchin monkeys, by contrast, scratching occurs so quickly that human observers often cannot perceive each single finger flexion during live observations; this is only possible from video records using slow motion playback (Uher et al., 2013a). Therefore, capuchin researchers commonly record occurrences of *episodes* of scratching that are defined by several consecutive finger flexions and that are demarcated from one other by a short break (Fragaszy, Visalberghi, & Fedigan, 2004).

The observers' possibilities to directly quantify behavioural events are generally limited to behaviours of very short temporal extension (called point or frequency behaviours) that occur in temporal and spatial proximity. Occurrences of behaviours with longer temporal extension (called duration behaviours) are often recorded in terms of their onsets and terminations that are encoded on binary scales in the raw data. This requires a continuous recording of events while observers focus on only one individual and his or her behaviours and interactions. Given the enormous effort involved such focal individual sampling continuous recording methods, duration behaviours are also often estimated from scan sampling instantaneous recording techniques, in which observers record whether at specified points of time defined kinds of duration behaviours do or do not occur, respectively. These time point samples allow for generating only crude quantitative estimates of behavioural durations, but they enable the collection of data on many individuals during the same observation period (as done in the primate studies reported below; Altmann, 1974; Lehner, 1998; Martin & Bateson, 2007).

From the data log files thus-produced, researchers can generate *post-hoc* (i.e., after the collection of raw data is completed) quantitative measures by recoding, transforming and further abstracting the raw data (e.g., by computing durations and latencies from the onsets and terminations recorded using behavioural coding software). From log files of observational data, scientific quantifications can be generated with the concept of time-relative probabilities.

Scientific quantification using the concept of time-relative probabilities

The TPS-Paradigm introduces the concept of *time-relative probabilities* to meet the algebraic requirement of scientific quantification for the momentary and fluctuating phenomena explored in individuals that often feature spatio-temporal units of variable extension, thus the phenomena of physiology and behaviour. It can also be applied to explore psychical phenomena (Uher, 2016). This concept relies not on space but on *time* as the physical standard units of measurement to which the occurrences of the defined events can be compared for generating scientific quantifications (Uher, 2013, 2015a).

Time-relative probabilities fundamentally differ from other concepts of probability because researchers of individuals, unlike physicists, cannot deal with random, equiprobable and mutually disjunctive events that are independent from one another and that could be experimentally repeated as in Laplacian theory. Rather, the units that can be identified in the phenomena explored in individuals often vary in their spatio-temporal extension so that demarcations and categorisations of events can be made in various ways. Moreover, different kinds of events may co-occur and even depend upon one another, in particular if they are functionally related (e.g., slapping others requires physical proximity, but both behavioural events do not always co-occur). Because of these peculiarities of living organisms, previous concepts of probability are not applicable (Uher, 2013, submitted).

To generate time-relative probabilities, nunc-ipsum records of the occurrences of defined events are accumulated over repeated occasions to derive post-hoc quantitative measurements. As momentary phenomena often fluctuate, these measurements can be only *probabilistic*. Time-relative probabilities are then obtained by relating these probabilistic measurements to the periods of time during which they were recorded and that are also precisely specified in terms of elements of the set *T* studied. Therefore, unlike other types of probability, time-relative probabilities always have a unit (of time) and their values are not constraint to values between 0 and 1 (but they cannot become negative; for details, see Uher, submitted, 2013, pp. 6-11).

The scientific quantifications thus-obtained are *ratio-scaled* because the international time standards provide equal units (e.g., minutes, hours) and because the non-occurrence of the events studied in the particular set *T* of occasions and periods of time considered in a study defines an absolute point of zero. For example, the aggressive behaviours of a particular child in his or her peer group during free play as measured in 10 hours of observation during 5 consecutive days could be scientifically quantified with an average of 40 seconds of expressing verbal insults to peers, no verbal insults to adults and two slaps to peers per hour. The measurement units thus-created (e.g., overall duration in seconds per hour, frequency per hour) can be understood in the same way all around the globe. Because data reflecting time-relative probabilities are ratio-scaled, they permit applications of all arithmetic operations and they can be directly compared across studies and disciplines (Uher, 2013, submitted). The concept of time-relative probabilities is therefore essential for comparing variations within and across individuals, groups and species.

Comparing variations within and between individuals, groups and species

The concept of time-relative probabilities enables scientifically quantified comparisons not only of *averages* but also of *variabilities* and *ranges* in the occurrences of events across time (e.g., day-to-day variabilities, longitudinal changes) within and between individuals, groups and species (Uher, 2015a,b,c). Exploring such patterns enables systematic contrasts with assessments that people provide on individuals and on differences between individuals, groups and species. Such contrast can shed a new light on the human tendencies to overestimate the magnitude of minor variations between individuals for differentiating highly similar individuals and to homogenise within-group differences and to exaggerate between-group differences for differentiating individuals from different groups and communities.

The TPS-Paradigm provides comprehensive methodological frameworks for enabling such explorations. In these frameworks, concepts from "personality" psychology, differential psychology, cross-cultural psychology and cross-species comparative psychology are systematically integrated and extended by novel ones (Uher, 2008a,b, 2011a,b).

Important insights about patterns of behavioural variations can be gained by comparing different kinds of variations with one another, such as by relating variations *within* particular samples of individuals to differences *between* particular samples. Different kinds of *samples* can be defined that are nested within each other, ranging from single individuals over various kinds of groups of (conspecific) individuals (e.g., of the same age, sex/gender, socio-economic status, level of education, nation, religion or language) up to species and groups of species. The following outlines basic concepts, focussing on individuals, groups and species as samples (see Table 1).

Data reflecting time-relative probabilities can be explored for patterns of within-individual variability around within-individual averages[6], for example, an individual's activity levels can be explored for day-to-day variability (de Weerth, van Geert, & Hoitink, 1999; van Geert & van Dijk, 2002). This allows for quantifying an individual's range of behavioural possibilities in terms of his or her average, minimum and maximum probability to show particular kinds of behaviours in particular kinds of situations (cf. the related concepts of individual density distributions of act frequencies or daily activity states; Buss & Craik, 1985, Fleeson, 2001). Studying within-individual variability is of particular importance for exploring the dynamics and processes of individual change and development (Thelen & Smith, 1993).

[6] Such approaches are often called ipsative-normative (Lazarus, 2000), sometimes also ideographic-nomothetic (Conner, Barrett, Tugade, & Tennen, 2007; Shoda, Mischel, & Wright, 1994); but because the connotations of these terms vary they are not used in the TPS-Paradigm.

Patterns of within-individual variability can be explored for commonalities and differences between individuals, such as between-individual differences in the day-to-day variability of individuals' activity (Uher, 2013). Patterns of within-individual variability can also be explored between the individuals of different groups, such as variability in daily activity patterns between individuals of different age groups (Table 1; for an overview of methods of analyses of variability, see van Geert & van Dijk, 2002).

Furthermore, individuals can be compared with one another in their averages. Differences between individuals' averages can be compared between different groups, such as between-individual differences in males with those in females. Averages of particular groups of individuals, in turn, can be explored for differences between groups, such as sex/ gender differences (e.g., Mehl, Vazire, Ramírez-Esparza, et al., 2007; Table 1). Between-group differences can be set in relation to differences between higher-order groups, such as by comparing sex/gender differences between different nations, amongst others, as studied in cross-cultural differential psychology (Heine et al., 2002; Leung & Bond, 1989; van de Vijver & Poortinga, 2002).

Research on nonhuman species opens up many further opportunities for comparing behavioural variations. For example, patterns of within-individual variability can be compared between species, such as within-individual variability in daily activity patterns between cats and dogs (e.g., Piccione, Marafioti, Giannetto, et al., 2014). Species can also be compared with regard to their between-individual differences or the between-individual differences of particular groups (e.g., sex differences in between-individual variations between three macaque species; Sussman, Ha, Bentson & Crockett, 2013, see also below) as is done in cross-species comparative differential and "personality" psychology (Uher, 2008a,b). Biologists frequently compare the averages of particular groups between species, such average age, sex/gender and social status differences between chimpanzees and bonobos (e.g., Boesch, Hohmann, & Marchant, 2000; Table 1).

Table 1 *Basic concepts for comparing variations within and between individuals, groups and species*

Differences between	Variations within		
	Individuals	**Groups**	**Species**
Individuals	*Between-individual differences in within-individual variations* (e.g., day-to-day variations around each individual's average activity level; Figure 1)	/	/
Groups	*Between-group differences in within-individual variations* (e.g., patterns of day-to-day variability compared between individuals of different age groups)	*Between-group differences in within-group variations* (e.g., individual differences in males compared with those in females)	/
Species	*Between-species differences in within-individual variations* (e.g., individual day-to-day variabilities in weeper capuchins compared to those in rhesus macaques; Table 2)	*Between-species differences in within-group variations* (e.g., individual differences in female bonobos compared with those in female chimpanzees)	*Between-species differences in within-species variations* (e.g., individual differences or average sex/gender differences in mandrills compared with those in toque macaques; Table 6)

Note. Patterns of behavioural variations can be explored by comparing different kinds of variations within and across different sample levels that are nested within each other, such as by relating *within-sample variations* to *between-sample differences.* The table specifies such comparisons, focussing on single individuals, groups of (conspecific) individuals and species as samples.

Applications of such comparative analyses can be demonstrated exemplarily with data from four nonhuman primate species. Individual behaviours were observed in 9 weeper capuchin monkeys (also called wedge-capped capuchins, *Cebus olivaceus*), 8 mandrills (*Mandrillus sphinx*) and 12 toque macaques (*Macaca sinica*) housed at the Berlin Zoological Garden and in 7 rhesus macaques (*Macaca mulatta*) housed at the Berlin animal shelter (Germany). The individuals[7] of each species lived together in one social group. Capuchins are

[7] The sample consisted 8 mandrills (4 males, 4 females), 12 toque macaques (5 males, 7 females), 9 weeper capuchins (3 males, 6 females) and 7 rhesus macaques (3 males, 4 females). It comprised individuals of all age groups; in the weeper capuchins, mean age was 6 years (*Mdn* = 3 years; range 1-21 years), in the mandrills, mean age was 9.75 years (*Mdn* = 8 years; range 1-26

endemic to South-America, mandrills to Africa and macaques to Asia. All four species live in multi-male multi-female groups but their behavioural and social systems differ (e.g., the dominance behaviours of mandrills and rhesus macaques are described as "despotic", whereas those of capuchins and toque macaques are described as "egalitarian" (Fragaszy et al., 2004; Thierry, 2007; Otovic, Partan, Bryant, & Hutchinson, 2014).

Analyses of between-individual differences in within-individual variations and averages can be illustrated by observational data on the behavioural activities of the 7 Rhesus macaques. Three behaviours representing different degrees of physical activity were differentiated on the basis of observable properties and were encoded in three mutually exclusive categories, thus on a nominal scale. Resting and not moving was encoded as "sit", moving on the spot but not changing the location was encoded as "move" and moving about, thus changing location as "run". Using nunc-ipsum methods and scan sampling instantaneous recording, the observers recorded (amongst others) the activity state of each individual in the group in 20-minute intervals starting from the end of the last scan. On average, data were collected on 14.8 scan sample occasions per day (*Mdn* = 14; range 12-16) from 10 a.m. to 5 p.m.; observations occurred on 12 days within a 4-week period (3 days per week).

These binary encoded raw data were post-hoc accumulated over all scans within each day and then divided by the number of scans collected on each given day. The ratio-scaled data thus-generated for each day reflect each individual's time-relative probabilities for showing the three activity behaviours at a randomly selected moment during the times of the day studied. Hence, these data allow for estimating each individual's daily time-budgets with regard to his or her physical activity. Figure 1a depicts the individuals' daily time-relative probabilities for showing activity states categorised as "move" (upper graphs) and as "run" (lower graphs); thus, the difference between each individual's daily sum of these scores to 1.0 represents his or her daily time-relative probability for resting ("sit"; not depicted).

The activity levels of the 7 Rhesus macaques varied considerably within each individual from day-to-day over the 12 days of observation (Figure 1a). The patterns of within-individual variability and individuals' averages over these 12 days (shown as continuous horizontal lines across each individual's graph) differed between individuals. The time-relative probabilities for moving about of the first individual, the male Rh_2P20, were similar to those of the second individual, the female Rh_1S07. But his average time-relative probabilities for moving on the spot were much lower than those of that female. In fact, his average was lower than the average of all Rhesus individuals studied (shown as dotted line across the graphs of all individuals), whereas her average was higher than the Rhesus average. But his within-individual variability in moving on the spot, thus

---

years); in the toque macaques, mean age was 4.69 years (*Mdn* = 4 years; range 0.25-13 years) and in the rhesus macaques, mean age was 17.68 years (*Mdn* = 20 years; range 7-31 years).

his range of behavioural probabilities for showing moderate activity levels was much higher than hers.

Figure 1 *Between-individual differences in within-individual variabilities and averages in the physical activity of seven rhesus macaques*

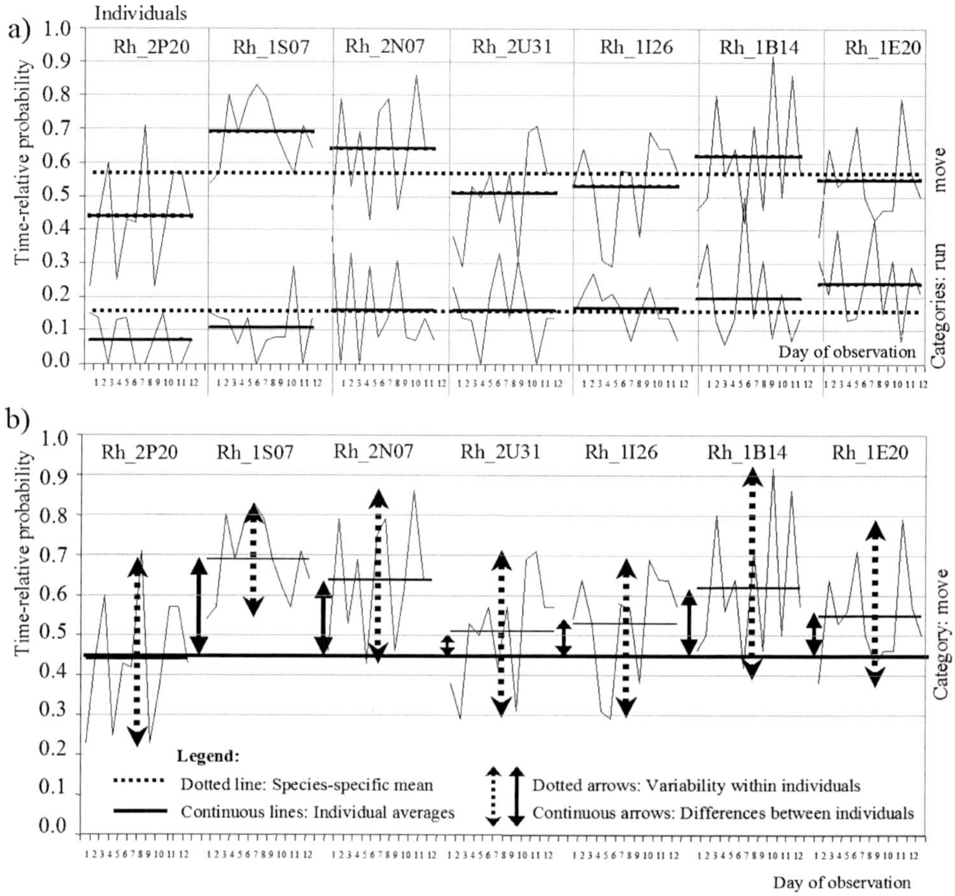

Note. The estimated time-relative probabilities of 7 rhesus macaque individuals for showing activity states categorised as "move" (i.e., moving on the spot; upper graphs) and "run" (i.e., moving about and changing location; lower graphs); the difference between each individual's daily sum of these scores to 1.0 thus indicates his or her time-relative probability for resting ("sit"; not depicted). The graphs show each individual's daily averages of his or her time-relative probabilities across 12 days of observation carried out within a 4-week period. *a)* Individuals' averages over these 12 days are shown as continuous horizontal lines across each individual's graph; the averages of all 7 rhesus individuals over the 12 days are shown as dotted lines across the graphs of all individuals. *b)* The day-to-day variability within individuals was much higher than the average between-individual variability as highlighted by the dotted and continuous vertical arrows for the individual variations in moving. Statistically seen, this is due to the higher reliability of the aggregated measurements generated at higher sample levels. But this broad range of individuals' behavioural possibilities shows that individual differences in behavioural patterns as they occur in everyday life are much less pronounced than those that can be extracted statistically from data or abstracted mentally from past observations.

The within-individual day-to-day variability was generally much higher than the average between-individual variability as highlighted by the dotted and continuous vertical arrows in Figure 1b for the individual variations in moving on the spot. These findings are in accordance with robust findings from cross-cultural psychology indicating that "within-unit variance overwhelms between-unit variance whatever the unit—individual, family, or culture" (Shweder & Sullivan, 1990, p. 412). Statistically, these differences in magnitude between within-sample variability and between-sample variability can be explained by the higher reliability of the aggregated measurements generated at higher sample levels. But importantly, this broad range of individuals' behavioural possibilities[8] illustrates that individual differences in behavioural patterns—as they occur in everyday life—are much less pronounced than those that can be extracted statistically from data or that can be abstracted mentally from observations made in the past.

Comparative analyses using nunc-ipsum recorded behavioural data therefore enable insightful contrasts to be applied with findings obtained from assessment studies, which are inherently based on strong aggregation (see below). Such contrast allow for exploring the human abilities to quickly form impressions of individuals and to develop for this purpose socially shared socio-cognitive categories in which observable variations are represented in either exaggerated or oversimplified ways. Given the enormous variability that can occur within and between individuals, such analyses presuppose metatheoretical and analytical concepts that enable scientists to disentangle patterns that are specific to particular individuals from those that are common to all of them (Uher, 2011a,b, 2015a).

Disentangling the specific from the common

Comparing individual variations requires the identification of what is specific to a particular individual, group or species and what is common to all individuals of the particular sample considered. Given that in research on individuals the basic ontological entity is the individual, the concept of individual-specificity is of central importance.

Individual-specificity: Metatheoretical concepts and methodological implications

In momentary and fluctuating phenomena like behaviours in which within-individual variations are often pronounced, patterns in the occurrences of

[8] The daily time-relative probability scores for physical activity shown in Figure 1 were also derived from aggregation over all on average 14.8 data points collected on each given day, which in turn are only time samples from the whole range of behavioural variability that occurred in these individuals.

events that can be empirically obtained for individuals can only be *probabilistic*. To be specific to an individual, these probabilistic patterns must differ between individuals, thus be *differential*. To make sure that these probabilistic between-differences reflect not just random variations derived from the dynamic fluctuations of behaviours, these patterns must also be stable for at least some amount of time, thus be *temporally stable* (Uher, 2011a).

Hence, individual-specificity is an abstract theoretical construct denoting the coincidence of differential and temporal patterns and, in momentary and fluctuating phenomena, also of probabilistic patterns in the occurrences of events. It was shown that the idea of individual-specificity is elementary to all definitions of "personality" and that definitions differ in the particular phenomena considered, which depends on the particular philosophical presuppositions made by the authors (Uher, 2013). For enabling transdisciplinary research, the TPS-Paradigm therefore conceives of "personality" as individual-specificity in *all* of the various kinds of phenomena explored in individuals (Uher, 2015a,b,c).

Importantly, neither differential, nor temporal nor probabilistic patterns can be directly observed in any given moment. Instead, to identify individual-specificity, (non-)occurrences of defined behavioural events must be recorded using nunc-ipsum methods and repeatedly across many occasions. The nominal-scaled behavioural raw data must be accumulated over time within each individual to generate post-hoc ratio-scaled scientific quantifications of *individual patterns* using the concept of time-relative probabilities. These individual patterns must then be compared between individuals to identify *differential patterns*.

But direct comparisons of scores within and between individuals are hindered because, in any given sample, different kinds of behaviours generally occur with different frequencies (cf. the differences in the average occurrences of behavioural activities coded as "moving" and "running" in Rhesus macaques; see the dotted horizontal lines in Figure 1). Even the same kind of behaviour commonly occurs with different frequencies across different kinds of situations. Differential analyses therefore require that the individuals' time-relative probabilities for showing a particular behaviour are statistically standardised across all individuals within each kind of situation studied and within the time periods for which the scores are determined (Uher, 2011a, 2013). Time-relative probability scores can be differentially standardised, for example, by using *z*-standardisation in which the deviation of individual scores from the mean score of all studied individuals is divided by their standard deviation (same time units provided).

Differential standardisation transforms scientific quantifications of *absolute* individual scores into scores reflecting *relative* between-individual differences. Therefore, differentially standardised time-relative probabilities have no time units. But as they were generated in specified steps of data processing rather than implicitly as is the case when people generate "personality" assessments, the absolute time-relative probabilities from which the differential time-relative probabilities were derived can always be traced when needed for interpretation, analyses and comparisons with other sets of individuals (as demonstrated below). Differential standardisation also enables direct comparison of scores between variables with different time units (e.g., frequencies, durations) both within and between individuals. It also enables statistical aggregations of different variables into composite or summary variables as required for computing construct measures (see below).

To identify individual-specificity, the differential patterns thus-identified must be shown to be stable across time periods longer than those in which the measurements were first ascertained and in ways that are considered to be meaningful (e.g., defined by the strength of statistical correlations over specified time periods). Thus, temporal patterns are to be explored in patterns that are in and of themselves defined by a certain temporal stability. To consider the effects of aggregation on the reliability of measurements, comparisons between individuals presuppose that the number of occasions and the lengths of the time periods considered for estimating individuals' time-relative probabilities are comparable and at best identical between the individuals being compared (Uher, 2013; Uher et al., 2013a).

Such analyses of individual-specificity can be illustrated by observational data on the rhesus macaques studied at the Berlin animal shelter and the weeper capuchins, mandrills and toque macaques studied at the Berlin Zoological Garden. Three constructs of individual-specificity describing social behaviours were studied. *Social orientation* was operationalised with grooming others and three proximity measures indicating different distances to the target individuals (i.e., body contact, arm length distance and 1m distance). *Aggressiveness* was operationalised with behaviours of contact aggression and non-contact aggression. *Dominance* was operationalised with dominant behaviours (i.e., displacing others) and behaviours of subordination (i.e., be displaced by others, subordinate to others) as indicators of low dominance.

The specific perceptible forms of these behaviours slightly varied between these four species also because they differ morphologically from one another to some extent. For example, mandrills are much larger than capuchins and the macaques. Mandrills have one of the greatest sexual dimorphisms of all primates, whereas in the other three species studied, the differences between males' and females' body sizes are still pronounced but much less than in the mandrills; Fragaszy et al., 2004; Thierry, 2007; Otovic et al., 2014). Therefore, it was the observers' task to abstract from this perceptible variability of these species' behaviours and to demarcate and categorise events that can be considered functionally comparable across the species studied. The inter-observer reliability in encoding the occurrences of these 9 different behaviours in the different species was high[9], demonstrating intersubjective agreement between two persons in the encoding of behavioural occurrences in the raw data.

[9] Inter-observer reliability in the binary scaled encoding of the (non-)occurrences of all 9 behaviours at specified times was studied across all species with Cohen's κ, which was also used as a very

In each of the three species observed at Berlin Zoo, the duration behaviours grooming and proximity were recorded using scan sampling instantaneous recording every 15 minutes starting from the last scan. The frequency behaviours of aggression and dominance generally occur less frequently and were therefore recorded using event sampling event recording, in which the observers recorded these events whenever they occurred in the group during a 5-minute time sample directly after completing the scan sampling records in the given species. On average, data were collected on 21 scan sample occasions and 21 event sample occasions per day and species (*Mdn* = 23; range 11-26) between 9 a.m. and 5 p.m. In the Rhesus macaques observed at the Berlin animal shelter, the same behaviours were recorded using the same behavioural categories and encoding scheme. But a slightly different time sample scheme was used. Scan sampling occurred only every 20 min, enabling the recording of on average 13.8 scan sample occasions per day (see above). Event recording of aggressive and dominant behaviours occurred during 20 minute time samples on 11 occasions on average per day.

For enabling direct quantitative comparisons between all four species, individuals' time-relative probabilities were standardised in two different ways so that the data represent exactly the same time units and the same situational conditions. First, the data obtained from the different time sample schemes were made directly comparable with one another by converting them into the same basic time samples. Thus in both studies, the binary raw data of the scan sample records were accumulated over all scan occasions within each day and then divided by the number of scans collected on each given day. The same was done for the binary raw data of the event samples in the zoo study. In the animal shelter study, the event sample data were accumulated over all 20-minute event samples collected within each day and then standardised to a time sample of 5 minutes, which corresponds to the basic time sample used in the zoo study. Otherwise, the frequencies of the event behaviours (i.e., aggression and dominance) in the Rhesus macaques would be significantly overestimated.

The ratio-scaled data thus-generated for each day reflect each individual's absolute time-relative probabilities for grooming when observed at a randomly selected moment and for showing each of the aggression and dominance behaviours during a randomly selected time sample of 5 minutes (during the times of the day studied). The proximity data reflect the average number of conspecifics in different distances to the target individual when observed at a randomly selected moment. Hence, the data thus-obtained are standardised with regard to the time units that they reflect. For example, an individual may have an absolute time-

strict measure for testing agreement between two observers in encoding the number of conspecifics located at different distances to the target individual. Inter-observer reliability computed over 621 single observations was high (κ_m = .87, ranging from κ =.74 to .99). For comparison, mean Pearson-correlations were r_m = .95** (computed using *r*-to-*Z* transformation), ranging from *r* = .81 to .99.

relative probability of 0.18 (i.e., an 18% probability) for showing contact aggression within 5 minutes of observation and it may be in arm-length distance to on average 0.23 conspecifics when observed at a randomly selected moment.

Second, for enabling direct quantitative comparisons of social interaction behaviours between individuals from social groups of different sizes, individuals' absolute time-relative probabilities were also standardised to a hypothetical number of 10 potential interaction partners within each group. The data thus-standardised reflect the average number of conspecifics in proximity and the average time-relative probabilities for showing the particular behaviours studied if 10 potential partners were available for each individual studied.

Observations in the zoo were carried out on 15 days, 5 days per week each in the first two weeks (t_1 and t_2) and in the last week (t_3) of a 5-week period. The 12 days of observation in the animal shelter were carried out within a 4-week period, thus in a time-span comparable to the time period covered by t_2 and t_3 of the zoo study. For temporal analyses, the data from the animal shelter study were therefore divided into two 2-week periods of 6 days each and assigned to the time periods t_2 and t_3 of the zoo study. This schedule enables temporal analyses over a 2-week period (t_1-t_2; in the zoo study), a 4-week period (t_2-t_3) and a 5-week period (t_1-t_3; in the zoo study). Overall, each individual of the three species studied at the zoo was observed for 80 hours, 26.5 hours on average per study period; each Rhesus individual was observed for 60 hours in total and 30 hours on average per study period. Hence, despite the different time sample schemes used in the zoo and in the animal shelter, the time periods used for estimating individuals' time-relative probabilities are comparable, thus enabling direct comparisons of the data between all four species.

To explore whether the individuals' absolute time-relative probabilities obtained from this observation scheme reflect individual-specific patterns, the between-individual variations of each behaviour category were analysed for temporal stability between the three study periods. This was done for each species separately by computing (Pearson) test-retest correlations of the rank-order of individuals' scores for each behavioural variable (i.e., using variable-oriented analyses; Bergmann & Trost, 2006; Uher, 2011a). Rank-order stability was explored in both individuals' averages (using individuals' means within each study period) and their within-individual variations (using the corresponding standard deviations). For an exemplary demonstration, some categories describing functionally related behaviours were summarised into more abstract categories; therefore, the individuals' scores on some more specific behavioural variables were added into scores on summary variables (i.e., the three different proximity measures, the two aggression measures and the two subordination measures; see Table 2). These *summary scores* still reflect *absolute* time relative probabilities (e.g., for showing any kind of aggressive behaviours in a randomly selected 5-minute time sample), which helps to demonstrate basic principles on which the subsequent steps of analyses are based.

In all behavioural (summary) scores, between-individual variations in individuals' *averages* were test-retest reliable over most study periods and in most species (except for the Subordination score SU in the toque macaques over 4-week and 5-week periods and in the weeper capuchins; see Table 2). These findings provide evidence for individual-specific patterns (considering the limited power of these analyses due to the small sample sizes). By contrast, between-individual variations in within-individual *variabilities* tended to be less test-retest reliable. In some behavioural scores, the test-retest reliability was low over some study periods and in some species; in the Proximity summary scores (PX) it was low over all study periods and in all species. This indicates that within-individual variability was pronounced and sometimes not differentially stable, in and of itself, despite the temporally stable and thus individual-specific patterns shown in within-individual averages (Table 2).

Table 2 *Temporal stability of between-individual differences in within-individual averages and variabilities over 2, 4 and 5 weeks: Evidence for individual-specific patterns within each species*

Behaviours xx Species	Within-individual averages (*m*) 2 weeks t_1-t_2 *r*	*p*	4 weeks t_2-t_3 *r*	*p*	5 weeks t_1-t_3 *r*	*p*	Within-individual variabilities (*sd*) 2 weeks t_1-t_2 *r*	*p*	4 weeks t_2-t_3 *r*	*p*	5 weeks t_1-t_3 *r*	*p*
GR Grooming score												
Weeper capuchins	**.72***	(.030)	**.96****	(.000)	**.71***	(.034)	.60	(.090)	**.87****	(.002)	**.74***	(.023)
Mandrills	.70	(.056)	**.91****	(.002)	**.72***	(.045)	.63	(.096)	**.74***	(.036)	**.90****	(.002)
Toque macaques	**.93****	(.000)	**.81****	(.001)	**.86****	(.000)	.46	(.129)	.54	(.070)	.43	(.162)
Rhesus macaques	-	-	.66	(.089)	-	-			.52	(.228)		
PX Proximity summary score												
Weeper capuchins	**.81****	(.009)	**.94****	(.000)	**.78***	(.012)	-.26	(.492)	.17	(.659)	.46	(.212)
Mandrills	**.89****	(.003)	.67	(.068)	.52	(.184)	-.19	(.647)	-.27	(.512)	-.25	(.543)
Toque macaques	**.92****	(.000)	**.95****	(.000)	**.94****	(.000)	.28	(.374)	.38	(.217)	.08	(.815)
Rhesus macaques	-	-	.64	(.125)	-	-			-.17	(.719)		
AG Aggression summary score												
Weeper capuchins	**.93****	(.000)	**.92****	(.000)	**.88****	(.002)	**.81****	(.008)	**.71***	(.034)	.65	(.058)
Mandrills	.68	(.064)	**.73***	(.039)	**.97****	(.000)	**.71***	(.048)	.69	(.056)	**.96****	(.000)
Toque macaques	**.72****	(.008)	**.78****	(.003)	.54	(.071)	.27	(.387)	**.59***	(.044)	.30	(.351)
Rhesus macaques	-	-	.71	(.077)	-	-			-.08	(.863)		
DI Displacement score												
Weeper capuchins	**.98****	(.000)	**.96****	(.000)	**.99****	(.000)	**.94****	(.000)	**.92****	(.000)	**.99****	(.000)
Mandrills	**.92****	(.001)	**.85****	(.008)	**.93****	(.001)	.50	(.204)	.11	(.787)	**.86****	(.007)
Toque macaques	**.92****	(.000)	**.85****	(.001)	**.95****	(.000)	**.59***	(.045)	.35	(.267)	**.76****	(.004)
Rhesus macaques	-	-	**.78***	(.038)	-	-			.38	(.399)		
SU Subordination summary score												
Weeper capuchins	.31	(.421)	.51	(.160)	-.23	(.562)	.45	(.219)	.63	(.068)	-.14	(.718)
Mandrills	**.89****	(.003)	**.82***	(.012)	**.82***	(.013)	**.89****	(.002)	**.86****	(.006)	**.83***	(.010)
Toque macaques	**.80****	(.002)	.44	(.149)	.08	(.811)	.07	(.830)	**.65***	(.022)	-.01	(.968)
Rhesus macaques	-	-	**.89****	(.007)	-	-			.73	(.065)		

Note. * $p < .05$; * $p < .01$. Variable-oriented analyses of the test-retest reliability of between-individual differences within each species (weeper capuchins, $N = 9$; mandrills, $N = 8$; toque macaques, $N = 12$; rhesus macaques, $N = 7$) using Pearson correlation *r*. The temporal stabilities of individuals' averages were calculated using the mean scores of individuals' absolute time-relative probabilities for showing a given behaviour and the mean scores of the number of conspecifics in proximity, respectively. The temporal stabilities of individuals' corresponding patterns of day-to-day variability were computed using the standard deviations. The summary scores represent more abstract categories of encoding and were derived by summarising the scores of more specific behavioural variables: The Proximity summary score summarises the three proximity measures, the Aggression summary score summarises contact and non-contact aggression, and the Subordination summary score summaries the categories being displaced by others and subordinating to others. The Grooming score and the Dominance score are no summary scores; they reflect grooming and displacement of others, respectively. For more direct comparisons between samples of different sizes, the correlations of each given sample (e.g., species) should be weighted by the sample sizes studied (not done in these exemplary demonstrations).

Exploring individual variations from three interrelated viewpoints: Specificity/ uniqueness, comparability and universality/ typicality

The concept of individual-specificity highlights that exploring individual variations involves three inter-related viewpoints—*specificity (i.e., uniqueness), comparability* and *universality (i.e., typicality)*. It shows that *specificity* can be determined and quantified only in relation to other individuals of the same kind. This implies that individuals can be compared with one another, thus *comparability*. The determination of both specificity and comparability depends on the particular set *I* of individuals considered (i.e., the reference population), which, in turn, determines the specifications of *universality* (Uher, 2008a,b).

In research on individual-specificity ("personality"), universality always refers to *populations* of individuals (e.g., groups or species) but not to single individuals because patterns that all individuals of particular a group or species show in the same way cannot be individual-specific. Individual patterns that are universal for all individuals of particular groups or species are explored in other fields of research (e.g., general psychology, biology, anthropology).

Importantly, the highest possible level for determining individual-specificity is the species level because species are considered the smallest biological populations that differ distinctively and not just continuously from another due to intrinsic barriers that prevent interbreeding (Campbell & Reece, 2005; Uher, 2008a,b). Thus, same-species individuals share essential organismal properties and are therefore similar to considerable extent. It is the variations occurring within this essential similarity of same-species individuals that are explored in research on individual-specificity (e.g., differential psychology, "personality" research). In the analyses presented above for illustrating these principles, the temporal patterns of individual differences were therefore analysed separately for each of the four primate species studied (Table 2).

The concepts of specificity, comparability and universality can be applied for explorations of individual variations across all sample levels. For example, if particular kinds of between-individual or between-group variations in humans are found only in a particular cultural community, then they are culture-specific. If all cultural communities exhibit these variations in similar ways, then these variations are universal to the human species (Kluckhohn, Murray, & Schneider, 1953). If particular kinds of variations are shown only by humans but not by any other species, then these variations are human-specific (or uniquely human). If several species show comparable kinds of between-individual or of between-group variations, then they can be considered universal for this particular group of species, for example, variations may be universally primate, universally mammalian or perhaps even universally vertebrate (Uher, 2008b). If the focus lies on comparisons between groups of species that do not exhibit a particular kind of variation, this variation can be, for example, primate-specific, mammal-specific and so on.

The pivotal point of such explorations is the concept of comparability being applied and the ways in which it is methodologically implemented in a given study.

Principles for establishing comparability

In a strict sense, no individual of whatever group or species is exactly like another, even if the differences are only small. Between-individual variability is pervasive—and it is essential for evolution (Darwin, 1859). Individuals from different groups and, to a much greater extent, individuals from different species often differ from one another in significant ways, such as in their morphology, behaviours and the behavioural situations they encounter in their lives as well as in the functions and meanings that these phenomena may have for these individuals (e.g., head-shaking and nodding signalling agreement or non-agreement; Uher, 2008a,b, 2013). Specifying the perceptible properties on which the demarcations of events can be based makes painfully clear that establishing comparability is *always* a matter of decision and abstraction on the parts of human individuals, whether explicitly or implicitly.

The more diverse the perceptible properties of the phenomena under study are, the more abstract the levels of abstraction need to be in order to establish comparability. Phrased differently, the more abstract the level of consideration, the more comparable will the properties considered appear to be. The particular kinds of abstractions on which observations of individual behaviour are based differ from those required in assessments.

Essential differences between observations and assessments

Observers are confronted with the heterogeneous properties of the fluctuating and dynamic phenomena of behaviour that can be directly perceived in the particular situations and time periods of observation. Observers must accomplish the difficult task to demarcate and abstract from this diversity particular kinds of events that can be considered to be identically repeatable at least to some extent. Thus, observers must establish *comparability between particular perceptible properties* to identify commonalities and differences between them in order to demarcate, abstract and categorise behavioural events. Observers must do this in systematic and standardised ways and in the given moments in which the events occur. To achieve this, observers are instructed and trained to focus their perception on particular properties specified in the encoding schemes, which are specifically developed for this purpose and tested for their viability using scientific principles.

Assessments also rely on people's perceptions of the complex properties of behaviours—yet on perceptions that they have made in the past without having been instructed or trained to focus on particular properties and to demarcate and categorise events in particular ways. In their everyday lives, people rely on intuitive abstractions often using the socio-cognitive categories that are encoded in everyday language. Assessment methods capitalise on this everyday knowledge by wording the statements to be assessed in everyday language and by using abstract and global everyday terms that are applicable to diverse kinds of properties and phenomena yet without specifying any particular ones.

But unlike scientific categories, everyday categories are not explicitly defined, well structured and disjunctive; rather, they are often fuzzy and context-sensitive, thus allowing for flexible demarcations (Hammersley, 2013). The words denoting everyday categories are used for making perceivably different properties subjectively comparable. Moreover, words are often erroneously assumed to directly reflect the phenomena that they denote (called the *fallacy of misplaced concreteness*; Bentham in Ogden, 1932; Whitehead, 1929). But this is possible only for words denoting concrete phenomena that can be directly perceived but not for words denoting abstract ideas that can be derived only by mental *construct*ion—such as words that denote individual-specific behaviours or "personality" (Uher, 2015b,c).

As a result, the particular elements of the sets *B* of behaviours, *S* of situations, *T* of time and *I* of individuals to which particular everyday words and statements may refer for particular individuals in particular situations (e.g., when generating assessments) will necessarily vary. In fact, it was already shown that the meanings that raters construct for the standardised item statements of established assessment instruments often vary considerably both within and between raters (Arro, 2013; Rosenbaum & Valsiner, 2011). This variability in people's interpretations of descriptors and statements about individual behaviours may also derive from the fact that everyday categories reflect not only abstractions from perceptible properties but also abstractions and categorisations that are made on the basis of implicit assumptions about the functions, meanings and values that particular behavioural events may have for particular individuals, thus on assumptions about their *functional comparability*.

In contrast to the forms of particular events and phenomena, the particular functions and meanings that they may have for particular individuals depend on complex constellations and can seldom be directly perceived or straightforwardly inferred. Assumptions about functions and meanings of behaviours therefore vary between groups of individuals, such as between different sociocultural and language communities (e.g., the particular behaviours considered "insulting" and "aggressive"). These different assumptions are implicitly contained in the sociocognitive categories and pertinent vocabularies that are established and used by human communities in their everyday lives. Therefore, the everyday words of different sociocultural communities may reflect different abstractions and categorisations of observable properties and phenomena.

Consequently, the apparently greater and more direct comparability of assessments of individual behaviours as compared to pertinent observational data solely derives from the much higher levels of abstraction on which everyday categories are based and should therefore not be mistaken as an indicator of higher data quality as this is the case in many fields of psychological and "personality" research (Uher, 2011b, 2015a,b,c). On the contrary, assessment methods fail to fulfil the requirements of scientific quantification because they specify neither the particular elements to be quantified nor the principles used for establishing comparability between particular elements nor the algorithms used for generating quantitative data on the empirical occurrences and interrelations of the elements considered (Uher, submitted). Comparability cannot be established by simply using identical words and statements in assessments because words are only signs that are used for encoding properties of the actual phenomena under study.

Establishing functional comparability of behavioural and situational categories

The TPS-Paradigm emphasises that comparability between kinds of events that differ in their perceptible properties can be established only on the basis of the known or assumed functions and meanings that they may have for the individuals of the different groups or species that are compared with one another (Uher, 2013, 2015a). Functional commonalities and dissimilarities between different kinds of events specify the *theoretical interrelations* of the studied elements within and between the sets *B, S, I* and *T*, which is prerequisite for empirical analyses (see below; Uher, submitted).

A systematic theoretical framework for establishing comparability in a behavioural study can be developed on the basis of a category system describing the known or assumed functions and meanings of the particular kinds of behaviours and behavioural situations studied on different levels of abstraction. In such frameworks, abstract functional concepts (e.g., survival) are broken down stepwise into more specific ones (e.g., finding food, finding shelter, defence against attacks from others; cf. Uher, 2008a). On lower levels of abstraction, the functional categories can be systematically linked with abstract categories of the perceptible properties of the behaviours studied (e.g., different modes of communication) and of the different kinds of phenomena that are comprised by a given behavioural situation (e.g., physical properties of objects or behavioural properties of other individuals present in a situation).

For example, a theoretical framework of functional categories of social contact behaviours may comprise specific categories that may each describe functions for establishing, maintaining and ending proximity to others, for keeping and increasing distance to others, etc. Each of these functional categories, in turn, may comprise more specific categories comprising the particular vocal, facial, gestural or postural behaviours shown by the individuals of the particular groups or species under study.

Statistical analyses of configurational comparability: Construct equivalence and patterning effects

Theoretical frameworks specifying the known or assumed functional interrelations between the events studied are prerequisite for analysing the *empirical interrelations* of their occurrences, such as to explore the statistical comparability of construct measures. For systematic explorations, scientists develop an empirical framework comprising the particular measurement variables that are used in a given study to operationalise the constructs that are specified in the theoretical framework. Systematic linkages within and between the theoretical and the empirical frameworks are specified using the concept of *nomological networks* (cf. Cronbach & Meehl, 1955).

For the primate studies used for illustrating the basic concepts, a theoretical framework was established specifying the three behavioural constructs of individual-specificity studied (Social orientation, Aggressiveness and Dominance) and the theoretical interrelations of the behavioural categories that each construct comprises. An empirical framework was defined specifying for each of the behavioural categories specific behavioural variables (e.g., different proximity measures for physical proximity) that were used in the encoding schemes for generating the data. This nomological network comprising the theoretical and the empirical framework guided the computation of composite measures of both the constructs and the behavioural (summary) scores as well as the analyses of their configurational comparability between species as shown below.

Statistical analyses of the configurational comparability of construct measures between different groups or species can draw on analytical concepts from cross-cultural "personality" psychology (Uher, 2008b), such as on the statistical concepts and methods for exploring *structural or construct equivalence* (van de Vijver & Leung, 1997a,b; van de Vijver & Poortinga, 1997). Configurational comparability in the empirical interrelations of composite measures across different constructs in terms of their latent structures (as described, e.g., in taxonomic "personality" models) can capitalise on the concepts and methods used for exploring *patterning effects* (Leung & Bond, 1989; Uher, 2008a,b).

Limitations and fallacies of assessment-based comparative analyses

The concepts and methods needed for such statistical analyses were primarily developed in assessment-based research where they are used to explore the empirical comparability between sets of data obtained for different groups of individuals (e.g., national, cultural or linguistic communities). These analyses are based on the widespread idea that comparability of measurements could be established by using the same assessment instruments or translated versions of it (van de Vijver & Tanzer, 2004)—an idea that cannot withstand critical analysis from a philosophy-of-science perspective. Assessment data are generated (mostly by lay people) on the basis of unspecified rules for demarcating, abstracting, converting and encoding information from the properties and phenomena to be assessed. Hence, it remains unspecified what particular properties and events the data thus-generated actually reflect and on what particular considerations the raters may have actually based their assumptions of comparability between observable properties (Uher, 2015b,c). Functionally comparable behaviours need not—and often do not—have spatio-temporal forms that are identical across the different samples studied.

Independent of this, construct measures are commonly derived by aggregating or adding together the raw scores across several measurement variables, thus across different scales. Although it is well known that ordinal-scaled units do not permit such arithmetic operations, these practices are widespread in psychology and the social sciences. Their application is commonly justified by assuming that inferences can be made from the statistical properties and structures of the empirical data (e.g., distribution patterns, latent factors) to the properties of the phenomena that these data are meant to represent. Therefore, metric properties that can be found in assessment data are widely assumed to constitute the ultimate evidence that the phenomena toward which they are targeted could have metric properties as well (cf. Michell, 2011, 2012). But importantly, such inferences are possible only if the ways in which the *data* were generated in the first place fulfil the requirements of scientific measurement (Uher, submitted).

The frequent finding that assessment data meet the assumptions of sophisticated statistical theories merely results from the rigorous selection of only those particular measurement variables that allow for generating sets of data that meet these particular assumptions and from discarding all those variables that do not meet them. This procedure radically matches the data generation to statistical theories rather than to the properties of the actual phenomena under study that therefore cannot be explored in data thus-produced (Uher, 2015b,c). In addition to these limitations derived from the ways in which assessment data are generated, further limitations and fallacies must be considered in the statistical analyses that are commonly used in assessment-based comparative research.

Limitations and fallacies of redundancy-based statistical analyses

The statistical analyses that are most frequently used for exploring configurational structures within and between construct measures (e.g., factor analysis, cluster analysis) rely on similarities and dissimilarities in the co-variations of scores of different measurement variables. Given that co-variation reflects redundancies (Uher, 2015b,c), this allows for the parsimonious description of the empirical variation contained in the data in aggregate scores on more abstract composite variables (Kaplan & Saccuzzo, 2008). It is widespread practice in many fields of research to reduce sets of variables solely on the basis of their empirical patterns of co-variation and to interpret the composite variables thus-created (e.g., factors, clusters) as reflecting meaningful phenomena. These practices are increasingly applied also to observational data, in particular in animal "personality" research.

But actually what does it mean if particular kinds of behaviours happen to occur in a given sample of individuals in similar ways over a specified period of time even if these behaviours are functionally unrelated or do not occur in spatio-temporal proximity? Researchers of individuals commonly interpret such kinds of overall empirical co-variation as reflecting "common underlying mechanisms" (cf. Allport, 1937; Cattell, 1946). But analyses of *between*-individual variations cannot yield results that are generalisable to the understanding and explanation of *within*-individual variations—much less of internal mechanisms or even their dynamics (Block, 2010; Cervone et al., 2001; Omi, 2012; Molenaar, 2004; Toomela, 2011; Uher, 2014, 2015b,c; van Geert & van Dijk, 2002). This type of fallacy, called *ecological fallacy* (Robinson, 1950), occurs in different forms in all fields of research (Pollet, Tybur, Frankenhuis, & Rickard, 2014; Subramanian, Jones, Kaddour, & Krieger, 2009; Uher, 2015c). It occurs, for example, when researchers erroneously project onto each other patterns of within-individual and between-individual variations (Moolenaar, 2004; Toomela, 2011), patterns of between-individual and between-group variations (Thorndike, 1939) or patterns of between-individual and between-culture variations (Hofsteede, 2001). Analogous fallacies also occur in cross-species comparisons.

When behavioural events functionally depend on one another (e.g., in primates, grooming involves body contact but not every body contact is due to grooming), then their empirical occurrences necessarily co-vary on the sample level. For example, the occurrences of body contact and grooming were moderately correlated in the weeper capuchins ($r = .28, p < .05$), the mandrills ($r = .20$; $p < .10$), the toque macaques ($r = .47$; $p < .01$) and the rhesus macaques ($r = .21$; $p < .05$). But such overall co-variations may not be found if functionally similar behaviours are assumed to differ in their functional intensity (e.g., if, in a particular situation, one act of contact aggression may fulfil the same function like three acts of non-contact aggression). In fact, empirical occurrences of functionally similar behaviours often show only low to moderate, sometimes even zero consistency across individuals (Uher, 2011a,b, 2015b; Uher et al., 2008, 2013a). Behavioural scientists studying humans have also reported repeatedly that the factors emerging from factor-analyses accounted for only low to moderate percentages of the variance in behavioural data (Blurton Jones, 1967, 1972; Smith, 1973; Smith & Connolly, 1972, 1980). The analyses revealed "intrinsic statistical inadequacies in the statistical treatment of consistency" in behavioural data (Allport & Vernon, 1933, p. 47).

The TPS-Paradigm therefore questions the utility of redundancy-based reduction principles for studies that are targeted towards exploring real-life issues (Uher, 2015b,c). Far more illuminative than explorations of redundancies between behavioural events are, for example, analyses of their spatio-temporal interrelations. This requires statistical context-based reduction principles that enable explorations of temporally and situationally contextualised behavioural data (amongst others; for details, see Uher, 2015b). Such data cannot be obtained with assessment methods. For exploring configurational comparability, function-based reduction principles are therefore needed as explored now.

Statistical explorations of configurational comparability

Constructs are abstract concepts denoting complex entities that are only *construct*ed by human minds and that therefore cannot be directly perceived (e.g., "personality"; intelligence; Cronbach & Meehl, 1955). As a consequence, the analysis of configurational comparability is primarily a theoretical task and only secondarily an empirical one.

Exploring configurational comparability using function-based reduction principles and ratio-scaled time-relative probabilities

The TPS-Paradigm provides a two-step function-based reduction principle in which the behavioural raw data are first statistically reduced according to the known or assumed functions of the behaviours studied regardless of potentially moderate or even low consistencies in the empirical occurrences of functionally related behaviours. In a second step, the functionally defined composite measures thus-derived, rather than the behavioural raw data, are statistically analysed using redundancy-based or context-based reduction principles (as demonstrated below). This function-based reduction principle corresponds to people's intuitive categorisations of behaviours in everyday life that are primarily based on the meanings attributed to behaviours rather than on their actual empirical occurrences (Uher, 2015b; Uher et al. 2013a,b).

To statistically explore the configurational comparability of functionally defined constructs, scientists also have to decide what kinds of empirical patterns they consider to be comparable between the particular groups or species studied. Specifically, researchers must decide if they weight functionally similar behaviours equally in their meaning as indicators of a particular construct or if they weight them differently in a particular study. These decisions cannot be made on the basis of mere statistical patterns; instead, they must be made on the basis of theoretical assumptions and with regard to the particular research question posed. In fact, these decisions precede statistical analyses because they determine the analytical algorithms that are used for computing composite measures. These algorithms influence the empirical results on the configurational patterns that can be identified in the behavioural variations of the different groups or species studied—and thus, the results on their configurational comparability.

The necessity of making such decisions does not become apparent in assessment-based research because people implicitly consider the different functions and meanings that they attribute to particular behaviours and may therefore implicitly weight the occurrences of particular behaviours differently when generating the raw data. In the primate studies used for illustrating these principles, all behavioural categories assigned to the same construct were attributed equal meanings. The corresponding behavioural variables were therefore weighted equally in the algorithms used for generating the composite measures of the three constructs studied. To consider that different behaviours generally occur with different frequencies in the same sample, all behavioural variables were first differentially standardised[10] (using z-standardisation). The z-standardised scores were then averaged across variables into a mean score per construct, thus weighted equally. Alternatively, some behaviours could also be considered to be more meaningful than others with regard to a given construct so that, for example, in the computation of the composite measures of Social Orientation, grooming and body contact could be weighted higher than arm-length and 1m proximity to others.

At the bottom of statistical analyses of the configurational comparability of construct measures and of patterning effects between groups and between species, respectively, are data reflecting individuals' *absolute* time-relative probabilities. This is because differential standardisation removes the information of absolute differences between individuals, groups and species, which are in the focus of these analyses. Therefore, configurational comparability across different sample levels is explored using three kinds of analyses that were developed for between-group comparisons in cross-cultural assessment-based research (Leung &

[10] The behavioural (summary) scores (cf. Table 2), by contrast, were derived by adding scores together across variables, thus without considering differences in the behaviours' general occurrences.

Bond, 1989). Analogous analytical methodologies can be derived for comparisons between species on the basis of scientific quantifications using time-relative probabilities as shown now.

Exploring configurational comparability across different sample levels demonstrated by the example of species comparisons: Species-specific, universal and species-comparative analyses

In *species-specific analyses*, individuals' absolute time-relative probabilities are differentially standardised within each species. The species-specific construct measures derived from averaging these scores can then be explored for individual-specific variations and their configurational patterns. The results of these analyses are collected in matrices consisting of the separate species' co-variation scores of measurements of behaviours that are known or assumed to be functionally comparable between the species studied (e.g., internal consistencies, intercorrelations, test-retest reliabilities, see Tables 3 and 4).

In *universal analyses,* individuals' absolute time-relative probabilities are differentially standardised across the entire sample of all individuals ignoring their species membership. Averaging the differential time-relative probabilities thus-standardised therefore leads to construct measures in which individual variations are confounded by species-typical variations. Such universally standardised measures allow for exploring species-specific variations but not for exploring individual-specific variations ("personality") because species is the highest sample level for identifying individual-specificity. However, universal analyses can be applied to study individual-specificity when there is no evidence for systematic mean level differences between the species studied (as shown, e.g., in methodological studies on small samples of individuals of four great ape species; Uher, 2011b, Uher et al., 2008). Moreover, when species-specific analyses provide evidence for individual-specificity within each species studied and for configurational comparability of the given constructs between these species, then universal analyses can be used to explore the individual-specific variations that are shared by these species for mean-level differences between species (as explored below). The results of universal analyses are collected in matrices comprising the common co-variation scores of measurements of behaviours that are considered to be functionally comparable between the species studied.

In *species-comparative analyses*, individuals' absolute time-relative probabilities are averaged within each species to derive species-specific means of absolute time-relative probabilities for each given behavioural variable. Species-specific means of construct measures are derived by averaging individuals' time-relative probabilities that are first differentially standardised in universal analyses across all individuals of all species studied. By contrast, differential time-relative probabilities derived from the species-specific analyses (i.e., that are differentially standardised within each species) cannot be used because *z*-

standardisation sets the species' means to zero. The results of species-comparative analyses are collected in the same kind of matrices as those collected for the results from the species-specific and the universal analyses.

The species-specific, universal and species-comparative matrices containing various kinds of co-variation scores form the basis of the comparative analyses of the configurational and temporal patterns identified. The degree of between-species comparability of the empirical configurations of (behavioural) scores within each construct measure (i.e., construct equivalence), the empirical configurations of composite measures across multiple constructs (i.e., patterning effects) and the test-retest reliability of measurement variables and construct measures can be analysed statistically. Suitable methods are, for example, factor congruence coefficients (van de Vijver & Leung, 1997a,b; van de Vijver & Poortinga, 2002) and multi-group confirmatory factor analysis and structural equations modelling, which enable simultaneous tests of the same correlational or latent structure across species or group while keeping each sample distinct (Byrne, 1994; Byrne, Shavelson, & Muthén, 1989; Vandenberg & Lance, 2000).

Applications of these three kinds of analyses for exploring configurational comparability across different sample levels can be exemplarily demonstrated by data on the social behaviour of the four primate species. The left part of Table 3 presents the results on the internal consistency of the construct measures generated for the three functionally-defined constructs; the right part presents the results on the intercorrelations between these construct measures. From top to bottom, the table contains the three different kinds of matrices used for cross-level comparative analyses. Part *1)* contains the species-specific matrix of the within-species findings on the internal consistency and the intercorrelations between the three construct measures. Part *2)* contains the results from the corresponding universal analyses across the joint sample of all individuals of all four species. Part *3*) shows the results from the corresponding species-comparative analyses performed on the species-specific mean scores (Table 3).

Table 3 *Configurational comparability: Species-specific, universal and species-comparative analyses of construct equivalence and of patterning effects*

Kind of analysis		**Construct equivalence (Internal consistency)**						**Patterning effects (Intercorrelations)**					
xx **Species**	*n*	SO-Index		AG-Index		DO-Index		SOi-AGi		SOi-DOi		AGi-DOi	
		r_m	[a]	*r*	*P*	*r*	*p*	*r*	*p*	*r*	*p*	*r*	*p*
1) Species-specific analyses of individual differences													
Weeper capuchins	9	**.51**	[a]	**.95****	(.000)	-.51	(.165)	-.15	(.709)	-.13	(.774)	**.98****	(.000)
Mandrills	8	-.13	[a]	**.96****	(.000)	-.29	(.487)	.21	(.618)	.47	(.244)	.60	(.119)
Toque macaques	12	.18	[a]	**.95****	(.000)	-.49*	(.103)	.08	(.794)	-.07	(.833)	**.70****	(.012)
Rhesus macaques	7	.03	[a]	**.56****	(.188)	-.28	(.624)	.03	(.942)	.12	(.804)	-.01	(.977)
2) Universal analyses of individual differences													
All species	36	.05	[a]	**.69****	(.000)	.14	(.404)	.04	(.838)	.08	(.668)	**.55****	(.001)
3) Species-comparative analyses of species-specific means													
All species	4	-.05	[a]	.27	(.726)	**.99****	(.000)	.33	(.672)	.17	(.833)	.51	(.495)

Note. * $p < .05$; * $p < .01$. *n* The number of individuals or species, respectively, studied in each given kind of analysis. [a] Mean correlations were computed using *r*-to-*Z* transformation; therefore, *p*-values cannot be reported. Exemplary demonstrations of analyses of configurational comparability of the three functionally-defined constructs in the four primate species studied: The *Social Orientation Index (SOi)* is based on grooming and the number of conspecifics in body contact, arm-length and 1m distance; the *Aggressiveness Index (AGi)* is based on non-contact aggression and contact aggression, and the *Dominance Index (DOi)* is based on displacing other, being displaced and subordinate to others (the latter two were a priori summarised into one variable because subordination occurred only rarely). Computations are based on individual means and species means of absolute time-relative probabilities, averaged across study periods t_2 and t_3 in which data from all four species are available. Construct measures (indices) were computed as mean scores of differentially standardised behavioural variables (using *z*-standardisation). In the *species-specific analyses*, *z*-standardisation was performed for each species separately before construct measures were computed. In the *universal and species-comparative analyses*, *z*-standardisation was performed on the individuals of the joint sample of all four species before individual construct measures and species means were computed. Universal and species-comparative analyses are used to explore whether the between-individual and between-species differences are comparable across the different sample levels. Construct equivalence was analysed in terms of the internal consistency of the composite measures using Pearson correlation *r*. Intra-class correlation could not be used because the internal consistency of the Social Orientation Index was low and tended to be negative and because the two measures summarised by the Dominance Index have opposite meanings (displace others and subordinate), thus resulting necessarily in negative co-variations. Patterning effects were analysed in terms of Pearson correlations *r* between the species-specific, universal and species-comparative measures of all three constructs.

The findings, although limited by the small sample sizes, illustrate basic principles. The species-specific internal consistencies of the Social Orientation Index (SOi) were generally low, except for the weeper capuchins (Table 3; left columns). The internal consistencies of this construct were also low in the universal analyses and in the species-comparative analyses. In psychometrics, it is common practice to discard measurement variables that yield only low internal consistency (Block, 2010). Such redundancy-based reduction principles were developed in assessment-based research that inherently relies on language, in which redundancies can be created at low cost and are therefore widespread (cf. Lahlou, 1996). But in behaviour, redundancies are rare and may be even constraint because they are too costly in ecological and evolutionary regards (Uher, 2015b; Uher et al., 2013a). Given the shared function and meaning of grooming and proximity to others, there is no reason to discard any of these behavioural measurements or even the construct just because the empirical occurrences of these behaviours do not co-vary on the sample level.

Species-specific internal consistencies of the Aggressiveness Index (AGi), by contrast, were high in three species and moderate in the rhesus macaques (Table 3). This is interesting because in some previous studies, occurrences of contact and non-contact aggression were not associated (e.g., in 21 tufted capuchins, *Cebus apella*; Uher et al., 2013a). High internal consistency of the Aggressiveness Index was also found in the universal analysis performed on the joint sample of all individuals from all four species. But in the species-comparative analysis performed on the species-specific mean scores, consistency was only moderate. These findings indicate absence of mean-level differences between the species as explored below.

The internal consistencies of the Dominance Index (DOi) showed inverse patterns (Table 3). The species-specific internal consistencies were only moderate in all four species, the universal internal consistency was low and the species-comparative internal consistency was high. The Dominance index comprises behaviours with opposite meanings (i.e., displace others and subordinate to others). Therefore, species-specific internal consistencies were negative as expected. But despite the opposite valences of these behaviours with regard to the construct Dominance, their occurrences in individuals are not mutually exclusive (e.g., because individuals may show both kinds of behaviours but to different social partners). This may explain the only moderate internal consistencies found within each species. The low but positive internal consistency found in the universal analysis and the high internal consistency found in the species-comparative analysis therefore indicate the presence of mean-level differences in the occurrences of these behaviours between at least some of the species studied as explored below.

The intercorrelations between these construct measures showed much more coherent patterning effects across the different levels of analysis (Table 3, right columns). The Social Orientation and Aggressiveness indices were not associated within and across the species. This is interesting because in a previous study on crab-eating macaques the behaviours described by these construct were associated (e.g., $r = .75$, $p < .001$, $n = 61$; Uher et al., 2013b). Likewise, the Social Orientation and Dominance indices were not associated on any level of analysis, except for the mandrills in which low to moderate species-specific associations occurred. The Aggressiveness and Dominance indices, by contrast, were substantially associated within three of the four species (except for the rhesus macaques) as well as in the universal analyses. The species-comparative analysis indicated similar associations.

In larger samples, the results collected in the three kinds of matrices could now be explored statistically for the degrees of construct equivalence and the degrees of similarity in the patterning effects between the different species studied and within and across the different sample levels explored. For the purposes of the present study and considering the small sample sizes, the similarities between the three matrices shall be sufficient to assume that the three constructs are configurationally comparable between the four species studied.

Additional evidence for this assumption is provided by results on these construct measures' temporal reliability derived from species-specific, universal and species-comparative analyses. The three matrices containing the corresponding test-retest correlations between all three study periods are shown in Table 4, which is structured identically to Table 3. The high temporal reliabilities shown in all species-specific analyses over 2 and 4 weeks for all constructs and over 5 week periods for most constructs provide evidence that the construct measures reflect individual-specific patterns in each of the four species. Temporal reliabilities were also high in all universal analyses. But universal analyses can yield high temporal stabilities even in absence of individual-specific variations because they are confounded by species-typical variations. First indications for systematic mean-level differences between the species therefore derive from high variable-oriented temporal stability of the species-comparative analyses as shown in Table 4.

Variable-oriented analyses explore the rank ordering of scores on the variables studied; thus without mean-level differences between the species, high temporal reliability cannot be found in species-comparative analyses. Therefore, the high test-retest reliabilities of the Social Orientation index across all study periods indicate the possible presence of mean-level differences between species, whereas the varying and low temporal reliabilities of the Aggressiveness and Dominance indices indicate the possible absence of temporally stable between-species differences. The TPS-Paradigm elaborates basic principles that allow for scientifically quantifying mean-level differences between groups and species as described in the following.

Table 4 *Species-specific, universal and species-comparative analyses of the temporal stability of individual behavioural variations over 2, 4 and 5 weeks: Evidence for individual-specific variations within and across species*

Kind of analysis			**Test-retest reliability of construct measures**					
			2 weeks		4 weeks		5 weeks	
Construct	**Species**	**n**	t_1-t_2		t_2-t_3		t_1-t_3	
			r	*p*	*r*	*p*	*r*	*p*
1) Species-specific analyses of individual differences								
SO-Index	Weeper capuchins	9	**.73***	(.026)	**.95****	(.000)	**.80****	(.010)
	Mandrills	8	**.73***	(.041)	.61	(.108)	.20	(.642)
	Toque macaques	12	**.92****	(.000)	**.90****	(.000)	**.93****	(.000)
	Rhesus macaques	7	-	-	**.60**	(.153)	-	
AG-Index	Weeper capuchins	9	**.80****	(.009)	**.89****	(.001)	.66	(.051)
	Mandrills	8	.68	(.065)	**.72***	(.043)	**.97****	(.000)
	Toque macaques	12	**.67***	(.017)	**.76****	(.004)	.55	(.062)
	Rhesus macaques	7	-	-	.73	(.065)	-	
DO-Index	Weeper capuchins	9	**.86****	(.003)	**.86****	(.003)	**.78***	(.010)
	Mandrills	8	**.93****	(.001)	**.86****	(.006)	**.87****	(.005)
	Toque macaques	12	**.85****	(.000)	**.74****	(.006)	**.70***	(.012)
	Rhesus macaques	7	-	-	**.79***	(.036)	-	
2) Universal analyses of individual differences								
SO-Index	All species .	36	**.91****	(.000)	**.86****	(.000)	**.84****	(.000)
AG-Index	All species	36	**.65****	(.000)	**.59****	(.000)	**.87****	(.002)
DO-Index	All species	36	**.92****	(.000)	**.80****	(.000)	**.82****	(.000)
3) Species-comparative analyses of species-specific means								
SO-Index	All species	4	**.97***	(.030)	.89	(.106)	.92	(.077)
AG-Index	All species	4	.72	(.277)	.37	(.630)	.74	(.262)
DO-Index	All species	4	.74	(.261)	-.67	(.330)	-.15	(.846)

Note. * $p < .05$; * $p < .01$. SO Social Orientation, AG Aggressiveness, DO Dominance. Variable-oriented analyses of the test-retest reliability (using Pearson correlation *r*) of between-individual differences across different sample levels. *n* The number of individuals or species, respectively, that were studied in each given kind of analysis. Computations are based on individual means and species means of differential time-relative probabilities, averaged across study periods t_2 and t_3 in which data from all four species are available. In the *species-specific analyses*, *z*-standardisation of the behavioural variables comprised by the construct measures was performed for each species separately. In the *universal and species-comparative analyses*, *z*-standardisation was performed on the individuals of the joint sample of all four species before individual construct measures and species means were computed. But importantly, only species-specific analyses can be used to identify individual-specificity ("personality") because species is the highest population level for determinating individual-specificity. Universal and species-comparative analyses are used to explore whether the individual-specific variations identified are comparable across the different sample levels as well as possible mean-level differences in these variations between species.

Statistical analyses of mean-level differences between groups and species: Positioning effects

Constructs describing individual-specific variations that are considered to be functionally and configurationally comparable between particular groups or species also allow for exploring quantitative differences between the groups or species studied. Such mean-level differences along shared dimensions of between-individual differences are also referred to as *positioning effects* (Leung & Bond, 1989; Uher, 2008a,b).

Scientific quantifications of positioning effects on the level of variables must be based on individuals' absolute time-relative probabilities; pertinent explorations on the construct level must be based on individuals' time-relative probabilities that are differentially standardised across the joint sample of individuals from all groups or species studied (i.e., in universal analyses). The TPS-Paradigm emphasises that scientific quantifications of behavioural mean-level differences between individuals, groups and species depend on the particular behavioural situations studied.

The role of situations for scientific quantifications of behavioural variations within and between individuals, groups and species

Given that behaviours are functionally mediated by other external phenomena that are present in the moments of their occurrence, analyses of mean-level differences require that relevant properties of the studied behavioural situations are known or assumed to be functionally and quantitatively comparable between the particular groups or species studied. Therefore, these situations need not—and often cannot—be nominally identical. Rather, comparability of behavioural situations must be established on higher levels of abstraction.

Higher levels of abstraction are also required because the functional relevance of situational properties varies also between individuals of the same group (Bandura, 1986; Mischel & Shoda, 1995; Rotter, 1954, 1981). In fact, it is well known that situational properties are directly related to individual variations. The concept of *weak situations* describes constellations of situational properties in which individual differences emerge in a given sample; such constellations have high power to discriminate between individuals. But there are also constellations of situational properties in which individual differences do not occur, thus resulting in floor or ceiling effects in the distribution of empirical scores. Such constellations do not discriminate well between individuals and are therefore referred to as *strong situations* (in the sense that they restrict the emergence of individual variations; Mischel, 1977; Tett & Guterman, 2000; Uher, 2011a,b).

The particular quantitative properties of behavioural situations that differentiate well between individuals and that result in comparable distribution patterns may vary between groups or species. For example, in some nonhuman species, most individuals may flee from unfamiliar objects sized 10% of their body size, whereas in other species most individuals may do so only if unfamiliar objects are sized 25% their body size. This in itself reflects quantitative differences between the particular groups or species studied. The concept of situational strength clarifies that statistical comparisons of behavioural scores without considering the particular properties of the behavioural situations in which they were obtained may bias findings on mean-level differences between individuals, groups or species.

In observational studies, situational properties that are considered to be relevant can be quantified and controlled for in the empirical analyses; for example, activity patterns may be weighted against the space available to each individual of the social groups studied. Experimental studies additionally allow for making adjustments and targeted manipulations of particular situational properties; for example, quantitative situational properties in novel object tests can be made comparable by using equal object-size–to–body-size ratios (e.g., what may be a small object for chimpanzees can be life-sized for mice). In the primate studies used here for illustrating the comparative methodologies, situational properties relevant for social behaviours were made quantitatively comparable between the species (and thus between social groups of different size) by weighting individuals' time-relative probabilities for showing particular behaviours against the total number of individuals in each social group to account for differences in the number of potential interaction partners available (see above).

Individual-specific and species-specific situation-behaviour profiles

Individuals' time-relative probabilities to display particular behaviours often vary across different behavioural situations. In addition to such general shifts in the occurrences of behaviours across situations in a given sample, there are often pronounced between-individual differences in these cross-situational variations that are relatively stable over time. If such individual-specific patterns emerge in a given sample, then the *cross-situational consistency* of the between-individual variations in the occurrences of this particular behaviour can be only moderate (Mischel, 1968; Uher, 2011a,b; Uher et al., 2008, 2013a; Wright & Mischel, 1987).

The cross-situational variations that are specific to particular individuals can be illustrated with *individual-specific situation-behaviour profiles* (sometimes called if…then…profiles; Mischel et al., 2002). In these profiles, an individual's time-relative probabilities to show a particular kind of behaviour are plotted against the particular kinds of situations in which they were measured. For direct comparisons of individual-specific scores between different situations, individuals' scores are differentially standardised within each situation. This allows for exploring, for example, in which kinds of situation a given individual has the highest time-relative probabilities to show a given behaviour and in which ways this may differ between the individuals studied (Uher, 2011a,b; Uher et al., 2008, 2013a).

The TPS-Paradigm extends the concept of individual-specific situation-behaviour profiles to the levels of groups and species for enabling scientific quantifications of mean-level differences in individual-specific behavioural variations between groups and between species. Figure 2a illustrates this concept using the hypothetical example of four species labelled A, B, C and D; the single letters represent single individuals of these species. The individuals' scores of time-relative probabilities to show a particular behaviour are plotted against three kinds of behavioural situations that are assumed to be functionally and quantitatively comparable between these species. Importantly, the scores are differentially standardised across the joint sample of all four species within each situation, thus using universal analyses.

The average scores of the individuals of species A vary across the three situations; the average is the lowest in situation 1 and much higher in situations 2 and 3. As the scores are differentially standardised across the joint sample of individuals from all species, these shifts indicate situation-specific variations in the averages of species A relative to the situation-specific variations in the averages of the other species studied. The averages of the species B, C and D also vary across the three study situations yet in different ways. These differential shifts in species-specific averages can be illustrated as *species-specific situation-behaviour profiles* as shown in Figure 2a.

Figure 2 *The concept of species-specific situation-behaviour profiles and its relations to the concepts of species-discriminative and species-nondiscriminative universal dimensions and species-specific dimensions of individual-specific behaviours*

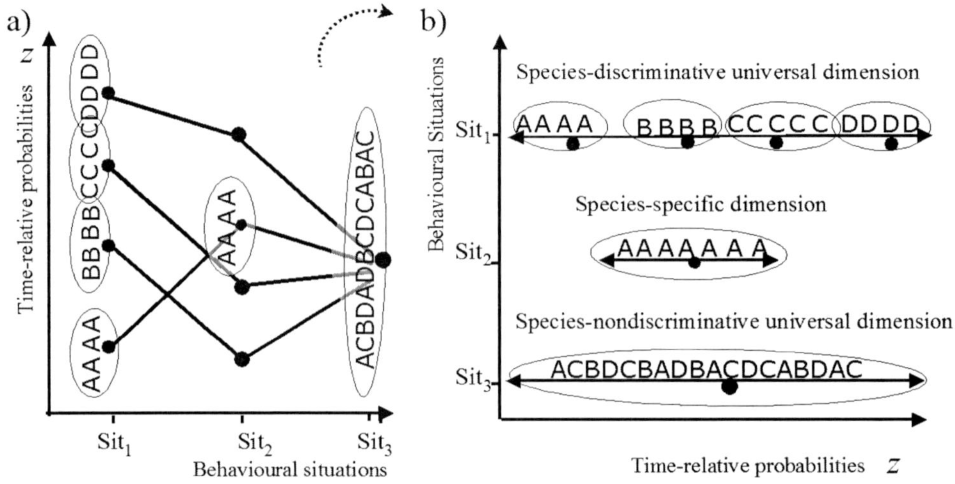

Note. *a)* The concept of species-specific situation-behaviour profiles for enabling scientific quantifications of mean-level differences in individual-specific behavioural variations between groups and between species, illustrated by a hypothetical example of four species labelled A, B, C and D; the single letters represent single individuals of these species. The individuals' scores of time-relative probabilities to show a particular behaviour are plotted against three kinds of behavioural situations and are differentially standardised across the joint sample of all four species within each situation, thus using universal analyses. The average scores of each given species vary across the three situations yet in different ways for each species as indicated by their different profile shapes across the different situations. Situation 1 allows for exploring both between-individual differences and between-species differences. Situation 2 allows for exploring only between-species differences; between-individual differences can be explored only in species A but not in the three other species. Situation 3, in turn, allows for exploring between-individual differences within each species but not between-species differences. b) Seen from an orthogonal view on Figure 2a, continuous dimensions of individual behavioural variations within each of the three kinds of situations studied become apparent that constitute prototypes. Species-specific constructs describe kinds of individual-specific variations that occur only in a particular species but not in other species under study. Universal constructs describe kinds of individual-specific variations that occur in various species in comparable ways. Species-discriminative universal constructs describe kinds of individual-specific variation that differentiate also between species. Species-nondiscriminative universal constructs describe kinds of individual-specific variation that do not differentiate between species.

In each kind of situation, the scores of the individuals of species A vary around the species' average. This illustrates the fact that an individual's score always reflects both individual variations and species-typical variations—unless individuals' scores are differentially standardised within each species as done in species-specific analyses (Uher, 2011a,b). In the species B, C and D, between-individual variations occur only in situations 1 and 3 but not in situation 2. Hence for these three species, situation 2 constitutes a strong situation in which all individuals behave in highly similar ways so that between-individual variations do not occur. Situations 1 and 2, by contrast, constitute weak situations for the species B, C and D because there are pronounced between-individual variations within each species (Figure 2a).

But situations 1 and 3 also differ from one another. Between-species differences occur only in situation 1, whereas the species' averages fall together in situation 3. Analogous to the concept of weak situations established for comparisons of between-individuals within a given sample (Mischel, 1977), the situations also differ in their power for discriminating between species. Situation 1 allows for exploring both between-individual differences and between-species differences. Situation 2 allows for exploring only between-species differences; between-individual differences can be explored only in species A but not in the three other species. Situation 3, in turn, allows for exploring between-individual differences within each species but not differences between species (Figure 2a).

Species-specific, species-discriminative universal and species-nondiscriminative universal variations of individual-specific patterns

An orthogonal view on Figure 2a reveals continuous dimensions of individual behavioural variations within each of the three kinds of situations studied (Figure 2b). Three kinds of between-species variations of individual-specific patterns can be distinguished that constitute prototypes.

Three prototypes of variations of individual-specific patterns within and across species

Situation 2 allows for discriminating between the four species only in terms of their averages but not in terms of between-individual differences. Such kinds of species differences are irrelevant for explorations of individual-specificity[11] (i.e., "personality") but they may be relevant for other fields of research (e.g., biology, anthropology). In cross-cultural psychology, variations in the averages of sociocultural groups in absence of between-individual variations are referred to as cultural dimensions (Leung & Bond, 1989). Between-individual differences and thus, individual-specificity can be identified in Situation 2 only in species A. Such kinds of variations are described in cross-species comparative research by constructs of *species-specific dimensions* (Uher, 2008a,b), derived from analogous constructs of *emic dimensions* in cross-cultural research (Leung & Bond, 1989).

Situation 3 allows for discriminating between individuals within each of the four species studied but not for discriminating between species. In cross-species comparative research, such kinds of variation are described by constructs of

[11] This vital point is mistaken in some animal "personality" or temperament studies (e.g. Clarke & Boinski, 1995; Herrmann, Hare, Cissewski, & Tomasello, 2011).

weak universal dimensions (Uher, 2008a,b), derived from analogous constructs of *weak etic dimensions* in cross-cultural research (Leung & Bond, 1989).

Situation 1 allows for discriminating both between-individual variations within all four species and mean-level differences between species. In cross-species comparative research, such kinds of variation are described by constructs of *strong universal dimensions* (Uher, 2008a,b; cf. also Capitanio, 2004), derived from the analogous constructs of *strong etic dimensions* in cross-cultural psychology (Leung & Bond, 1989).

The various meanings of "weak" and "strong" in comparative concepts may cause confusion. In the concept of situational strength from "personality" psychology, the terms refer to constraints that situations may impose on individuals' behaviours; thus, "strong" indicates absence of variations. In the cross-cultural and cross-species comparative concepts, by contrast, the terms refer to discriminative power; thus, "strong" denotes presence of variations.

The TPS-Paradigm therefore applies a more descriptive terminology. Kinds of individual-specific variation that occur only in a particular species but not in other species under study are called *species-specific*. Those kinds of individual-specific variations that occur in various species are called *universal* for the particular group of species considered. Universal kinds of individual-specific variation that also differentiate between species are called *species-discriminative* and those that do not differentiate between species are called *species-nondiscriminative*. Analogous concepts for comparisons within and across groups of conspecific individuals describe group-specific, group-discriminative and group-nondiscriminative universal variations of individual-specificity.

Empirical demonstration of the comparative methodologies for exploring differences between species

These concepts are directly related to the three different kinds of analyses used for exploring variations within and between groups and species. This can be illustrated by the empirical data on the four primate species. The various species-specific analyses of the three construct measures (cf. Tables 3 and 4) provided evidence for configurationally comparable individual-specific variations in all four species; thus, none of these variations are species-specific. The universal analyses suggested that the three constructs describe individual-specific variations that are universal for these species. Species-comparative analyses indicated stable mean-level differences in the Social Orientation index between at least some of the four species, i.e., species-discriminative universal variations, and absence of stable between-species differences in the Aggressiveness and Dominance indices, i.e., species-nondiscriminative universal variations of individual-specificity.

These indications were statistically tested using One-way ANOVAs on the individuals' averages across study periods t_2 and t_3 for the three construct measures, which reflect differentially (z-)standardised scores, and for the more specific behavioural (summary) scores, which reflect absolute-time relative probabilities. The magnitude of the between-species differences was estimated using Cohen's effect size d on pooled standard deviations. This effect size can also be interpreted in terms of the percent of non-overlap of the score distributions between the two groups contrasted (Cohen, 1988). Given the small sample sizes, post-hoc power analyses were conducted using G*Power software (Faul, Erdfelder, Lang, & Buchner, 2007) to explore which of the results are likely to replicate.

Significant species-differences occurred in the Social Orientation index (SOi), $F_{SOi}(3, 32) = 8.274$, $p = .000$. Bonferroni tests indicated that the weeper capuchins ($M = -0.41$; $SD = 0.27$) scored significantly lower than the mandrills ($M = -0.04$; $SD = 0.16$), toque macaques ($M = 0.19$; $SD = 0.38$) and rhesus macaques ($M = 0.13$; $SD = 0.21$) with effect sizes ranging from $d = -1.6$ to 2.2 (73-85% non-overlap in the score distributions and .88-.98 achieved power of detecting such a difference; see Table 5, upper part). Hence, the Social Orientation index has a high power to discriminate weeper capuchins from the three other species but not for discriminating between these three species.

These species differences were further explored by analysing the proximity summary score (PX) and the grooming score (GR) that the Social Orientation index comprises. Weeper capuchins ($M = 0.75$; $SD = 0.25$) stayed in proximity to significantly fewer conspecifics than toque macaques ($M = 1.36$; $SD = 0.47$) but not significantly fewer than mandrills ($M = 1.01$; $SD = 0.17$) and rhesus macaques ($M = 0.99$; $SD = 0.15$), $F_{PX}(3, 32) = 6.430$, $p = .002$ (using Tamhane's T2 test; see Table 5, lower part). Hence, the proximity summary score (PX) had high power only for discriminating the capuchins from toque macaques but not from the two other species. The time-relative probabilities for grooming did not differ between weeper capuchins ($M = 0.03$; $SD = 0.03$) and Mandrills ($M = 0.03$; $SD = 0.29$), but both species groomed significantly less often than toque macaques ($M = 0.09$; $SD = 0.05$) and rhesus macaques ($M = 0.10$; $SD = 0.04$); the two macaque species did not differ from one another; $F_{GR}(3, 32) = 8.408$, $p = .000$ (using Bonferroni tests). Thus, the grooming scores had high power for discriminating between these two groups of species ($1\text{-}\beta > .90$; see Table 5).

Table 5 *Mean-level differences between species: Evidence for positioning effects in the construct measures and the behavioural (summary) scores*

Species		**Construct measures (universally standardised)**											
contrasted		**SO-Index**			**AG-Index**			**DO-Index**			**DI+SU-Index**		
Sp_1	Sp_1	d_{sp}	$\%_{NO}$	$1\text{-}\beta$	d_{sp}	$\%_{NO}$	$1\text{-}\beta$	d_{sp}	$\%_{NO}$	$1\text{-}\beta$	d_{sp}	$\%_{NO}$	$1\text{-}\beta$
Cw	Md	**-1.6**	**73**	**.88**	-0.4	27	.12	0.0	0	.05	**-2.2**	**85**	**.99**
Cw	Tq	**-1.8**	**77**	**.97**	-0.2	15	.06	0.1	7	.05	**-1.7**	**75**	**.98**
Cw	Rh	**-2.2**	**85**	**.98**	0.1	8	.06	0.1	7	.05	-0.3	21	.15
Md	Tq	-0.8	47	.38	0.3	21	.10	0.0	0	.05	**1.5**	**70**	**.95**
Md	Rh	-0.9	52	.36	0.5	33	.17	0.0	0	.05	**2.1**	**83**	**.99**
Tq	Rh	0.2	15	.07	0.5	33	.17	0.0	0	.05	**1.6**	**73**	**.93**
		Behavioural (summary) scores (absolute time-relative probabilities)											
		PX			**GR**			**DI**			**SU**		
Sp_1	Sp_2	d_{sp}	$\%_{NO}$	$1\text{-}\beta$	d_{sp}	$\%_{NO}$	$1\text{-}\beta$	d_{sp}	$\%_{NO}$	$1\text{-}\beta$	d_{sp}	$\%_{NO}$	$1\text{-}\beta$
Cw	Md	-1.2	62	.64	0.1	7	.05	-1.4	68	.79	-1.2	62	.64
Cw	Tq	**-1.6**	**73**	**.93**	**-1.5**	**71**	**.95**	-0.8	48	.38	-1.2	62	.71
Cw	Rh	-1.2	62	.57	**-2.0**	**81**	**.98**	-0.3	21	.08	0.1	7	.05
Md	Tq	-1.0	55	.54	**-1.6**	**73**	**.90**	1.0	55	.53	0.9	52	.45
Md	Rh	0.1	8	.06	**-2.1**	**83**	**.96**	1.4	68	.70	1.2	62	.56
Tq	Rh	1.1	59	.55	-0.2	15	.07	0.7	43	.27	1.1	58	.56

Note. d_{Sp} Effect sizes Cohen's *d* for differences between species; bold effect sizes reflect species differences for which the given construct measures have a high test power ($1\text{-}\beta > .88$) in the samples studied and that are thus more likely to replicate in larger samples. $\%_{NO}$ Percentage of non-overlap of the score distributions of the two species compared. $1\text{-}\beta$ test power achieved in the given sample sizes. Sp_1 and Sp_2 indicate the species contrasted; their order in the table is relevant for interpreting the direction of the mean-level differences between them such that a negative effect size indicates that the scores of Sp_1 are lower than those of Sp_2. Cw weeper capuchins, Md mandrills, Tq toque macaques, Rh rhesus macaques. Construct measures (upper part of the table) reflect individuals' differential time-relative probabilities and were computed in universal analyses as the means of standardised behavioural scores that were z-standardised across the individuals of all species. Behavioural (summary) scores (lower part) reflect individuals' absolute time-relative probabilities to show particular kinds of behaviours (summary scores and were computed by adding together the scores from the more specific related behavioural variables). Computations are based on individuals' averages across study periods t_2 and t_3 in which data from all four species are available. Results on the aggression summary scores (AG) are not shown because were virtually identical to those of the Aggressiveness index (AGi), which were derived from the same variables yet using a slightly different algorithm. The Dominance index (DOi) was computed from individuals' displacement scores and their inverted (*z*-standardised) subordination scores to reflect individuals' dominance relationships within their social group and thus within each species; therefore, the Dominance index cannot reflect species-differences. For enabling species comparisons, the DI+SU-Index was computed from non-inversed (*z*-standardised) subordination scores; thus the DI+SU-Index reflects the differential occurrences of *any kind* of dominance-related behaviours, i.e., dominant and subordinate.

In the Aggressiveness index (AGi), the mandrills scored the highest (*M* = 0.24; *SD* = 0.99) but not significantly higher than the weeper capuchins (*M* = -0.08; *SD* = 0.64), toque macaques (*M* = 0.00; *SD* = 0.38) or rhesus macaques (*M* = -0.15; *SD* = 0.20); $F_{AGi}(3, 32) = .612$, $p = .612$. The aggression summary scores (AG) were virtually identical because they were derived from the same variables yet with a slightly different algorithm (Table 5, upper part). Both kinds of measures had no power for discriminating between any of the four species.

The Dominance Index (DOi) did not reflect species-differences, $F_{DOi}(3, 32) = .002$, $p = 1.000$; but the strikingly similar mean-scores of the four species, weeper capuchins (*M* = -0.01; *SD* = 0.11), mandrills (*M* = 0.00; *SD* = 1.11) toque macaques (*M* = 0.00; *SD* = 0.42) and rhesus macaques (*M* = 0.00; *SD* = 0.10; Table 5, upper part), indicated the possibility of a methodological artefact derived from the algorithm used for its computation. The Dominance index comprises two behavioural variables with opposite meanings (i.e., displace and subordinate) and was therefore computed from the inverted (*z*-standardised) scores of one of these variables (i.e., subordinate) so as to reflect individuals' dominance rank within each social group. Dominant individuals seldom display subordinate behaviours and subordinate individuals seldom display dominant behaviours. Therefore, possible species differences in the overall occurrences of both behaviours cannot be reflected in the index.

This issue was further explored by analysing the two behavioural summary scores that the Dominance index comprises and that reflect individuals' absolute-time relative probability scores. Displacement (DI) occurred in the mandrills (*M* = 0.25; *SD* = 0.23) more often than in the weeper capuchins (*M* = 0.02; *SD* = 0.03) and in the rhesus macaques (*M* = 0.02; *SD* = 0.02), but the displacement score had only moderate power for detecting such differences in the given samples (Table 5, lower part). Mandrills also displaced conspecifics more often than did the toque macaques (*M* = 0.08; *SD* = 0.11); but the power of these scores for discriminating between these species was only low. Given the unequal variances, none of these differences were significant as Tamhane's T2 tests showed, $F_{DI}(3, 32) = 6.116$, $p = .002$. Subordination (SU) also occurred in the mandrills (*M* = 0.27; *SD* = 0.30) more often than in the weeper capuchins (*M* = 0.02; *SD* = 0.01), toque macaques (*M* = 0.08; *SD* = 0.07) and rhesus macaques (*M* = 0.02; *SD* = 0.03), $F_{SU}(3, 32) = 5.357$, $p = .004$, but also not in significant ways as Tamhane's T2 tests showed. The power of the subordination score for discriminating between the species was only moderate (Table 5, lower part).

To account for the opposite meanings of displacement and subordination behaviours and for the resulting different distribution patterns of these behaviours within each species, an alternative construct measure was computed using non-inversed (*z*-standardised) subordination scores. This DI+SU-index thus reflects the differential occurrences of *any kind* of dominance-related behaviours, i.e., displace and subordinate. In this index, the mandrills (*M* = 0.87; *SD* = 0.83) scored significantly higher than the weeper capuchins (M = -0.42; SD = 0.08) and the rhesus macaques (M = -0.39; SD = 0.09) but not than the toque macaques (M = -0.08; SD = 0.26), and the toque macaques scored significantly higher than the weeper capuchins and the rhesus macaques; $F_{PX}(3, 32) = 16.595, p = .000$ (using Tamhane's T2 tests); $F_{DI+SUi}(3, 32) = 16.596, p = .000$. Despite the small sample sizes, the DI+SU-index had high power to discriminate between the species except for discriminating between weeper capuchins and rhesus macaques (see Table 5, upper part)

These positioning effects are illustrated in Figures 3a-c in which individuals' differential time-relative probabilities (standardised across all individuals from all species in universal analyses) from study period t_2 are plotted against those from study period t_3. Hence, the graphs depict the temporal stability of the between-individual variations described by the three construct measures that were explored within and across species. As these variations were also stable within each species (see Table 4), they reflect both individual-specific variations (i.e., "personality" differences) and—in some cases—mean-level differences in the species' mean scores around which these individual-specific variations occur. The individuals of all four species vary along the dimensions of individual-specific variations described by the three constructs and that are thus universal for these species.

Figure 3 *Empirical evidence for species-discriminative and species-nondiscriminative universal variations of individual-specific behaviours*

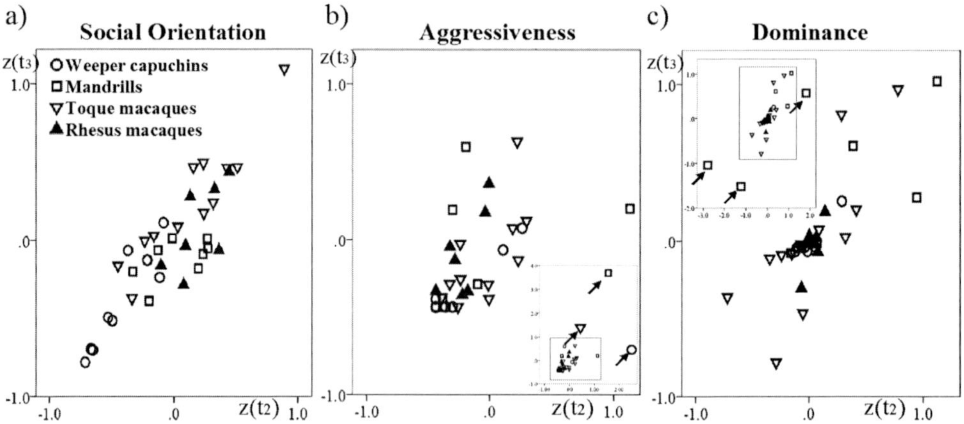

Note. Empirical demonstrations of the concepts of species-discriminative and species-non-discriminative universal dimensions of individual-specific variations and the species' positioning effects. Individuals' differential time-relative probabilities (standardised across all individuals from all species in universal analyses) from study period t_2 are plotted against those from study period t_3. The individuals of all four species vary along the dimensions of individual-specific variations described by the three constructs, thus they are universal for these species. For more direct comparisons between the constructs, the three graphs are all scaled such that each axis spans about two standard deviations (z = -1 to +1). The small graphs inserted in the Figures 3b and 3c are scaled differently. In Figure 3b, the x-axis is scaled from z = -1.0 to 2.5 and the y-axis from z = -1.0 to 4.0; the three outliers are the Capuchin alpha male $z(2.6;0.4)$, a mandrill female $z(1.4; 3.6)$ and the alpha male of the toque macaques $z(0.5;1.4)$. In Figure 3c, the x-axis is scaled from z = -3.0 to 2.0 and the y-axis from z = -2 to 1.0); outliers are three mandrills, two low-scoring females $z(-1.2; -1.5)$ and $z(-2.7;-1.1)$ and the alpha male scoring high in study period t_2 $z(1.8; 0.5)$. *a)* The Social Orientation index describes a species-discriminative universal dimension of individual-specific variants with regard to weeper capuchins as compared to the three other species but a species-nondiscriminative universal dimension if only mandrills, toque macaques and rhesus macaques are considered. Thus, the two prototypes of species-discriminative and species-nondiscriminative universal variations merge together in this construct (cf. Figure 2a,b). *b)* The Aggressiveness index describes a species-nondiscriminative universal dimension of individual-specific variants; individuals of all for species vary along this dimension but there are no mean-level differences between species. c) The Dominance-index describes a universal dimension of individual-specific variations in which species differences did not emerge in the species' averages but in their between-individual *variabilities*. The average within-species variabilities of the mandrills (M_{SD} = .83) were much higher than those of toque macaques (M_{SD} = .26) that in turn were higher than those of the weeper capuchins (M_{SD} = .08) and rhesus macaques (M_{SD} = .09), which did not differ from one another.

In the Social Orientation index (Figure 3a), the scores of the weeper capuchins (depicted as circles) were distributed at the low end of the dimension and those of the two macaque species (depicted as white and black triangles) were distributed toward the high end. Mandrills (depicted as squares) were distributed more in the middle of the dimension. Hence with regard to the weeper capuchins as compared to the three other species, this construct describes a species-discriminative universal dimension of individual-specific variants with only 15-27% overlap in the score distributions between the weeper capuchins and the three other species. If only mandrills and the two macaque species are considered, the construct describes a species-nondiscriminative universal dimension of individual-specific variants. Thus in this construct, the two prototypes of species-discriminative and species-nondiscriminative universal variations merge together (cf. Figure 2).

In the Aggressiveness index (Figure 3b), the scores of the individuals from all four species were distributed along the same dimension. The more scattered distribution patterns reflect the slightly lower temporal stability of these between-individual variations (cf. Table 4). The mixed distribution of the scores from the different species across the entire dimension reflects the absence of species differences. Hence, the Aggressiveness index describes a species-nondiscriminative universal dimension of individual-specific variants.

For more direct comparisons between the constructs, the three graphs are scaled in exactly same way so that the ranges of individuals' score distribution span about two standard deviations (z = -1 to +1). The small graph inserted in the bottom right corner of Figure 3b, by contrast, is scaled differently and shows the distribution of all Aggressiveness scores including three outliers (a weeper capuchin, a mandrill and a toque macaque) with scores up to 4 standard deviations higher than the individuals at the low end of the Aggressiveness dimension.

In the Dominance-index, individuals' scores also varied along the same dimension. The graph shows that the ranges of the within-species variabilities of the mandrills and toque macaques were much higher than those of the weeper capuchins and rhesus macaques. Three mandrills scored up to three standard deviations lower and two standard deviation higher, respectively, than the average individual from all four species (see the small differently scaled graph inserted in the left upper corner of Figure 3c). Interestingly, these pronounced within-species deviations from the joint average of all species occurred in both directions. This explains the absence of mean-level differences between species. That is, in the mandrills (and some extent also in the toque macaques) there were some individuals who showed displacement significantly more often and subordination significantly less often than the average of all four species, thus who behaved extremely dominant, and other individuals who showed the reverse pattern, thus who behaved very submissively. This suggests that the mandrills' dominance hierarchy was much steeper than those of the other species. This is commonly referred to as a "despotic" dominance style as opposed the more "egalitarian" styles of other species (Otovic et al., 2014).

Hence, the Dominance-Index describes individual-specific variations in which species differences did not emerge in the species' averages but in their between-individual *variabilities*. Species-comparative analyses of the species' variabilities (using standard deviations of their between-individual differences) yielded high temporal stabilities across all study periods of $r_{t1\text{-}t2} = .99$ ($p < .032$, $n = 3$), $r_{t2\text{-}t3} = .98$ ($p < .022$, $n = 4$), $r_{t1\text{-}t3} = .96$ ($p < .181$, $n = 3$) that contrast with the varying and partly absent temporal stability of the species' averages (see last row in Table 4). Across the study periods t_2 and t_3 depicted in Figure 3c, the average within-species variabilities of the mandrills ($M_{SD} = .83$) were much higher than those of toque macaques ($M_{SD} = .26$) that in turn were higher than those of the weeper capuchins ($M_{SD} = .08$) and rhesus macaques ($M_{SD} = .09$), which did not differ from one another. Consequently, the Dominance-Index describes universal individual-specific variations that are species-discriminative with regard to the species' variabilities but species-nondiscriminative with regard to the species' averages.

Empirical demonstration of the comparative methodologies for exploring between-group differences within and across species

Analogous analytical methodologies can be applied for comparisons of groups of individuals within and across species (see Table 1). An example of such analyses is provided in Table 6 containing tentative findings from species-specific analyses of sex differences in the four primate species using the behavioural (summary) scores, which reflect absolute time-relative probabilities. Given the small samples sizes, sex differences were explored only using Cohen's effect size *d* yet without testing for significance. Post-hoc power analyses were conducted to explore which of the results are likely to replicate. Sex differences were largely absent in all species with two exceptions. In the toque macaques, females tended to stay in proximity to more conspecifics than males ($M_F = 1.61$, $SD_F = 0.43$; M_M

= 1.02, SD_M = 0.29) and in the rhesus macaques, females groomed others twice as much as males (M_F = 0.12, SD_F = 0.01; M_M = 0.06, SD_M = 0.02).

Table 6 *Sex differences within each species based on absolute time-relative probabilities*

Behavioural (summary) score	Weeper capuchins (n = 6/3)			Mandrills (n = 4/4)			Toque macaques (n = 7/5)			Rhesus macaques (n = 4/3)		
	$d_{F\ vs.\ M}$	$\%_{NO}$	*1-ß*	$d_{F\ vs.\ M}$	$\%_{NO}$	*1-ß*	$d_{F\ vs.\ M}$	$\%_{NO}$	*1-ß*	$d_{F\ vs.\ M}$	$\%_{NO}$	*1-ß*
GR	0.9	52	.19	1.8	77	.59	1.1	59	.38	**4.0**	**2**	**.98**
PX	0.3	21	.07	-1.0	55	.21	**1.6**	**73**	**.70**	0.2	15	.05
AG	-0.5	33	.10	0.6	38	.11	-0.6	38	.16	-0.4	27	.08
DI	-0.6	38	.12	0.0	0	.05	-1.3	65	.51	0.9	52	.16
SU	1.2	62	.29	1.7	75	.51	0.8	47	.22	-0.7	43	.12

Note. d_{Sp} Effect sizes Cohen's *d* for differences between females (F) and males (M); positive scores indicate that females score higher than males. Bold effect sizes reflect sex differences for which the given construct measures have a moderate or high test power, respectively (*1-ß* > .70) in the samples studied and that are thus more likely to replicate in larger samples. $\%_{NO}$ Percentage of non-overlap of the score distributions of the two sexes compared. *1-ß* test power achieved in the given sample sizes. Behavioural (summary) scores reflect individuals' absolute time-relative probabilities to show particular kinds of behaviours (summary scores were computed by adding together the scores from the more specific related behavioural variables): GR Grooming score, PX Proximity summary score, AG Aggression summary score, DI Displacement score, SU Subordination summary score. Computations are based on individuals' averages across study periods t_2 and t_3 in which data from all four species are available.

The present findings are in accordance with previous findings from a study on 26 tufted capuchins living in four social groups, in which sex differences in individual-specific behaviours were absent in 18 out of 20 different constructs studied (Uher et al., 2013a). These studies, although limited in sample sizes, showed that in five group-living species of nonhuman primates with pronounced sexual dimorphisms in body size, individuals did not exhibit pronounced sex differences in individual-specific behaviours as is often assumed for our human ancestors by evolutionary psychologists (e.g., Buss, 1999).

These findings contrast with findings from assessment-based studies that frequently report on sex and gender differences in "personality" in both nonhuman primates and humans (e.g., King, Weiss, & Sisco, 2008; Soto, John, Gosling, & Potter, 2011). But in lack of systematic contrasts to differences that can actually be observed in individuals' behaviours, it is still largely unknown to what extent assessments reflect socio-culturally shared beliefs, ideas and values. A previous study on 104 crab-eating macaques (*Macaca fascicularis*) and their 99 human observers with Dutch language-background has already demonstrated systematic attribution biases in the observers' assessments of these monkeys' individual-specific behaviours. These attribution biases were likely derived from the observers' socioculturally shared stereotypical beliefs about of sex/gender, age and status differences in *human* individuals—thus, anthropomorphic biases (Uher et al., 2013b).

Summary

This research applied the Transdisciplinary Philosophy-of-Science Paradigm for Research on Individuals (TPS-Paradigm) to elaborate comprehensive metatheoretical and methodological frameworks for quantitative comparisons of individual variations within and across situations, groups and species. These frameworks, basic principles and concepts were elaborated using behavioural phenomena as examples. Their applications were demonstrated empirically using behavioural data from four nonhuman primate species. These principles and concepts were also used to critically analyse the quantifications of individual variations that can be obtained from standardised assessments and to highlight serious methodological deficiencies of assessment methods that are not well considered.

First, the chapter introduced a metatheoretical definition of behaviour that highlights the functionally mediating role of the behavioural situations in which behaviours occur. Particular spatio-temporal properties that can be conceived for behaviours (i.e., external to individuals' bodies, momentary and immaterial physical) were specified and used to derive various methodological implications (e.g., nunc-ipsum methods). Then the chapter outlined some basic concepts of the philosophy-of-science foundations that the TPS-Paradigm provides for scientific measurement and quantification (e.g., the set-theoretic and algebraic requirements, definitions of data, methods of data generation, the concept of time-relative probabilities). Their applications for generating scientific quantifications of individual variations in behaviour were demonstrated empirically by the example of behavioural studies in various primates. The philosophy-of-science foundations were also used to highlight fundamental differences to standardised assessment methods, which, unlike observational methods, do not allow researchers to fulfil the requirements of scientific quantification.

In the second part, the chapter applied these foundations to elaborate systematic metatheoretical and methodological frameworks for comparing individual variations within and across different sample levels using individuals, groups and species as examples. These frameworks were developed on the basis of concepts from "personality" psychology, differential psychology and cross-cultural and cross-species research that were systematically integrated into coherent frameworks and complemented by concepts for comparing individual-specific variations (i.e., "personality") between species.

Then concepts for disentangling specific from common variations were elaborated highlighting three interrelated viewpoints that are involved in any comparative exploration of individuals (i.e., specificity/ uniqueness, comparability, universality/ typicality). The chapter discussed basic principles for establishing the functional comparability of behavioural and situational categories that allow researchers to consider that individuals from different groups and species often show different behaviours and encounter different situations and thus cannot be studied with identical variables as is done in assessment-based research.

Using these concepts and principles, methodologies for the statistical analyses of the configurational comparability (i.e., equivalence and patterning effects) of constructs within and across different sample levels, originally developed in cross-cultural psychology, were discussed and generalised to concepts for cross-species comparisons (e.g., species-specific, universal and species-comparative analyses). The chapter introduced basic principles for enabling such explorations on the basis of function-based approaches and time-relative probabilities that can help researchers to overcome the limitations of assessment-based methods (e.g., subjective quantifications generated on the basis of unknown encoding rules, redundancy-based principles, ecological fallacies). Applications of these principles and analytical methodologies were demonstrated empirically in explorations of three constructs of individual-specific behaviours (Social Orientation, Aggressiveness and Dominance) that were shown to be configurationally comparable between the four primate species studied.

Finally, analytical methodologies needed to scientifically quantify mean-level differences between groups and species were explored (i.e., positioning effects). The chapter introduced the concept of species-specific situation-behaviour profiles that demonstrates the ways in which situational properties are related to quantitative differences between individuals, groups and species. Using these methodologies, the three studied constructs were shown to describe species-discriminative and species-nondiscriminative universal variations of individual-specific behaviours. Applications of the analytical methodologies for comparing groups of individuals within and across species were demonstrated by exploring sex-differences in the individual-specific behaviours described by the three constructs and that were shown to be largely absent in all four species studied.

Implications

Given the complex issues involved in comparative analyses of individual variations as explored in this research, how realistic is it to assume that people can accurately assess individual-specific variations (i.e., “personality”)? And how realistic is it to assume that standardised assessments methods enable people provide quantifications on differences between individuals, groups and species that correspond to patterns that can be identified in observable events?The meta-theoretical and methodological frameworks elaborated in this research enable systematic contrasts to be applied with assessments that people provide on individuals and on differences between individuals, groups and species. Such contrast allow for exploring the human abilities to quickly form impressions of individuals and to develop and use socially shared socio-cognitive categories and pertinent everyday vocabularies.

Such contrast can shed a new light on the human tendencies to overestimate the magnitude of minor variations between individuals for differentiating highly similar individuals and to homogenise within-group differences and to exaggerate between-group differences for differentiating individuals from different groups and communities—and species. A better understanding of these tendencies can help to explore the mechanisms and processes underlying stereotypical beliefs and biases, to investigate their impact on assessments of individuals and to develop methodologies that enable researchers to minimise such biases in empirical comparisons of individuals.

Scientific quantifications of observable individual behaviours could also provide important evidence supporting the findings from cross-cultural psychology that "it is almost as if the full range of human diversity reproduces itself at every level of organization" (Shweder & Sullivan, 1990, p. 412). Exploring this diversity will be important for exploring real world issues in the increasingly pluralistic societies of our times.

Acknowledgements

I thank the editors for their invitation to contribute this chapter to this volume. I also thank Dr. med. vet. André Schüle and Heiner Klös from Berlin Zoological Garden for their support of the study on the weeper capuchins, mandrills and toque macaques and Rishi Kumar for carrying out the observations at the zoo. Furthermore, I thank Dr. Michael Begall and Uwe Hehmann from the Berlin Animal Welfare Federation (Tierschutzverein für Berlin und Umgebung Corporation e.V.) for their support of the study on the rhesus macaques at the animal shelter Tierheim Berlin e.V. and Anja Pfadenhauer and Melanie Büchner for carrying out the observations. A previous version of this chapter was entitled "An integrative meta-theoretical framework for research on individual behaviour in context—situations, populations, species". This research was funded by a grant from the German Research Foundation (DFG; UH-249/1-1).

15 Beneficial Effects of Pet Ownership on Human Health: The Influence of Caretakers' Attachment Style and Personality as well as Dog's Personality and Behavior

Corinna Buderer, Verena Schreiner and Rainer Wohlfarth

Key Words: *Human-animal interaction, dog-caretaker relationship, attachment, personality, health Dog, big five, personality traits, dog's behavior problems, canine behavior, quality of life*

Abstract

The current situation of studies indicates positive effects of dog-human interaction regarding human health. The aim of the present study was to examine the influence of the caretakers′ attachment style and personality in conjunction with the dog-caretaker relationship quality on caretakers′ self-rated health. Furthermore, the influences of the subjectively reported personality characteristics and behavior problems of the dogs on the relationship and on self-rated health have been surveyed due to a lack of research regarding these factors so far. The study was an online survey with a sample size of 281 female dog caretakers. For data collection self-rating measures were used (SF-36, SCL-14, MDORS, MCPQ-R and C-BARQ modified). The Results show that neither attachment-style nor personality in conjunction with attachment-quality has had a significant effect on self-rated health. Only the two factors attachment and perceived emotional closeness to the dog showed a significant interaction effect. Significant correlations between behavior problems and personality characteristics of the dog with self-rated health of the caretakers were found. However, effect sizes turned out to be small in most of the cases. Across analysis neuroticism showed a significant correlation with self-rated health, especially self-assessed mental health. The results and potential limitations are being discussed.

1. Introduction

In the last decades literature has revealed a substantial amount of studies indicating positive health benefits as an outcome of human-animal interactions. The positive effects for the caretakers are found on psychological as well as on physiological health and can be induced throughout short-term interactions e.g.

animal based therapies or long-term interactions as pet caretaker ship (Wells, 2009; Julius, Beetz, Kotrschal, Turner & Unvas-Moberg, 2013). The physical interaction with a companion animal or the mere presence of it can reduce the heart rate and blood pressure of the caretaker (Allen, Blascovich, Tomaka & Kelsey, 1991; Wells, 2009). From a psychological point of view companion animals can serve as catalysts for social relations, are able to reduce loneliness, isolation, depression and anxiety and can help increasing self-confidence and self-esteem (Wells, 2009; Julius et al., 2013; Hart, 2010). Studies in this context point out the exceptional role dogs take on (Headey, Na & Zheng, 2008; Headey & Grabka, 2007; Serpell, 1991). Considering stress as a potential mediator of physical and psychological illness, interactions with companion dogs were found to reduce the stress hormone cortisol and to decrease the heart rate of the involved person. Furthermore, the hormone oxytocin, which is known to stimulate social interactions, reducing anxiety and producing calm and serenity, is thought to be released while interacting with companion dogs (Odendaal & Meintjes, 2003; Nagasawa, Kikusui, Onaka, & Ohta, 2009; Handlin et al., 2011; Beetz et al., 2011). The dog´s ability to reach humans on three different levels, the physical, emotional and social, can be seen as one of the reasons for their exceptional position among pets (Mende & Mende, 2011). Furthermore, dogs are willing to learn, flexible and adaptive. More than other companion animals they are able to initiate communicative interactions, understand some of human gestures and recognize simple forms of visual attention (Miklosi, 2007). Although studies reinforce the thesis that companion animals are good for human health, a causal conclusion cannot be drawn (Wells, 2009). The lack of evidence leads back to methodological problems in many studies, such as sample sizes, which are too small, not representative and heterogeneous, and the absence of a control group (Kruger & Serpell, 2010). Further, the impact of confounding variables has been neglected in former studies (Julius et al., 2013). Studies point to a range of different variables which should be taken into consideration. Besides socio-demographic data, the intensity of the human-animal bond, personality and attachment style of the caretaker as well as the dog´s personality and behavior may influence whether the human-animal interaction leads to a positive health outcome or not (Julius et al., 2013). This study has taken into account these facts by including all mentioned confounding variables. In doing so, the study tried to contribute to a better understanding of the underlying mechanisms in human-animal interactions.

Attachment Style and Personality Characteristics

Bowlby (1969, 1979) and Ainsworth (1963, 1972) provide the theoretical framework to explain and investigate close and long-term relationships between humans. According to the theory there are mainly the different styles: secure, insecure-ambivalent, insecure-avoidant and disorganized attachment style. The attachment style which is influenced by parental bonding seems to be an essential factor for physical and mental health in adulthood (Enns, Cox, & Clara, 2002; Maunder & Hunter, 2008). The attachment theory can be transferred to human-animal bonds (Julius et al., 2013).

When investigating personality characteristics, the most common categorical system used to illustrate personality dimensions are the big five. The five factors neuroticism, extraversion, openness, conscientiousness and agreeableness are found across cultures and are useful to describe personality traits and differences in personality traits between people (Asendorpf & Neyer, 2012). The following explications about the interrelation between attachment style, personality and health benefits of the human-animal interaction give a short outline about the current state of studies.

Colby and Sherman (2002) point out that depending on the attachment style in elder people, differences in mood can be found after a short-time interaction with a dog. Beetz and co-workers (Beetz et al., 2011) revealed in their study that children with an insecure and disorganized attachment style have a greater benefit from a dog as social supporter than from a toy dog or a friendly person in a stressful situation. Secure attached children on the other hand also profited from the friendly person and therefore showed lower levels of cortisol as a physiological indicator of stress in both investigated conditions. Julius et al. (2013) conclude that companion animals are able to serve as secure attachment figures. Thus, they take over the role of social support, which is known to be an important contribution to human health.

With respect to personality traits, studies revealed differences in dog-human relations and therefore varying impacts on human health may be assumed. Kotrschal and coworkers (Kotrschal, Schöberl, Bauer, Thibeaut & Wedl 2009) found that caretakers of dogs with high scores on the dimension neuroticism showed a stronger relation to their dogs, gave their dogs more attention and saw them as social support. Compared to them, caretakers with high scores on the dimension extraversion saw their dogs as companions for joint activities rather than social support. The results of this study may indicate a different quality of human-dog relationships with respect to the caretaker's personality. Thus, personality traits should be investigated in the context of human-animal interaction and health as well.

The Dogs 'Personality' and Behavior

As far as we know there has been no research investigating the dogs´ personality and behavior and its impacts on human health so far. Serpell (1991) found in his study that caretakers with a weak relationship to their dogs described themselves as less satisfied with behavioral aspects of the dogs like anxiety, agitation, lack of obedience and hyperactivity. As there is an impact of the dogs´ personality and behavior on the quality of the human-dog relationship it can be assumed that human health is influenced as well. Furthermore, a consensus can be found on some prerequisites which should be fulfilled for health beneficial effects. Keeping animals must be species-appropriate as only then do they attain a degree of well-being and are treated as social partners (Beetz & Kotrschal, 2012). The mere presence of a dog is not enough to cause beneficial health effects. The relationship to the animal must be positive, which includes a positive physical contact as well (Julius et al., 2013).

Aims

According to previous research findings, we hypothesized that there are correlations between the personality and the attachment style of the caretaker and the subjective perceived quality of the dog-caretaker relationship (hypothesis 1). Furthermore we expected relations between the subjective perceived quality of the relationship and the reported health of the caretakers (2). We assumed that insecure attached caretakers with a good reported quality of the relationship rate their health better than those with a relationship quality reported as being worse. For secure attached caretakers, we hypothesized that differences in the perceived quality of the relationship do not show an impact on their self-rated health (2a). Exactly the same direction of effects we assumed for the personality trait neuroticism. Caretakers with high scores on this dimension were expected to rate their health better if the subjective perceived quality of the relationship was good. For those with low scores, we did not assume an impact of the reported relationship quality self-rated health (2b).

Besides caretaker traits we supposed that the dogs' behavior, particularly behavior problems, and personality characteristics influence the caretakers′ self-rated health (3). If the dog were to show behavior problems we assumed a poorer self-rated health. Furthermore, we expected to detect personality characteristics which related to the subjective perceived health of the caretaker. Also, we supposed that there is a correlational relation between the caretaker-dog relationship and the dogs' behavior problems as well as with the personality characteristics of the dog (4).

2. Method

The protocol and procedure employed for the present study has been performed in accordance with the ethical standards delineated in the 1964 Declaration of Helsinki. Participants were approached via social media, online dog forums and a data base from a previous study in Germany. Except for requiring a minimum age of 18 years and living together with the dog for at least half a year, there were no further prerequisites for participation. The study was realized online with the software Unipark. To enhance the willingness to participate, 20 vouchers with a value of 20 Euros each were given as payment. The duration of the participation was between 30 and 45 minutes. The survey was conducted anonymousl. Globalpark as the supplier of the software Unipark guaranteed the privacy and personal security of the data. Initially, participants were informed about the purpose of the study, duration, anonymity and payment.

Participants

The sample consisted of 296 dog-owners. Only 15 participants (5.1%) were male, 281 (94.9%) were female. To ensure the interpretability of the data, only the female participants were included in the analysis. They had a mean age of M = 40.6 years (SD = 11.4 years) with a range from 18 to 68 years. 29.2% stated that they were living in a relationship, 40.2% were married, 28.8% single and 1.8% widowed. Their professional state differed between employed (48%), self-employed (20.6%), Students (8.9%), retired persons (5.3%), without employment (3.6%) and apprentices (0.4%). 13.2% did not categorize their professional state. 81 (28.8%) persons indicated that they were chronically ill.

Among the 281 dogs 119 (42.3%) were male and 162 (57.3%) were female. The dogs´ age ranged from 1 to 17 years (M = 5.8 years, SD = 3.56). 159 (60.1%) dogs were neutered and 80 (28.5%) dogs were from an animal shelter. 259 (92.2%) persons indicated that they were mainly the caretaker of the dog.

With respect to self-rated health our sample showed scores on the SF-36 questionnaire in line with the norm sample of the German population from 1998 (Ellert & Bellach, 1999). On the scale ´physical functioning´ they had $M = 93.42$ ($SD = 10.82$), on ´role-physical´ $M = 86.03$ ($SD = 29.33$), on ´bodily pain´ $M = 76.00$ ($SD = 18.63$), on ´perceived health´ $M = 34.69$ ($SD = 13.65$), on ´vitality´ $M = 59.11$ ($SD = 18.49$), on ´social functioning´ $M = 87.41$ ($SD = 21.21$), on ´role-emotional´ $M = 82.44$ ($SD = 31.75$) and on the scale ´mental health´ $M = 73.96$ ($SD = 17.43$). The same arose for the scores on the SCL-14, for which a valid norm sample only exists for the general severe index (Hessel et al., 2001). Our sample differed with $M = .46$ less than a quarter standard deviation from the norm.

For the neuroticism scale of the NEO-FFI and the insecure attachment scale of the RSQ we bisected the sample by median. Thus, 129 of the caretakers rated themselves with lower scores and 152 with higher scores on the dimension ´neuroticism´. For the attachment style the bisection revealed 129 caretakers with a more secure attachment style and 152 participants with a more insecure attachment.

No comparison with a norm sample was possible for the results of the MDORS. For the scale ´dog-caretaker interaction´ our sample showed $M = 52.49$ ($SD = 4.84$), on ´perceived emotional closeness´ $M = 22.04$ ($SD = 6.85$) and on ´perceived costs´ $M = 39.15$ ($SD = 5.11$). Here we also bisected the sample by median, which revealed 165 caretakers scoring high on ´dog-caretaker interaction´ and 116 scoring low. Furthermore 156 caretakers indicated a stronger ´perceived emotional closeness´ than the other 122 participants and 159 of the caretakers scored higher on ´perceived costs´ than the other 122 caretakers.

Due to a lack of the norm sample for the MCPQ-R we compared the personality descriptions of the dogs to an Australian sample (Ley et al., 2008) with which they resembled and didn´t differ more than half a standard deviation on each scale (extraversion *M* = 54.83, *SD* = 14.35; amicability *M* = 70.43, *SD* = 16.34; training focus *M* = 82.26, *SD* = 12.75; motivation *M* = 75.55, *SD* = 16.81 and neuroticism *M* = 45.30, *SD* = 17.23).

For comparing behavior problems of the dogs which resulted from the C-BARQ modified, neither a norm sample nor another study was accessible. Our sample scored on ´stranger-directed aggression´ *M* = 1.11, *SD* = .32; ´owner-directed aggression´ *M* = 1.59, *SD* = .65; ´stranger-directed fear´ *M* = 1.40, *SD* = .69; ´non-social fear´ *M* = 1.51, *SD* = .7; ´dog-directed fear or aggression´ *M* = 2.0, *SD* = .84; ´separation-related behavior´ *M* = 3.14, *SD* = .87 and ´attachment or attention-seeking behavior´ *M* = 1.52, *SD* = .76.

Instruments

Questionnaires to assess socio-demographic data, subjective health, personality traits and attachment style of the caretakers, personality traits and behavior of the dogs and the perceived quality of the relationship between the dogs and caretakers, were provided online in German versions.

Neo-Five-Factor-Inventory

We used the multidimensional Personality Inventory from Costa and McCrae (1992), the NEO-FFI, which is seen as the state of the art in assessing personality traits (Hahn, 2013). The five personality dimensions 'neuroticism', 'extraversion', 'openness for new experiences', 'agreeableness' and 'conscientiousness' are investigated by questions, given a five-point scale answer format from strong disagreement to strong agreement (Borkenau & Ostendorf, 2008).

Relationship Scale Questionnaire

With the RSQ (Griffin & Bartholomew, 1994), we assessed the attachment styles of the participants. The RSQ also uses a five-point rating scale asking the participants for their level of agreement or disagreement. On the basis of the scores the four dimensions result: 'fear of separation', 'fear of closeness', 'missing trust' and 'wish for independence'. They correspond with the four attachment styles mentioned above (Steffanowski et al., 2001). High scores on the dimensions ´fear of separation´ and ´fear of closeness´ indicate an 'insecure attachment style' and a low score a 'secure attachment style' (Steffanowski et al., 2001).

SF-36 Health Survey

The SF-36 (Bullinger & Kirchberger, 1998) with the eight dimensions 'physical functioning', 'role-physical', 'bodily pain', 'general health', 'vitality', 'social functioning', 'role-emotional' and 'mental well-being' was used to assess health related quality of life. There are two factors underlying these dimensions, physical and mental health. The answers of the questionnaire are in different formats and relate to the health experiences of the previous week.

Symptom-Checklist-14

The SCL-14, as the short version of the SCL-90, served to indicate symptoms of physical and mental illness. The SCL-14 gives a 'general severe index', showing a general mental load, and the subscales 'depression', 'somatization' and 'phobic anxiety' (Hessel, Schumacher, Geyer & Brähler, 2001). The participants were asked 14 questions related to their experiences of the previous seven days.

Monash Dog Owner Relationship Scale

The MDORS (Dwyer, Bennett & Coleman, 2006) were used to assess the attachment and intensity of the relationship between the dog and his caretaker. 28 questions with five-point scale answers revealed the three subscales 'dog-caretaker interaction', 'perceived emotional closeness' and 'perceived costs', which can be interpreted separately or as parts of one overall scale.

Monash Canine Personality Questionnaire – Revised

To assess the personality of the dogs we used the MCPQ-R (Ley, Bennet & Coleman, 2008). The questionnaire consisted of 26 items, containing dog describing adjectives, which the participants had to rate with a score from one (describes my dog not at all) to a six (describes my dog exactly). The five dimensions 'extraversion', 'amicability', 'training focus', 'motivation' and 'neuroticism' resulted from the questionnaire.

Canine Behavioral Assessment and Research Questionnaire – Modified

We modified the C-BARQ (Hsu & Serpell, 2003) to investigate behavior problems of the dogs. Due to our research topic to detect tendencies of behavior problems rather than to classify them, we shortened the questionnaire to 22 items. The five-point scale answer format was maintained, as well as the seven dimensions, which turned out to be clinically relevant. Namely, these are 'stranger-directed aggression', 'owner-directed aggression', 'stranger-directed fear', 'non-social fear', 'dog-directed fear or aggression', 'separation-related behavior' and 'attachment or attention-seeking behavior'.

Data Analysis

Data were analyzed with SPSS 21.00. A Kolmogorov–Smirnov test indicated that dependent measures were not normally distributed. The F test is robust to non-normality, if the non-normality is caused by skewness rather than by outliers. Visual inspection shows that there were some outliers, which were removed.

We dichotomized the continuous variables 'insecure attachment style' and the subscales of the dog-caretaker relationship quality ′emotional closeness′, ′dog-caretaker interaction′ and ′perceived costs′ by median split. Then, we performed univariate two-way ANCOVAs on mean of SF-36 scales with attachment style (secure vs. insecure) and with each of the three MDORS subscales ′emotional closeness′ (low vs. high), ′dog-caretaker interaction′ (low vs. high) and ′perceived costs′ (low vs. high) as the between-subject factors. We included ′age′ and 'neuroticism' as covariates. Thus, we tested group differences in caretakers′ attachment style and quality of the dog-caretaker relationship and their impact on the caretakers′ mental and physical health. We did the same analyses to examine group differences in caretakers′ neuroticism characteristic and quality of the relationship and their impacts on caretakers′ health. Therefore, the between subject effects on mental and physical health were tested with univariate two-way ANCOVAs with neuroticism (secure vs. insecure) and the three relationship quality scales each at a time (low vs. high) as factors. We included age as a covariate. For estimating effect sizes we used partial eta-square and evaluated those referring to Cohen (1988): η^2 = .10: small effect, η^2 =.24: medium effect, η^2 = .37: larger effect.

As most of the used scales were not normally distributed correlational analyses were done by Spearman′s Rho. A significance level of p = .05 was adopted for all tests.

3. Results

Personality, Attachment Style, Relationship Quality and Caretakers Health

Table 1 displays the correlational coefficients for all subscales calculated. Significant correlations were found between personality traits and the dog-caretaker relationship. The subscale 'perceived costs' showed a significant correlation with 'extraversion' (r_{rho}=.14, p<.05) and 'agreeableness' (r_{rho}=.14, p<.05), and a highest significant correlation with 'conscientiousness' (r_{rho}= .21, p<.001) and 'neuroticism' (r_{rho}= -.32, p<.001). Furthermore, there was a highest significant correlation between the subscale 'perceived costs' and an insecure attachment style (r_{rho}= -.25, p<.001). The subscales 'interaction with the dog' and 'emotional closeness' showed a significant correlation with the personality trait 'openness for experiences' (r_{rho}=.12, p<.05). A highest significant relation also arose between an insecure attachment style and 'neuroticism' (r_{rho}=.56, p<.001).

With respect to health, highest significant correlations were found between the subscale 'perceived costs' and 'physical health' (r_{rho}=.16, p< .001), as well as with 'mental health' of the SF-36 (r_{rho}=.42, p<.001). No significant correlations were found between self-reported health of the SF-36 and the other subscale 'emotional closeness' and 'dog-caretaker interaction'. Furthermore, regarding self-reported health according to the SCL-14, there were highest significant correlations between the scales 'perceived costs' and the 'general severe index' (r_{rho}= -.35, p< .001).

Table 1. *Correlations between perceived dog-caretaker relationship (MDORS) and personality (NEO-FFI), attachment style (RSQ) and self-rated health (SF-36, SCL-14) of the caretakers*

	IS	N	E	O	A	C	MH	PH	GSI
IA	.00	-.02	-.03	.12*	.10	.06	.05	.01	.05
EC	-.08	-.08	.00	.12*	-.05	.01	.04	-.04	.01
PC	-.25***	-.32***	.14*	.00	.14*	.21***	.42***	.16***	-.35***

Note: * significant for p<.05; ** significant for p<.01; *** significant for p<.001.IA: dog-caretaker Interaction; EC: Emotional Closeness; PC: Perceived Costs; IS: Insecure Attachment style; N: Neuroticism; E: Extraversion; O: Openness; A: Agreeableness; C: Conscientiousness; MH: Mental Health; PH: Physical Health; GSI: General Severe Index.

Attachment Style and Dog-Caretaker Relationship Impacts on Self-Rated Health

The ANCOVA revealed a significant interaction effect $F(1, 273) = 4.371$, p=.037, η2=.02 between the two between-subject factors attachment style and 'emotional closeness' (Figure 1). Both continuous variables were dichotomized by median split. Secure attached caretakers, who reported a high emotional closeness to their dogs rated their physical health on the SF-36 consistent better (M= 89.34), compared to all other combinations of the two factors mentioned above. Lowest scores on the scale 'physical health' were shown by caretakers with a weaker perceived 'emotional closeness' to their dogs (M= 82.48). The influence of the covariates age $F(1, 273) = 13.661$, $p<.001$, $\eta^2=.05$ and 'neuroticism' $F(1, 273) = 17.687$, $p<.001$, $\eta^2=.06$ became significant.

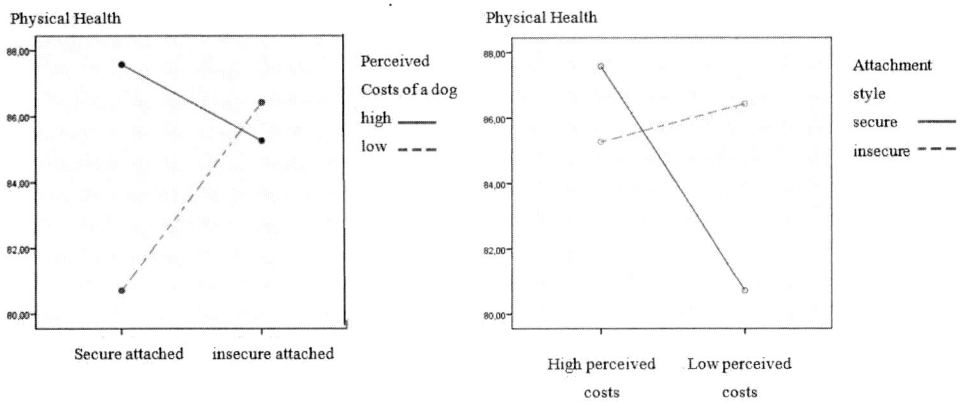

Figure 1. *Interaction between attachment style and perceived costs as a subscale of the perceived dog-caretaker relationship on physical health of the caretakers.*

With respect to mental health on the SF-36 a significant main effect for the dichotomized subscale 'perceived costs' was found F(1, 273) = 7,799, p =.006, η^2= .03. Thus, caretakers with less reported costs rated their mental health consistent better (M= 82.70), compared to caretakers who reported high perceived costs (M= 70.39). 'Neuroticism' showed again a significant confounding effect F(1, 273) = 114,394, p<.001, η^2=.30. No significant effects were found for the attachment style and the other two scales ′emotional closeness′ and ′interaction′ on mental health.

Neuroticism and Dog-Caretaker Relationship Impacts on Self-Rated Health

No interaction effects were found for the between-subject factors 'neuroticism' and the dog-caretaker relationship subscales (dichotomized in low vs. high category). However a significant main effect for 'neuroticism' was found throughout all calculations with the subscales. For the calculation with 'perceived costs' $F(1, 273) = 5.868$, $p=.016$, $\eta^2=.02$, 'interaction with the dog' $F(1, 273) = 6.970$, $p=.009$, $\eta2=.03$ and 'emotional closeness' $F(1, 273) = 7.356$, $p=.007$, $\eta^2=.03$. Therefore caretakers with low 'neuroticism' reported a better 'physical health' on the SF-36, compared to caretakers with high 'neuroticism'. Age as a covariate became significant for all calculations $F(1, 273) = 11.537$, $p=.001$, $\eta^2=.04$. With respect to mental health on the SF-36, the same picture was found. For all calculations with the dichotomized subscales of the dog-caretaker relationship a significant main effect for 'neuroticism' was found. The results were for 'perceived costs' $F(1, 273) = 29.742$, $p<.001$, $\eta^2=.10$, for 'interaction with the dog' $F(1, 273) = 31.804$, $p<.001$, $\eta^2=.10$ and for 'emotional closeness' $F(1, 273)= 34.695$, $p<.001$, $\eta^2=.11$. As a consequence caretakers with low 'neuroticism' also reported a better 'mental health', compared to those with high 'neuroticism'. Furthermore, the results showed a significant main effect for 'perceived costs' $F(1, 273) = 10.423$, $p=.001$, $\eta^2=.04$. Therefore caretakers who perceived <u>fewer</u> costs rated their mental health better (M=82.70) than those who reported high 'perceived costs' (M= 70.39). Attachment style as a covariate also became significant $F(1, 273) = 11.170$, $p=.001$, $\eta2=.04$. Finally, regarding the general severe index, the calculations showed the same pattern. A significant main effect for 'neuroticism' was found for all scale, 'perceived costs' $F(1, 273) = 28,279$, $p<.001$, $\eta^2= .09$, 'interaction with the dog' $F(1, 273) = 28.604$, $p<.001$, $\eta^2= .10$ and 'emotional closeness' $F(1, 273) = 30,253$, $p<.001$, $\eta^2= .10$. Hence, caretaker with low 'neuroticism' reported less severe symptoms (M= 0.728) than caretakers with high 'neuroticism' (M= 0.201). Attachment style again showed a significant confounding effect $F(1, 273) = 18.507$, $p<.001$, $\eta^2=.06$.

Self-Rated Health, Reported Behavior Problems and Personality Traits of the Dogs

We investigated a correlative relation between the General Severe Index of the SCL-14 and the seven behavior dimensions of the C-BARQ, as well as with one overall behavior problems factor. Significant correlations were found for 'stranger-directed aggression' (rrho = .123, $p< .05$) and 'attachment-seeking behavior' ($r_{rho}= .151$, $p< .05$). Highest significant correlations appeared for 'non-social fear' ($r_{rho}= .256$, $p< .001$), 'separation-related fear' ($r_{rho}= .222$, $p< .001$)

and 'general behavior problems' (r_{rho}= .304, $p < .001$). With respect to the dogs personality traits significant correlations arose for 'training focus' (r_{rho}= -.132, $p < .05$) and 'amicability' (r_{rho}= -.146, $p < .05$) and a highest significant correlation with 'neuroticism' (r_{rho}= .189, p< 001).

Self-rated health measured with the SF-36 showed highest significant correlations between the subscales 'non-social fear' and 'mental well-being'. For the 'general behavior problems' factor highest significant correlations were found with 'vitality', 'social function' and 'mental well-being'. With respect to reported personality traits of the dogs the results showed highest significant correlations for 'amicability' and ´neuroticism' with the subscale 'mental well-being'. All results are displayed in Table 2.

	OA	SA	SAN	DA	NF	SB	AB	BP	E	M	TF	A	N
KÖFU	-.030	-.069	.121*	.023	-.064	.002	-.020	-.057	.067	-.070	.084	-.032	-.002
KÖRO	-.123*	-.025	.033	.059	-.053	-.083	-.034	-.078	.053	-.039	.105	-.038	-.011
SCHM	-.142*	-.020	-.072	.018	-.025	-.065	-.066	-.081	.041	-.077	.113	.052	.026
VITA	-.091	-.064	-.052	-.116	-.181	-.142*	-.162**	-.266***	.031	.105	.188**	.154**	-.169**
SOFU	-.133*	-.091	-.078	-.037	-.140*	-.188**	-.141*	-.224***	-.021	-.003	.025	.101	-.093
EMRO	-.109	-.055	-.065	.009	-.148*	-.192**	-.120*	-.200**	.025	.054	.027	.113	-.122*
PSYC	-.113	.108	-.102	-.063	-.227***	-.200**	-.175**	.498***	-.085	.087	.074	.225***	-.216***
GSI	.108	.123*	.084	.079	.256***	.222***	.151*	.304***	.080	-.009	-.132*	-.146*	.189**

Table 2. *Correlations between self-rated health (SF-36, SCL-14), dogs´ behavior problems (C-BARQ) and dogs´ personality traits (MCPQ)* **(↓)**

Note: * significant for p<.05; ** significant for p<.01; *** significant for p<.001.KÖFU: physical functioning; KÖRO: role-physical; SCHM: bodily pain; VITA: vitality; SOFU: social functioning; EMRO: role-emotional; PSYC mental well-being; GSI: General Severe Index; OA: Owner-directed aggression; SA: Stranger-directed aggression; SAN: Stranger-directed fear; DA: Dog-directed fear; NF: Non-social fear; SB: Separation-related behavior; AB: Attachment-seeking behavior; BP: Behavior problems; E: Extraversion; M: Motivation; TF: Training focus; A: Amicability; N: Neuroticism

Perceived Dog-Caretaker Relationship and Reported Behavior Problems and Personality Traits of the Dogs

Our correlational calculations revealed significant relations between the subscale 'dog-caretaker interaction' and 'extraversion' (r_{rho}= -.145, p< .05) and 'amicability' (r_{rho}= -.131, p< .05). Highest significant correlations were found with 'training focus' (r = -.189, p< .001) and 'attachment-seeking behavior' (r_{rho}= -.207, p< .001). The subscale 'emotional closeness' showed a high significant correlation with 'amicability' (r_{rho}= -.160, p< .01) and highest significant correlations with 'training focus' (r_{rho}= -.369, p< .001) and 'attachment-seeking behavior' (r_{rho}= -.264, p< .001). For the subscale 'perceived costs' we found a significant correlation with 'neuroticism' (r_{rho}= -.152, p< .05) and high significant correlations with 'dog-directed fear or aggression' (r_{rho}= -.176, p< .01), 'non-social fear' (r_{rho}= -.167, p< .01) and 'separation-related behavior' (r_{rho}= -.171, p< .01). Highest significant correlations were found for 'training focus' (r_{rho}= .385, p< .001), 'amicability' (r_{rho}= .287, p< .001), 'owner-directed aggression' (r_{rho}= -.206, p< .001) and 'general behavior problems' (r_{rho}= -.262, p< .001). All results are displayed in Table 3.

Table 3. *Correlations between perceived dog-caretaker relationship (MDORS), reported behavior problems (C-BARQ) and personality traits (MCPQ) of the dogs*

	OA	SA	SAN	DA	NF	SB	AB	BP	E	M	TF	A	N
IA	.080	-.021	-.032	.004	.039	-.095	-.207***	-.068	-.145*	-.048	-.189**	-.131*	-.070
EC	.063	-.069	.010	.026	.075	.048	-.264***	-.067	-.011	-.034	-.369***	-.160**	.016
PC	-.206**	-.055	-.048	-.176**	-.167**	-.171**	-.056	-.262***	-.076	-.015	.385***	.287***	-.152*

Note: * significant for p<.05; ** significant for p<.01; *** significant for p<.001.IA: dog-caretaker Interaction; EC: Emotional Closeness; PC: Perceived Costs; OA: Owner-directed aggression; SA: Stranger-directed aggression; SAN: Stranger-directed fear; DA: Dog-directed fear; NF: Non-social fear; SB: Separation-related behavior; AB: Attachment-seeking behavior; BP: Behavior problems; E: Extraversion; M: Motivation; TF: Training focus; A: Amicability; N: Neuroticism

4. Discussion

With respect to our first hypothesis, we have only found a relation between 'perceived costs′ and the attachment style of the caretaker. Thus, there is a relation between an insecure attachment style and a perception of an amount of negative aspects and personal limitations, which appear as a result of the dog-caretaker relationship. We could not find any relation between dog-caretaker interaction as well as 'emotional closeness' and the attachment style. Therefore, our results did not support other findings from previous studies, which proposed a benefit for insecure attached persons from dogs as social support (Beetz et al., 2011).

Second, we found a relation between caretakers who characterized themselves as more neurotic and higher perceived costs of the factor taking care of a dog. A relation to interaction behavior and 'emotional closeness' were not found. Furthermore, the results gave evidence that different personality traits are associated with a different perception of the dog-caretaker relationships quality. But once more, our results did not support previous findings which postulated a stronger dog-caretaker relationship if the caretaker scored high on neuroticism (Kotrschal et al., 2009).

Third, investigating the relationship between the quality of the dog-caretaker relationship and the self-rated health of the caretaker, the results revealed relations only for the negative aspects of taking care of a dog which was associated with a worse reported mental and physical health. Positive aspects such as interacting with the dog and emotional closeness did not show substantial correlations with self-rated health. Therefore, the data do not support the assumption that a good relationship with the dog can be seen as a resource for the caretakers′ health.

For our second hypothesis that insecure attached caretakers with a good relationship to their dogs would report a better health than insecure attached caretakers with a worse relationship, we failed to find any evidence. On the contrary, secure attached caretaker with strong emotional bond to their dogs rated their physical health best compared to secure attached caretaker with a weaker emotional bond. Insecure attached caretaker reported a better health if their relationship to the dog was weaker, than those with a stronger bond. But the interaction effect showed a marginal effect size ($\eta 2=.02$) which, according to Cohen (1988) cannot be seen as a small effect.

With respect to 'neuroticism' in relation with the relationship quality, as the second part of our second hypothesis, we couldn′t find evidence for an impact on the reported health. However, in our calculations 'neuroticism' and the caretakers′ age showed repeated confounding effects, but didn′t meet the criteria of a small effect. The negative impact of 'neuroticism' on physical health corresponds with other studies which for instance showed a higher morbidity (Maas & Spinath, 2012), or vulnerability for stress and coronary heart diseases (Wittchen & Hoyer, 2006) in relation to neuroticism as a personality trait. Equally, neuroticism has been discussed as a protective factor, because people may notice physical warning symptoms earlier and therefore receive treatment faster. These contrary sides of the mechanisms could offer an explanation for the very small effect sizes found in this study. Furthermore, we have to take into consideration that we exclusively used subjective measures. The results might give a different pattern using objective measures.

The third hypothesis, that caretakers rate themselves as less healthy if the dog shows behavior problems, could be supported by the results of our study. We found a positive relation with a medium effect size between the 'general severe index' as a global indicator of a general psychic strain and reported problem behavior of the dogs. Furthermore, the results revealed a negative relation with a medium to large effect size between self-rated mental well-being and reported problem behavior. Small effects were found for a negative relation between reported behavior problems with all subscales of mental health (SF-36). These negative finding were expected due to previous studies showing positive influences of dogs on mental health (Wells, 2009). A dog's well-being would be a prerequisite for that (Beetz & Kotrschal, 2012), which cannot be assumed when a dog shows behavior problems. Relations between physical health and behavior problems were not found in our data. Results of other studies postulating positive impacts of dogs on physical health (Headey & Grabka, 2007; Headey et al., 2008; Serpell, 1991) cannot be supported by our study. A negative relation would have been expected when dogs showed behavior problems.

A similar pattern was found for the relation between reported personality traits of the dogs and self-rated mental health. A general mental strain of the caretaker was related to lower 'training focus', less 'amicability' and higher 'neuroticism' scores of the dog. Also, these personality traits of the dogs showed the same relations with self-rated 'vitality'. High reported 'neuroticism' scores of the dogs were given by caretakers with a worse self-rated 'mental well-being' and higher scores on 'emotional role'. On the other hand caretakers who described their dogs as high amicable reported a better 'mental well-being'. Again, impacts on physical health could not be found and the findings showed only small effect sizes.

Our last hypothesis, concerning the relation between the dog-caretaker relationship and reported behavior problems and personality traits were supported by the data and correspond therefore with findings from previous studies (Serpell, 1996). A better quality of the relationship was associated with a better 'training focus' and 'amicability'. Also, the results showed an association between higher 'perceived costs' and reported 'neuroticism' of the dog. Reported 'extraversion' of the dog related to more intense dog-caretaker interaction. All effect sizes were small, except that concerning the relation with 'training focus'. For reported 'behavior problems' relations with small effects were found for 'perceived costs'. Caretakers perceiving rather negative aspects of taking care of their dogs reported a higher 'owner-directed aggression', higher 'aggression against other dogs', higher 'non-social fear' and more 'separation related behavior' of their dogs. Reported 'attachment-seeking behavior' was associated with more 'dog-caretaker interactions' and a stronger 'emotional closeness'. This may lead to the assumption that caretaker did not see attachment-seeking behavior as an undesirable problem.

Limitations

The validity of the results is limited by the fact that in many cases we found only small correlational effect sizes. Medium effect sizes were found in few relations, these were highlighted in the section above. Furthermore, the quasi-experimental setting did not allow drawing causal conclusions, only correlational relations could have been disclosed. Thus, we could not investigate the mechanisms of action. Also, external validity was limited because we exclusively examined women, and our sample showed a heterogeneous structure regarding the age of the participants. Although we could not find any impact of age on self-rated health in our study, possible effects should be considered based on other studies, which found a benefit of a dog particularly for elder people and children (Julius et al., 2013).

Further limitations were given by the fact that we exclusively used questionnaires and therefore obtained only subjective data. Particularly, the assessment of behavior problems is mentioned being very subjective (Wells & Hepper, 2000). Unacceptable behavior of a dog could mean for some caretakers normal behavior and is therefore not evaluated as a behavior problem. Dog related questionnaires are on the one side reliable measures (Fratkin et al., 2013), but on the other side show a lack of validity. Furthermore, it has to be emphasized that the personality of a human being, as well as of animals is much more complex than it could be reflected by a few personality dimensions. Health related questionnaires referred to a time frame of one to two weeks before the survey, and may lead to the same lack, not reflecting the real state of health. .

Finally it has to be mentioned that despite the fact of including many possible confounding variables, we have to take others into account not included precisely because of the complexity of the topic.

5. Conclusion

The results of our study can contribute to a more far-sighted approach in this complex field of study. Many aspects have to be taken into consideration investigating dog-human interactions. Due to our results a general conclusion that dogs are good for peoples´ health, cannot be drawn. Furthermore, individual aspects must be considered. Future studies should examine homogenous samples with control groups, use objective measures and control for many relevant variables as possible. Studies with a longitudinal character should be preferred.

Part 5:

Altered States of Conciousness

16 How does Hypnosis Heal? Change in an Ego-Free Status

Dirk Revenstorf

Translated by **David Emmans**

This is the abbreviated version of an article appearing in German, in full, with a complete reference list in the DGH website: www.dgh-hypnose.de

Key Words: Erickson hypnosis, direct suggestion, indirect induction, trance depth, DMN, suggestibility

Abstract

Meta-analyses of almost 10,000 patients published in controlled studies demonstrate that hypnotic therapy is highly effective in spite of occasionally very brief treatment times, in widely differing fields of intervention, and that this impact can reach the level of katamnesis in some studies. To explain these effects, referral will be made to the fact that hypnosis represents a changed state of consciousness. Recent neurobiological work with imaging techniques has yielded results which show that hypnosis induces a state of "hypo-frontality" (that is, a change in the functioning of the dorso-lateral prefrontal and the orbitofrontal cortices with a lowering of one's ability for critical review and a concomitant enhancement of one's degree of suggestibility). At the same time, the hypnotic trance represents, in a certain sense, an "ego-free" state, inasmuch as those regions of the brain involved in a person's self-image (in particular the precuneus and certain medio-prefrontal areas) are deactivated. This means that a patient, while in hypnotic trance, can accept suggestions without controlling for their compatibility with his or her everyday personality. With the help of clinical case studies this chapter will show how patients can abandon their everyday self-image with the help of post-hypnotically effective suggestions.

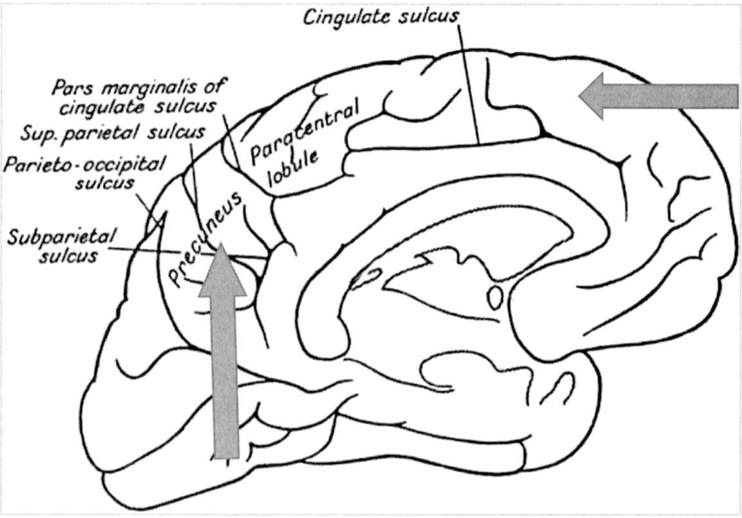

Figure 1: *Cerebral regions of the default mode network (from Wikipedia)*

1. Hypnosis: The Deactivation of the DMN

Changes in the so called default mode network (DMN) are viewed as an indicator for the state of a hypnotic trance. The DMN includes the medial prefrontal cortex (MPFC) and the medioparietal cortex, consisting of the precuneus (PCu) and the posterior cingulate cortex (PCC). The DMN is involved in various processes such as, for example, integrating cognitive and emotional processes, making decisions, evaluating the social consequences of behavior, sustaining attention, the feeling for time, planning actions, developing initiatives and the evolvement of one's will. It is involved among other things in complex interpersonal decisions such as evaluating and then approving social behavior, moral judgments, abstract thinking, self-reflection and self-images.

In phases of initial task orientation and subsequent concrete action planning, the DMN is deactivated while other areas specifically concerned with the function are correspondingly aroused. But interestingly for our topic, the same DMN is also deactivated under conditions of a hypnotic trance but without generating activity in any other areas: Although hypnosis may be introduced by means of a prior phase of relaxation or quiescence in which the DMN is clearly at work, the cerebral working mode starts distinguishing itself from that of the relaxation phase as soon as a hypnotic trance has established itself. The DMN-typical un-directed, "rambling" attention and self-referential thinking is "downsized" when hypnosis is successfully initiated. As opposed to a mere relaxation exercise, the deactivation of the DMN in a neutral ("suggestion-free") hypnosis (without any specific therapeutic suggestions) only occurs in persons easily influenced by suggestions and, importantly, without any reduction in the thalamic indicators of alertness. In the case of low-suggestible persons the DMN remains active even after trance induction and the thalamic signs of alertness or vigilance diminish, meaning that after hypnotic induction non-suggestible persons merely enter a relaxed phase.

That the activity of the DMN is suspended here is viewed as indicating that in a hypnosis in susceptible persons spontaneous cognitive activity does not develop that would otherwise stimulate reflecting on one's own personal identity, an evaluation of one's self-image and a consolidation of memory content. This would well explain the frequent occurrence of post-hypnotic amnesia. Likewise, this suspension of DMN activity induces a loss of empathy for other persons, which in turn offers an explanation for socially inacceptable behavior after some cases of stage hypnosis.

Hypnotized persons react to suggestions and associated images to a certain extent in an "ego-less" manner, that is, without consulting their established self-image (their everyday ego) and without evaluating their ensuing actions for future consequences or their effects on others with the criteria of empathy, that is, without checking these actions with memories of semantic and emotional-episodic contents. They refrain from rating and evaluating with such judgments as: "I can't do that," "I mustn't do that" or "That's not what I am". This explains why being in a state of deep relaxation and merely imagining possible actions or absolutely willing, desiring to do something in normal everyday thoughts is different from hypnosis whereby hypnosis allows for suggesting an alternate self-Image with different perceptual and behavioral possibilities, disconnecting the usual self-images from everyday thinking and their limitations which otherwise would impede actually performing the hypnotic suggestions.

A different hypothesis on the other hand assumes that the relationship to the hypnotist plays the essential role and that the bonding hormone oxytocin is released through the situation-specific intimate nature of the bond to the hypnotist which stimulates the person to fulfill his demands.

2. Posthypnotic Suggestions: An Ego-Free Behavior

The assumption that the everyday ego is in fact circumvented by hypnosis makes some forms of therapeutic changes feasible which are otherwise rejected due to more traditional paradigms of thinking. The possibility of such circumvention can be shown in rather simple cases of the use of direct suggestions in trance.

Posthypnotic suggestions are convincing examples that persons execute behavior which was suggested to them while in trance after the hypnosis has been concluded but which they themselves would not have considered possible, instead calling it ego-syntonic and basically rejecting the idea that they would ever even contemplate such behavior. Apparently, the persons fail to engage in this fatal syntonality assessment while in trance and such an omission has consequences post-hypnotically. For this reason posthypnotic suggestions are simple cases which demonstrate the validity of the deactivation theory of self-referential thinking (that is, the default mode) through a change in the modulation of the precuneus-frontal brain (that is, hypofrontality).

In their short-term and middle-range effects, posthypnotic suggestions have been documented impressively. Scholz (2008) identified several parameters for effectively designing posthypnotic suggestions: the short and cogent formulation of the final ability desired in the form of a concise slogan ("Work quickly and precisely!"), the association with action-relevant internal or external cues ("When the clock reaches 10 P.M., turn the TV off automatically and get up from your sofa!") and the visually concrete description of the whole scene. Consider the following examples:

1. Chocolate: An obese woman usually ate several bars of chocolate a day and she hid them in her bureau drawers. After going into a trance, she heard the instructions: *"I will only eat a single piece of chocolate an hour, meaning eight a day."* Next session she reported that for a whole week and for some unknown reason she only ate a single piece of chocolate an hour and put the rest back in the drawers. For the next three weeks she ate no chocolate at all, and when a year later she was asked about her craving she said with a slight stammer that she had given up chocolate altogether: "I don't need chocolate any more, I'm into cookies now."

2. Marital quarrelling: A couple going through a serious marital crisis arrived for their final session without any hopes of solving their daily problems. Their coping styles in the crisis remained just too different and partly even complementary: The woman was quick-thinking, efficient and very critical, the husband was relaxed, flexible and very easily hurt. The basic needs of the two remained chronic and in fact mutually unrecognized: The woman wanted support and the man wanted appreciation. After entering trance (sitting back to back so that neither had the feeling of being watched and instead both could better concentrate on his or her own inner feelings), they heard the direct suggestions: *"Whenever Mr. A. you experience your wife getting angry, you will only see her as a young girl in need of being hugged close, and you will feel the overwhelming desire to hold her tight."* And: *"Whenever Mrs. A. you experience your husband getting angry, you will only see him as the man you love and you will feel the overwhelming desire to tell him what a wonderful man he truly is."* Both reported a week later that they felt very fond of each other that week and had in fact been relatively free of any conflicts, without even addressing the topic of separation at all.

These may not be clinically relevant examples, but that is not so important at the moment: The essential fact is that the persons involved changed something disturbing in their behavior: something which they engaged in habitually and which they absolutely thought beforehand was impossible to change. The two cases following do have clinical relevance and make the point again:

1. Falling asleep: A woman who was unable to fall asleep next to her husband out of fear that he could start snoring at any moment heard the simple instruction: "As soon as you have turned your light off at night for sleeping, imagine, while breathing in, a mountain and, while breathing out, 'Immovable like a mountain'" She later reported: "Since Sunday I've been able to sleep 'like a mountain'. Today my husband had to wake me up because I was doing the snoring!"

2. Allergy for oranges: A woman physician had an allergy for oranges and in a trance she was given the instruction to imagine a pre-allergic reaction, as when she was on Crete, to then sense the feeling in her body of well-being while drinking a glass of orange juice, to call that feeling by a name of some color which could finally recall the trance state afterwards. In addition she heard an anecdote in which the sentence came up: "The war is over." Later the woman related: "As I was told, before drinking a glass of orange juice I recalled the feeling from my past on Crete by using the words 'let green come'. The test that followed was pretty demanding: There was a pitcher with half a liter of orange juice and two tasty whole oranges to drink and eat right after that! All I had was a slight reaction in the skin a few hours later, and I reacted to that by saying: 'The war is over!'. Otherwise I had no reaction whatsoever."

Examples 1 and 2 treat habits (such as eating or quarreling) which one engages in and interrupts voluntarily (even though it may not be so easy for the couple in the quarrel where both would have to want to stop at the same time). But example 3 concerns a behavior of the autonomic nervous system which is not under voluntary control (falling asleep). Similarly, example 4 describes a reaction of the endocrine system (an allergy) which is also not under direct conscious control.

The common denominator in these cases of posthypnotic suggestion, as in many others, is the fact that the persons involved, without transition or any prior practice possibilities or effort of their will power behave in a manner that they considered impossible up to then. The exact behavior or the physical reaction was basically always within the full range of their potential behavior, and to be exact for well before the hypnotic intervention. It may have properly belonged to their repertoire, but it was as yet inaccessible. Under hypnosis it was simply claimed, merely stated, that the reaction (rejecting sweets, falling asleep, eating allergens without their usual sensitizations) is possible. In standard discourse in each and every case the objection would certainly come up that such behavior had not been possible as of yet and therefore would still not be so at the moment. It is precisely this bothersome matching-up of a possible, but as yet unpracticed behavior against previous memories that is deactivated in hypnosis.

Instead, some other, earlier or perhaps even innate self-image is evoked here, which is fully accepted in the state of trance, and adopted without being scrutinized: un the case of the allergic woman it is the woman from out of her non-allergic past enjoying oranges; in the case of the patient suffering from insomnia it is the simple image of an immovable mountain as a metaphor for her other ego-images. In the case of the couple in marital crisis, each was instructed to see in the other that person he or she loved. This possibly means very well ignoring conflict-laden aspects inherent in the situation: anger at the inconsiderate snoring husband, the frustration which could only be overcome with the help of chocolate, or maybe even an original traumatic experience that lead to the allergy in the first place.

3. Discussion: Hypofrontality and Hypnotic Compliancy

Physiological studies on the brain using differing methodology have shown that in trance, on the one hand, a right-hemispheric and occipital activation occurs which in turn facilitates visual and concrete thinking. On the other hand, a neutral hypnosis, without specific tasking, deactivates the DMN which is responsible for "rambling" self-referential thinking.

Within the DMN, different regions are inhibited during a hypnotic trance, and we suspect that access to semantic and emotional memories is thus reduced, the feeling for time and sustained attention are curtailed and action planning is impaired. Simultaneously, attention is narrowed down, either to an object, a mental image or even just the voice of the hypnotist. When a trance is accompanied by tasks such as posthypnotic suggestions there is a change in the connectivity between the precuneus and the prefrontal cortex which is interpreted as meaning that executive control has been modulated.

The resulting change in the state of consciousness is, compared to normal, everyday thinking, rather expanded because it now gives free reign to one's visual processing and imagination and is not much bothered by rational criteria or principles of morality. This has decided advantages for divergent problem solving and for times when a particular objective experience is supplemented by later constructions and suggestions. A limited access to prior emotional experiences and their final appraisal (positive, negative, etc.) prevents on the one hand classifying momentary behavior according to its temporal perspective. This could explain the gullibility (or even seducibility) and the lack of personal feelings of shame seen in some participants at hypnosis shows, participants who for all intents and purposes willingly submit to someone else in front of the public and accept being humiliated. Feelings such as shame or guilt are basically experienced only when a behavior can be matched up against earlier experiences or against expectations of coming consequences. Instead of that, the attention of persons under hypnosis is fully concentrated on the here and now: All are laughing, so the poor victim laughs too: at himself.

The changes in information processing discussed above, however, would also offer an explanation for "obediency" or compliance with intra- and posthypnotic suggestions which in the context of stage hypnosis can have fatal effects while in a therapeutic context they are productive. The following summary now presents a view of the state and reactions of subjects in hypnotic trance based on data increasingly validated from the field of brain physiology.

4. Summary

The hypnotized person is relaxed but not sleepy (non somnolently relaxed) but instead focused on the coming suggestion expected and on mental images. Performing hypnotic behaviors or suppressing them apparently does not function on the basis of having some reactions or sensations become blocked off or obstructed, but rather through a change in one's self-image or self-representation that can be externally suggested and more easily accepted under hypnosis than in normal everyday consciousness. Under this condition, other self-images, including interfering ones, can be inhibited. An evaluation or estimation of the social consequences (that is, the relationship to one's everyday-ego, or feelings for empathy) is deferred. Just which role the bonding hormone oxytocin plays here has not been fully determined as of yet. If it in fact has a mediating function (and augments confidence and cooperational readiness both within and outside the hypnotic trance environment) then the presence of the hypnotist (as opposed to an anonymous CD) and the application of bodily closeness, physical touching and a qualitative voice modulation are major factors. Erickson's slogan "My voice accompanies you everywhere" thus appears once again in a new light. Furthermore, all elements supporting the regression will be relevant to the bonding.

The question of therapeutic ethics comes up here: Does the therapist want to help an uncritical patient reach a change in behavior or perception for his or her own good, even if doing so means an unreflected acceptance of the therapist's views, or is empowerment of the person the goal? Is the therapist striving for an enlightened patient and an interventional method that is at all times transparent or is he satisfied with making use of the patient's ability for dissociation while under hypnosis to overcome mental blocks? My reaction to such questions is to say they are wrongly put, because experiential preferences, once freed of a particular blockade, mean both an extension of some resources and at the same time an extinction of other, irrelevant perceptions.

17 State after Removal of a Meningeoma. Mental Rehabilitation with the Support of Hypnosis: Case Study

Hans Riebensahm and Francesca Scarpinato-Hirt

Key Words: rappor, therapeutic alliance, brain tumor, frontal lobe, declining organic brain syndrome, explosive disorder, trance, dream, metaphor, metamorphosis, anosmia

Abstract

The 61-year-old patient had suffered from a meningioma, which was removed by surgery. After successful surgery the patient would come out in aggressive outbursts whenever he saw someone disregarding society's generally accepted rules of behavior. His objective was to regain control of his impulses and affects. Following 34 sessions of a course of therapy involving trances, dreams and suggestions and with the help of many exceptional resources the patient arrived at a satisfactory result: He at last felt balanced and enjoyed a good quality of life. The major importance of good rapport (= "therapeutic alliance") is evident here.

1. Preliminary Remarks

When I was invited to make a contribution to the present publication, I initially felt greatly honored, but then I also saw myself under the obligation of having to produce a scientific case study. As I am a practical psychotherapist, not a scientist, I took some days to think about how I could fulfill this expectation. A scientific case study would have involved taking an objective approach towards the patient, the interactional process and also towards myself. To describe a therapeutic process in an objectifying, scientific language might well have omitted important aspects of subjective assessment and perception. That would go against my preference of a process-oriented therapy. So I am going to describe the mental rehabilitation process from my – of course subjective – first-person perspective. During preparation of this manuscript I was fortunate to have my highly competent colleague Francesca Scarpinato-Hirt by my side. I have learned so much from the friendly expert discussions with her and would now like to thank Francesca for offering me her time, creative ideas and feedback.

I am furthermore convinced, that an approach of well-meaning support is more important for effective therapy than collecting a complete set of information. Later on in this essay I will describe how I – fortunately only once –

endangered the rapport by trying to obtain more objective and complete information about the patient. We were luckily then able to restore mutual confidence and the rapport between ourselves.

2. My Initial Contact with the Patient

When Herbert*) called me at the beginning of January 2014, he told me that he had suffered from a brain tumor, known as a meningeoma, which had been removed in March 2013. After surgery he was offered inpatient rehabilitation and underwent psychological testing. As a result of these tests he was recommended for a course of psychotherapy in a psychosomatic clinic. However, as he told me, he would prefer to undergo psychotherapy near his home, not in a hospital far away.

When I asked him why he had chosen me as his psychotherapist (by that time I was already retired), Herbert answered he had asked a friend whether he knew of an older, experienced male psychotherapist. As this friend had been my patient some years ago, he recommended me and gave Herbert my telephone number. I had in fact decided (despite my age) to take up my profession of psychotherapist once again, I told Herbert I would be willing and able to work with him.

I had never before treated a patient who had undergone surgery for the removal of a meningeoma. I therefore might well have refused to treat Herbert. But when talking with him, Herbert somehow awakened my curiosity and sympathy and I felt confident of being able to support him here.

While talking with him, I remembered a case study which I had read just a few months earlier. In his book "Descartes' Error" (Damasio 1994) the author described the fate of a patient named "Elliot" who also had a meningeoma. It was removed by surgery, and, as Damasio reported, "The surgery was a success in every respect" (p. 36). But then unfortunately after a while this patient underwent a personality change, to adverse effect. The process already started in the course of his physical recovery and astonished both family and friends. "In many ways ... Elliot was no longer Elliot." The changes mainly concerned his social behavior and his ability to evaluate the benefits and risks involved in decisions. Finally Elliot was obliged to take up residence in a care home. (p. 34-51).

Although I of course had the case of Elliot in the back of my mind while talking with Herbert, I did not mention it. Nor did I mention other possible symptoms and risks, which are described also by Förstl (2005) (p. 84-99,) because I first and foremost aspired to stimulate positive expectations instead of suggesting fears.

---

*) All names of the patient and family members are pseudonyms; some biographical data have also been changed.

3. Herbert's Personal Background

At our first personal meeting on January 9th, 2014 Herbert gave me two MRT scans of his meningeoma and some medical reports, which had been prepared by his surgeon and his neurologist at the University Hospital of Göttingen.

When asked, Herbert told me his life story as follows:

He was born just seven years after the Second World War (1952) and grew up in a small town in northern Germany. As a boy he lived with his parents and an older sister. Herbert describes his parents as being strict and emotionally rather cool. But with one of his grandfathers (paternal grandfather) he enjoyed a warm and trusting relationship. Whenever he had a problem in his childhood, he could expect Grandpa's sympathy. But when Herbert was 14 years old, his beloved grandfather died, and Herbert, felt he had lost his greatest supporter. It may well have taken some time to overcome this traumatic experience.

Herbert's own father was a banker (manager of a savings bank) while also being a member of the marching band of the local shooting club. Such shooting clubs belong to the customs of many rural areas in Germany: In particular many medium-sized towns still have one. Dignitaries as for example, the head of the local savings bank of course are expected to join their local club. Once a year, when the club organized its shooting festival, Herbert as a boy was allowed to march along with his father's band. Naturally he was very proud of this and enjoyed both the music and also being part of this official ceremony. For Herbert even today, his memory of these events makes him well up. But possibly the tears I noticed in his eyes while he was telling his memories do not express consciously felt emotions but are merely symptoms of his current disease.

After Herbert graduated from high school, he would initially have preferred to study history of art, but on his father's recommendation, he decided to study economics at the University of Göttingen. But even while studying economics, as Herbert told me, he still seized every opportunity to visit exhibitions of painting and sculpture. Whenever he attended conferences on economics or other symposia, e.g. in Munich, Zurich or Vienna, he was on the lookout for information about local art exhibitions. But years later, when employed at the university, he no longer took time to visit expositions or paint for himself as he had once done while a schoolboy. Finally he completed his studies and took a doctorate in economics.

He was fortunate to then be offered employment as a lecturer at the Faculty of Economics in Göttingen. There he had to organize academic teaching, to conduct seminars, prepare lectures, and assist the chairholder. At the beginning of his academic career Herbert felt a high level of job satisfaction, partly because both students and the chairholder appreciated his achievements, something that made him proud. And he also liked dealing with the subject of economics. In retrospect Herbert felt that it had been the right decision to study economics instead of history of art.

In his thirties, Herbert told me that he fell in love and had a relationship with a woman called Anna. This relationship was comparatively short, lasting only a few years. But nevertheless Herbert and Anna had a son, Max, who is now (2014) 23 years old and is studying architecture elsewhere in Germany. Herbert emphasized, that in spite of separating from Anna, he is still on good terms with both, Anna and their son. To me this seemed plausible, because, by chance, I met Herbert, Anna and Max together during the interval of a theater performance. Herbert introduced me to both of them and we had a brief talk.

4. Turn for the Worse

Unfortunately, some years later, Herbert's situation at work then changed. The former chairholder had retired, and his successor seemed to dislike writing articles for publication or, as Herbert suspected, was less capable in this regard. Whatever the situation, Herbert was asked several times to write passages for one of the chairholder's publications. But instead of receiving recognition for his work, Herbert observed that his superior had amended Herbert's precise writing style (something he is especially proud of) into a style that is not sufficiently precise for such a complex topic. But after some discussion about the differences in opinion between Herbert and the chairholder, Herbert then avoided such debate.

But finally Herbert had to recognize, so he told me, that he was in a less favorable position than his colleagues, who received promotion earlier than himself. Herbert complained about this circumstance and requested equal treatment for himself. Superficially the chairholder seemed to agree, but failed to do what he had promised. Finally, in spite of several reminders, the chairholder even "forgot" to sign the application. The relationship with his superior of course deteriorated to an increasing extent, along with Herbert's attitude towards him. I assume the two men progressively developed at least a mutual dislike. This process of deterioration ended for Herbert one day when he was directly summoned by the Dean of the Faculty of Economics.

Regarding his conduct in previous years Anna described Herbert as always behaving very correctly, being conscientious, and displaying a groomed appearance and a well structured style of work. Herbert himself remembered being a "control freak". He would have tried to perform all his activities in exactly the right manner. "But now", he added, "I have left that behind me. I must no longer be perfect!"

The Dean then confronted Herbert with numerous individual complaints from students and colleagues, claiming for example that he had come to his lectures late several times or had even been absent altogether instead of teaching. Herbert tried to justify himself, arguing that complaints concern only the past turn and he had decided to take things easier. In the past he always had met his obligations and now felt he had the right to slow down.

These and other utterances and strange behavior of Herbert since the summer of 2012 seemed to indicate a major change in Herbert's personality. The Dean insisted that Herbert should undergo neurological testing. With the support of Anna and Herbert's general physician Herbert then – more or less voluntarily – agreed to undergo the requested neurological examination at Göttingen's University Hospital, although Herbert himself rejected the idea of his being sick.

But it was not only Herbert's superior, colleagues and students who supposed him to be ill: His previous partner Anna had noticed unusual behavior as well. Here I would like to include just a few items out of a list of more than twenty or so items, which were observed and listed by Anna before the Dean requested a neurological exam. The observation period extended from summer 2012 until March 2013. Herbert himself mentioned the existence of this list, and when asked for it, he agreed that I might use the list for the purpose of the present case study. But when he delivered it to me, he commented that he himself did not want to read it. Nor did he want to believe what Anna had listed. Despite this comment, when I asked him how he remembered that period, Herbert only reported some health complaints, e.g. long-term fatigue, an almost complete loss of energy and a significant weight increase as well.

Anna had additionally noted behavior disorders such as staying in the bathtub for hours and refusing to get out, refusing to consult a physician, sleeping and eating disorders and others. As his therapist I have intentionally avoided confronting Herbert with Anna's list of symptoms or insisting on subsequent questions as I did not want to possibly trigger bad feelings or reactance that might disturb our good rapport. Moreover, I do not believe that confronting Herbert with these negative experiences would help him in any way. On the contrary: I feared that Herbert might feel ashamed or even guilty because of the trouble he had caused. In this specific case, I find it perfectly natural to help him to forget this difficult experience.

5. Turn for the Worst?

Finally, the magnetic resonance imaging (MRI) scan clearly revealed a large meningeoma about 8 cm in diameter. The neurological audit revealed anosmia, optic atrophy on the left side and changes in psychomotor performance.

The tumor was situated in the frontal lobe in the midline area just above the nasal cavities above the plane formed by the roof of the eye sockets. The diagnosis was made on March 21st, 2013. Surgery was deemed to be essential and took place just five days later. According to the operation protocol the surgeon (University Hospital of Göttingen) adopted a microsurgical approach, both to minimize tissue trauma and to ensure predictable tissue maintenance. It was possible to remove the meningeoma completely without damaging parts of the frontal lobe tissue.

Surgery was of course followed by rehabilitation and checkups. Although a postoperative CT scan showed normal proportions, the patient's neurological status has remained unchanged. Herbert still suffers from anosmia and from deficits on the left side of the visual field, and these deficits will most probably remain.

Not entirely unexpectedly two new symptoms occurred firstly, – most disturbingly – aggressive outbursts, even in public whenever Herbert was faced with someone, who – from Herbert's point of view – was ignoring some generally accepted rule of behavior. For example, whenever Herbert observes cyclists using the sidewalk instead of the road or cycle path. He then started yelling at them for minutes, even when the bikers have already disappeared. Afterwards Herbert was very ashamed, but, so he told me, in such situations he felt unable to stop yelling. The second symptom was less disturbing for him, but nevertheless upsetting for others: he had to weep for no reason at all, sometimes even sobbing so tears flow from his eyes. Fortunately this happened mainly when he was alone or together with close friends, relatives or while talking with me. He welled up for example when he was listening to music or talking about his grandfather or when he was telling me a dream about being in his grandfather's garden.

At this time (November 2013) Herbert's physical condition was diagnosed by his neurologist (University Hospital of Göttingen) as "declining organic brain syndrome and depression". Herbert reported he also was suffering from intermittent explosive disorder (according to DSM IV).

6. Herbert's own View of his Situation

After Herbert had told me his life story so far, I asked him how he himself would feel about his current personal and professional situation. "The meningeoma marks an undeniable turning point in my life," he said. Not having worked at the university for almost the entire year, he said that economics went more or less completely out of his mind. Today he was no longer interested in this subject and felt he was in transition to an entirely new period of his life. He would not want to go back to teaching economics. He emphasized that he thought of his meningeoma as an earthquake, something caused by natural forces. He had to now deal with it instead of asking himself, "Why did this happen to me of all people?" I congratulated Herbert on taking this approach, because, I added, this attitude would provide a stable basis for future satisfaction with his life.

During recent months Herbert reported that he had rediscovered his love of the arts, especially for classical music. He liked to listen to CDs of such music or attend a live performance of the Göttingen Symphony or Academic Orchestra. He had also again started painting pictures with watercolors, in oil or acrylic paint. And whenever he finished a picture and believed it to be particularly successful, he would feel deep satisfaction, pride and happiness."

"Great", I said, because someone at the clinic had told Herbert he might generally lose his ability to feel emotion. What Herbert had told me about the change in his interests led me to assume that he might find a way back to his previous passion for the arts. In the context of his life story he had told me that he had studied economics mainly on the advice of his father, and not history of art as he himself would have preferred.

I was very pleased to hear this and also felt empathically that Herbert (unlike Elliot, Damasio's patient), does really feel emotion – not just joy and happiness but also disgust and anger (albeit still not expressed in the proper manner). And he is obviously not depressiv as he previously was diagnosed at the university hospital in 2013.

On the contrary I repeatedly felt surprised by the new resources Herbert was reporting: He told me he likes hiking in the countryside around Göttingen, on his own or with a friend, sometimes for two hours without a break. He also enjoys painting pictures, taking photographs of nature and landscapes, listening to music, reading books and magazines and visiting exhibitions. Herbert is obviously interested in current events all over the world, in history, philosophy, technology, especially in aviation and space technology. With this wide range of interests, Herbert has broad general knowledge.

I then asked Herbert what objective he wants to achieve through our therapeutic efforts. He answered that above all he wanted to learn to control again his emotions and behavior. "I can well understand that you wish to control your emotions and behavior," I answered. "That's natural and at the same time not easy to realize. You have already seen this. It is not easy because, since the removal of the meningeoma, only your unconscious mind was controlling your emotions and to a certain extent, also your impulsive behavior. What do you think about telling your unconscious mind to stay calm when you see someone breaking social conventions or rules? Or why not suggest to your unconscious mind that it should only trigger tears when your conscious mind agrees as well? "Yes, why not?" Herbert responded.

7. Proposal of Hypnotherapy Accepted

So I proposed to use hypnotherapy on Herbert. Because, as I told him, the method of hypnotherapy is aimed at communication between the unconscious and the conscious levels of experience. I would therefore expect, I said, that through hypnotic trances his unconscious mind could help him to achieve his objectives. I asked Herbert how he felt about my proposal. Herbert told me he was always interested in learning something new and did not know anything about hypnosis. I told him a bit about it and gave him numerous examples and metaphors of how his unconscious mind might work – not only during a state of trance in a formal hypnotherapeutic setting but also often surprisingly non-formal situations during his daily life.

I also asked him, whether he could already remember any experiences similar to any of the examples I had given him just before. Herbert said, "Yes, indeed". He remembered the time when he was writing his doctoral dissertation. For him it had been an interesting, agreeable and satisfying experience because his unconscious mind had helped him with it. He then described in detail how this had happened while he had been dreaming. Before going to sleep, he had been thinking about how to continue the next part of his text. Of course he did not dream the entire text in detail, he said, but worked out the thrust of the text, his flow of thoughts while asleep. In this way he was able to easily complete his dissertation in a relative short period of time.

I was of course very much impressed and pleased to hear Herbert's detailed description I was convinced that he and his unconscious mind might have sufficient resources to utilize and thereby to achieve his goals.

I have been working as psychotherapist for around 40 years, but as mentioned above, have never before had a patient from whom a meningeoma had been removed and who felt it necessary to enter a new phase in his life and was planning to do so. In particular, I had never before had to treat a patient with "declining organic brain syndrome".

But fortunately, from the very start of my training in hypnotherapy (1978), I have been greatly interested in its neurobiological aspects. Over the years I have read extensively in the field of neuroscientific literature, for example (it goes without saying) Halsband (2004), Damasio (1994), Dehaene (2014), Kandel (20124), Roth & Strüber (20154) and others.

The majority of researchers in this area seem to agree on the fundamental assumption that any mental process is based on biological processes. Metaphorically speaking, mind and body are an inseparable pair, and only death will separate them. That means that these processes interact in a very complex manner. As an example here, Halsband (2004) confirmed that trance inductions in fact lead to plastic changes in the brain. Moreover, inspired by Roth and Strüber (2015), I assume that rapport*) as an unspecific factor whose psychotherapeutic effectiveness has already been proven, will of course affect processes in the brain.

I thus felt encouraged to hope (albeit not to expect or even predict!) that a series of trance inductions might help Herbert's brain to reconstruct certain functions and possibly also even restore his sense of smell.

---

*) Overall, the quality of a therapeutic alliance (= rapport) arguably is the most effective factor of every course of psychotherapy (p. 331 (German edition)).

8. Probatory Sessions

Before officially embarking on a course of psychotherapy, we conducted five so-called probatory sessions. During these five hours we undeniably established a sustainable therapeutic alliance. Herbert then asked his health insurance to cover the costs of therapy. The insurer gave written approval to reimburse the costs for 40 sessions of psychodynamic psychotherapy. I believed this amount of psychotherapy would be sufficient to assist Herbert in regaining an at least acceptable level of impulse control and quality of life.

What puzzled me was that Herbert reported positive results after only the second or third probatory session, namely he had already sometimes succeeded in staying calm in situations when he previously would have exploded. One day for example, he had a difference of opinion with his son Max. Afterwards, Max commented to his father that Herbert's behavior in this discussion had shown remarkable improvement.

When Herbert had told me about this initial success, I of course expressed my delight. But simultaneously I recommended taking as much time for changes as were necessary. "Not so fast, Herbert!," I warned. And I reminded him that every process of learning, healing and regenerating needs a certain amount of time. By the way, I tend to include and repeat such suggestions on numerous occasions so as to generally avoid putting patients under pressure to perform, something that may unintentionally cause reactance.

After a comprehensive anamnesis and reciprocal provision of information I also told Herbert that I had been invited to write a paper about our work on the planned therapy: The paper was to be a contribution to a publication dedicated to Ulrike Halsband for her 60th birthday. I of course also told him that Ulrike Halsband is a well-known scientist in the field of neuropsychology at the University of Freiburg. I then asked him whether he agreed to this paper being published as an anonymized report in this commemorative volume, and Herbert gave his consent.

9. Herbert's First Formal Trance Experience on January 16th, 2014

Although we were still conducting a probatory session at this time, I asked Herbert whether he might now be ready to experience a hypnotic trance. As he agreed, I started with the following verbal trance induction while Herbert was sitting in a very comfortable armchair with an adjustable footrest.

Once Herbert had spontaneously closed his eyes, I then began, speaking slowly and pacing my words with the rhythm of his breathing:

"You don't need to do anything special, you don't need to feel anything special, or to think anything special. The only important thing is to let yourself be as comfortable as possible. Your thoughts can come and go as they want – like

your feelings and emotions, too; they just come and go. Just watching, just listening, just feeling. As you relax further in this comfortable armchair, as you continue to hear my voice and my words, you may not consciously understand what I am saying, although your unconscious mind understands everything I say to you. Every time you exhale, your body will sink a bit deeper into the armchair – deeper and deeper. When this happens, sooner or later certain muscles will relax. And you will notice how your limbs become heavier – or lighter, depending on what you prefer. It is quite possible you will feel both heaviness and lightness at the same time. And this is an interesting experience, too.

I don't know in which part of your body you will primarily notice any changes. In your right hand on the right thigh? Or in your left hand on your left thigh? Heaviness or lightness of your legs on the footrest? Greater or lesser contact with the seat? Contact with the backrest or the headrest? And other processes inside your body will also begin to change. The rhythm of your breathing will become gentle and even – your heart rate will slow down too. Other bodily processes will also change. Your blood pressure will fall very slightly, whereas your head region will remain well supplied with blood.

These changes take a bit of time, they are not so fast. They take time like all changes; all healing processes, all regeneration and all learning takes time. And you can take all the time you need, all the time in the world. With each exhalation you can let yourself be carried away further and further on the stream of time, further and further.

And now in this altered state, in this trance, your unconscious mind, is right now in close contact with that huge pool of your past experiences, including experiences which your conscious mind barely remembers; close contact with your entire knowledge, especially your intuitive knowledge, which rises up with images, and your unconscious mind is now in close contact with all of your abilities and skills, even hidden abilities, which your conscious mind does not yet know of.

And I don't know which of your experiences, which images and which of your skills and abilities your unconscious will utilize for healing and learning...."

From this point, I do not think it is essential to quote here the entire trance induction. The induction used here is only an example of a pattern that I employ in a multitude of variants, guided by my own intuition and related to our therapeutic goals and what Herbert and I had talked about beforehand. In addition, I myself sometimes go into a trance while speaking. I intersperse these inductions with especially or generally supporting suggestions. Such a trance induction normally takes about twenty to thirty minutes.

After Herbert had come back from his first formal trance in my office, he soon spontaneously began to tell me about a dream he has had during the trance state. What he said surprised me in several regards. I now quote Herbert's own words (translated from German), as he had originally described the dream in a dream protocol (which I had asked him to write it at home and then send to my email address).

Herbert wrote:

"This is my first session of hypnosis, and I do not yet have any idea what to expect. I can relax quite easily and quickly. I fall into a daydream in which I'm riding in a modern sailplane. At the beginning I am sitting in the closed cockpit under a glass cover and am waiting for the plane to be started by winch. While the towing rope becomes taut, I hear Mr. Riebensahm's invitation to relax. This invitation makes me smile because right now it's time for maximum concentration. The winch is running at full speed, and after a few seconds I feel myself catapulted into the sky. The rope is released, and I am flying in wide-open circles over the beautiful sunny countryside. On the ground woodland areas alternate with farmland and meadows. I can fully enjoy this from my bird's-eye view, because the machine doesn't require any attention from me. It is flying automatically as I want. I'm just listening to the sound of the wings, which have small winglets. The trance ends while I'm still flying – not by me landing to complete the flight."

Herbert N.

Not only was I surprised by Herbert's detailed description of his perceptions and experiences while dreaming of riding in a sailplane, but also by how realistically he described the starting process and flight of a glider. During my schooldays, when I was about 17 years old, I myself had tried to learn to fly a glider. I could therefore compare Herbert's description with my own real-life experience. When I asked Herbert whether he had ever been in a glider in his youth, he said, "No, never, but I had wished to do so with all my heart!" "And you never did?" I asked him. Herbert told me that his mother had explicitly forbidden him to join the flying club because his mother's former husband was a pilot in the German Airforce during the war and had crashed. His mother didn't want to lose her only son as well. At the time Herbert had accepted this prohibition, but, as he told me, he had collected every piece of information about flying sailplanes that he could get. And he had of course often flown sailplanes in his imagination.

After Herbert told me about these connections, I got an idea of why Herbert had possibly asked for an older male therapist. Was Herbert (and still is?) looking for a trustworthy father figure, a surrogate or even a grandfather substitute (I am now 79)? However, I didn't bring up this question explicitly: I thought that would not be necessary unless Herbert himself wanted to talk about it, or it becomes self-evident.

There was another aspect to his trance dream which caught my attention: the metaphorical aspect. Could this ride in a sailplane not be seen as a metaphor for Herbert's healing process? Or at least as part of it? While being pulled up by the towing rope and the winch Herbert is feeling relaxed yet at the same time highly concentrated. He can enjoy the process because it does not request any (conscious) attention from him. The process then stopped, and the landing (end of therapy) has not yet taken place. So are further such dreams to be expected?

When I vaguely expressed my view of seeing his dream as a metaphor, Herbert did not disagree. For me this seems another good reason to expect positive results from the course of therapy.

10. What is going to happen to the psychotherapy?

Herbert's course of psychotherapy began formally on February 13th, 2014. About three months later, after a trance session on May 29th, 2014 Herbert reported another dream, which also used the topic of "flying an airplane" as a metaphor. Here the metaphorical character of the dream is even clearer than in the first dream in trance when he had ridden a glider. Herbert reported the following:[12])

"Suddenly I am captivated by the experience of sitting in the cockpit of a combat jet, which is flying at a high altitude over the Pacific Ocean. I am wearing an olive-colored uniform with a helmet and oxygen mask. In the seat of the machine I feel somewhat trapped but safe. Moments later I recognize an aircraft carrier far down in the sea, which from this altitude seems to be tiny. But as I well know, I can land only on the carrier, and this seems very difficult. I circle around the landing point counterclockwise several times. After some hesitation I decide to descend, very slowly. For a moment I lose sight of the carrier. When I reach the right altitude for landing, I realize that the machine and also I myself have been transformed. Instead of a combat jet, I now am sitting in an old-fashioned sailplane, dressed like a tennis player from the 1930s: a white shirt with big, open collar, white pleated-front trousers with wide legs. Flying slowly I once again circle the giant steel aircraft carrier and then tumble down without making a crash landing. When I get out, two guides with their signal discs come up to me. They look confused. I also feel completely out of place, but nevertheless know I am safe and have finally arrived at the right place."

Each session lasted approximately 50 to 60 minutes or sometimes longer, depending of the process and topics of communication. We usually began with a "normal" conversation about any especially good experiences occurring during the previous week. Other topics might include dreams of a previous night, contact with Anna, Max or friends, any other experiences with music at a concert, experiences with his own paintings; sometimes we also talked about philosophical, political or historical issues of special interest.

These conversations normally lasted on average about 10-15 minutes. Then Herbert or I myself asked for a trance induction. I induced a trance state

---

[12] original text in German, translation by the author

during 14 of the in-all 34 sessions. Every time he was in a trance, Herbert had a dream, and on awakening, Herbert reported the particular dream. We talked about it, and I additionally asked him to send me a protocol of that dream for the purposes of this study. The reader can find all these protocols (in the original German) in the appendix to this manuscript.

On July 23rd (2014) Herbert was invited to attend the University Hospital to undergo examination by his surgeon. This revealed stable conditions. No relapse was found, but the wound cavity was still filled with liquor.

I was myself a bit disappointed. I had hoped the cavity would have at least shrunk slightly. After obtaining Herbert's permission to meet with his surgeon in person, I made an appointment to learn the surgeon's view of the process and stage of rehabilitation. He told me that he too had expected to find the cavity smaller in size. But each case has its own special features and in this regard the findings were normal. He however did not now expect the cavity to shrink or refill with brain tissue or any undergo other visible alteration. Too much time had passed since removal of the meningeoma.

During the subsequent therapy session I again induced a trance. According to spontaneous intuition, I included suggestions such as, "I am wondering, Herbert, if this cavity in your head, until now still filled with liquor, might not discharge the fluid, drop by drop, through your blood vessels and kidneys like a dripping tap".

On waking up from the trance, Herbert reported the following dream:

"I find myself in a nice little bay on the Mediterranean. The sun is shining. Towards the land the bay is bound by an edge of ground with multicolored stripes. Over the sea I can see as far as the horizon. I am the only person in the bay. I go into the water and I am diving. (Herbert emphasizes, "I really can dive!") To start with, it is still bright. The ground is close to me. There is then a step, and the bottom of the sea is now also deeper. The light becomes fainter, the sun can't get through. I am diving deeper, that's easy. Also I can easily breathe under the water. That seems to be quite normal. I look around and find a cave. I swim into the cave without any fear. I feel completely safe. Farther in, the cave turns into a tunnel. At the end of the tunnel the light is bright. I swim towards the brightness and finally come out of the cave, the tunnel. I again find myself on a beach, but different one. The beach is filled with people. They are celebrating, holding a barbecue party. Everyone is in white, including me. I am welcomed in a friendly manner. Some people smile at me, but I don't understand anything they say. They are using a language I don't know. I suppose it's Greek, because they are drinking retsina. They give me a little bottle of retsina as well, a bottle shaped like a cone. It reminds me on a vacation I took in Greece some years ago. Strangely, the bottle has a crown cap. I open the bottle but don't drink. I set the bottle aside and wait until the right time to drink. Then the dream ends. "Very pleasant!"

I don't know whether my suggestion and/or the subsequent dream will have any effect on processes in Herbert's brain, and if so, what the result will be. Nobody knows. At the moment I only can hope and wish things might improve for Herbert.

In spite of this uncertainty the dream is obviously – at least semantically – related to the previous suggestion. And this one too, like the first dreams (flying a glider and combat jet) can be seen as a self-produced metaphor for a process of metamorphosis.

Since having a heart attack 4 years ago, I go dancing once a week at a club for people of all ages. Most surprisingly I ran into Herbert there together with a woman who was not Anna. We only said hello. But at our next session I told him I had been very surprised to see him there dancing. He will undoubtedly benefit from dancing (as I do myself). I have now already met him there three times, and to me this does not look like depression.

At another session Herbert surprised me by saying he now has embarked on a new project. In the past he had already built a number of model aircrafts, some even with battery-powered engines and gliders as well. He also experiments a lot, trying out different sizes of plane and various materials. He had for example discovered a new material, known as Depron, which is lighter than balsa wood, resistant to moisture and easier to work with. Next time he showed me a small piece of Depron, and during the entire session we talked in detail about many aspects of aerodynamics. We are of course both experts in the field of aerodynamics, although at an amateur level.

11. A Critical Incident

On October 16th, 2014 Herbert underwent neurological and neuropsychological examination at the University Hospital of Göttingen. The written report contains generally satisfying results. Psychologically, the patient was described as being alert, clear, fully oriented and focused in a friendly manner. No neuropsychological abnormalities were observed. The patient also reported, subjectively, that his levels of concentration and memory have now improved.

When Herbert delivered this report to me, I asked him whether I could contact his former partner Anna to also find out what changes she had observed in Herbert's behavior since January 2014. Herbert agreed and sent me her address and phone number after he had told Anna and asked for her permission to do so.

When I called Anna, she was very friendly and approachable. She told me that over the past year Herbert has clearly changed in a positive way. In particular he now – unlike in the past – makes it pretty plain if he really dislikes something. At the end of our telephone conversation I asked her to send me some Key words: by email so I could recall our conversation more easily, and she promised to do so.

I would have liked to have got more concrete data as proof of the success of this therapy, especially by means of neuropsychological testing. I therefore sent Herbert an email, telling him that I would like to talk with the neuropsychologist who had tested him on October 16th, 2024. In my email I used the words: “subject to your agreement”.

The following day I received a response via email in which Herbert wrote: “Dear Mr. Riebensahm, in your last email you assumed that I would agree to your request regarding the result of my neuropsychological test. On this point I have to emphatically correct you. I hereby explicitly forbid you to collect further information about myself. The large amount of data you have already collected about me involves so many facts that I now feel uneasy at the thought of being permanently under observation. I feel forced into the role of a servile patient. For this reason I also asked Anna not to tell you any more about my Character and not to write down the Key words: she has already told you. ...”

I likewise responded by email: “Dear Mr. N., as you may well imagine, I am shocked at your change of mind. But I nevertheless respect your request not to seek further information concerning yourself. I can understand that the mass of data I have collected makes you feel uncomfortable. But I must assure you that any data that might enable a reader of the planned article to identify you will be heavily disguised. I would like to apologize for have provoked doubts and discomfort on your part!”

During the subsequent session we of course undertook a ‘critical incident debriefing’. And I was naturally very much relieved when Herbert not only accepted my apologies, but also explicitly stated, that his former feelings of discomfort had dissipated, and that there was no longer any obstacle to continuing the course of therapy. In this context I told Herbert, that Anna had recently reported on the phone that Herbert would now give clear feedback, unlike than in the past.

Herbert thereupon confirmed this and told me an anecdote about the time when he had to move out of his office at the university.(In the meantime he had been relieved of his position, as he had wished). Anna and Max were helping him to sort out his books and papers. But after a few minutes he realized that Anna and Max were conducting the entire process while ignoring his opinion. Herbert became angry and said (without being very aggressive!), “Thank you very much for helping me! I couldn't do it on my own. But this office is my ship, and I am the commander. I am the one to decide which books go into the garbage and which ones I’m taking home!” They both accepted his objection, and this outcome was a success.

12. Final Phase of Therapy

At the end of November 2014 Herbert told he wanted to end his therapy with the 34th session, in order to keep a 5 or 6 therapy sessions in reserve should he need any psychotherapeutic help at some time in the future. I not only agreed but also told him I would have made the same suggestion. We therefore then scheduled our last session for February 12th, 2015.

In the beginning of our penultimate session on January 29th, 2015 Herbert reported a dream he had had the night before: Some people, well known to Herbert, were sitting around in front of a barn that they had just repaired as a team effort. They now wanted to have breakfast together to celebrate the completion of their work. It is warm, the sun is shining, the yard is flanked by hedges with "young green bushes" (emphasized by Herbert). As Herbert goes up to the buffet to take his favorite bitter orange marmalade, another man on the other side grabs at it. For a moment Herbert feels anger rise up in him. He is looking into his opponent's face, and his opponent likewise into his. But they both burst into laughter at the same time and then share the marmalade between them. Both are satisfied with this solution.

To me this dream seems to be a charming metaphor for a happy end to the therapy. But this session nevertheless ended with a surprise for both of us: Herbert once again reported a very special dream after being in a trance. Although I had performed the induction without any special suggestion, Herbert told me about an experience in which he found himself in a pine grove three times in just one dream. There he was aware of an intensive smell of pine trees. And he greatly enjoyed this experience of smelling the pines in his dream. A surprising experience for a man with anosmia!

After Herbert came out of the trance, we talked over his new dream experience of enjoying a sense of smell. Herbert told me how, a few days before Christmas, he had walked around the Christmas market. There he had called to mind the smell of mulled wine and other spices. I then told Herbert the story of Milton Erickson – a tale very familiar to hypnotherapists. As a boy Milton was lying paralyzed in his bed and over and over again tried to remember the feeling in his toes when he had still been able to move them. Very, very slowly Milton learned to move his toes again in tiny steps thanks to a long-term training program of this kind. . In the end he was able to move almost his entire body, – although he could only walk with crutches.

"Why not smelling with the crutches of your memory?" I asked.

So to date, February 12th, 2015 we have undertaken 34 therapy sessions out of the forty which had been approved by the health insurer.

Each time Herbert arrived on the dot every Thursday afternoon at 4.00 pm. At the start we met once a week. In July Herbert told me he would like to extend the intervals between sessions from seven to fourteen days. These intervals were sometimes longer depending on factors such as vacation, sickness or other reasons. Once for example Herbert traveled to Switzerland to spend some days with his son Max, who was undergoing training there at the time. I assessed this activity as yet another step towards a positive outcome to the therapy.

At our last session on February 12th, we reviewed our work together over the past year. Herbert said he was feeling happy and satisfied by the results of his therapy. In particular he had found an inner balance again and is now looking forward to the next period of his life.

In a few days we will be meeting once more. I will give him a copy of this article and will talk about it with him. I am curious to hear his opinion.

13. Epilog

Today is February 16th, 2015, and I had my last therapeutic session with Herbert four days ago. On awakening this morning at about 6.00 am, I again fell into a trance or daydream which concerned Herbert. While in trance I remembered the death of the man that Herbert's mother had years ago chosen to be father of her son. But he died just a few weeks before the Second World War ended. I suddenly also remembered my own brother's death a few weeks before the end of World War Two. He was a boy of 17, and would normally still have been at school, but he was called up for service, becoming (as we would see it today) a child soldier. He died in March 1945. I had loved and admired him: He was literally my 'big brother'. Once, when a member of the 'Hitlerjugend' he took me with him to demonstrate flying a model sailplane he had built. But since my first contact with Herbert one year ago, I had never consciously thought of my brother.

Transference and countertransference: If Herbert saw me as a father or grandfather figure, I saw him as my brother. I like this idea.

Acknowledgements:

I would like to thank Herbert for his cooperation and permission to use his experiences to write the present article. I also appreciate his creativity and his willingness to share his thoughts and feelings. Last but not least, I appreciate how Herbert, from our very first meeting, again and again gave me the kind of feedback that encouraged me to look forward hopefully to a "happy end" to our work. Many thanks, my brother in mind, if not in body!

18 The Science of Consciousness: Basics, Models, and Visions

Thilo Hinterberger

Key Words: consciousness, neuroscience, perception, subjectivity

Summary

As a basis for scientific discourse in the field of Applied Consciousness Sciences I would like to present a few models of the phenomenon *consciousness* emerging from modern neuroscience.

A first model is based on the dynamics of information processing in the brain. Using the properties of evoked electric brain potentials the hierarchical sequence of functions leads to conscious perception ranging from attention, pattern recognition, categorisation, associations and onwards to judgments and complex thoughts. Another model treats conscious perception as a process of internalisation leading to the "self" as conscious observer. As a consequence every conscious perception can be seen as a reduced and already interpreted observation of an inner representation of an outer or imagined "world".

The distinction between functions of consciousness and subjective qualities of conscious perception illustrates that most functions can be thought as being implemented in the brain as a neurobiological computer. In contrast, subjective experience offers properties which can only be experienced from inside and cannot be made objective. The basic values of humanity can be derived from these subjective qualities such as responsibility, love, compassion, freedom, and dignity.

Therefore, in contrast to the Natural Sciences, the Science of Consciousness is additionally challenged to deal with those subjective qualities, emphasizing the resulting influence on health, social interactions, and the whole society.

Introduction

Questions about the concept of consciousness are still a current topic in our scientific advanced age. Specifically, the ontology of this phenomenon is regarded as one of our great but still unsolved riddles even though our thoughts and feelings which are held as expressions of consciousness are tightly connected to us. What is the reason for this? What is it that makes this phenomenon so special? And which scientific disciplines may be privileged to find a solution? In the last few years hope was increasingly placed in the field of neuropsychology for providing clarification on this issue (Crick & Koch, 2003). And although it is neuropsychology that feels most likely obligated to the phenomenon of consciousness, it becomes an interdisciplinary task especially through contributions from psychology, philosophy, the social sciences and physics.

One difficulty already arises in defining the concept of consciousness. Therefore, neuroscientists try to avoid this term in order to more specifically address the different functionalities of consciousness such as attention, perception, cognition, memory functions, emotions and intention. Based on developments in neuropsychology the 'philosophy of mind' (see, for example, Searle, 1992) arose, representing the world view of a biological naturalism. Neuropsychology as well as neurophilosophy (for example, Metzinger, 2005) both aim at a basic theoretical clarification of the phenomenon around consciousness through integration of the recent level of knowledge. Accordingly, consciousness is frequently regarded as a neuronal emergent and therefore as a generated phenomenon of the first person perspective. Even the "self", representing a reference to our existence as an observant being, is hence debunked as an illusion. However, the attempt at reducing phenomena of consciousness to neurobiological mechanisms leaves questions unanswered so that the riddle of consciousness should not be regarded as solved through our recent world view. Since spiritual issues and questions are also discussed with increasing interest in modern neuropsychology, one can even suspect some sincerity among scientists to seek a higher level synthesis of scientific results and individual experiences. This is highlighted by an increasing number of scientific conferences with consciousness, spirituality and neuropsychology as range of topics. The research field of Applied Consciousness Sciences would like to join this trend as well.

Yet, for a science of consciousness it is only one side of the coin to fathom the phenomenon of consciousness. The other side constitutes the meaning of consciousness for us humans in the most different areas of our lives. Consciousness in and of itself does not want to solely be investigated but also to be lived and mastered, because consciousness is not just a peculiarity of mankind but a virtue, a virtue of experience, which decides on the quality of our lives. By reason of this guiding principle, the Applied Consciousness Sciences want to address the development of consciousness not only by discussing and further developing the knowledge deriving from consciousness science but also by returning it to humankind so that it can bring about changes and help.

In this chapter I first want to present some models of consciousness which emphasize the phenomenon and its properties. These models are not primarily intended to explain consciousness but rather to establish a basis for discussion on which a science of consciousness can then be set up. Then, in that case, science no longer needs to be perceived as an opponent of phenomena of subjectivity or individual spirituality because both of them are expressions representing the substance of our common reality.

1. Properties of a Phenomenon

2.1 Consciousness as a Process

First of all, I want to emphasize the temporal aspect of consciousness, in other words its process-related qualities. Terms like the flow of consciousness suggest that consciousness is more comparable to a process than a state. From this, one can derive important knowledge about the experience of different states of consciousness. In the following, this statement will be exemplified by the brain's information process that normally occurs when stimuli are perceived. Hence, we will first look at event-related potentials (ERPs) of the EEG (electro-encephalogram) derived from electrodes connected to the brain via the scalp. The ERPs are analyzed by averaging many temporal response signals from events resulting in a typical response curve. Figure 1 shows a series of response curves of visual stimulus events (for example, a picture that is being viewed) at time 0. The consecutive signal peaks can roughly be categorized into the following phases: Components arising about 100 milliseconds predominantly represent the activation of primary sensory areas. A subsequent component around 200 milliseconds after stimulus onset is assigned to attention control (Rugg & Coles, 1995). Hence, there is a process taking place that determines which part or aspect of the event is considered as being relevant for the resulting observation. This process is autonomous and still preconscious. After about 300 milliseconds measurable signals indicate processes which can be assigned to a higher conceptual processing. Here, one can find the so called P300-components which are associated with novelty and memory processes (Mangun et al., 1995). The stimulus is analyzed and compared to as well as associated with familiar patterns, concepts arise and, finally, the stimulus is perceived in terms of the resulting interpretation process. Therefore, one can say that an event becomes conscious not until some hundred milliseconds have passed; however, since our brain automatically dates the event back in time, an experienced "now" is formed.

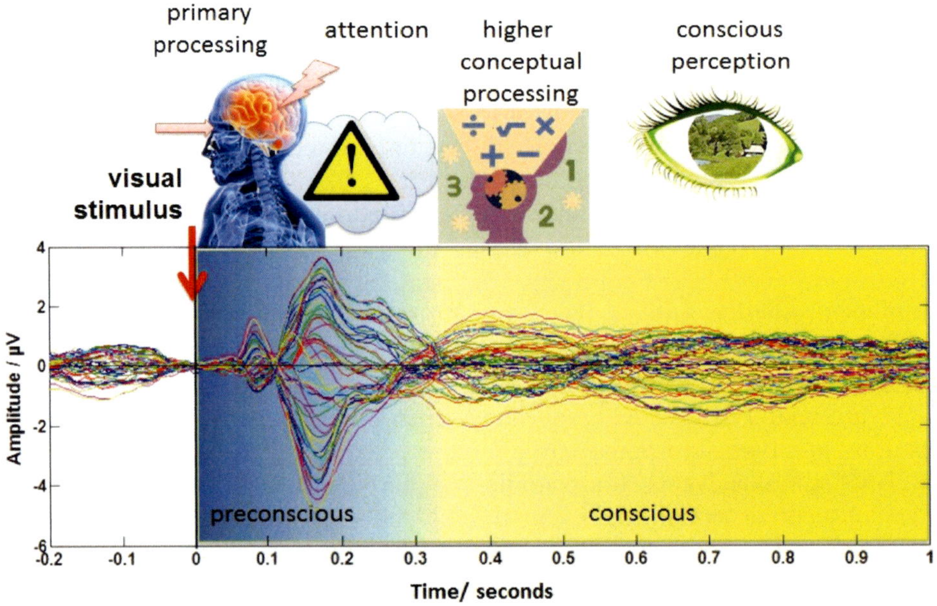

Figure 1. *Event related electrical signals offer insight into the various steps of the process of capturing and processing visual information in the brain. Accordingly, an event requires several hundred milliseconds until we become consciously aware of it.*

1.2 Consciousness is Interior Space

I want to contrast the above presented model of the measurable electrical neurophysiological information process as an indicator of becoming aware of something with a second model. This model treats information processing as a process of internalization resulting in conscious perception. Comparable to Figure 1 an image of the external world is processed as a stimulus. In order to become aware of the world, sensory information passes through the eyes via the optical chiasm to the primary visual areas located in the occipital region of the brain as shown in Figure 2a. From there, they are sent through different signal paths into various brain areas which are responsible for functions like spatial representation, pattern recognition, memory, association, information processing, or movement control. Eventually, a first order neuronal map is generated due to synchronous activation of these different areas. This neuronal map, which on the functional level is dynamic neuronal network activation per se, is not necessarily conscious. Consciousness can be interpreted as the observation of this internal representation that could be realized by a process that creates a second layer representation interrelating these two layers. This picture is described by Damasio (2002). The internal copy of the world outside is available to conscious perception. Thus, consciousness is not observing the world but rather observing an internal representation of a world which does not have to correspond to the objective one, necessarily. The processes for generating the internal image or (re-)presentations are the focus of intensive research in neuropsychological science. The difficult problem however, (that is in our picture the relationship between the functional aspects that form the inner (re-)presentations and the resulting *inner observer* who experiences qualia) is still subject to speculation. As the observer and the inner image are mostly not separated from each other the inner image is usually not perceived as such, but the observer has the impression of seeing the world outside. Metzinger (2011) refers to the transparency of the representation meaning its invisibility to the observer. However, the world outside can never be perceived directly but always needs an inner, individual image which is clarified more thoroughly in the following. To sum up here: All experiences are observations within an internal space.

Figure 2. *Models of conscious perception. The functional level (a) can be described by neuroscience while the subjective level of conscious experience requires a different model (b). The difficult problem of consciousness addresses the relationship between those two*

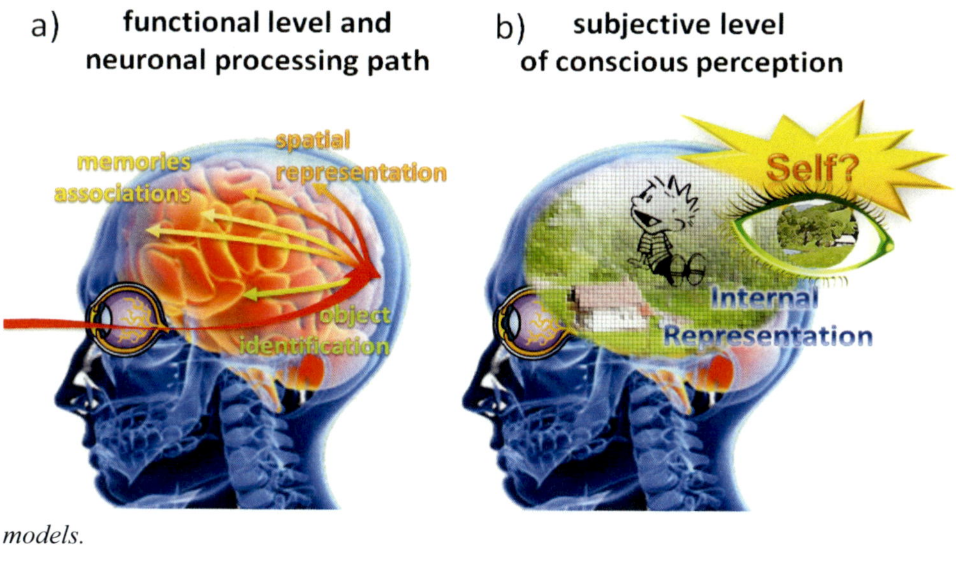

models.

1.3 Consciousness and Dreaming

While dreaming, our brains prove their stunning capability for presenting the world and its scenery to our consciousness that can be generated without any sensory input. Here, the internal representation has no correspondence to a sensory image of an external world but seems to be an autonomously and spontaneously generated inner world characterized by a considerably high degree of coherence. A special form of dreaming is lucid dreaming. Lucid dreamers sometimes even report clarity of consciousness which even may transcend that of waking consciousness. Furthermore, the lucid dreamer is not only an observer of his dream but also knows that he is dreaming, is able to develop a self-image and behave in a deliberate way in the dream (Tholey, 1997). Such lucid dreams are not so rare as many might expect: Many persons are familiar with them from their own experience. According to Schredl and Erlacher (2004) people characterized by a high capacity for absorption, imagination, and openness for new ideas show a significant positive correlation with the frequency of lucid dreams. Weak self-boundaries seem to favor lucid dreaming, whereas neurotic tendencies do not correlate with lucid dreaming. Studies on exercising lucid dreaming have shown that around 75% of the participants are able to learn lucid dreaming (La Berge, 2009). Since many brain areas are similarly activated in dreaming and especially lucid dreaming compared to sensory experience in waking consciousness, one can even consciously practice learning processes, just like motor tasks, inside of the dream.

1.4 Knowledge Which We do not Know

Since inner dream worlds as such are not consciously planned and generated it is obvious that the construction of an inner representation is a preconscious process offering only limited access to deliberate and hence manipulative acts. This lack of freedom in the initial 'perception' is used, for example, when applying the Rorschach Test as a psycho-diagnostic tool in order to gain insight into a personality structure (Rorschach, 1921; Bohm, 1951). Libet's experiments with slow event-related EEG-signals also show this lack of freedom with respect to the 'initial will' because brain signals can be used to forecast later decisions even before a decision is consciously perceived (Libet, 1985, 2004, Jo et al., 2014). These experiments have long been the reason for speculation about the non-existence of free will as such. I am using the term "initial" since freedom can be experienced when being able to agree or disagree on a consciously perceived decision act. Libet himself called this the veto-possibility of will. However, this veto-process is not a real argument for a freedom of will as the veto-process itself is driven by probabilistic aspects, cognitive ones or again unconscious ones. Therefore, we are at the mercy of our organism's and psyche's partly highly 'intelligent' but blind autonomous dynamics with regard to every subconscious or unconscious process.

The realm of the unconscious has different aspects. In the field of depth psychology it represents, for example, all those mental contents which are not directly accessible to consciousness. Unfortunately, due to its manifold application, the term unconscious has become a general term for everything unknown in the psychic field. This will be differentiated in the following.

All those processes in the brain that are executing functionalities of consciousness without being consciously perceived by the subjective observer will be called *unconscious perception*. One example for this is the phenomenon of blindsight, a form of blindness in which not the eye but the primary visual cortex is damaged. These patients actually cannot see consciously, in other words, there is no internal representation appearing to them, but their brain is still capable of processing the perceived stimuli so that it can respond to them in a specific way. Obviously, our brains can perform sophisticated information processing even without involving a conscious observer.

In addition, *implicit and procedural knowledge* is referred to as unconscious as well. This knowledge needs not to be "thought" of in a linguistic or other kind of symbolic way in order to be used. It rather arises from a complex bio-cybernetic control system (Polanyi, 1969).

Further, I want to refer to a domain I call the *'causally unconscious'*. It is the source of creativity which should not be confounded with its creative product, though. How did a freely improvised composition evolve? Or where did the world of a dream come from which appears quite bizarre after awakening? This composition and this realm of dreams presumably do not 'exist' until they are "thought" and "felt". They need an organism to unfold, to become explicit and there is little or no reference of their existence beforehand. Probably, the impulses generating creative mental products which I call the causal unconscious are quite faint and poor in information compared to the resulting conscious appearances. But they may be essential for the result. However, where do these causal impulses come from? One answer would be that they come from sensory input similar to the construction of a mental space in waking consciousness. Another option is that they are implicitly generated out of the organism's activity itself. Furthermore, there are phenomena called *extrasensory perception* such as telepathy, clairvoyance, precognition, and other transpersonal phenomena. Despite 100 years of parapsychological science, the mechanisms behind those forms of extrasensory perceptions are still not unraveled, and a replicable confirmation of their existence has not yet even been given. However, rudimentary models do exist. Therefore, there are still implications for not viewing the brain as a closed but rather an open system, i.e. a system that possesses (aside from the classical sensory paths) still other possibilities for being influenced.

1.5 I and Self

After all, there is the search for a physiological process of 'becoming conscious' that transforms a causal impulse into a conscious observation. But the question regarding the observer also still seems unsolved. This observer seems to be closely connected to the notion of the "self". Both concepts, self and observer, are characterized by individuality, i.e. our minds have to split up into subsystems, so that the observer experiences the world as a counterpart or in other words as "not-self".

Damasio (2002) for example distinguishes between several types of 'self'. He calls the instantaneous representation of the organism or an object via neuronal patterns the *proto-self* which is not consciously accessible. As mentioned above, one can become conscious only after a secondary order representation is generated out of the changes in the proto-self, and this forms the so called *core-self*. Furthermore, he refers to an '*autobiographical self*' constructed by the activation of memory contents (Damasio, 2002, pp. 211ff). As shown in Figure 2b, the autobiographical self creates the construct of 'I' as a mental formation which is similar to other objects. Therefore, in Figure 2b the autobiographical self becomes an object in the inner representation space. Damasio attributes an important characteristic to the core-self: Since it results from changes in the representation, it is generated anew with every attention impulse. Therefore, consciousness is a phenomenon of changes whereby phenomena of habituation as well as increased consciousness (after directing attention on something novel) become plausible. Thus, consciousness would be linked to a dynamic neuronal map of secondary order. Damasio used this model predominantly to describe emotions and their conscious perception precisely because the latter results from secondary order representations. Hence, according to Damasio the self is a result of neuronal activity which represents processes in the organism. Trehub (2007) also takes the approach of the theory of self-models and emphasizes that this model requires the existence of a core-self. D'Aquili and Newberg (1999) localize the self in the superior-posterior parietal cortex. In those areas the integration and interpretation of various perceptions takes place generating the quality of experiencing oneself as an observer.

As a consequence of the models presented above the self seems to be no separate entity supporting a dualistic world view but rather a characteristic inside the one physical world which performs the act of separation through taking an inward position inherent to the system. Thus, while dualists assume a generic separation between body and soul, the model presented here suggests the 'self' resulting from a process generating an intrinsic duality that can be perceived as being dual from the perspective of the conscious observer.

However, there seems to be a singular source of consciousness which can be anticipated or even experienced in meditation when being able to abstain from the (autonomous) separating mechanism which might require long-term practice but which could also occasionally happen (Hinterberger et al., 2014). Spiritual experiences of oneness, connectedness and transcendence result from overcoming this separation process.

2.6 The Role of the Observer

One might still ask: Is the observer more than just a subjective illusion in an objective world? Here, I want to present the idea that even the phenomenon of an objective world can be interpreted as an illusion of a subjective observer. So let us turn to physics and consider the fact that both great theories of modern physics, the theory of relativity and the theory of quantum mechanics, imply a special reference to the observer phenomenon. The theory of relativity postulates that the physical properties of space and time are invariant with respect to the observer's reference system. Each observer constitutes his or her own reference system to which the same universal law of the constancy of the speed of light applies, so that all dependent measures such as space and time appear individually and relatively. This means that all physical properties solely exist in reference to an observer.

The same applies to quantum theory: The observation itself determines the properties in which quantum states are realized. Here, the terms 'measurement' and 'observation' can be treated synonymously, yet according to the Copenhagen interpretation a measurement device is characterized as something that forms a describable subsystem. Measuring thus means defining subsystems which are able to extract information from the overall system. Without measurement, i.e. without interaction, the system stays in a 'superposition of wave functions', in other words in a state of unrealized possibilities. However, by defining subsystems, quantum physics appears to be paradox since one has to isolate parts in the 'one world' which are not treated as quantum systems with the aim of learning something about the world. In doing so, the categories of the information that can be finally depicted are defined by the design of a measurement device. The question arises: Is there a physical process that separates the world? Even today, it is still being discussed how this act of separation is accomplished or whether it is merely an illusion. E.g., the so-called 'collapse of the wave function' which is another term for this separation might just be a concept of our (mis-)interpretation. [13]

Yet, this links to our question regarding the conscious observer. Conscious observers experience themselves as part of the world and through the process of attention-control they choose the categories of their perception in which information manifests itself, therefore becoming aware and conscious. By reason of the close link to basic physical processes the question regarding the nature of consciousness is still a serious topic for discussion in quantum physics (Zeh, 2010; Jaeger, 2009). If the physical observation process shares the same principles which the observing 'self' underlies, then the 'self', formerly eluding scientific accessibility, will become a system-theoretically essential physical concept.

[13] The interested readers might find help regarding this topic in the discussions on the Heisenberg-cut, the collapse of wave functions and decoherence.

Hence, the result would be that conscious observation creates a partitioning in subsystems so that states become concrete (this is the hypothetical collapse of the wave function).

Thus, according to Figure 2b, the representation as well as its underlying micro-conditions would not be defined a priori but would exist as a non-local and complex superposition that could be expressed by wave-function. Creating facts would then be an act of our 'self's' attentional focus to transform it to a 'here and now'. A neuronal network, however, is actually such a non-local and complex superposition of possible mental formations which are realized through the network activity so that each mental representation is an attractor state of the network. This view would not link directly to quantum physics but would just offer similar phenomena. Quantum physical systems and neuronal networks would then be metaphorically comparable by showing similar properties. Therefore, it would be desirable to continue discussing this approach and to further investigate it empirically.

3. Functions and Qualities of Consciousness

3.1 Functions of Consciousness

Let us return to neuroscience. In the light of the phenomenology of consciousness just presented, the question now concerns the implementation of these properties inside the brain's neuronal structure. In order to give us some ideas about this it will be explained briefly:

Essential functions of consciousness such as those of perception, memory or recognition can be explained plausibly by the model of the brain as a great neuronal network. That is because abstract mathematical models of neurons incorporate the properties such as virtual storage of a wide range of patterns in a holographical fashion within the neuronal network as well as recognition of patterns through the presentation of similar patterns to the network.

Indeed, there are mathematical models of attentional processes but they are descriptive rather than explanatory (see the model of attention by Bundesen, 1990). In the same way, measurements using EEG or functional magnetic resonance imaging (fMRI) contain no information about the 'how' but solely about the 'what' and 'where' something happens. Nevertheless, attempts are being made to discover the way different contents in brain dynamics could form a homogeneous perception and conscious experience (D'Aquili & Newberg, 1999; Singer, 2001). Thoughts cannot be captured as such but solely as correlates. However, the attempt at differentiating various thoughts with respect to mental representations using EEG has only been successful in a rudimentary way. Using these methods a computer, for example, could distinguish at most only around five or six mental representations (Lee et al., 2010; Anderson et al., 2007).

Although it is difficult objectifying emotions, Damasio (2002, p. 339) refers to them as somatic reactions whose changes result in *feelings*. While certain basic emotions are regarded as being inherent patterns of reactions, feelings are seen as the results of mental evaluation mechanisms (Birbaumer & Schmidt, 1999).

Since it is possible in neuropsychology to describe every process and interaction as chains of stimulus and reaction, behavioral neurobiology offers quite mechanistic traits and has introduced a probabilistic description of facts and predictions sorely needed because of the plurality of unknown processes. Here, statistical probabilities in psychophysiology are of a completely different nature than quantum-physical probabilities. Nevertheless, the fact that the brain is a probabilistic system challenges research more than many other scientifically investigated systems.

3.2 Qualia: How is Subjectivity Generated?

One of the many discussed questions regarding the peculiarities of consciousness is the question of the experiences of qualia. 'Qualia' refers to the qualities of subjective experience whereupon color vision is one of the most popular examples. How could the subjective experience of the color blue be explained?

Such an explanation relies first on showing how the process of perception, with special regard to visual perception, is linked to several changes of categories. Blue light can be physically described as an electromagnetic wave with a wavelength of about 420 nanometers. This radiation reaches the retina inside our eyes, is absorbed and stimulates cones which are sensitive to blue. Thus, photons are transformed into neuro-electrical impulses; thus, a first categorical transformation has happened. Blue is not a property of light anymore since even an artificial stimulation of visual cells would end up in experiencing the color blue. Afterwards, the neuronal impulses are passed on to the visual areas of the brain. Here again, the color blue changes its category. The color blue can be achieved by the activation of a complex cerebral pattern within parietal and occipital areas (area V2 and V4). Hence, one could elicit the imaginative experience of a blue light by targeted stimulation of the visual areas, for example, via transcranial magnetic stimulation (TMS). Dreams demonstrate (color) vision's autonomy without sensory stimulation of optical nerves. However, the neuronal correlates of such conscious perception are distributed over wide areas of the cortex. Whether a visually perceived event becomes conscious or not is essentially dependent on the paths of information processing in the brain (see the phenomenon of blindsight given above).

Finally, in order to consciously perceive the color blue one more essential transformation has to occur, namely that from the objectivity of events and activation patterns to the subjectivity of the conscious observer. For understanding this transformation, one would have to leave the descriptive level of processes and instead take a view within the neuronal information processing itself. This is the point where the debate around qualia begins: What are the properties of a system that experiences its own information processing? This question is addressed in a metaphysical theory called *endophysics*. O.E. Rössler (1998) formulated essential thoughts in his book "*Endophysics – The World as an Interface*". Principally, we are all inside our own world and our commonly experienced world. Nobody can escape and take the position from outside. However, we have found methods that help to take so-called exo-perspectives for investigating subsystems. And we know from the laws of quantum mechanics that properties are different for endo- and exoperspectives. Thus, qualia might be a category that only exists in the endo-domain of our brain and can never be a phenomenon in the exo-perspective which is taken by neuroscience.

Many functions of consciousness can be put into practice in machines (for example computer systems) which are based on deterministic-mathematical algorithms. Even a camera possesses the ability for representation and in some digital cameras there are algorithms implemented for face-recognition. Such systems would be described as intelligent at best but not yet conscious. So, what would be needed for a computer to be conscious in our way of thinking? One possible answer could be: the inner observation. And in order to truly understand its subjectivity one would have to change one's viewpoint from the external perspective to the inner perspective of the information process itself. Since such a change is actually impossible, we can hardly make statements about such a system's consciousness for now. However, we ourselves are in the inner perspective of our brains. Therefore, I would dare the hypothesis of a '*basic self*' as being an emergent property of neuronal functions transforming the inner perspective into subjective experience. There still remains the topic as to whether this change of perspectives is really sufficient for creating the experience of qualia.

3.3 On the Physics of Subjectivity

The experienced qualities are not completely indescribable. I would like to maintain that even qualia are based on several physical rules and laws by using the example of listening to music. While reading the descriptions of subjective sound qualities in journals for music and audio one can notice that terms like sharp, voluminous, smooth, bright, black, etc. are frequently used. These synesthetic attributes originate from the sound's spatial representation in our mind. Physically it is well understood which shapes are created inside of us in this process. High tones for example have small wavelengths. Therefore, they can be easily located and accordingly they form small mental structures which are described as *sharp* or *fine resolved*. In contrast, bass tones seem to fill the room because of their long wavelength and are thus barely localizable so that they are characterized as voluminous. Following this, a fraction of subjective quality is determined. Those who are well schooled in music theory know that our tonal system is based upon a mathematical system. Integer ratios of frequencies are experienced as harmonies and along with personal associations an inner *mood* is generated. Thus, qualia might be describable, but even the most detailed description still cannot represent and hence cannot replace conscious experience. However, knowing the laws of qualia could enable us to create a specific experience. Many great musicians used and still use this knowledge – some of them intentionally and others implicitly or intuitively.

3.4 A Two-Dimensional Working Model

Based on the former observations, one may construe a model now in which two dimensions of consciousness result from the generic self: (1) A conceptual dimension describing the process of consciousness and (2) a dimension for the mental space of consciousness. The conceptual dimension represents the degree of complexity regarding information processing. Thus, the source which I want to call *basic* or *pure consciousness* originates in a domain free of concepts and categories. Yet, this realm is speculative and requires scientific debate. But in this dimension more and more complex processing mechanisms can be arranged such as the dynamics of generating a second order map, the mental operation of creating time, planning, empathic functions, etc. The second dimension describes the inner space and originates from the intrinsic activity creating the individual mental space and ranges to the outside, i.e. those mental formations which are tightly organized through sensory impressions and interactions with the environment. These two dimensions may be classified into four quadrants to which different aspects of psychological aspects can be assigned (see Figure 3 below). Moreover, each of these aspects can be associated with distinct fields of research.

1. Complex processing of external stimuli

The bottom right quadrant refers to everyday consciousness which is essentially characterized by a high amount of external sensory perception (i.e., of the environment but also of one's own body). Many tasks and interactions require complex mental processing. We perceive, represent, evaluate and think about the constantly changing information flow we are exposed to while driving, working, listening to lectures, etc. Most experiments in cognitive neuroscience refer to this field.

2. Complex processing within the intrinsic and subjective space

The realm of externally triggered mental activities constantly interacts with intrinsic inner processing, namely individual cognitive and emotional processes which are located in the bottom left quadrant. As shown above, complex information processing does not require external stimuli. Thoughts, imaginations, fantasies, feelings, or dreams can either be triggered merely by the environment or even self-induced. E.g., when reading a book, only a few words might be sufficient to unfold entire mental sceneries. Also feelings are reactions to perceptions taking place inside the body.

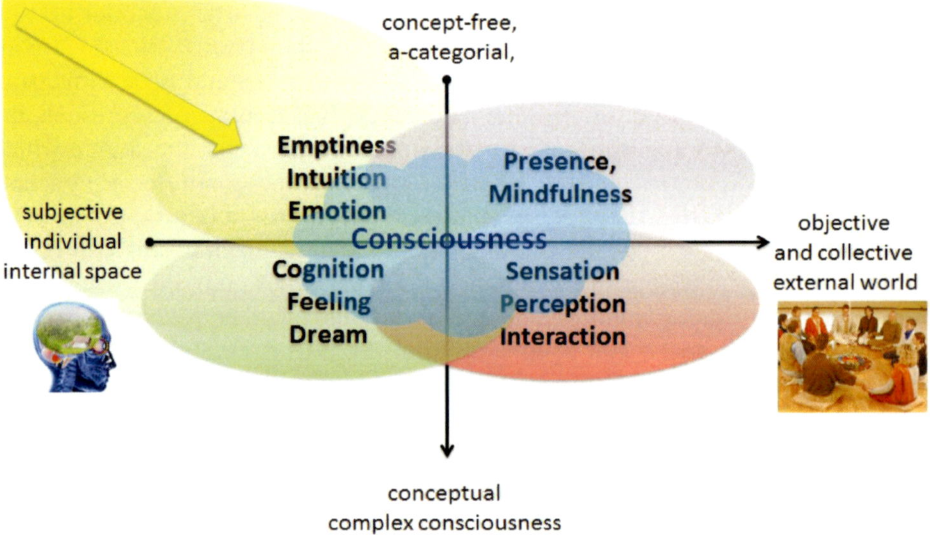

Figure 3. *Working model of a consciousness field which is spanned by a categorical dimension and a dimension of internal versus external space. Thus, four different fields of states of consciousness can be distinguished.*

3. Non-conceptual processing of external stimuli

The top-right field addresses minimal categorization and conceptualization while being interconnected with our senses to the environment or our own body. This field constitutes a state of mindfulness as it is practiced in mindfulness meditation (Kabat-Zinn, 1990). Kabat-Zinn defines mindfulness as a state of a non-judgemental wakeful presence. By directing the focus of attention to one's own breath or an external object, one is continuously connected to the physical environment including the physical body. However, as the perceived content should not be evaluated or interpreted, and should not lead to a stream of thoughts, the state desired is ideally non-conceptual or a-categorical. It is a state of presence and acceptance. There is increasing interest in psychophysiological research on mindfulness and meditation.

4. **Non-conceptual processing within the intrinsic and subjective space**

A special and mostly unexplored area is located in the upper left field. Still on a physiological level, emotions can be experienced as perceptions which are initially free of concepts. Viewed from a purely mental perspective, this quadrant presents the realm of intuition and creativity and possibly the initial impulse of a will. In precisely that corner we can place the causal unconscious impulses which precede and initiate mental formations. Here one can find states of emptiness and silence which meditators experience when not attached to any sensory stimuli. The yellow arrow in the top-left corner represents the source of vitality and indicates the causal direction of an intrinsic impulse that provides us with the mental power for well-being, optimism, joy, love, peace. This however, is a hypothesis which well worth being investigated as an essential goal in sciences of consciousness. Despite many people intuitively agree with this metaphor, to my knowledge there is only little scientific research regarding this phenomenon up to now. It is beyond what is addressed in many meditation studies. Moreover, it remains to be considered just which methods and approaches would be productive for this kind of research.

3.5 Objectification of Subjectivity

One ambition in consciousness science is the objectification of subjectively experienced human observations. This targets unambiguous assignments of subjective experiences of consciousness to external physical measures as documented in EEG or fMRI. Modern neuropsychology assumes the identity between neuronal activity and a corresponding subjective experience. In this case one could theoretically draw conclusions from neuronal processes about personal experience. Such assignments are made for example by the cognition detection system we developed in order to make statements about cognitive abilities and processing in coma patients (Hinterberger et al., 2005). However, while dealing with those patients we have to remain honest. Even if we can measure certain processes as taking place in the brain it is not mandatory that the patient consciously perceives his or her 'understanding'. Or vice versa: Even if it seems that there is no information processing detectable it is still speculative to assume that the patients would be unconscious as long as they are not able to communicate it to us or as long as we do not have enough cases of reports related to a certain EEG pattern. Though neuronal activity may indicate certain brain processes usually related to consciousness, conscious experience still remains the observer's secret. As mentioned, the qualia of experience are a privilege of the observer. Finally, the best suited method for measuring subjectivity is offered by verbal communication. Basically, our language has developed itself in a direction to objectify and externalize subjective experiences so that the content of personal experiences can be shared and understood. Therefore, in psychology questionnaires are the most valid measuring device for contents of consciousness.

4. Final Thoughts

Science's approach is based on the objectification of phenomena and therefore prefers methods which make properties independent from subjective descriptions through the act of measurement. In this process the subjective content is eliminated. However, by ignoring our own individual experiences we might not promote them anymore. As a consequence, the common 'objective' world we live in will change itself so that the human being's lively expression is threatened with extinction. Hence, in order to observe and understand the world as a whole, science has to integrate even those subjective fractions which cannot be objectified but which determine objectivity. This means that the science of consciousness should feel obliged to investigate subjective experience in particular.

In this context, a first step consists in creating an awareness for noticing that each social system is not only built up by but also for humans whose life quality essentially results from individual inner world experiences. As diagnoses for burnout symptoms are rapidly increasing, a humanist science of consciousness has enormous importance and possibly burnout symptoms can at least be partly attributed to the ongoing neglect of the inner life impulse as presented in the top-left of Figure 3. Fostering this holistic form of consciousness in society means to develop ways for enabling humans to appreciate, (re)discover, cultivate and finally apply their subjectivity in concordance with the objective and rational world for designing an environment worth living.

This chapter is an attempt to equip this understanding with a scientific basis. It tries to synthesize science and personal experience in which the experience of pleasure, love, freedom, encounter, spirituality and transcendence form an integral part of each individual as well as the whole society.

Part 6:

History of Experimental Psychology and Clinical Neuroscience

19 Wilhelm Wundts Neuropsychologie

Jochen Fahrenberg

Key Words: Apperzeption/-psychologie, Assoziationspsychologie, Aufmerksamkeit, Bewussteseinspsychologie, Lokalisationstheorien, Neuropsychologie, Wilhelm Wundt

Summary

Wilhelm Wundt was a neurophysiologist, psychologist and philosopher. He is considered to be the founder of the first laboratory for experimental psychology with an explicit research program as well as the founder of psychology itself as a scientific discipline. He became reknown especially through his publication Grundzüge der physiologischen Psychologie (1874; 6th edition: 1908-1911). However, empirical psychology is not a natural science although in General Psychology it relies, when possible, on physiological methods: for examining sensation (psychophysics), concentration/vigilance and apperceptive processes (mental chronometry) and emotional expression (psychophysiology). Wundt's textbook is especially characterized by unusually extensive and in the following editions expanded chapters on the status of anatomy and the functional principles of the CNS.

Wundt's concept of physiological psychology, however, was subjected to a misunderstanding that can scarcely be changed even today, something Wundt himself consciously attempted to avoid by writing „physiological psychology" and precisely not „Physiological Psychology" in the German text, revealing his intention to emphasize that he was working with physiological instruments, with a good measure of interest in psychophysiological relationships, but was emphasizing from the very beginning that psychology could not be reduced to physiology, something he considered to be impossible (1896, p. 21).

Wundt's arguments are especially intriguing because he has been recognized for his neurophysiological research publications and at the same time he is considered to bet he most famous psychologist of his day. But work on Wundt's ideas can be rewarding from another perspective: He developed a psychological concept of conscious processe and associated them with a (neurophysiologically formulated) hypothetical apperception center in the frontal cortex. In a highly differentiated manner his psychology of apperception describeshow the synthesis (integration) of sensory, motor, autonomic, cognitive, emotional and motivational processing components could function/develop, in the terms of that initial phase of neuropsychology. Wundt's plea for the necessary cooperation between psychologists and physiologists is revealing, as he himself had a command over the interdisciplinary approach and research competency.

Two themes in Wundt's neuropsychology stand out:

(1) Critique of elementary localization theory.
(2) The theory of apperception.

Taking intelligence as a particular example, Wundt explained why he rejected the idea represented by Meynert, Hitzig, Ferrier and Flechsig that intelligence could be localized in the frontal lobe. Rather than examining intelligence as being a collective term for quite variegated phenomena all subsumed under that one concept, he recommended „dissecting intelligence into its elementary processes as far as possible, processes with which a lucid and simple psychological concept can be associated which then finally reveals the relationship to a correspondingly simple physiological correlative concept" (p. 381). Such an elementary concept could be seen, he theorized, when someone was concentrating, here he assumed that we can see an alternation between activating and inhibiting processes. Wundt favored the idea that experimentation on localisation of the higher central nervous functions should depend on PR and psychologically founded research hypotheses given the fact that major questions could not be satisfactorily resolved merely on the basis of the anatomical and physiological levels (compare the comments by Ziche, 1999). For Wundt, the topics of attention/concentration and its navigation were perfect examples of the association he was calling for between experimental-psychological and physiological research. (Summary translated by David Emmans.)

Abstrakt

Wilhelm Wundt war Neurophysiologe, Psychologe und Philosoph. Er gilt als der Gründer des ersten Labors für experimentelle Psychologie sowie der Psychologie als Disziplin. Bekannt wurde Wundt vor allem durch seine *Grundzüge der physiologischen Psychologie* (1874; 6. Auflage 1908-1911). Die empirische Psychologie ist keine Naturwissenschaft, aber sie stützt sich, wenn möglich, in der Allgemeinen Psychologie auch auf physiologische Methoden: bei Sinnesempfindungen (Psychophysik), Aufmerksamkeit und apperzeptive Prozesse (mentale Chronometrie) und Gefühlsausdruck (Psychophysiologie). Wundts Lehrbuch zeichnet sich durch ungewöhnlich ausführliche und später noch erweiterte Kapitel über den Stand der funktionellen Neuroanatomie und der Physiologie des ZNS aus. Dazu gehört eine kritische Diskussion der zeitgenössischen Lokalisationstheorien und allgemeiner Funktionsprinzipien. Wundt plädiert dafür, die neuroanatomischen und -physiologischen Fragestellungen an prägnanten psychologischen Konzepten auszurichten. Diese Konzeption einer interdisziplinären

Neurowissenschaft ist heute Allgemeingut, doch wird Wundts Beitrag zu dieser Entwicklung kaum noch erinnert.

Aufmerksamkeit und Aufmerksamkeitssteuerung bilden für Wundt ein herausragendes Beispiel der wünschenswerten Verbindung experimentalpsychologischer und physiologischer Forschung. Noch wichtiger sind ihm die höheren integrativen Prozesse, die er sehr differenziert und mit den in seinem Labor verfügbaren psychologischen Methoden beschreibt. Als allgemeines Bezugssystem entwirft er seine Apperzeptionstheorie, die – in heutiger Terminologie – sensorische, kognitive, emotionale, motivationale, auch die phänomenal-bewussten und die hypothetischen neurophysiologischen Funktionen zusammenfasst. In dem aufmerksamen und gerichteten Bewusstseinsprozess werden Empfindungen und Vorstellungen apperzeptiv mit typischen Gefühltönen verbunden, auf verschiedene Weise assoziiert und kombiniert, auch mit motorischen und vegetativen Innervationen verknüpft, nicht bloß „verarbeitet“, sondern auch „schöpferisch synthetisiert“.

Dieser Prozess ist vorrangig durch die aktive Aufmerksamkeit und willentliche Steuerung bestimmt und wird im Unterschied zu heute verbreiteten Forschungsansätzen nicht systematisch in kognitive, emotionale und volitionale Partialprozesse aufgespalten. Wundts Heuristik eines *Apperzeptionszentrums* im Frontalcortex ist als Leitidee eines primär psychologisch orientierten Forschungsprogramms über die höchsten integrativen Prozesse gemeint. In der späteren neurowissenschaftlichen Forschung wurde diese Konzeption nicht angenommen. Die Funktionen werden weitgehend isoliert, d.h. nicht als zusammengehörige Prozesskomponenten untersucht – auch wegen der Schwierigkeiten der Methodik. Gegenwärtig scheint das Interesse an multimodalen Konvergenzzonen auf verschiedenen Ebenen der zentralnervösen Organisation zuzunehmen. Wundts Konzept des multimodalen Apperzeptionszentrums ist heute fast völlig vergessen, die Heuristik bleibt aktuell.

1. Einleitung

Die Neurowissenschaft ist eine interdisziplinäre Aufgabe – diese Einstellung ist heute selbstverständlich. Wenn es um die höheren zentralnervösen Funktionen geht, sind außer den neuroanatomischen und physiologischen auch psychologische Konzepte und Methoden unverzichtbar. Allerdings gibt es auch die Einstellung des extremen Reduktionismus, Bewusstsein sei nur ein „Schatten der Hirnphysik“, doch selbst dieser Epiphänomenalismus ist auf Heuristiken aus der Introspektion und Bewusstseinspsychologie, zumindest auf verhaltenspsychologische Begriffe und Methoden angewiesen.

In den Anfängen, d.h. in der zweiten Hälfte des 19. Jahrhunderts, war dieser Perspektivenwechsel keineswegs selbstverständlich. Einige der einflussreichen Neuroanatomen und Neurophysiologen jener Zeit waren aufgrund ihrer naturwissenschaftlichen Grundüberzeugung nicht geneigt, psychologischen Konzepten grundsätzlich eine heuristische oder gar gleichberechtigte Bedeutung in der Forschung zuzubilligen. Es fehlt letztlich der naturwissenschaftliche Erklärungswert. Die vier Physiologen (Physiker und Mediziner) Ernst von Brücke, Emil Du Bois-Reymond, Carl F. Ludwig und Herrmann von Helmholtz bildeten um 1845 einen Zirkel, der sich gegen den zeitgenössischen Vitalismus, d.h. Ideen über eine eigentümliche, nicht genau fassbare „Lebenskraft", wendete und ausschließlich physikalisch-chemische Kräfte im Organismus gelten lassen wollte.* Mit der Abwehr vitalistischer Auffassungen verband sich wohl eine Reserviertheit gegenüber der zeitgenössischen Psychologie, die z.B. in der Rede von Helmholtz (1878) über *Die Tatsachen in der Wahrnehmung* deutlich wird. Der Psychiater Paul Flechsig (1896, S. 11) meinte, dass „die Erforschung des Gehirns den Schlüssel zu einer wissenschaftlichen Erforschung des Seelenlebens bringen werde, und die heutige medizinische Psychologie will in der Tat nichts anderes sein, als ein Abschnitt der Lehre von den Hirnfunktionen. Welche Hirnteile sind in Tätigkeit, wenn wir denken oder fühlen; welcherlei chemische und physikalische Vorgänge sind hierbei beteiligt?"

Auch Wilhelm Wundt forderte die strikte Unterscheidung der Naturkausalität der Physiologie von der kategorial grundverschiedenen Bewusstseinspsychologie mit ihrem Subjektbezug, Willenstätigkeit (Zweckprinzip), Wertbezug, und mit anderen eigenständigen Erkenntnisprinzpien. Er forderte jedoch, dass sich die Versuche zur morphologisch-funktionellen Lokalisation von höheren zentralnervöser Funktionen nach psychologischen Konzepten richten sollten. Auf der physiologischer Ebene allein sind die Fragestellungen nicht hinreichend zu präzisieren. Wundts Argumente sind von besonderem Interesse, da er durch neurophysiologische Forschungsarbeiten ausgewiesen war und zugleich als der bekannteste Psychologe seiner Zeit gilt. Sich mit Wundts *Neuropsychologie* zu befassen, lohnt noch aus einem zweiten Grund: Er entwickelte eine psychologische Konzeption der Bewusstseinsprozesse und bezog diese auf ein – neurophysiologisch formuliertes – hypothetisches Apperzeptionszentrum im Frontalcortex. Seine Apperzeptionspsychologie beschreibt in sehr differenzierter Weise wie die Synthese (Integration) sensorischer, motorischer, vegetativer, kognitiver, emotionaler und motivationaler Prozesskomponenten ablaufen könnte – in den Begriffen jener Anfangsphase der Neuropsychologie. Wundts Auffassung über die notwendige Kooperation von Psychologen und Physiologen ist bemerkenswert, denn er verfügte in herausragender Weise bereits über diese interdisziplinäre Einstellung und Forschungskompetenz.

1.1 Wundts Werk und neue Wissenschaftskonzeption der Psychologie

Wilhelm Wundt (1832-1920), Physiologe, Psychologe, Philosoph, gilt als der Gründervater der *Psychologie im Sinne einer eigenständigen Disziplin* an den Universitäten. In heutigen Lehrbüchern und geschichtlichen Darstellungen der Psychologie wird Wundt (nach Gustav Theodor Fechner) als einer der ersten Experimentalpsychologen anerkannt, während seine Kulturpsychologie (Völkerpsychologie) weitgehend und seine Neuropsychologie fast völlig vergessen zu sein scheinen. Wundts akademischer Lebenslauf lässt erkennen wie er sich vom Neurophysiologen zum Psychologen entwickelte. Nach seiner Promotion zum Dr. med. 1856 mit den „Untersuchungen über das Verhalten der Nerven in entzündeten und degenerierten Organen" verbringt er ein Forschungssemester in Berlin bei Johannes Müller und Emil Du Bois-Reymond. Nach der Habilitation 1858 in Heidelberg ist er bis 1865 Assistent von Hermann Helmholtz in der Physiologie; anschließend außerordentlicher Professor für Anthropologie und medizinische Psychologie in Heidelberg. Im Jahr 1874 wurde er Professor für induktive Philosophie (philosophische Wissenschaftslehre) in Zürich, dann 1875 Professor für Philosophie an der Universität Leipzig. In der Heidelberger Zeit publiziert Wundt 10 Arbeiten zur Physiologie und Neurophysiologie (u.a. Muskelphysiologie, Augenbewegungen, Nervenleitung, Curare), ein *Lehrbuch der Physiologie des Menschen* (1865, 4. Aufl. 1878) und ein *Handbuch der Medizinischen Physik* (1867). Er verfasste ca. 70 Rezensionen über aktuelle Publikationen auf den Gebieten Neurophysiologie und Neurologie, Physiologie, Anatomie, Histologie.**

Wundts (1862) *Beiträge zur Theorie der Sinneswahrnehmung* entstanden seit 1858 in der Physiologie, während die *Vorlesungen über die Menschen- und Tierseele* (1863, 6. Aufl. 1919) bereits seine Lehrtätigkeit in Anthropologie und medizinischer Psychologie und den breiten Horizont seiner Forschungsinteressen widerspiegeln. Sein bekanntestes Lehrbuch *Grundzüge der physiologischen Psychologie* (1874, 7. Aufl. 1923) entstand noch in Heidelberg. In Leipzig gründete Wundt das erste Laboratorium für Psychologie mit einem expliziten Forschungsprogramm der experimentellen Psychologie. Diesem Programm folgte er über mehr als 50 Jahre in intensiver Weise. Unter Wundts 183 Doktoranden waren 70 Ausländer, davon 18 Amerikaner (Meischner-Metge, 2003). Zu seinem Werk gehören auch Bücher zur Philosophie (Erkenntnistheorie, Metaphysik, Logik, Ethik) in vielen Auflagen. Eine adäquate Biographie Wundts existiert nicht, auch keine edierte Werkausgabe; mehrere wesentliche Bücher und Aufsätze sind nicht ins Englische übersetzt.

Wundts Forschungsprogramm erstreckte sich von der Allgemeinen Psychologie, d.h. Psychophysik der Sinnesempfindungen, Hauptthemen der Bewusstseinspsychologie, Psychophysiologie der Emotionen u.a., bis zur Sprach-psychologie und Kulturpsychologie. Er entwickelte eine umfassende Wissenschaftskonzeption und Wissenschaftstheorie der Psychologie. Dazu gehört die Ableitung von Prinzipien und Entwicklungsgesetzen, die als erste *spezielle Kategorien- und Prinzipienlehre der Psychologie* verstanden werden kann. Seine Konzeption ist multi-perspektivisch und schließt sowohl das experimentelle Paradigma als auch das interpretativ-vergleichende Paradigma ein (Fahrenberg, 2012). Die Psychologie muss zwar die physiologischen und biologischen Grundlagen einbeziehen, ist jedoch keine Naturwissenschaft, sondern „empirische Geisteswissenschaft". Die Trennung von der Philosophie würde nur dazu führen, dass jeder Psychologe seiner eigenen Metaphysik folge statt die ontologischen und erkenntnistheoretischen Voraussetzungen gemeinsam und kritisch zu diskutieren.

Wundt wird für die Sicht der Psychologie als Naturwissenschaft in Anspruch genommen, doch er hat diese Definition strikt abgelehnt. In dieser einseitigen und oft verzerrten Rezeption seines Gesamtwerks gingen Wundts Kulturspsychologie und Wissenschaftstheorie, sein „anderes Erbe" (Jüttemann, 2006) weitgehend verloren. Gegen wissenschaftliche Programme, in denen psychologische Konzepte interpretiert werden als ob sie naturwissenschaftliche wären, müsste Wundt auf die kategoriale Eigenständigkeit der Psychologie verweisen und den heute verbreiteten Reduktionismus und dessen Kategorienfehler kritisieren.

1.2 Psychologie kann nicht auf Physiologie reduziert werden

„Die Physiologie gibt über jene Lebenserscheinungen Aufschluss, welche sich durch unsere äußeren Sinne wahrnehmen lassen. In der Psychologie schaut der Mensch sich selbst gleichsam von innen an und sucht sich den Zusammenhang derjenigen Vorgänge zu erklären, welche ihm diese innere Beobachtung darbietet" (1874, S. 1). „Mit zureichender Sicherheit lässt sich wohl der Satz als begründet ansehen, dass sich nichts in unserem Bewusstsein ereignet, was nicht in bestimmten physiologischen Vorgängen seine körperliche Grundlage fände. Die einfache Empfindung, die Synthese der Empfindung zu Vorstellungen, die Assoziation und Wiedererweckung der Vorstellungen, endlich die Vorgänge der Apperzeption und der Willenserregung sind begleitet von physiologischen Nervenprozessen. Andere körperliche Vorgänge, wie insbesondere die einfachen und komplizierten Reflexe, gehen an und für sich nicht ein in das Bewusstsein, bilden aber wesentliche Vorbedingungen der bewussten oder im engeren Sinne psychologischen Tatsachen" (1874, S. 858 f). Der *physiologischen Psychologie* weist Wundt die Aufgabe zu: „*erstlich* diejenigen Lebensvorgänge zu erforschen, welche, zwischen äußerer und innerer Erfahrung in der Mitte stehend, die gleichzeitige Anwendung beider Beobachtungsmethoden, der äußeren und der inneren, erforderlich machen, und *zweitens* von den bei der Untersuchung dieses Gebietes gewonnenen Gesichtspunkten aus die Gesamtheit der Lebensvorgänge zu beleuchten und auf solche Weise wo möglich eine Totalauffassung des menschlichen Seins zu vermitteln" (1874, S. 2).

Wundt erfuhr ein offensichtlich kaum noch zu beseitigendes Missverständnis, das er durch die Kleinschreibung des Adjektivs vermeiden wollte: die *physiologische* Psychologie bezieht sich zwar auch auf physiologische Aspekte, aber ist gerade *nicht* als eine Psychologie aus physiologisch-naturwissenschaftlicher Sicht gemeint. „Das Attribut ‚physiologisch' will nicht sagen, dass sie [die physiologische Psychologie] die Psychologie auf Physiologie zurückführen wolle – was ich für ein Ding der Unmöglichkeit halte –, sondern dass sie mit physiologischen, d.h. experimentellen Hilfsmitteln arbeitet und allerdings mehr, als es in der sonstigen Psychologie zu geschehen pflegt, auf die Beziehungen der psychischen zu den physischen Vorgängen Rücksicht nimmt" (1896, S. 21). Seine Auffassung des psychophysischen Parallelismus ist nicht ontologisch gemeint, sondern als Heuristik in erkenntnistheoretischer und methodologischer Hinsicht. Wundt unterstreicht später die „relative Unzulänglichkeit des heuristischen Parallelprinzips", denn die Aufgabe erschöpfe sich ja nicht darin, nur den Zusammenhang der psychischen und der physischen Prozesse aufzuzeigen. Die Hilfsmittel der Physiologie bleiben nicht nur vorläufig, sondern grundsätzlich unzureichend für die Aufgabenstellung der Psychologie. Ein solches Beginnen sei ergebnislos, „weil es dem Zusammenhang der psychischen Vorgänge selbst verständnislos gegenüberstehen würde, auch wenn uns der Zusammenhang der Gehirnvorgänge so klar vor Augen stünde wie der Mechanismus einer Taschenuhr" (1911, S. 754).

1.3 Mögliche Missverständnisse der Terminologie und der Wissenschaftstheorie

Im Rückblick können sich leicht begriffliche Missverständnisse ergeben. Zum Beispiel meint Wundts Begriff Element in der Regel eine kleinste unterscheidbare Funktionseinheit in einem Ganzen, wobei die Zergliederung von der allgemeinen Betrachtungsebene abhängt, d.h. aus psychophysischer Sicht wird auch das Gehirn als „zentrales Element" bezeichnet. Wenn Wundts Psychologie von Psychologiehistorikern als mechanistische „Elementenpsychologie" dargestellt wird, ist das ein grundsätzliches Missverständnis dieser – empirisch-analytisch unumgänglichen – Differenzierungen eines Ganzen und übersieht völlig Wundts Prinzipienlehre. Ein Beispiel seiner Erkenntnisprinzipien ist das „*Prinzip der schöpferischen Synthese*" (Wundt, 1863, 1, S. 435; siehe Fahrenberg, 2011, 2013, S. 263 ff), das inhaltlich dem späteren Begriff „Übersummativität" der Gestalttheorie entspricht und heute *Emergenzprinzip* genannt wird (vgl. Fahrenberg, 2013). Er verlangt die *koordinierte Doppelbetrachtung* nach dem naturwissenschaftlichen Kausalprinzip der Physiologie und nach den eigenständigen Kategorien und Prinzipien der Bewusstseinspsychologie.

Wundt unterscheidet Sinnesempfindungen, Vorstellungen, Gefühle und Affekte sowie Willenstätigkeit. Seine deskriptiven Begriffe sind mit den heute gängigen, Kognition, Emotion und Volition (Motivation), nur ungefähr zu treffen. Für Wundts Menschenbild sind die Syntheseleistung der Bewusstseinsprozesse und die willentlichen Komponenten wesentlich. Der Kontrast zu Johann Friedrich Herbarts Psychologie (1825), die primär auf einer Theorie der Vorstellungen aufbaut und Willensvorgänge als deren Wirkungen interpretiert, ist groß. Wundt (u.a. 1911, S. 322) kann der „Mechanik der Vorstellungen" in dieser „intellektualistischen" und spekulativ-mathematischen Psychologie nicht folgen. Bereits im theoretischen und methodischen Ansatz widerspricht er dieser Separierung von kognitiven, emotionalen und motivationalen Teilfunktionen der zentralen Prozesse und betont deren prozessuale Verbindung in seiner Apperzeptionstheorie

Wichtige Leitgedanken Wundts, d.h. die Unterscheidung zwischen Perzeption und Apperzeption, der psychophysische Parallelismus und auch der perspektivische Denkstil, sind primär von Gottfried Wilhelm Leibniz beeinflusst. Wundt unterscheidet aber zwei in *kategorialer* Hinsicht grundverschiedene Bezugssysteme (Betrachtungsweisen), und verlangt eine sich wechselseitig ergänzende, koordinierte Doppelbetrachtung, die in ihrer Meta-Relation dem später von Niels Bohr vorgeschlagenen Komplementaritätsprinzip ähnlich ist. Beide Betrachtungsweisen der psychophysischen Einheit sind gleichberechtigt und unverzichtbar. Der Begriff des *Verhaltens* für eine dritte Perspektive neben Bewusstsein und Hirnphysiologie war zu Wundts Zeit noch unüblich; zwar wurden im Labor Verhaltensmerkmale beobachtet und gemessen, doch fehlte die bereits durch Immanuel Kant (1798) mit seiner Methodenkritik der Introspektion angebahnte Explikation der Verhaltensebene (siehe Fahrenberg, 2015).

Der heutige Ausdruck „Neuropsychologie" für Wundts Konzeption ist problematisch, es sei denn, dass seine epistemologisch strikte Unterscheidung der neurophysiologischen und der bewusstseinspsychologischen Perspektive bedacht ist und dabei reflektiert wird, was aus Wundts Sicht gravierende Kategorienfehler sind. Den Begriff „Neuropsychologie" hätte Wundt wohl kaum noch gewählt, nachdem er die groben Missverständnisse seiner „physiologischen Psychologie" wegen der Reihenfolge in diesem Wortpaar erfahren hatte. Die ihm vorrangige Perspektive innerhalb der an sich gleichberechtigten Doppelbetrachtung der zentralen *psychophysischen* Prozesse würde der Begriff *Psychophysiologie* ausdrücken. Vielleicht kannte er den von dem Psychiater Christian Friedrich Nasse (1822) eingeführten Begriff nicht oder wollte ihn nicht übernehmen. Erwähnt wurde Nasse ebenso wenig von Hans Berger (1921), der noch vor seiner Entdeckung des EEG, die *Psychophysiologie* in dem modernen Sinne zweier gleichberechtigter Forschungsperspektiven bestimmte.

Hier sind nur Hinweise möglich und nur eine Skizze von Wundts Neuropsychologie. Vielleicht wird dabei deutlich, weshalb in der Folgezeit den weitaus einfacheren Assoziationstheorien und den spezialisierten Richtungen der kognitiven oder emotionalen Neuropsychologie der Vorzug gegeben wurde, statt Wundts Apperzeptionspsychologie mit ihrer Absicht konzeptueller Integration weiterzuführen. Seine von der Aufmerksamkeitsteuerung ausgehende Theorie der Apperzeption betrifft die höchsten Prozesse der Synthese (Integration) und verbindet sensorische, emotionale gedankliche und willentliche Teilprozesse, auch motorische vegetative Symptomen des Gefühlsausdrucks.

Diese Zusammenhänge machen die Interpretation von Wundts anspruchsvoller Gesamtkonzeption zu einer komplizierten Angelegenheit. Hinzu kommt, dass Wundt diese parallelistische Wissenschaftskonzeption über mehr als ein halbes Jahrhundert, von seinem Lehrbuch der Physiologie (1865) bis zu seiner Wissenschaftslehre (in der Logik, 1919-1921) schrittweise aufbaute, ohne jedoch neben seinen zahlreichen anderen Werken ein systematisches Lehrbuch der Wissenschaftstheorie und Methodologie der Psychologie zu verfassen. Es gibt Entwicklungsschritte in Wundts Auffassungen, begriffliche Inkonsistenzen und einzelne Widersprüche zwischen den Werken und ihren Auflagen, aber keine grundsätzlichen Revisionen. Wundts Stil und Satzbildung können für heutige Leser schwierig sein. Außerdem fehlten damals noch einige wichtige Begriffe der heutigen Wissenschaftstheorie und Methodologie. Anspruchsvoll ist der häufige Perspektiven-Wechsel zwischen physiologischer und psychologischer Argumentation, die jeweils für den Experimentalpsychologen Wundt auch methodische und für den Wissenschaftstheoretiker Wundt kategoriale Konsequenzen haben.

Die Rezeptionsforschung ergab, dass Wundts Wissenschaftskonzeption, auch seine Neuropsychologie, nur sehr geringe Resonanz fanden, vielleicht kaum verstanden wurden. Bereits die meisten Schüler Wundts klammerten seine Neuropsychologie, seine Kulturpsychologie, seine Tierpsychologie, und nicht nur seine Ethik, sondern in der Regel auch seine Wissenschaftstheorie aus (Fahrenberg, 2011). Der unbestrittene Gründervater der empirischen Psychologie als Disziplin ist insofern ein Außenseiter geblieben. In dem Rückblick auf Wundts „Neuropsychologie" kommt es hier auf seine Programmatik und auf die Ideengeschichte an. Sind Konzepte zu erkennen, die heutigen Vorstellungen nahe stehen, Trends vorwegnahmen oder spätere Defizite und eventuell wieder aktuelle Sichtweisen aufzeigen?

2. Themen der Neuropsychologie

Zwei Themen in Wundts Neuropsychologie ragen hervor: (1) seine Kritik der elementaren Lokalisationslehre, die durch die Vorstellung multipler Repräsentation abzulösen sei, verbunden mit dem Vorschlag, von *psychologisch* begründeten Forschungshypothesen auszugehen; (2) die neuropsychologische Konzeption der Apperzeptionstheorie, die ein Bezugssystem für die höchsten integrativen Prozesse geben soll. Das erste Thema wurde von Ziche (1999) in *Neuroscience and psychology in the work of Wilhelm Wundt* so ausführlich dargestellt, dass ihm mit wenigen Ergänzungen und Literaturhinweisen zu folgen ist. Ziches Interesse richtet sich vornehmlich auf die Beziehung zwischen physiologischen und psychologischen Konzeptionen in der Anfangsphase der entstehenden Neurowissenschaften. Er diskutiert: (1) Wundts kritische Ansichten über die zeitgenössische Reflexlehre und die Lokalisationslehre; (2) die Auffassungsunterschiede über die Bedeutung psychologischer Konzepte für die physiologische Forschung; (3) nur sehr knapp Wundts Apperzeptionstheorie; und (4) mögliche Gründe, weshalb Wundts kritische Argumente kaum aufgenommen wurden. Ziches Beitrag wird hier übersichtsartig referiert; anschließend steht Wundts Apperzeptionstheorie mit ihren neuropsychologischen Aspekten im Zentrum. Eine adäquate Rekonstruktion dieser anspruchsvollen Bewusstseinstheorie einschließlich ihrer epistemologischen und methodologischen Grundlagen würde mehr Raum beanspruchen; sie ist offenbar bisher nie versucht worden.

Verwendet werden die *Grundzüge der physiologischen Psychologie* in der 6. Auflage (1908-1911), die auch Ziche heranzog. Der Band 1 enthält den umfangreichen Hauptabschnitt *Von den körperlichen Grundlagen des Seelenlebens* mit den Kapiteln: Bauelemente des Nervensystems, Physiologische Mechanik der Nervensubstanz, Formentwicklung der Zentralorgane, Verlauf der nervösen Leitungsbahnen. Das Kapitel 6 *Physiologische Funktion der Zentralteile* umfasst drei neuropsychologisch interessante Abschnitte: Funktionen der Großhirnhemisphären, Beispiele psychophysischer Analyse komplexer Großhirnfunktionen und Allgemeine Prinzipien der zentralen Funktionen (1908, S. 335-397). Wundts *Apperzeptionstheorie* steht im Abschnitt über die psychophysische Analyse komplexer Großhirnfunktionen (S. 360-385) mit dem „Schema der hypothetischen Verbindungen des Apperzeptionszentrums" (S. 383, siehe Abbildung 1). Außerdem gibt es, vor allem im Band 3 (1911), systematische physiologische Hinweise in den Kapiteln über die Sinnesempfindungen, das Reflex- und Willkürverhalten, die Ausdrucksbewegungen und die körperliche Seite der Affekte (Emotionen). Nach der Anzahl der Seiten eingeschätzt besteht Wundts Lehrbuch zu knapp einem Viertel aus dem sinnesphysiologischen, neuroanatomischen, neurophysiologischen und biologischen Grundwissen seiner Zeit. Das ist im relativen Anteil mehr als in einem anderen Lehrbuch der *Allgemeinen Psychologie*, damals oder heute.

Abbildung 1: *Schema der hypothetischen Verbindungen des Apperzeptionszentrums (Wundt, 1908, S. 383).*

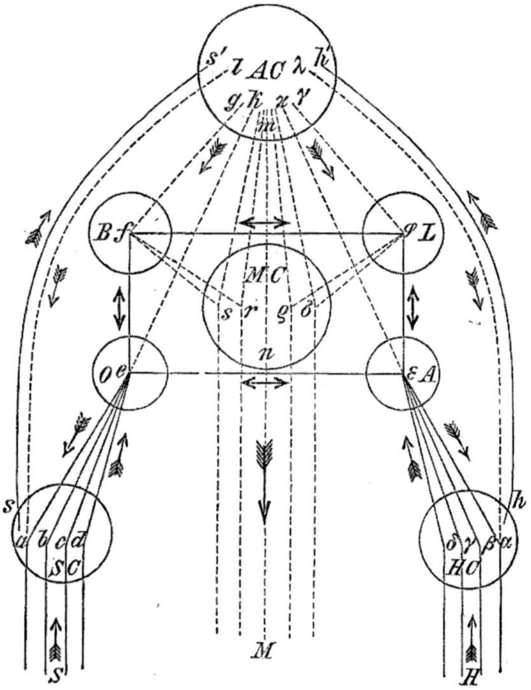

Fig. 105. Schema der hypothetischen Verbindungen des Apperceptionscentrums. *SC* Sehcentrum. *HC* Hörcentrum. *S* centrale Sehnervenfasern. *H* ebensolche Hörnervenfasern. *A*, *O* sensorische, *L*, *B* motorische Zwischencentren. *MC* directes motorisches Centrum. *M* motorische Centralfasern. *AC* Apperceptionscentrum. *s s'*, *h h'* centripetale Bahnen zu dem letzteren, *l a*, *g f* u.s.w. centrifugale Verbindungen desselben.

3. Wundts Kritik der Lokalisationslehren und der unzulänglichen Forschungskonzeption

Als Hintergrund dieser Kontroversen referiert Ziche die *Allgemeinen Prinzipien der zentralen Funktionen.* Dazu gehören nach Wundt *vier Prinzipien* zu Verlauf und Funktion der Leitungsbahnen und *fünf Prinzipien* über die zentralen Funktionen; Wundt folgt hier Meynert, Munk, Ramón y Cajal u.a. Autoren. Neben dem Prinzip der mehrfachen Vertretung [multiple Repräsentation] sind das

Prinzip der zentralen Verknüpfung räumlich getrennter Funktionsgebiete und die Theorie der Kreuzungen, das Prinzip der Übung und Anpassung, das Prinzip der Stellvertretung sowie das Prinzip der relativen Lokalisation hervorzuheben (1908, S. 275-291). Wundt stellt die peripheren und die zentralen Nervenfunkionen einander gegenüber und schließt, dass die *zentralen* Phänomene nicht als Analogien zur Physiologie der motorischen Reflexbögen verstanden werden könnten. Der Kritik an solchen damals verbreiteten Reflexlehren (Reflexologie) folgt die Diskussion von Ausfallserscheinungen und eine ausführliche Kritik an zeitgenössischen Lokalisationslehren (S. 341 ff).

Wundt wendet sich gegen „Dogmen der älteren Nervenphysiologie", wenn er schreibt: „Anzunehmen mit der Existenz eines zentralen Elementes [Gehirn] sei der spezifische Inhalt einer Empfindung von selbst gegeben, oder mit der ‚Projektion' des Netzhautbildes auf eine zentrale Sinnesfläche sei der Sehakt vollendet, oder das ‚Wortgedächtnis', die ‚Intelligenz' usw. seien so, wie sie in der populären Psychologie als ungeteilte Begriffe figurieren, auch in fest abgegrenzten Hirnregionen lokalisiert, – alles dies anzunehmen, ist natürlich sehr viel einfacher, als die Konsequenzen zu ziehen, die sich aus den oben aufgestellten Prinzipien ergeben. Aber, abgesehen davon, dass jene Vorstellungen den Tatsachen widerstreiten, sind sie schon deshalb unmöglich, weil sie auf einer gänzlich unhaltbaren Psychologie, auf unzulänglichen physiologischen Begriffen und im Grunde selbst auf einer antiquierten Auffassung vom Bau des Nervensystems beruhen" (S. 397).

Am Beispiel der Intelligenz begründet Wundt, weshalb er die verbreitete, von Meynert, Hitzig, Ferrier und Flechsig vertretene, Auffassung als verfehlt ansah, die „Intelligenz" im Stirnhirn zu lokalisieren. Statt solche unter einem unbestimmten Sammelnamen zusammengefassten Erscheinungen zu untersuchen, empfiehlt er, diese „möglichst in solche elementare Vorgänge zu zerlegen, mit denen sich ein klarer und einfacher psychologischer Begriff verbinden lässt, der eventuell die Beziehung auf einen entsprechend einfachen physiologischen Korrelatbegriff möglich macht" (S. 381). Ein solcher Elementarbegriff sei der Zustand der Aufmerksamkeit. Wundt vermutet, dass mit dem Stärker- und Schwächerwerden einer Empfindung die Zu- und Abnahme bestimmter physiologische Erregungs- und Hemmungsvorgänge einhergehen. Dagegen sei es „ein aussichtloses Unternehmen, für den verwickelten Begriff der ‚Intelligenz' überhaupt irgendwelche bestimmt begrenzte physische Substrate aufzusuchen" (S. 382 f).

Das allgemeine *Prinzip der relativen Lokalisation* formuliert Wundt, indem er sich ausführlich mit dem damaligen Wissensstand einschließlich der Methodik und speziell mit Meynerts (1871) und Munks (1881) Argumenten auseinandersetzt. In Wundts Kritik sind mit Ziche (S. 421 ff) zwei Ebenen zu unterscheiden: auf der Ebene der neurophysiologischen Forschung widerspricht Wundt Meynerts Unterscheidung von Projektionszentren und Assoziationszentren mit neurophysiologischen Argumenten und auf der psychologischen Ebene wendet er ein, dass Meynert mit seiner Annahme eines Assoziationszentrums anatomisch-physiologische Strukturannahme und psychologische Konzepte vermische.

3.1 Wundt zur Bedeutung psychologischer Konzepte für die Physiologie

Wundt hielt den Cortex von allen Strukturen des Gehirns für am besten untersucht aufgrund der damals verfügbaren Techniken, d.h. experimenteller Läsion und Ablation, neuroanatomischer und histologischer Untersuchungen der Bahnen sowie der direkten Stimulation des Cortex (Fritsch, Hitzig). Jedoch könnten selbst die fortgeschrittensten Arbeiten Meynerts die Hirnfunktionen nicht erklären, weil ein Konzept fehle, welcher Art diese Funktionen wären. Ziche referiert die Kontroverse zwischen dem Sprachwissenschaftler Steinthal (1874) und Fritsch und Hitzig, die neurologisch über die Innervation des Sprechapparates forschten, aber kaum an Sprache interessiert waren (Ziche, 1999, S. 417 f; siehe auch Breidbach, 1997, S. 125 ff; Hagner, 1997, S. 279-288). Wundt äußert sich ähnlich wie Steinthal, dass die Physiologen kaum wüssten, was sie sehen und messen (Ziche, 1999, S. 417).

Wundts Diskussion der Lokalisation, so Ziche (S. 426), sei charakteristisch für seine Idee einer physiologischen Psychologie. Wundt beziehe sich auf die enge Korrelation beider Betrachtungsweisen, lehne aber *grundsätzlich* physiologische *Erklärungen* psychischer (geistiger, bewusster) Ereignisse ab. Ziche sieht außerdem zwei Hauptargumente: (1) die Komplexität der Probleme (welche künftig überwunden werden könnte) und (2) die Notwendigkeit, genau zu wissen, was man in der Physiologie untersuchen wolle. In dieser Hinsicht zeige sich die Physiologie grundsätzlich begrenzt, denn kein Fortschritt der Physiologie könne klären, welches die relevanten Funktionen des Gehirns sind.

„Die Gehirnphysiologie hinwiederum kann sich der Einsicht nicht länger verschließen, dass sie viel mehr Fragen an die Psychologie zu stellen hat, von deren Beantwortung die Deutung ihrer eigenen Befunde abhängt, als dass sie imstande wäre, die psychologische Analyse selbst zu ersetzen." ... „Man kann die Konstruktion einer Maschine nicht verstehen, ohne genau zu wissen, was die Maschine zu leisten hat. Im gleichen Sinne setzt die Erkenntnis der Funktionen eines Organs die Analyse dieser Funktionen voraus, und das natürlich um so mehr, je komplizierter sie sind" (Wundt, 1913, S. 197).Die Sinnesphysiologie kann den Psychologen über die relevanten Grundlagen geistiger Prozesse informieren, aber nur die Psychologie vermag die adäquaten Fragen zu stellen, die durch die Physiologie des Sehens und Hörens zu beantworten sind. Wundt (1921, S. 222) betont die notwenige Arbeitsteilung beider Disziplinen. An anderer Stelle hat Ziche (2008) die *Wissenschaftslandschaften* untersucht und ist dabei ausführlich auf Wundts allgemeine Überlegungen zu einer neuen Klassifikation der Wissenschaften in der zweiten Hälfte des 19. Jahrhunderts eingegangen. Die physiologischen Forschungsarbeiten, so Wundt, reichen allein nicht aus, die Funktionen des Gehirns zu begreifen, im nächsten Schritt müssten physiologische und psychologische Betrachtungsweisen kombiniert werden, da „jedes dieser Gebiete selbständig für sich besteht, insofern es in keiner Weise jemals auf das andere zurückgeführt werden kann. In der Tat vermögen wir ebenso wenig die Mechanik der Nervensubstanz aus den Verbindungen unserer Empfindungen und Gefühle, wie umgekehrt die letzteren aus jener abzuleiten" (1908, 1, S. 143). Die Warnung vor einem Reduktionismus verbindet Wundt mit dem Strategievorschlag: zuerst die psychologischen Aspekte genauer zu bestimmen und sich dann eingehend der Physiologie zuzuwenden (1908, S. 381 f).

Wundt tritt, so Ziche, für eine strategische Trennung von Physiologie und Psychologie ein, da die Physiologie wie in der Kontroverse über Lokalisation unter einem schweren Defizit leide; in vielen Fällen könne nur die Psychologie die richtige Art Bezugsrahmen geben in dem die physiologische Forschung fortschreiten könne, trotz der Unsicherheiten, wie die physiologischen Grundlagen sind, habe doch die Psychologie eine leitende Funktion, zumindest für die wichtigsten strukturellen Tatsachen der Sprache, des Sehens und der Apperzeption. Die Funktionen des Gehirns können nicht allein durch die Physiologie erforscht werden. In der Forschungspraxis bedeutet es sogar, den Gebrauch physiologischer Elemente in psychologischen Kontexten zu eliminieren (Ziche, 1999, S. 427).

Vor diesem Hintergrund ist Wundts Kommentar an der zu einfachen „Gleichung Geisteskrankheit gleich Gehirnkrankheit" zu verstehen. Er kritisiert den von bekannten Physiologen und Anatomen (er nennt Meynert, Flechsig, Hitzig, Munk) unternommenen Versuch, „die Ätiologie ausschließlich in die physischen Bedingungen der begleitenden Hirnerkrankung zu verlegen" (1911, S. 652 f). Wundt hält die Auffassungen seines zeitweiligen Mitarbeiters Emil Kraepelin und ausdrücklich auch Sigmund Freuds Ansatz für aussichtsreicher. Erwähnenswert sind Kraepelins 1882 bis 1883 im Leipziger Labor und mit Ratschlägen Wundts begonnenen experimentalpsychologischen Untersuchungen über die Wirkungen von Alkohol, Kaffee und Tee, sowie Chloroform, Morphium u.a. Substanzen, die auch in methodischer Hinsicht als die Pionierarbeiten der Pharmakopsychologie an Gesunden anzusehen sind (Müller, Fletcher & Steinberg, 2006).

3.2 Mögliche Gründe fehlender Rezeption

Ziche führt aus, dass die Mehrzahl der herausragenden Neurophysiologen und Neuroanatomen jener Zeit keineswegs eine interdisziplinäre Gemeinschaftsaufgabe erkannt haben (Helmholtz, Hitzig, Meynert, Munk u.a.; siehe Hagner, 1996). Sie hätten von der psychologischen Perspektive wenig Erklärungswert erwartet, und man war bereit, sozusagen im Alleingang, auch die höheren Funktionen aufzuklären. Auf der anderen Seite zeigte sich in der Hauptströmung der Psychologie zwar ein zunehmendes Interesse an der Experimentalpsychologie, jedoch nur ausnahmsweise ein neuropsychologisches (oder psychophysiologisches) Forschungsinteresse, obwohl die Doppelperspektive des psychophysischen Parallelismus relativ häufig akzeptiert wurde.

Für den Neurophysiologen Wundt mit seinen zunehmenden psychologischen und philosophischen Interessen ergab sich dagegen eine fundamentale wissenschaftstheoretische und methodologische Herausforderung. Ziche zufolge lautet Wundts zentrales Argument: die Neuroanatomen arbeiten bei ihren Ablations- und Stimulations-Prozeduren, und ähnlich die Neurophysiologen, zwar naturwissenschaftlich genau, verfügen aber jenseits der elementaren Begriffe über keine theoretische Konzeption, welche *funktionellen* Zusammenhänge und Leistungen erklärt werden sollten. Hier fehlen primär psychologische Begriffe und geeignete Methoden. Diese Beurteilung sei von den Physiologen nicht akzeptiert oder auch nur gewürdigt worden, auch nicht von medizinisch interessierten Psychologen wie Oswald Külpe. So hätten Physiologen wie Munk oder Sherrington in Wundt nur den Physiologen gesehen und nicht dessen psychologische Argumente aufgenommen. Wundt sei es offensichtlich nicht gelungen, zu zeigen, dass Psychologie unerlässlich für die physiologische Forschung über das ZNS sei. Es fehlte die Übertragung von der Psychologie zur Neurophysiologie. Ziche meint den Grund darin zu sehen, dass es nur wenige zentrale Begriffe gab, die sowohl in Wundts Psychologie als auch in der Physiologie Platz hätten. Wundt habe sein Konzept für eine Lokalisierung der apperzeptiven Strukturen neuroanatomisch nicht wirklich diskutiert und die übliche Redeweise von psychischen Prozessen als „Funktion" oder „Wirkung" physiologischer Vorgänge abgelehnt.

Die künftige Neurowissenschaft, so hätte Ziche in heutiger Formulierung noch anschließen können, ist auf interdisziplinäre Zusammenarbeit, wesentlich auch auf bewussteins- und verhaltenspsychologische Konzepte angewiesen; umgekehrt ist für die Psychologie das Wissen über die neurophysiologischen Grundlagen und Erklärungsweisen von Bewusstsein und Verhalten notwendig. Mit solchen „Brückenkonzepten" hat sich Wundt theoretisch und experimentalpsychologisch eingehend befasst: unter anderem in der *Neuropsychologie der Aufmerksamkeit* und in der *Psychophysiologie der Gefühle (Emotionen)*. Dass Wundt als Neurophysiologe verstand, worum es ging und gerade die Beziehungen zu psychologischen Fragestellungen wesentlich fand, steht außer Frage. Wenn Ziche hier die mangelnde Bereitschaft der genannten Physiologen meint, sich in die eigenständigen Begriffe und Methoden der Psychologie hineinzudenken, trifft seine Einschätzung wohl zu. Tatsächlich zitiert Sherrington (1906) an sechs Stellen Wundts Forschung über Reflexe, auch aus den weithin bekannten *Grundzügen* (Wundt, 1874), aber nirgends einen psychologischen Begriff.

Auch ohne psychologische Konzepte würden zweifellos von der Neuroscience-Forschung noch fundamentale naturwissenschaftliche Forschungsergebnisse als Basis bestehen bleiben. Aber eine Theorie der höheren integrativen Prozesse *ohne psychologische* Konzepte, d.h. ohne Fragestellungen, die wesentlich auch in Begriffen und Methoden der Bewusstseins- und Verhaltenspsychologie präzisiert sind, ist solche Neuroscience unmöglich – das meinte schon Wundt. Die weitere Entwicklung lief auf Wundts Auffassung zu, denn aus heutiger Sicht scheint die interdisziplinäre Verfassung der Neurowissenschaften selbstverständlich zu sein. Genauer ist jedoch zu überlegen, bei welchen Fragestellungen genuin psychologische Konzepte und Methoden notwendig sind, um eine adäquate Forschung zu leisten. Anzumerken ist, dass Wundt zwar oft den Ausdruck „subjektiv" oder „innere Erfahrung" verwendet, jedoch keineswegs nur die trainierte Selbstbeobachtung im psychologischen Experiment meint (naive Introspektion lehnt er energisch ab). Am Leipziger Institut wurden umfangreiche Experimentalreihen zur Chronometrie apperzeptiver Prozesse durchgeführt, außerdem vegetative Korrelate von emotionalen Reaktionsverläufen registriert.

4. Neuropsychologische Apperzeptionstheorie

Wundt entwickelt mit seiner Apperzeptionstheorie die wichtigste Leitidee seines gesamten Werks. *Apperzeption* bedeutet zunächst, dass im Vergleich zu den elementaren und passiven Assoziationsvorgängen aktive und selektive Prozesse stattfinden, beispielsweise die willentliche Aufmerksamkeitssteuerung. Wundt entwickelt ein kompliziertes Annahmengefüge. Er folgt nur teilweise der Assoziationspsychologie der englischen Autoren John Locke, David Hartley, David Hume, Thomas Brown und Alexander Bain und bezieht sich ausdrücklich auf den von Gottfried Wilhelm Leibniz in die Philosophie eingeführten Begriff *Apperzeption.* Dieser Begriff hat zwei Bedeutungen: Erstens eine klare Vorstellung gegenüber einer dunklen, bloßen Perzeption, und, zweitens, die Aufnahme einer Vorstellung in das Selbstbewusstsein. Kant und Herbart meinen mit Apperzeption hauptsächlich eine an das denkende Selbst gebundene „Synthesis" bzw. Einheitsfunktion (zur langen philosophischen Ideengeschichte vgl. Janke & Hermann, 1971; Lüdtke, 1911; zu Aufmerksamkeit vgl. Neumann, 1971). Demgegenüber strebt Wundt zunächst „eine rein empirisch-psychologische Bestimmung" an, möchte die Beziehung zum Selbstbewusstsein völlig bei Seite lassen und von Leibniz nur das erste Merkmal, die relative Klarheit der Bewusstseinsinhalte, übernehmen und zum alleinbestimmenden Merkmal machen (1911, S. 322 f). An anderer Stelle greift Wundt (1911, S. 354) jedoch die zweite Bedeutung auf, indem er die Apperzeption mit den an sie gebundenen Gefühlen und Vorstellungskomponenten als die „Hauptträgerin des Selbstbewusstseins" bezeichnet und dieses Selbstbewusstsein als Ich und als die individuelle Persönlichkeit" bezeichnet (in einem *psychologischen* und nicht philosophisch-idealistischen Sinn).

4.1 Bewusstsein und Aufmerksamkeit

Unter Bewusstsein versteht Wundt den gesamten Inhalt der unmittelbaren Erfahrung, d.h. die Bildung von Vorstellungen aus Sinneseindrücken, in dem „Kommen und Gehen der Vorstellungen und Gefühle" (1911, S. 297). Indem Wundt Psychisches als *aktuellen* Prozess definiert, verlässt er den ontologischen (philosophischen oder religiösen) Substanzbegriff der „Seelenwissenschaft" und der traditionellen Psychologie. Die alte philosophische Idee, Bewusstsein als *Synthese* psychischer Tätigkeiten zu bestimmen, erhält durch Wundt eine experimentalpsychologische und neurophysiologische Fassung.

„Den Eintritt einer Vorstellung in das innere Blickfeld wollen wir die Perzeption, ihren Eintritt in den Blickpunkt (oder das Aufmerksamkeitsfeld) die Apperzeption nennen" (1874, S. 718; 1911, S. 307). Es gibt zwei hauptsächliche Bestimmungsmerkmale: die Klarheit der Apperzeption und die verschiedenen Grade (Schwellen und Stufen) des Bewusstseins.

Das Klarerwerden eines bestimmten Bewusstseinsinhaltes ist im „Zustand der Aufmerksamkeit" mit einem typischen Gefühl verbunden (1908, S. 381). Die Zuwendung der Aufmerksamkeit ist zunächst Bewusstseinssteigerung, verbindet sich apperzeptiv mit Gefühlstönen von zunehmender Klarheit und Spannung und tendenziell mit anderen Gefühlstönen und willentlichen Vorgängen. Psychologische Untersuchungen und auch Messungen sind geeignet, die Spannweite der Aufmerksamkeit, äußere und innere Störungen der Aufmerksamkeit, Oszillationen der Aufmerksamkeit, Erwartung und Ermüdung, Überadaptation und Unteradaption zu beschreiben (1908, S. 579 ff).

4.2 Assoziation und Apperzeption

Wundt kritisiert die Assoziationspsychologie und meint, dass für die Verknüpfung von gleichförmigen Bewusstseinselementen nicht hauptsächlich die Wiederholungshäufigkeit maßgeblich ist; er hält die „vier alten Assoziationsprinzipien" [d.h. Ähnlichkeit, Kontrast, Kontiguität, Wiederholung] für viel zu einfach und ungenügend. Als Hauptformen der *assoziativen Verbindungen* unterscheidet Wundt Verschmelzungen, Assimilation, Komplikationen, d.h. die Verbindung von Vorstellungen und Gefühlen disparater Sinnesgebiete, assimilative und sukzessive Erinnerungsassoziationen. Demgegenüber nennt er als Hauptformen der komplexen *apperzeptiven Verbindungen* die synthetischen, analytischen und kombinierten Apperzeptionen. Wundt differenziert diese Aspekte noch weiter, gestützt auf Daten und Methoden aus Leipziger Experimentalforschung

(1911, S. 500-554) und beschreibt: verbindende und zerlegende Funktionen, Agglutination von Vorstellungen, Verschmelzungen, insbesondere bei Sprachformen, wobei es zwei Folgen geben kann: „die Verdichtung und Verschiebung der Vorstellungen“ (1911, S. 545). Solche Verbindungen sind reichhaltiger durch Stellvertretung eines Begriffs, zerlegende Funktionen der Nachbildung, der Neuerzeugung in Phantasietätigkeit und begrifflicher Vermischung. ***

Am Beispiel der Sprache erläutert Wundt das Schema der sprachlichen Assoziation einer vollständigen Wortvorstellung, d.h. von Schriftbild und Artikulationsbewegung, in beiderlei Richtung mit veränderlicher, individuell übungsbedingter Stärke und Richtung des Assoziierens und er weist auf das begleitende Tätigkeitgefühl hin. Wundt grenzt beide Typen *psychischer Verbindungen* wegen der fortwährenden Übergänge assoziativer und apperzeptiver Prozesse nicht scharf voneinander ab bzw. hat seine frühere Begriffsbildung relativiert. Während bei dem Vorgang der einfachen Assoziationen, elementare Inhalte verbunden werden (geschriebener Buchstabe und Laut) verknüpft werden, sind mit Apperzeption höhere Integrationsprozesse gemeint. Es sind also Unterschiede der Komplexität, denn in die apperzeptiven Prozess gehen auch Erwartungen ein, und es kommt zu einer „schöpferischen Synthese“ von Elementen zu Gebilden mit neuen Attributen (Emergenzprinzip). Die Apperzeptionsverbindung ist ein Prozesse höherer Stufe gegenüber den Assoziationen und baut sich aus diesen auf, jedoch nicht in einem einfachen additiven Sinn. „Vielmehr ist auch sie ein neues Gebilde, dessen Charakter wesentlich durch die Beziehungen bestimmt werden, in denen die einzelnen in sie eingehenden assoziativen Prozesse zueinander stehen, und die sie zu anderen apperzeptiven Gebilden des gleichen Bewusstseins darbieten (1911, S. 500). Der gesamte Apperzeptionsvorgang lässt sich nach Wundt in Teilvorgänge zerlegen, von denen drei wesentlich sind: (1) Klarheitszunahme einer bestimmten Vorstellung oder Vorstellungsgruppe verbunden mit dem für den ganzen Prozess charakteristischen Tätigkeitsgefühl; (2) Hemmung anderer disponibler Eindrücke oder Erinnerungsbilder; und (3) subjektive Begleiterscheinungen im Verlauf der Spannungs- und Lösungsgefühle. „So ist „die Apperzeption gleichzeitig elementarer Willensakt und konstituierender Bestandteil aller Willensvorgänge“ (1911, S. 316).

In den Apperzeptionsprozess können die reflektorischen „Ausdrucksbewegungen“ der Gefühle integriert werden, d.h. die mimischen Bewegungen und vor allem die respiratorischen und vasomotorischen Symptome (1911, S. 370). Im Unterschied zu den nur reflektorischen Vorgängen der niederen Zentren wie der Medulla, werden respiratorische und vasomotorische Vorgänge dann zu Symptomen von Gefühlen, wenn sie von Vorgängen in den Sinnes- und Apperzeptionszentren begleitet sind, Wundt erläutert am Beispiel der vagalen Innervation des Herzens einerseits die Effekte aufgrund physiologischer Selbststeuerung oder neurophysiologischer Stimulation, andererseits den vom Apperzeptionszentrum ausgehenden Einfluss mit einer Korrelation erregender und hemmender Innervationen in dem entstehenden Symptombild (unter Bezug auf seine dreidimensionale psychophysiologische Gefühlstheorie und zeitgenössische Experimente von Lehmann und Störring im Leipziger Labor sowie Lange, Weber u.a. (siehe Fahrenberg, 1967, S- 109 ff): Es gebe charakteristische Veränderungen bei Erregung und bei Gefühlen der Spannung und Lösung sowie Gefühlen der Lust und Unlust: u.a. kardiosvaskuläre Indikatoren in der Höhe der Pulswellen und in der Anzahl der Pulsschläge (1911, S. 370 f). Spannungs- und Lösungsgefühle haben eine besondere Stellung, denn sie sind Bestandteile der allgemeinen Apperzeption der Bewusstseinsinhalte, d.h. des notwendigen Aufmerksamkeitsfaktors. Sie sind „an die zentraleren Bestandteile jener einfachen Bewusstseinsvorgänge gebunden, deren subjektive Komplemente die einfachen Gefühle bilden" (1910, S. 346).

4.3 Konzeption des Apperzeptionszentrums

Die Betrachtungen über die *physiologischen Substrate* der Apperzeption seien ausschließlich auf die psychologische Analyse der Funktionen gestützt, während „von der physiologischen Seite, abgesehen von der dürftigen Analogie der Reflexhemmung, nur die allgemeinen Gesichtspunkte der Nervenmechanik zu Gebote stehen" (1908, S. 383). Die Heuristik dieses Ansatzes möchte Wundt jedoch mit einer ausführlich erläuterten schematischen Darstellung veranschaulichen (siehe Abbildung 1, seine Seite 383).

(Knotenpunkte bedeuten intermediäre Zentren) in Verbindung mit: einem zentripetalen System, das ihm die Sinneserregungen aus Sehzentrum, Hörzentrum u.a. Sinneszentren (nur in dem relativen Sinn von „Zentrum" gemeint), zuleitet, und einem zentrifugalen System, das den untergeordneten Zentren die hemmenden Impulse zuführt. „Je nachdem solche Impulse an Sinnes- oder Muskelzentren übertragen werden, erfolgt dann entweder die Apperzeption von Empfindungen oder die Ausführung von Willensbewegungen, indem im ersten Fall andere Empfindungen, die durch äußere oder innere Reize entstehen, im zweiten Fall ebensolche motorische Impulse zurückgedrängt werden." Wundt räumt eine Analogie mit dem Reflexvorgang und der Reflexhemmung ein, dennoch entferne sich seine Auffassung weit von diesem Schema. Im Unterschied zum zwingenden Reflexmechanismus „lässt sich bei der Apperzeption und bei der Willensbewegung nur von einem regulierenden Einfluss der stattfindenden Erregungen reden, womit eben angedeutet wird, dass zahlreiche, unserer näheren Nachweisung entgehende Zwischenglieder auf das Endresultat den entscheidenden Einfluss ausüben" (1908, S. 383). Die physiologische Natur dieser Zwischenglieder sei vollkommen unbekannt, aus psychologischer Erfahrung sei zu schließen, dass aufgrund der generellen und individuellen Entwicklung bestimmte Dispositionen entstehen und die Vorgänge bestimmen. Die weiteren Verbindungen im Schema erläutert Wundt an den sprachlichen Funktionen, d.h. den psychologischen Aspekten und den hypothetischen physiologischen Zwischengliedern der sprachlichen, visuellen und motorischen Assoziationen und Apperzeptionen, betont jedoch, dass in diesem Schema andere Aspekte außer Betracht bleiben: die Festigkeit und Richtung des Assoziationen, die ständigen Einflüsse der Übung und Stellvertretung und alle – jeder schematisierenden Darstellung unzugänglichen – Einflüsse, „welche psychologisch die Konstellation des Bewusstseins, physiologisch der Gesamtzustand der nervösen Dispositionen auf die jeweils stattfindende Assoziationen und Perzeptionen ausübt" (1908, S. 385).

Den experimentalpsychologischen Zugang, zumindest zu einem kleinen Ausschnitt apperzeptiver Prozesse, sah Wundt in der Methodik, die heue als mentale Chronometrie bezeichnet wird. Zuvor war es Helmholtz gelungen, die Leitungsgeschwindigkeit in peripheren Nerven zu messen, und Wundt war natürlich mit diesem Ansatz im Labor vertraut. Von der Methode der holländischen Physiologen Donders und de Jaager angeregt wurden in Leipzig die sog. Reaktionsmethoden weiterentwickelt, um die Reaktionszeiten bei verschiedenen, insbesondere bei komplex zusammengesetzten Aufgaben in ihre Komponenten zu zerlegen: die Reizwahrnehmung, die zentrale Verarbeitungszeit sowie die Dauer der physiologischen Leitungs- und Bewegungsvorgänge, u.a. für die die motorische Vorbereitung und das Niederdrücken der Taste. Durch Subtraktion werden u.a. berechnet: die reine Dauer der Apperzeption einfacher und auch zusammengesetzter Vorstellungen, der zusätzliche Zeitaufwand (gegenüber den einfachen Reaktionsaufgaben) bei Wahlreaktionen zwischen mehreren Reizen bzw. mehreren Reaktionsmöglichkeiten, aber auch „Unterscheidungs- und Willenszeiten" bei der Assoziation von Vorstellungen (Wontorra, 2009; Wundt, 1908-1911). Diese Chronometrie, damals schon auf Millisekunden genau möglich, war vor der Entdeckung des EEG *die Methode der Wahl*, denn es gab kaum einen anderen empirisch-analytischen Weg, sich dem Prozess der Apperzeption, anzunähern. Zugleich waren diese Reaktionsexperimente frühe Beispiele für die systematische Verhaltensmessung im Labor. Gundlach (1996) untersuchte detailliert die in Leipzig, u.a. von Friedrich, Kraepelin, Merkel durchgeführten Reaktionsversuche im Hinblick auf den Begriff der Willkürhandlung und die Argumente gegen die „intellektualistischen" Willenstheorien.

4.4 Quintessenz

Apperzeption ist die Bezeichnung für ein komplexes Annahmengefüge über den integrativen Prozess der Bewusstseinstätigkeit und zentralen (regulativen, willentlichen) Organisation. Der Prozess kann psychologisch *mehrdimensional* (multireferenziell) beschrieben werden: nach graduellen Unterschieden der Klarheit und der Bewusstseinsintensität, nach Umfang (Spanne) und nach Verbindungsformen. Die Aufmerksamkeit ist reaktiver Vorgang oder willkürlich gesteuerte Aufmerksamkeitszuwendung und entsprechenden Tätigkeitsgefühlen, mit Absichten und Gefühlstönen verbunden. In dem aufmerksamen und gerichteten Bewusstseinsprozess werden Sinnesempfindungen und Vorstellungen aktualisiert, akzentuiert, ausgewählt, analysiert, auf verschiedene und differenziert zu beschreibende Weise kombiniert und ausgedrückt, nicht bloß „verarbeitet", sondern auch „schöpferisch synthetisiert". Apperzeption sei eine zur passiven Assoziation besonders hinzukommende Tätigkeit, die eine sowohl willkürliche und auswählende als eine vorstellende und vergleichende sei, als apperzeptive Willenshandlung und apperzeptive Vorstellungsfunktion.

Wie dieser Prozess im Verlauf und in den emergenten psychischen Vorgängen zu differenzieren ist, und wie dieser zentrale Prozess methodisch-experimentell, zumindest teilweise, zugänglich zu machen ist, hat Wundt theoretisch und methodologisch intensiv beschäftigt. So unterscheidet er im Apperzeptionsprozess bestimmte Prinzipien, d.h. Relationsbegriffe wie Kontext, Kontrast, Interaktion, Emergenz, Reduktion, Selbstentwicklung. Sie bilden Wundt zufolge eigenständige psychologische Erkenntnisprinzipien. Die selektive Aufmerksamkeits-Steuerung und der komplexe Apperzeptionsprozess sind demnach zu interpretieren als eine kognitive, emotionale und volitionale Integrationsleistung als Vorstufe der Initiierung von Handlungstendenzen. Wundt versucht, in seiner Konzeption die Idee des Bewusstseins als *Synthese* psychischer Teilprozesse in empirische Begriffe und ansatzweise in Untersuchungsmethoden umzusetzen mit noch heuristischer Blickwendung auf die noch kaum zu bestimmenden Konzepte. Die behauptete willentliche Steuerung ist mit einer naturalistischen Sichtweise oder einer reduktionistischen Wissenschaftslehre der Psychologie nach dem Vorbild der Physik kaum zu vereinen. Andererseits wurde aus der Sicht zeitgenössischer Psychologen, von denen viele, wie Herbart, Lotze, Brentano oder Stumpf an dem metaphysischen Seelenbegriff festhielten, Wundts „Psychologie ohne Seele" und Wundts Menschenbild als „voluntaristisch" kritisiert. Wundt, der nur noch von aktuellen *Prozessen der Bewusstseinstätigkeit* sprach, hielt dagegen, diese Sichtweise sei ihm durch die empirische Psychologie nahegelegt (zur Wundt-Rezeption, Fahrenberg, 2011, 2013, 2015).

Wundts Apperzeptionstheorie bietet ein vorzügliches Beispiel, wie die Auffassungen eines bedeutenden Philosophen und Polyhistors, d.h. Leibniz' Gedanken über Perzeption und Apperzeption, über Bewusstsein und „Synthesis", über psychophysischen Parallelismus und Perspektivität des Denkens, von einem Psychologen und Neurophysiologen in empirisch psychologische Begriffe umgeformt und ansatzweise auch experimentalpsychologisch operationalisiert werden – auf dem Wege zum Verständnis der höchsten integrativen Bewusstseinsleistungen und willentlichen Verhaltenssteuerung.

5. Rezeption von Wundts Neuropsychologie

Wundts Argumente für eine *relative* Lokalisation und sein Plädoyer *gegen* eine ausschließlich physiologische Untersuchungsstrategie der höheren ZNS-Funktionen sind Allgemeingut geworden, ohne dass sein Anteil an dieser Entwicklung, zumindest sein ideengeschichtlich frühes Engagement, noch erinnert wird. Andere Psychologen, wie Ebbinghaus, Külpe, Stumpf oder Ziehen, scheinen durchaus bereit gewesen zu sein, solche einfachen Lokalisationen anzunehmen statt genauer nach den psychologischen Konstrukten zu fragen. Wundts Neuropsychologie ist nur von sehr wenigen Autoren rezipiert worden, doch haben sich die Neurowissenschaften inzwischen – im Sinne von Wundts Plädoyer – als interdisziplinäres Forschungsgebiet entwickelt.

Wundts multireferenzielle Beschreibung von Aufmerksamkeit und Aufmerksamkeitssteuerung wird in der Regel übergangen. Seine in psychologischen Begriffen hochdifferenzierte Apperzeptionstheorie, sogar der Begriff der *Apperzeption* im Unterschied zur Perzeption und zu den elementaren Vorgängen der *Assoziation* fehlen in heutigen Lehrbüchern, sogar in den Texten zur Geschichte der Neuropsychologie, völlig oder werden höchstens kurz erwähnt. Wundts Vorbild, den Prozess der Aufmerksamkeit zu einem relativ elementaren Brückenkonzept zu machen, d.h. als *psychologisch* begründete Fragestellung an die physiologische Forschung zu richten, ist zunächst nicht rezipiert worden. Zwei Hinweise auf spätere Forschungsprogramme sind angebracht: Durch das von Sokolov (1963) und anderen Autoren genauer entwickelte Konzept der *Orientierungsreaktion* wurde ein breites psychophysiologisches Forschungsinteresse mit multiparametrischen Studien gefördert. Es mangelte jedoch an einer parallelen Forschung über *spontane* bzw. *willentliche* Aufmerksamkeitssteuerung. Innovative Methodik hat hier neue Ansätze ermöglicht, beispielsweise in der Forschung über aufmerksame Blickbewegungen und elektrokortikale Korrelate (u.a. Klein, 2002), die heute mit portablen Systemen auch unter Alltagsbedingungen möglich wären. Aufmerksamkeitsstörungen sind im Hinblick auf die verbreitete Aufmerksamkeitsdefizit-Störung (ADS) zu einem bedeutenden Forschungsgebiet geworden.

Bereits Ziehen (1893) lehnt Wundts Psychologie grundsätzlich ab und will sich eng an „die sog. Assoziationspsychologie der Engländer“ anschließen und eine „exakte naturwissenschaftliche Psychologie“ verfolgen; Wundt verzichte dagegen auf „jede psycho-physiologische Erklärung“ (S. III). Ziehen weist Wundts Apperzeptionslehre, ohne sie überhaupt genauer zu referieren, als überflüssig ab. Wenn Wundt die willkürliche Aufmerksamkeitssteuerung hervorhebt und die psychische Verknüpfung der Empfindungen, Vorstellungen, Gefühle mit der Willenstätigkeit untersucht, sieht Ziehen darin die metaphysische Annahme eines „aktiven Subjekts“. Die von Wundt angenommene Lokalisation der apperzeptiven Funktionen im Frontalcortex lehnt Ziehen ab, denn das Stirnhirn habe diese Funktion nicht (S. 162). Demgegenüber reichen aus Wundts Sicht die elementaren Assoziationsgesetze nicht aus, um die komplizierteren psychischen Verbindungen, beispielsweise die emergenten Eigenschaften, zu erklären.

Bekannt ist die kompromisslose Forderung von Krech (1950), jedes Konstrukt der Psychologie müsse so angelegt sein, dass es einem neurologischen Konstrukt kongruent ist. Ob dieser „Neuroreduktionismus“ aufgrund einer Lektüre von Wundts Überlegungen differenzierter ausgefallen wäre? Sabat (1979) würdigt Wundt Beitrag zur physiologischen Psychologie bzw. Neuropsychologie streift aber die Themen und die Perspektiven nur kurz. Aus amerikanischer Sicht versucht Woodward (1982) einen Überblick über Wundts interdisziplinär angelegtes Programm der Psychologie zu gewinnen, wobei er auch Missverständnisse seitens Titchener und James erkennen lässt. Woodward gibt zwar das Schema des Apperzeptionszentrums wieder, jedoch ohne Kommentar oder Hinweise auf die Neuropsychologie. Charakteristisch ist die Sicht von Posner und DiGiorolamo (2000), für die eine Neuropsychologie eigentlich erst während er 1960er Jahre in den USA zu beginnen scheint, abgesehen von dem alten Problem der Aufmerksamkeit, für das James (1890) genannt wird, nicht etwa Wundt (1874). So werden gelegentlich Bemerkungen von William James (1980, S. 416) über focalization, concentration of consciousness u.a. zitiert (Sturm, 2008), nicht jedoch Wundts frühere und differenziertere Bestimmungen oder die speziellen Verbindungsformen der Apperzeptionspsychologie. Weder der an Hirnfunktionen interessierte Rohracher (1958), noch seine Schüler erwähnen Wundts Beitrag in den ersten deutschsprachigen Büchern zur Neuropsychologie (Guttmann, 1972; Haider, 1971). Markowitsch (1996, 1999) zeigt in einer Übersicht über Netzwerkmodelle Wundts Schema des Apperzeptionszentrums ohne Kommentar und weist stattdessen nur auf Ziehens Kritik hin.

Ausnahmen bilden Hagner (1996) und Breidbach (1997). Hagner macht jedoch aus dem hypothetischen Apperzeptionszentrum ein „Apperzeptionsorgan“ und schreibt zuvor, dass Wundt von Hughlings Jackson und dessen psychophysischem Parallelismus ausging – die historische Beziehung wäre mit Bezug auf Leibniz, wenn überhaupt, eher umgekehrt. Hagner meint, dass Wundt gegen Flechsig und andere einen funktionalistischen Lokalisationismus vertrat, dessen strategische Bedeutung jedoch in Wundts System „wesentlich relativiert“ sei, da physiologische Vorgänge diese Leistungen immer nur begleiten. Die damalige Kontroverse und Wundts Doppelperspektive sind hier nur unzureichend erschlossen. Hagners Einschätzung, Wundt habe „die Psychologie stets als Teil der Philosophie“ betrachtet und „ihr Komplement keineswegs in der Physiologie, sondern in der Völkerpsychologie“ gesehen (1996, S. 70) geht an Wundts Gesamtkonzeption und Wissenschaftstheorie vorbei. Breidbach (1997) überschreibt einen Abschnitt seiner Geschichte der Hirnforschung: *Wilhelm Wundt – Erste Konturen einer Neuropsychologie.* Er hebt Wundts (1874) breit angelegte Darstellung der neurophysiologischen und -anatomischen Grundlagen des menschlichen Verhaltens hervor, Wundt habe „die Essenz dieser einzelwissenschaftlichen

Aussagen für sein eigenes Forschungsprogramm – die Analyse der Grundstrukturen des Geistes – zu ziehen" gesucht. Breidbach meint sogar, Wundts Buch habe „einen modernen Reflex in der Arbeit *Neurophilosophy* von Patricia Churchland gefunden" (S. 171). (Wundt wird allerdings von Churchland (1986) nicht zitiert, und Breidbach kennt nicht die wichtigen späteren Auflagen der *Grundzüge*). – Wundts Prinzipien fehlen auch in neueren Büchern über Bewusstsein (z.B. Dennett, 1994, oder Metzinger, 1996), die primär an der amerikanischen Auffassung der *Philosophie des Geistes* interessiert sind und folglich diese Perspektive und Begrifflichkeiten übernehmen, ohne die Breite der neurophilosophischen Kontroversen und methodologischen Konsequenzen zu repräsentieren (vgl. Fahrenberg, 2008, 2015).

Goschke (1996) und Kuhl (1996) zitieren Wundts Apperzeptions- und Willenspsychologie nur nebenbei an zwei irrelevanten Stellen, aus den alten Auflagen, und ziehen spätere, insbesondere amerikanische Autoren vor, statt die Ideengeschichte anzuerkennen. So erwähnt Goschke nicht Wundts programmatische neuropsychologische Konzeption des hypothetischen Apperzeptionszentrums, wenn er über das Konzept des zentralen Exekutivsystems und über neuropsychologische Evidenz für ein *präfrontales Exekutivsystem* sowie die *Modularität kognitiver Subsysteme* schreibt. Ebenso fehlen Wundts Differenzierungen zwischen verschiedenen Formen der assoziativen und apperzeptiven Verbindungen (heute grob und unscharf: automatisch versus kontrolliert). Wenn Goschke einleitend in der Motivations- und Handlungsforschung sowie in den Kognitions- und Neurowissenschaften „nach kognitiver und emotionaler Wende" eine „volitional revolution" sieht und primär Autoren aus den 1980er Jahren zitiert (1996, S. 584), hätte diese moderne Perspektive auch einfacher lauten können: „zurück zu Wundt".

Wundts programmatische Prinzipien der Neuropsychologie und die Heuristik seiner Apperzeptionstheorie sind, falls man von den Bänden der *Enzyklopädie* und bekannten Lehrbüchern der Neuropsychologie ausgeht, fast völlig vergessen.

5.1 Neuere Perspektiven

Das Vergessen bereits erreichter Prinzipien und Heuristiken wäre verständlicher, wenn an die Stelle von Wundts Entwürfen eine fortgeschrittene psychologisch-neurophysiologische Konzeption der höchsten integrativen Leistungen, d.h. der Synthese der kognitiven, emotionalen und motivationalen Partialprozesse sowie ihrer Repräsentation im Bewusstsein vorzuweisen wäre.

Was die neuropsychogische Theoriebildung zur Aufmerksamkeit und Aufmerksamkeitssteuerung anbelangt, so scheint ein Teil der von Wundt gemeinten Facetten zu fehlen. Zwar werden *Intensitätsaspekte*, *Selektivitätsaspekte* sowie

Aspekte der visuell-räumlichen Aufmerksamkeit und Wechsel des Fokus unterschieden (siehe u.a. Sturm, 2008). Zitiert werden häufig Broadbents Filtertheorie, Posner und Snyder zur Unterscheidung *kontrollierter* Prozesse und *automatischer* Prozesse, Shallice u.a. Autoren zu kognitiven Schemata und Modulen. Aber wird *Aufmerksamkeit* prägnant als *multireferenzielles theoretisches Konstrukt* bestimmt und entsprechend operationalisiert? Die Zuordnung der Untersuchungsmethoden (Paradigmen), d.h. der zahlreichen einfachen und komplexeren Aufgaben, Wahlreaktionsaufgaben, standardisierten Tests und Fragebogen für klinische Störungsbilder scheint a-theoretisch konzipiert zu sein. Die Taxonomie dieser möglichen Indikatoren von *Aufmerksamkeit* wirkt unsicher. Neben den Fortschritten, die einzelne Facetten operational genauer zu definieren, fällt auf, dass die Prinzipien multipler Operationalisierungen, d.h. Multi-Trait-Multi-Method Analysen theoretischer Konstrukte und zweckmäßige Strategien der Multimodalen Diagnostik, nicht adäquat eingesetzt werden, wie das seit Jahrzehnten als Assessmenttheorie in der differenziellen Psychologie und Psychophysiologie (Stemmler, 1992) der Fall ist. Multivariate Forschungsstrategien sind noch kaum zu finden.

Das einseitige Interesse an der *reaktiven* Aufmerksamkeit scheint zu dominieren, denn die zweifellos gegebenen Merkmale der *Bewusstseinsqualität* und der *willentlichen* Selektion werden begrifflich durch den diffusen Ausdruck „kontrolliert" ersetzt, so dass die Frage nach der Instanz offen bleibt: ein anderes kognitives Schema? Einseitig reduzierend wirkt diese Einstellung auch, weil die charakteristischen Erfahrungen der subjektiven Klarheit, die emotionalen Tönungen und möglichen Ansätze von Reaktions- und Handlungstendenzen bei der Explikation der theoretischen Konstrukts *Aufmerksamkeitssteuerung* weitgehend entfallen sind. Wie werden diese Facetten oder Komponenten der Aufmerksamkeitsprozesse – und in welchen Relationen – wieder funktional zusammengeführt, so integriert wie Wundt es vorschlug? Ein theoretisches Annahmengefüge dieser Art (mit kognitiven, emotionalen, volitionalen Partialprozessen) scheint als forschungsorientierendes Bezugssystem noch zu schwierig zu sein – oder noch nicht benötigt zu werden. Wie sollen die separierten Verbindungen in anderen Teilgebieten der Psychologie in emotional-kognitiven oder als volitional-emotional-kognitiven Konzepten wieder zusammengesetzt werden? Wie werden *Cognitive Neuroscience* und *Affective Neuroscience* und *Volitional Neuroscience* einmal so integriert, wie es Wundt in seinem heuristischem Entwurf vorschwebte?

Nicht zu übersehen sind die philosophischen Vorentscheidungen, wenn Phänomene wie „bewusst" und „willentlich" in einer fast verschämt wirkenden Ausdrucksweise heute als „kontrolliert" bezeichnet werden, um den Eindruck mentalistischer oder voluntaristischer Irrtümer zu vermeiden. Aber gerade auf diesem Forschungsgebiet können, wie bereits Wundt hervorhob, bestimmte philosophische Postulate als absolute Voraussetzungen der Erkenntnis- und Wissenschaftstheorie maßgeblich für bestimmte Denkweisen, Themen und Methoden sein, aber auch Kategorienfehler zur Folge haben. Entsprechende *Manifeste*

(Braitenberg, 1992; Elger et. al., 2004) scheint es in dieser Form wohl in keinem anderen Forschungsbereich der Psychologie zu geben.[i]

Die folgenden Thesen bleiben *spekulativ*: Wundt wäre von der Flut empirischen Forschungsergebnisse der Neurowissenschaften überwältigt, würde jedoch forschungsstrategische Defizite feststellen: Erstens eine Tendenz zur *kognitivistischen Reduktion*, wenn die kognitiven Prozesskomponenten systematisch von den emotionalen und motivationalen Aspekten isoliert werden, in den Paradigmen und dann in den theoretischen Konzeptionen. Zweitens würde Wundt aus seiner perspektivischen („komplementären") Wissenschaftstheorie die Folgen und die Kategorienfehler des *naturalistischen Reduktionismus* nach dem Vorbild der Physik kritisieren, wenn die eigenständigen Kategorien der Psychologie übersehen und beispielsweise *bewusste* Aufmerksamkeit, *willentliche* Aufmerksamkeitssteuerung, *Klarerwerden und andere Gefühlstöne* zu einem bloß kognitiven Schema und „kontrollierter" Informationsverarbeitung vereinfacht werden.

Eine Übersicht von Peper (2008) lässt die gegenwärtig hohe Forschungsaktivität über die Regulation von Aufmerksamkeit, Aktivierung und Emotionen erkennen. Seit den älteren Modellen, wie dem Aufsteigenden Retikulären Aktivierungssystem von Moruzzi und Magoun oder Grays drei neurobehavioralen Systemen , sind hier von herausragendem Interesse: der limbisch-hypothalamische Komplex, Amygdaloider Komplex, Basales Vorderhirn, Hippocampus, die Funktionsschleifen des Präfrontalcortex mit seinen subkortikalen Verschaltungen. So gibt es Beiträge zum emotionalen Regulationsverhalten (u.a. von Rolls), zu höheren Aufmerksamkeitsprozesse und motivationalen Kontrollen.

Für Wundt wäre es hochinteressant, solche Forschungsergebnisse über kognitive Exekutivfunktionen im präfrontalen Cortex und über das zunehmende Forschungsinteresse an korrespondierenden „emotionalen Exekutivfunktionen" zu sehen. Leisten vielleicht die hypothetischen Konvergenzzonen der ventralen und der dorsalen Verbindungen im PFC und Konvergenzzonen auf anderen Ebenen bzw. die heteromodalen cortical-limbischen Netzwerke jene Integration, die Wundt meinte? Die erforderliche Methodik ist im Vergleich zu typischer Cognitive Science Forschung extrem komplizierter und verlangt wesentlich humanpsychologische Experimente mit einem erweiterten Repertoire psychologischer bzw. biobehavioraler Paradigmen. Dazu gehört auch die Weiterentwicklung des ambulanten Assessment: Neuropsychology in the real world (Peper & Loeffler, 2014).

Das zentrale Thema der Allgemeinen Psychologie Wundts scheint gegenwärtig noch zu anspruchsvoll und spekulativ zu sein, der komplizierte Begriff *Apperzeption* ist völlig verschwunden. Die Forschung scheint, trotz zunehmenden Interesses, noch weit davon entfernt zu sein, eine moderne Konzeption dieser höchsten Integrationsprozesse in ihrem psychischen und neurophysiologischen Zusammenhang zu vermitteln – so wie es Wundt anstrebte und zumindest in seiner neuropsychologischen Heuristik der Apperzeptionsforschung geleistet zu haben meinte.

Anmerkungen (Endnotes)

* In der von Emil Du Bois-Reymond überlieferten Formel lautete diese Überzeugung: „Brücke und ich, wir haben uns verschworen, die Wahrheit geltend zu machen, dass im Organismus keine anderen Kräfte wirksam sind als die gemein physikalisch-chemischen; dass, wo diese bislang nicht zur Erklärung ausreichen, mittels der physikalisch-mathematischen Methode entweder nach ihrer Art und Weise der Wirksamkeit im konkreten Falle gesucht werden muss oder dass neue Kräfte angenommen werden müssen, welche von gleicher Dignität mit den physikalisch-chemischen, der Materie inhärent, stets auf nur abstoßende oder anziehende Componenten zurückzuführen sind" (Vidoni, 1991, S. 44).

** Zu Wundts intellektuellem Umfeld in Leipzig gehörten Gustav Theodor Fechner (1801-1887) und der Philosoph und Arzt Rudolph Hermann Lotze (1817-1881) sowie u.a. die Physiologen Carl Ludwig und Johann Nepomuk Czermak , der Anatom und Physiologe Ernst Heinrich Weber, der Chemiker Wilhelm Ostwald, der Physiker und Astronom Karl Friedrich Zöllner, der Philosoph M. W. Drobisch und der Erkenntnistheoretiker Eduard Zeller, die Historiker Karl Lamprecht und Friedrich Ratzel. Mit einigen stand Wund im fachlichen Austausch, mit anderen war er befreundet. Als Mitarbeiter bzw. Assistenten (bis 1900) werden u.a. genannt: J. McK. Cattell, E. Kraepelin, H. Münsterberg, O. Külpe, E. Meumann, Ch. Spearman, E. B. Titchener, L. Witmer. Studierende bzw. Besucher mit später bekanntem Namen waren: Becheterv, Boas, Durckheim, Husserl, N. N. Lange, Malinowski, Mead, Sapir, Tönnies, Whorf, Wygotski. Bei der Mehrzahl der amerikanischen Psychologen der ersten und zweiten Generation steht Wundt im akademischen Stammbaum (Ben-David & Collins, 1966).

Ben-David, J. & Collins, R. (1966). Social factors in the origins of a new science: The case of psychology. American Sociological Review, 31 (4), 451-465.

*** Das Begriffspaar Verdichtung und Verschiebung, das bereits in der 2. Auflage der *Grundzüge* steht (1880; S. 310), verwendet auch Freud (1900) in seiner Traumpsychologie.

**** PSYNDEX und PsycINFO verzeichnen außerdem noch Manifeste von Neurowissenschaftlern zum Konnektionismus sowie über die Neurale Basis der kognitiven Entwicklung; in dieser Dichte sonst nur zu Kontroversen bei klinischen oder sozialen Problemen und Genderfragen.

Das Schriftenverzeichnis Wundts enthält 589 Titel. Wundt (The Virtual Laboratory Library Search Results), Max Planck Institute for the History of Science, Berlin. http://vlp.mpiwg-berlin.mpg.de/library/

20 The Role of Psychologists for the Clinical Neurosciences

Hans-Joachim Freund

Key Words: neuropsychology, psychology, neurology, brain lesions, neurological deficits, cognitive deficits, bridging specialties, single case observation

Psychology was previously regarded as a branch of philosophy, and the lack of quantification as a barrier towards the natural sciences (Kant, 1755). Helmholtz (1867) implemented the ophthalmoscope and the measurement of nerve conduction velocity, thereby providing early empirical data for applications in clinical medicine. This deep interest in the processes linking receptor physiology and perception was taken up by his student Wilhelm Wundt, who founded a laboratory for experimental psychology in 1879, the first of its kind in the world. Around the same time, William James founded an experimental psychology laboratory. Both contributed landmark textbooks such as *Grundzüge der Physiologischen Psychologie* (1874) by Wundt and *The Principles of Psychology* by William James (1890).

Jean Piaget and Edouard Claparede classified different stages of child development. Noam Chomsky drew special attention to the view that the genetic disposition for language must play a pivotal role thereby triggering the famous nature versus nurture debate on the development of language. Wernicke and Broca anticipated the localization of language functions well before the discovery of cortical cytoarchitectonics thus disclosing the association between regional structural specialization and different cortical functions.

The link between brain localization and elementary sensory and motor functions as well as cognition was then successively established by studies on the effects of focal brain lesions. This approach also initiated the interest in brain plasticity exemplified by the centennial contribution of Donald Hebb (1983) elucidating the mechanisms underlying neural plasticity during development. This issue was then extensively investigated by experimental studies opening a new field of research with particular impact for the clinicians. The exploration of these mechanisms in humans and particularly in the adult human brain disclosed the various mechanisms underlying functional recovery after brain lesions. The role of local reorganization for brain plasticity was elegantly revealed by the experimental studies of Merzenich and his colleagues (Wang et al., 1995) and network reorganization for complex functions such as neglect studied in the human by Mesulam (1981).

Lesion Studies

The Case of Memory Function

As a neurologist, I will preferentially concentrate in this chapter on a few centennial neuropsychological and clinical contributions to our knowledge of brain function derived from observations of neurological deficits in human patients. At a time when large cohort studies, having passed ethical committees, are the avenue to further progress these few examples may illustrate how much of our current knowledge derives from observations on single or a few cases.

The work of **Brenda Milner** (1957, 1958) is one example to illustrate this**.** She and her colleagues reported on the patient H.M., probably the most published patient ever. The patient suffered from drug resistant epilepsy and was selected for surgery. He was operated as a young adult. The neurosurgeons decided to remove both hippocampi. After the operation, the patient had full command of everything he had learned or experienced up to the time of the operation and therefore had a normal IQ. He could talk and interact normally. But he had completely lost the ability to learn anything new. Consequently, he had no recollection of anything that happened since the operation. Consequently he did not have any further access to his recent life history. This led to the concept that the hippocampus does not play a role in the preservation of memories but is pivotal for the formation of new ones. The final storage of once consolidated memories must therefore ensue in the cortex.

Subsequent work revealed that memory loss was restricted to declarative memory leaving implicit memory functions and conditioning unaffected. Thus, skill learning remained intact. Extensive experimental work led to a better understanding of the hippocampal physiology and pathophysiology. But as this example demonstrates, the comprehensive picture of hippocampal functioning did not emerge from experimental work but rather from this single clinical case observation representing a major breakthrough in our understanding of memory functions.

Observations on Lesions in Eloquent Motor Areas

Luria favored a more global view on the basis of his observations on patients with brain lesions anticipating later concepts of functional networks. Other prominent Neuropsychologists elaborated the effects of lesions on specific functions. **Hans Lukas Teuber** was specifically interested in the effects of brain lesions on perception, mainly visual perception, whereas the broader concept of eloquent cortex was elaborated by neurosurgeons and neurologists such as **Kleist (1934)**, a neurologist examining patients with gunshot wounds after World War II, and the neurosurgeons **Foerster (1936)** and **Penfield (1954)**. Both, Foerster and Penfield showed that some regions of the brain could be regarded as silent areas from a neurosurgical viewpoint because their excision demonstrated no obvious neurological or psychological deficits or obvious personality changes. Remarkably, both neurosurgeons performed frontal lobectomies anterior to premotor cortex. Penfield also performed bilateral frontal lobectomies, with barely detectable deficits in some post-operative cases. One patient was his sister. He was surprised to find out that the only observable deficits he could detect in her personality involved the difficulty in card sorting while playing bridge.

Such observations stand in obvious contrast to the devastating personality changes or neurological deficits seen in cases such as Phineas Gage who had suffered a perforant trauma of his forehead. Penfield attributed the poor outcome observed in some cases after frontal lobectomy to secondary effects such as scar formation and ischemia. But in particular Foerster, a well-trained neurologist who later decided to become a neurosurgeon, meticulously examined the effects of excisions of the eloquent cortex on function. Based on the observations of Broca and Wernicke on the effects of lesions affecting the areas critical for speech production and language understanding, Foerster meticulously elaborated the effects of damage of primary and premotor cortex and the sensory areas. He also implemented electrical stimulation of the motor and also sensory cortex for the sake of intraoperative localization, a method that had experimentally been established already in 1870 by Fritsch and Hitzig.

Woolsey et al. (1952) and Penfield and Welsh, (1949) recognized and defined the functional specificity of the medial part of the premotor cortex, which they termed the supplementary motor area (SMA). Bancaud and Talairach (1977) confounded the presumed role of the SMA for movement initiation and preparation in the human. They demonstrated that unilateral SMA lesions cause transient contralesional hemiakinesia, whereas bilateral SMA lesions cause permanent akinetic mutism. Subsequent studies in nonhuman primates by **Lawrence and Kuypers** (1968) revealed the anatomical organization underlying the clinical observations: unilateral damage of the pyramidal tract causes persistent hemiparesis on the contralesional side whereas unilateral SMA or pre-motor cortical lesions are transient. These differences depend upon this anatomical organisation, i.e. whether a projection system is mainly unilateral as in the case of primary motor cortex and the pyramidal tract or bilateral and thus more redundant, as in the case of the SMA, premotor cortex is (PMC) and cingulate motor cortex (CMA).

Split Brain Studies

An important chapter in disclosing the interplay between conscious and unconscious processes was the study of the different roles of the two hemispheres. **Sperry** (1967) laid the ground for novel vistas that soon were illustrated by the subsequent split brain operations severing the two hemispheres by cutting the corpus callosum (Gazzaniga, Bogen & Sperry, 1962).

To appreciate this revolutionary change it is important to realize that in the 1950s consciousness was envisaged as a centered brainstem reticular and centrencephalic mechanism. The neocortex was regarded as a relatively late operating stage for enhancing and elaborating the basic qualities of conscious experience as elaborated in the mesencephalic structures. As Sperry (1967) pointed out: "The long-standing questioning in philosophy here was whether consciousness was restricted to men or represent a more general property in other animals". But it was Sperry who also pointed out the more general aspects of the relation between neural activity and consciousness, a debate that continues to remain an unresolved issue in Neurobiology. He wrote that "conscious mental experience in our present interpretation is conceived to be a holistic merchant of brain activity, different from and more than the neural events of which it is composed, and a real phenomenon in its own right processing causal potency in brain function. At present more detailed or explicit description in objective terms is hardly possible but this will presumably be achieved with further advances in brain research". Consequently the mental events are not conceived as the mere consequences of brain activity but reveal the causal relation between the universal powers of the whole over its parts. This was of course at variance with the later prevailing view considering subjective phenomena as the emerging correlates of the neural events. It is interesting to look back at the writings of this pioneer on split brain studies in the light of the present debate on determinism. Roger Sperry wrote that "...among other things, the acceptance of inner mental experience as having a significant causal role in cerebral function has produced a changed picture of scientific determinism as applied to human behaviour and social action. The phenomena of subjective experience, including feelings and values of all kinds, must now be recognized as positive causal factors in the brain's decision-making process. The freedom thereby introduced into the causal brain sequence leading to a volitional choice far surpasses, in both degree and kind, the notions envisaged in the more mechanistic atomistic forms of the determinism that have excluded mental events. The present interpretation may be seen to set the human brain apart in respect to free will, placing it at an apex above all other known systems in the deterministic universe of science. Our new approach in mind- brain theory thus goes far to restore to human nature some of the personal dignity, freedom, inner creativity and responsibility of which it has long been deprived by behaviourism and by materialistic science generally" (Sperry, 1972). Determinism later received support by **Libet's** (1965) experiments with the readiness potential until later evidence from modified experiments conducted in Pauen's lab gave another turn to the debate (Herrmann et al., 2008). Their abstract states: "Benjamin Libet has demonstrated that the readiness potential precedes the time at which participants consciously decide to perform an intentional motor act, and suggested that free will is an illusion. We performed an experiment where participants observed a stimulus on a computer monitor and were instructed to press one of two buttons, depending on the presented stimulus. We found neural activity preceding the motor response, similar to Libet's experiments. However, this activity was already present prior to stimulus presentation, and thus before participants could decide which button to press. Therefore, we argue that this activity does not specifically determine behaviour. Instead, it may reflect a general expectation. This interpretation would not interfere with the notion of free will." This more recent evidence rings a bell with respect to the above cited passages from Roger Sperry and the different aspects of the debate about consciousness.

Whereas the dominance for language had already been established by Broca and Wernicke, another intriguing aspect of cerebral dominance was elucidated by subsequent studies on split-brain patients by Gazzaniga et al. (1962) When stimuli of any modality reached the minor hemisphere, the subject did not become consciously aware of them. Only the dominant hemisphere could accomplish conscious awareness. But surprisingly, the subconscious information processes in the minor hemisphere also determined behaviour.

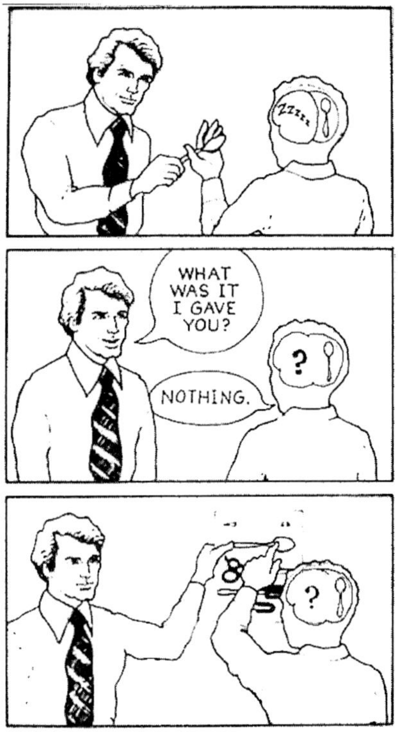

Figure 1: *Subconscious information processes in the minor hemisphere have an influence on behaviour. (Taken from Figure 6 from Gazzaniga and LeDoux, 1978.)*

This is illustrated in Figure 1: Here the left hemisphere of the patient was exclusively anesthetized by sodium amytal. When asked to identify a spoon given to his left hand with closed eyes he responded "nothing". But when asked to point to any of the set of objects presented to him he invariantly pointed to the objects given into his left hand. These results demonstrated that although the patient is not consciously aware of his active touch percept, his subconscious perception determined his actions. Experiments of this kind had far-reaching consequences. They also modified the classical doctrine put up by Wilhelm von Humboldt that thinking solely depends on the capacity of language. The split brain studies along with lesion studies demonstrated that thought without language is possible so that the two processes can be dissociated favouring the view that the development of language sub served communicative purposes and that the development of abstract thought and action control developed independently. Amongst the many examples underpinning all sorts of dissociations were reports on composers rendered aphasic after a left hemisphere stroke that were not compromised in their ability to compose music as before the stroke. The reverse example was also observed.

Conscious Experience and Neglect

Quite a different approach about the relation between conscious and subconscious experience emerged from the work of **Weiskrantz**, the mentor of Ulrike Halsband in Oxford as summarised in his book *Thought Without Language* (1988). His points of departure were observations on patients with hemianopia in whom stimuli applied to the blind hemi field were not consciously perceived. But when the patient was asked to point deliberately in a direction of his choice after stimulus presentation in the blind hemi-field the proficiency was far above chance level. These observations were of interest scientifically because they brought into play subcortical structures such as the superior colliculi. They also laid the ground for subsequent therapeutic approaches to train the unconscious brain to learn to use subconscious "knowledge" for action control. These observations showed a close resemblance to the results obtained in split brain patients in whom the conscious-subconscious dissociation took place between the major and minor hemisphere and the action targeted to the subconscious object was correct.

Motor Cognition

With the progress of experimental and clinical neuropsychology the discussion on the functional role of premotor-parietal circuitry has received major input from two sources: **Jeannerod's** (1994) hypothesis that *covert actions and overtly executed actions* represent a continuum in the sense that the state in which an action is simulated necessarily precedes execution of that action and the *mirror neurone concept* elaborated by **Rizzolatti** and co-workers (1996). The new field of motor cognition opened a new dimension to understand motor behaviour and its disorders making motor imagery a powerful new tool for the study of the representational aspects of motor behaviour. The novel methodology to consider mental states as real entities and the concept of motor representations set the scene for neuroimaging studies of covert mental states and for the elaboration of the functional anatomy of motor cognition. They showed that imagination, observation, imitation and the performance of movement all activate similar networks. Their functional equivalence is impressively illustrated by the various facets of higher motor disturbances as observed in apraxia **(Freund et al.**, 2005).

Since the cognitive aspects of motor behaviour that determine our conscious interaction with the environment are processed in parallel with the automatic processing streams, the resonance-based and the analytical operational modes may interact at multiple re-entrant levels. The study of such interactions will be a major challenge for future research about the close interplay between perceptive, motor, and cognitive processes. Perception appears to be embedded in the dynamics of action, becoming much more composite than used to be thought in the past.

Against this background the arbitrary divisions between perceptive, motor and cognitive processes were transformed into a more coherent picture, so that the different subsystems become bound by the acting brain into a pragmatic, preconceptual and pre-linguistic form of understanding, constituting the basis of cognitive abilities.

Prinz (2005) has introduced another major issue in this debate by pointing out one principal difference between perception and movement: Sensory and semantic analysis provides information about present and past. In contrast the motor systems are "anticipation engines ", conveying information about the future and forthcoming events and about the consequences of a given motor act. The cognitive aspects of our conscious, sensory interactions with our surroundings are processed in parallel to the automatic motor online processes anticipating the consequences of a given action. They further provide inferences about what the other is going to do next on the basis of the simulation processes that operate in real time.

The discovery of the mirror neurones by Rizzolatti and his colleagues in Parma (Rizzolatti *et al*., 1996) disclosed a novel operational principle employing a dual representational mode of action and action observation at the level of single neurones. Adding the investigative repertoire in the human, its significance for cognitive functions could be explored as well as the evolving implications for the social sciences and the humanities. The mirror neuron story and its presumed theoretical implications are summarized by Giacomo Rizzolatti and the philosopher of science Corrado Sinigaglia in their book *Mirrors in the Brain* (2008).

The mirror neurone concept was again based on simple observations on their monkeys, that premotor neurons did not discharge when the objects are seen, but only and selectively when trained monkeys performed specific movements like grasping that object. The surprising observation was that a similar discharge was elicited when the monkey observed the same gesture being performed by the experimenter or by another monkey. Similar selective relationship between movement and movement observation could be observed for different prototypical gestures such as holding, pointing and grasping. Thus the activation of the mirror neurons is typically seen in interactions between a body part and objects. These neurons were considered as primarily involved in the understanding of the meaning of actions performed by others. This matching hypothesis implicates the immediate recognition of specific types of action and the appropriate preparation. This multimodal recognition process is conceived as based on the motor knowledge and the vocabulary of motor acts in the brain of the observer. This resonance in turn enables the observer to interpret the intention of motor events.

The human data elaborated in functional imaging studies (Buccino et al., 2001, 2004) provided evidence that the mirror neuron system plays a key role in communication such as in pantomime, intransitive gestures and oro-facial communicative expressions. In their book, Rizzolatti and Sinigaglia even discuss whether the progressive evolution of the mirror neuron system is at the root of the formation of a neural substrate for communicative behaviour.

For language, the motor theory of speech perception (Liberman et al., 1967) has already implemented such an operational mode which became a pertinent theme in cognitive science during the past half century, although so far lacking any known neural substrate. The basic assumption is that listening to language directly activates those motor circuitries that would produce the same token. This can be considered as an early version of the mirror neuron principle. The concept that 'the acting brain is also and above all a brain that understands' introduces a complementary perspective.

Hemispherectomy: Shifting Language to the Other Hemisphere

In this context a fascinating relationship between motor skills and language lateralisation has been revealed by observations on patients who have undergone hemispherectomy. It is well known that the preferred use of the dominant hand determines the lateralization of language functions. In spite of this, it has been equally well established that the language areas are basically organized bilaterally. This has been shown by imaging studies activating both hemispheres during all sorts of language tasks. Correspondingly, neural recordings from the left temporal lobe language areas and their right hemisphere homologue during wake surgery in epilepsy patients demonstrated that neuronal activations could be observed on both sides (Creutzfeldt & Ojeman, 1989).

Clinically, this has been impressively demonstrated by hemispherectomies performed in children with epilepsy, substantial structural damage or progressive damage by Rasmussen encephalitis. Such operations are now performed up to the age around puberty. If the affected dominant left hemisphere has to be removed in the right-handed child, language functions remain partially preserved because the minor hemisphere compensates what is not possible in the adult. Individuals with left-sided, early-onset focal epilepsy often show atypical (i.e. bilateral or right-sided) language dominance. In a single case report Vargha Khadem (1997) reported that "Case Alex, with Sturge-Weber Syndrome affecting the left hemisphere, failed to develop speech throughout early boyhood, and his comprehension of single words and simple commands remained stagnant at an age equivalent of three to four years. But then, following left hemidecortication at age eight and a half years and withdrawal of anticonvulsants when he was more than nine years old, Alex suddenly began to acquire speech and language.... It is concluded that clearly articulated, well structured, and appropriate language can be acquired for the first time as late as age nine years with the right hemisphere alone." In larger patient populations it was observed that mild dysarthria is persistent after left or right hemispherectomy, irrespective of age at onset of hemiplegia. These results indicate incomplete functional re-organization for the control of fine speech motor movements throughout childhood, and provide no evidence of hemispheric differences" (Liégeois et al., 2010). In a review Vargha-Kahdem and colleagues concluded: "Only in regard to language processes is there a consensus regarding the differential effects of left and right hemidecortication, and here the differences are apparent only in the relatively subtler aspects of language. Thus, the isolated right hemisphere is at a significant disadvantage compared with the left in the comprehension of abstract, low frequency words, in phonetic feature analysis, and in the subtleties of grammar, such as the comprehension of passive negative constructions and the correct use of morphological markers in unfamiliar contexts (Vargha Khadem, 1992).

Taken together, these results provide new insights into the range of plasticity, in this case enabled by the bilateral organization of language areas, but also in the maladaptive influences exerted by deranged circuitries. In children, this provides a remarkably different perspective on the conventional view of the unique language capacity of one hemisphere. Why the dormant ability of the minor hemisphere cannot be used in the adult is presently not understood. Progress in this direction would be a useful step towards therapeutic implications.

Closing remarks

Ulrike Halsband worked experimentally with her mentors Richard Passingham and Lawrence Weiskrantz. She elaborated complex features of pre-motor neurons not related to direct motor function in the monkey as she later did in Düsseldorf in similar experiments with human patients suffering from premotor strokes. This was a major and important contribution to the study of structure-function relationships which became possible by the advent of high-resolution imaging methods (Halsband, 1990, 1993a,b). I will always be grateful for how Ulrike Halsband guided our group with her comprehensive experimental background about premotor cortex organisation thereby enabling our work in the human. Therefore she stands in the long role of psychologists contributing to the advance of Neurology.

References

Abel S, Weiller C, Huber W, Willmes K & Specht K. (2015). Therapy-induced brain reorganization patterns in aphasia. Brain 2015; 138:1097-1112. Epub, Feb 15.

Abrahams, S., Goldstein, L. H., Kew, J. J. M., Brooks, D. J., Lloyd, C. M., et al. (1996). Frontal lobe dysfunction in amyotrophic lateral sclerosis: A PET study. Brain, 119, 2105-2120.

Adam G (1998). Visceral Perception. Plenum Press, New York.

Adams, D. K. & Zener, K. E. (1935). Translators' preface. In K. Lewin (1935). A dynamic theory of personality. Selected papers. New York and London: McGraw Hill.

Addante, R. J., Ranganath, C., & Yonelinas, A. P. (2012a). Examining ERP correlates of recognition memory: evidence of accurate source recognition without recollection. Neuroimage 62, 439-450.

Addante, R.J., Ranganath, C., Olichney, J., and Yonelinas, A.P. (2012b). Neurophysiological evidence for a recollection impairment in amnesia patients that leaves familiarity intact. Neuropsychologia 50, 3004-3014. Aggleton, J. P. & Brown, M. W. (2006). Interleaving brain systems for episodic and recognition memory. Trends in Cognitive Sciences, 10(10), 455-463.

Addelston, H (1959). Child patient training. CDS Review, 38: 27-29.

Adolphs R (2002). Neural systems for recognizing emotion. Curr Opin Neurobiol 12:169-77.

Aggleton, J. P. & Brown, M. W. (2006). Interleaving brain systems for episodic and recognition memory. Trends in Cognitive Sciences, 10(10), 455-463.

Ainsworth, M. D. S. (1991). Attachment and other affectional bonds across the life cycle. In C. Parkes, J. Stvenson-Hinde & P. Marris (Eds.), Attachment across the life cycle (pp. 33-51). New York: Routledge

Akkal D, Bioulac B, Audin J, Burbaud P. (2002) Comparison of neuronal activity in the rostral supplementary and cingulate motor areas during a task with cognitive and motor demands. Eur J Neurosci. 15:887-904

Akkal D, Dum RP, Strick PL (2007) Supplementary motor area and presupplementary motor area: targets of basal ganglia and cerebellar output. J Neurosci 27: 10659-10673.

Albert MS, DeKosky ST, Dickson D, Dubois B, Feldman HH, Fox NC, Gamst A, Holtzman DM, Jagust WJ, Petersen RC, Snyder PJ, Carrillo MC, Thies B, Phelps CH (2011). The diagnosis of mild cognitive impairment due to Alzheimer's disease: recommendations from the National Institute on Aging-Alzheimer's Association workgroups on diagnostic guidelines for Alzheimer's disease. Alzheimers Dement., 7(3):270-279.

Alexander GE, Crutcher MD. (1990) Functional architecture of basal ganglia circuits: neural substrates of parallel processing. Trends Neurosci. 13(7):266-271.

Allen, K., Blascovich, J., Tomaka, J. & Kelsey, R. M. (1991). Presence of human friends and pet dogs as moderators of autonomic responses to stress in women. Journal of Personality and Social Psychology, 61, 582-589.

Allen, KD (2006). Management of children's disruptive behavior during dental treatment. In DI, Mostofsky, AG, Forgione & DB Giddon (Eds.), Behavioral dentistry (pp. 175-187). Blackwell Munksgaard, Ames (Iowa).

Allen, PF, McMillan, AS (2003). A review of the functional and psychosocial outcomes of edentulousness treated with complete replacement dentures. J Can Dent Assoc, 69: 662.
Allison T, Puce A, Mc Carthy G. (2000) Social perception from visual cues: role of the STS region. Trends in Cognitive Sciences. 4:267-278.
Allport, G. W. (1937). Personality: A psychological interpretation. New York, NY: Macmillan.
Allport, G. W., & Vernon, P. E. (1933). Studies in expressive movement. New York: Macmillan.
Altmann L.J.P., Saleem A., Kendall D., Heilman K.M., Gonzalez Rothi L.J. (2006). Orthographic directionality and thematic role illustration in English and Arabic. Brain and Language (In press).
Altmann, J. (1974). Observational study of behavior: Sampling methods. Behaviour, 49, 227-267.
Amador, S. C., Hood, A. J., Schiess, M. C., Izor, R., & Sereno, A. B. (2006). Dissociating cognitive deficits involved in voluntary eye movement dysfunctions in Parkinson's disease patients. Neuropsychologia, 44(8), 1475-1482.
Ament, P, Ament, A (1970). Body image in dentistry. J Prosthet Dent, 24: 362–366.
American Psychiatric Association Practice, G. (2001). Practice guideline for the treatment of patients with borderline personality disorder. American Psychiatric Association. [Guideline Practice Guideline]. Am J Psychiatry, 158(10 Suppl), 1-52.
Andersen RA, Asanuma C, Essick G, Siegel RM. (1990). Corticocortical connections of anatomically and physiologically defined subdivisions within the inferior parietal lobule. J Comp Neurol 296: 65-113.
Anderson, C. W., Kirby, M. J., Hundley, D. R. & Knight, J. N. (2007). Classification of Time-Embedded EEG Using Short-Time Principal Component Analysis. In: Dornhege, Guido (Ed.). Toward Brain-Computer Interfacing (pp. 261-277). Cambridge, Massachusetts: MIT Press.
Andrews, K., Murphy, L., Munday, R., & Littlewood, C. (1996). Misdiagnosis of the vegetative state: Retrospective study in a rehabilitation unit. British Medical Journal, 313, 13-16.
Annoni, G. M., Pegna, A., Michel, C., Estade, M., & Landis, T. (1998). Motor perseverations: a function of the side and the site of a cerebral lesion. European Neurology, 40(2), 84-90.
Ansari, D., Garcia, N., Lucas, E., Hamon, K. and Dhilil, B. (2005) Neural correlates of symbolic number processing in children and adults. Neuroreport, 16, 1769-1775
Ansari, D., Grabner, RH, Koschutnik, K., Reishofer, G. & Ebner, F. (2011). Individual differences in mathematical competence modulate brain responses to arithmetic errors: an fMRI study. Learning and Individual Differences, 21, 636-643.
Antoniades, C., Ettinger, U., Gaymard, B., Gilchrist, I., Kristjánsson, Á., Kennard, C., Leigh, J., Noorani, I., Pouget, P., Smyrnis, N., Tarnowski, A., Zee, D. & Carpenter, R.H.S. (2013). An internationally standardised antisaccade protocol for clinical use. Vision Research, 84, 1-5.
Antonowsky, A. (1979). Health, Stress and Coping. San Francisco and London: Jossey-Bass Publishers.
APA. (1994). Diagnostic and Statistical Manual of Mental Disorders. Washington, DC: American Psychiatric Association.

Arai, K., & Mardiyanto, R. (2011). Eyes based eletric wheel chair control system. Int. J. Adv. Comput. Sci. Appl, 2(12), 98-105.
Archibald, S. J., Mateer, C. A., & Kerns, K. A. (2001). Utilization behavior: clinical manifestations and neurological mechanisms. Neuropsychology review, 11(3), 117-130.
Arenaza-Urquijo EM, Landeau B, La JR, Mevel K, Mezenge F, Perrotin A, Desgranges B, Bartres-Faz D, Eustache F, Chetelat G (2013). Relationships between years of education and gray matter volume, metabolism and functional connectivity in healthy elders. Neuroimage, 83:450-457.
Arntz, A., Klokman, J., & Sieswerda, S. (2005). An experimental test of the schema mode model of borderline personality disorder J Behav Ther Exp Psychiatry (Vol. 36, pp. 226-239). United States.
Arro, G. (2013). Peeking into personality test answers: Inter- and intraindividual variety in item interpretations. Integrative Psychological and Behavioral Science, 47, 56-76. Bandura, A. (1986). Social foundations of thought and action: A social cognitive theory. Englewood Cliffs, NJ: Prentice-Hall.
Asendorpf, J. B., & Neyer, F. J. (2012). Psychologie der Persönlichkeit. Springer-Verlag.
Askay, SW, Patterson, DR, Sharar, SR (2009). Virtual reality hypnosis. Contemp Hypnosis, 26: 40-47.
Atkinson, R. C., & Shiffrin, R. M. (1968). Human memory: A proposed system and its control processes. In K.W. Spence and J.T. Spence (Eds.), The psychology of learning and motivation Advances in research and theory, vol. 2 (pp. 349-441). New York: Academic Press.
Awad, M., Warren, J. E., Scott, S. K., Turkheimer, F. E., & Wise, R. J. S. (2007). A common system for the comprehension and production of speech. Journal of Neuroscience, 27, 11455–11464.
Azari NP, Nickel J, Wunderlich G, Niedeggen M, Hefter H, Tellmann L, Herzog H, Stoerig P, Birnbacher D, Seitz RJ (2001) Neural correlates of religious experience. Eur J Neurosci 13: 1649-1652.
Baad-Hansen, L (2008). Atypical odontalgia - pathophysiology and clinical management. J Oral Rehabil, 35: 1-11.
Baba, K, Aridome, K, Haketa, T, Kino, K, Ohyama, T (2005). Sensory perceptive and discriminative abilities of patients with occlusal dysesthesia. Nihon Hoteshu Shika Gakki Zasshi, 49: 599-607.
Bader, R., Mecklinger, A., Hoppstädter, M., & Meyer, P. (2010). Recognition memory for one-trial-unitized word pairs: Evidence from event-related potentials. NeuroImage, 50, 772-781.
Baeuchl, C.*, Meyer, P. *, Hoppstädter, M., Diener, C., Flor, H. (in press). Neural correlates of configural processing during contextual fear conditioning using feature-identical contexts. * contributed equally. Neurobiology of Learning and Memory
Bakheit, A. M. O., Brennan, A., Gan, P., Green, H., & Roberts, S. (2013). Anarchic hand syndrome following resection of a frontal lobe tumor. Neurocase, 19(1), 36-40.
Baldo, J. V., Klostermann E. C., & Dronkers N. F. (2008). It's either a cook or a baker: patients with conduction aphasia get the gist but lose the trace. Brain Lang, 105, 134–140.
Baldry, PE (2005). Acupuncture, trigger points and musculoskeletal pain. (Third edition). Elsevier, Edinburgh - London - New York - Philadelphia - San Francisco – Toronto. 45-72.

Bálint, D. (1909). Seelenlähmung des "Schauens", optische Ataxie, räumliche Störung der Aufmerksamkeit. European Neurology, 25(1), 51-66.
Banks, G., Short, P., Martínez, A. J., Latchaw, R., Ratcliff, G., & Boller, F. (1989). The alien hand syndrome: Clinical and postmortem findings. Archives of Neurology, 46(4), 456-459.
Bar M, Neta M, Linz H (2006). Very first impressions. Emotion 6 :269-278.
Barabasz, Areed Franz (2004). Hypnose-Konzepte: Fragen und Durchbrüche in der Forschung. In: Hirn und Hypnose. Vol Hykog 21(1+2), 139-156.
Barash, S., Melikyan, A., Sivakov, A., Zhang, M., Glickstein, M., & Thier, P. (1999). Saccadic dysmetria and adaptation after lesions of the cerebellar cortex. The Journal of Neuroscience, 19(24), 10931-10939.
Barbieri, C., & De Renzi, E. (1988). The executive and ideational components of apraxia. Cortex, 24(4), 535-43.
Bartlett, F. C. (1932). Remembering: A study in experimental and social psychology. Cambridge, UK: Cambridge University Press.
Batsch EG. (1956). Die myeloarchitektonische Untergliederung des Isocortex parietalis beim Menschen. J Hirnforsch 2: 225-258.
Bauby, J.-D. (1997). Le scaphandre et le papillon (1 ed.). Paris: Editions Robert Laffont.
Bauer, G., Gerstenbrand, F., & Rumpl, E. (1979). Variables of the locked-in syndrome. Journal of Neurology, 221, 77-91.
Bauer, Joachim. (20132). Das Gedächtnis des Körpers. Wie Beziehungen und Lebensstile unsere Gene steuern. Frankfurt/Main: Piper.
Baumeister, R. F., Vohs, K. D., & Funder, D. C. (2007). Psychology as the science of self-reports and finger movements: Whatever happened to actual behavior? Perspectives on Psychological Science, 2, 396-403.
Baumgartner T, Knoch D, Hotz P, Eisenegger C, Fehr E (2011). Dorsolateral and ventromedial prefrontal cortex orchestrate normative choice. Nat Neurosci 14: 1468-1474.
Beaumont, J. G. (2008). Introduction to neuropsychology. Guilford Press.
Beck, A, Varga, G, Hermann, P, Fábián, G, Fejérdy, P, Fábián TK (2012) Methods for the treatment of denture induced psychogenic symptoms. In: T.K. Fábián, P. Fejérdy & P. Hermann (Eds.), Dentures. Types, benefits and potential complications (pp 165-197). Nova Science Publishers, New York.
Beetz, A. & Kotrschal, K. (2012). Gastbeitrag: Stand der Wissenschaft. Tiere und Gesundheit. In Mars Petcare GmbH (Hrsg.) Hund-Katze-Mensch. Die Deutschen und ihre Heimtiere. Verden: Mars Petcare Deutschland GmbH.
Beetz, A. Kotrschal, K., Turner, D., Hediger, K., Uvnäs-Moberg, K., & Julius, H. (2011). The effect of a real dog, toy dog and friendly person on insecurely attached children during a stressful task: An exploratory study. Anthrozoös, 24, 349-368.
Behrens TEJ, Hunt LT, Rushworth MFS (2009). The computation of social behaviour. Science 324: 1160-1164.
Bell V, Halligan PW, Ellis HD (2006) Explaining delusions: a cognitive perspective. Trends Cogn Sci 10: 219-226.
Bender, D. S., Dolan, R. T., Skodol, A. E., Sanislow, C. A., Dyck, I. R., McGlashan, T. H., Gunderson, J. G. (2001). Treatment utilization by patients with personality disorders. [Comparative Study Research Support, U.S. Gov't, P.H.S.]. Am J Psychiatry, 158(2), 295-302.

Bender, J., Tark, K.J., Reuter, B., Kathmann, N., Curtis, C.E. (2013). Differential roles of the frontal and parietal cortices in the control of saccades. Brain and Cognition, 83(1), 1-9.

Bennett K.M., Latto R., Bertamini M., Bianchi I., Minshull S. (2010). Does left-right orientation matter in the perceived expressiveness of pictures? A study of Bewick's animals (1753- 1828). Perception, 39, 970-981.

Bensing, J (2000). Bridging the gap. The separate worlds of evidence-based medicine and patient-centered medicine. Patient Education Counseling, 39: 17-25.

Bergendal, B (1989). The relative importance of tooth loss and denture wearing in Swedish adults. Community Dent Health, 6: 103-111.

Berger, H. (1921). Psychophysiologie. Jena: Fischer.

Berggren, U, Carlsson, SG (1984). A psychophysiological therapy for dental fear. Behav Res Ther, 22: 487-492.

Berggren, U, Meynert, G (1984). Dental fear and avoidance: causes, symptoms and consequences. J Am Dent Assoc, 109: 247-251.

Berggren, U, Carlsson, S, Hakeberg, M, Hägglin, K, Samsonowitz, V (1997/a). Assessment of patients with phobic dental anxiety. Acta Odontol Scand, 55: 217-222.

Berggren, U, Carlsson, SG, Hägglin, C, Hakeberg, M, Samsonowitz, V (1997/b). Assessment of patients with direct conditioned and indirect cognitive reported origin of dental fear. Eur J Oral Sci, 105: 213-220.

Berggren, U, Hakeberg, M, Carlsson, SG (2000). Relaxation vs. cognitively oriented therapies for dental fear. J Dent Res, 79: 1645-1651.

Bergman, L. R. & Trost, K. (2006). The person-oriented versus the variable-oriented approach: Are they complementary, opposites, or exploring different worlds? Merrill-Palmer Quarterly, 52, 377–389.

Beurze SM, de Lange FP, Toni I, Medendorp WP. (2007) Integration of target and effector information in the human brain during reach planning. J Neurophysiol. 97:188-99,Brinkman C. (1984) Supplementary motor area of the monkey's cerebral cortex: short- and long-term deficits after unilateral ablation and the effects of subsequent callosal section. J Neurosci. 4:918-929

Biesanz, J. C., & Human, L. J. (2010). The cost of forming more accurate impressions: Accuracy motivated perceivers see the personality of others more distinctively but less normatively. Psychological Science, 24, 589-594.

Binder, H, Binder, K (1989). Autogenes Training, Basispsychotherapeutikum. Deutscher Ärzteverlag, Köln.

Binder, J. R., Desai, R. H., Graves, W. W. & Conant, L. L. (2009). Where is the semantic system? A critical review and meta-analysis of 120 functional neuroimaging studies. Cerebral Cortex, 19, 2767–2796.

Binkofski F, Buxbaum LJ. (2013) Two action systems in the human brain. Brain Lang. 127(2):222-9.

Binkofski, F. C., & Buxbaum, L. (2013). Two action systems in the human brain. Brain Lang, 127(2), 222–229.

Binkofski F, Dohle C, Posse S, Stephan KM, Hefter H, Seitz RJ, Freund H-J (1998) Human anterior intraparietal area subserves prehension. A combined lesion and functional MRI activation study. Neurology 50: 1253-1259.

Biran, I., Giovannetti, T., Buxbaum, L., & Chatterjee, A. (2006). The alien hand syndrome: What makes the alien hand alien? Cognitive Neuropsychology, 23(4), 563-582.

Birbaumer, N. (2006). Breaking the silence: Brain-computer-interfaces (BCI) for communication and motor control. Psychophysiology, 43, 517-532.
Birbaumer, N., Cohen, L. (2007). Brain-Computer-Interfaces (BCI): Communication and Restoration of Movement in Paralysis. The Journal of Physiology, 579 (3), 621-636.
Birbaumer, N., Gallegos-Ayala, G., Wildgruber, M., Silvoni, S., Soekadar, S.R. (2014). Direct brain control and communication in paralysis. Brain Topography, 27, 4-11.
Birbaumer, N., Ghanayim, N., Hinterberger, T., Iversen, I., Kotchoubey, B., Kübler, A., Perelmouter, J.,Taub, E. & Flor, H. (1999). A spelling device for the paralysed. Nature, 398, 297-298.
Birbaumer, N., Piccione, F., Silvoni, S., Wildgruber, M. (2012). Ideomotor silence: the case of complete paralysis and brain-computer interfaces (BCI). Psychological Research, 76, 183-191.
Birbaumer, N., Ramos Murguialday, A., Cohen, L. (2008). Brain-Computer-Interface (BCI) in paralysis. Current Opinion in Neurology, 21, 634-638.
Birbaumer, N., Ruiz, S., Sitaram, R. (2013). Learned regulation of brain metabolism. Trends in Cognitive Sciences, 17 (6), 295-302.
Birbaumer, N. & Schmidt, R. F. (1999). Biologische Psychologie (4th Edition). Berlin: Springer.
Bisiach, E., Capitani, E., Luzzatti, C., & Perani, D. (1981). Brain and conscious representation of outside reality. Neuropsychologia, 19, 543-551.
Blaffer-Hrdy, S. (2009). Mothers and others: the evolutionary origins of mutual understanding. Cambridge MA: Belknap Press.
Blakemore, S. J., Wolpert, D. M., & Frith, C. D. (2002). Abnormalities in the awareness of action. Trends in cognitive sciences, 6(6), 237-242.
Block, J. (2010). The five-factor framing of personality and beyond: Some ruminations. Psychological Inquiry, 21, 2–25.
Blurton Jones, N. G. (1967). An ethological study of same aspects of social behaviour of children in nursery school. In D. Morris (Ed.), Primate ethology (pp. 347–368). London: Weidenfeld & Nicholson.
Blurton Jones, N. G. (1972). Categories of child-child interaction. In N. G. Blurton Jones (Ed.), Ethological studies of child behavior (pp. 97-127). London: Cambridge University Press.
Boesch, C., Hohmann, G. & Marchant, L. (2002). Behavioural diversity in chimpanzees and bonobos. Cambridge: Cambridge University Press.
Bognar, Zsuzsanna et al. (2002). The subjective experiences of both the hypnotist and the subjekt in the real-simulating paradigm. Hypnosis International Monographs 6, 125-128.
Bohland, J.W., & Guenther, F.H. (2006). An fMRI investigation of syllable sequence production. NeuroImage, 32(2), 821-841.
Bohm, E. (1951). Lehrbuch der Rorschach-Psychodiagnostik. Für Psychologen, Ärzte und Pädagogen. Bern: Hans Huber.
Bokde, A. L., Lopez-Bayo, P., Meindl, T., Pechler, S., Born, C., Faltraco, F., Hampel, H. (2006). Functional connectivity of the fusiform gyrus during a face-matching task in subjects with mild cognitive impairment. Brain, 129(Pt 5), 1113-1124. doi: awl051 [pii] 10.1093/brain/awl051

Boly, M., Coleman, M., Davis, M. H., Hampshire, A., Bor, D., et al. (2007). When thoughts become action: An fMRI paradigm to study volitional brain activity in non-communicative brain injured patients. Neuroimage, 36, 979-992.

Borkenau, P. & Ostendorf, F. (2008). NEO-FFI – NEO-Fünf-Faktoren-Inventar nach Costa und McCrae. Handanweisungen. Göttingen: Hofgrefe.

Borovsky, A., Saygin, A. P., Bates, E., & Dronkers, N. (2007). Lesion correlates of conversational speech production deficits. Neuropsychologia, 45, 2525–2533.

Borowsky R, Loehr J, Friesen CK, Kraushaar G, Kingstone A, Sarty G (2005). Modularity and intersection of "what", "where" and "how" processing of visual stimuli: A new method of fMRI localization. Brain Topogr 18: 67-75.

Botto, RW (2006) Chairside techniques for reducing dental fear. In: D.I. Mostofsky, A.G. Forgione & D.B. Giddon (Eds.) Behavioral dentistry (pp. 115–125). Blackwell Munksgaard, Ames (Iowa).

Botvinick MM. (2007) Conflict monitoring and decision making: reconciling two perspectives on anterior cingulate function. Cogn Affect Behav Neurosci. 7:356-366

Botvinick MM, Braver TS, Barch DM, Carter CS, Cohen JD. (2001) Conflict monitoring and cognitive control. Psychol Rev. 108:624-652

Bötzel, K., Rottach, K., & Büttner, U. (1993). Normal and pathological saccadic dysmetria. Brain, 116(2), 337-353.

Bourne, V.J. (2008). Examining the relationship between degree of handedness and degree of cerebral lateralization for processing facial emotion. Neuropsychology, 22, 350-356.

Boussaoud D, Wise SP. (1993) Primate frontal cortex: neuronal activity following attentional versus intentional cues. Exp Brain Res. 95:15-27

Bowlby, J. (1969). Attachment and loss. Vol.1: Attachment. New York: Basic Books.

Bowlby, J. (1979). The making and breaking of affectional bonds. London: Tavistock.

Bowles, B., Crupi, C., Mirsattari, S. M., Pigott, S. E., Parrent, A. G., Pruessner, J. C., et al. (2007). Impaired familiarity with preserved recollection after anterior temporal-lobe resection that spares the hippocampus. Proceedings of the National Academy of Sciences of the United States of America, 104, 16382-16387.

Boyer P (2003) Religious thought and behaviour as by-products of brain function. Trends Cogn Sci 7: 119–124.

Braak H, Braak E (1991). Neuropathological staging of Alzheimer-related changes, Acta Neuropathol (Berl), 82:239–259.

Braak H, Braak E (1997). Frequency of stages of Alzheimer-related lesions in different age categories. Neurobiol Aging. 1997, 18(4):351-357.

Braak H, Braak E, Yilmazer D, de Vos RA, Jansen EN, Bohl J. (1996) New aspects of pathology in Parkinson's disease with concomitant incipient Alzheimer's disease. J Neural Transm Suppl. 48:1-6.

Bradley, RM, Grabauskas, G (1998). Neural circuits for taste. Excitation, inhibition, and synaptic plasticity in the rostral gustatory zone of the nucleus of the solitary tract. Ann NY Acad Sci, 855: 467-474.

Brainin M, Seiser A, Matz K (2008) The mirror world of motor inhibition: the alien hand syndrome in chronic stroke. Journal of Neurology, Neurosurgery and Psychiatry 79(3), 246–52.

Braitenberg, V. (1992). Manifesto of Brain Sciences. In: A. Aertsen & V. Braitenberg (Eds.). Information processing in the cortex (S. 473-477). Berlin: Springer.

Braun, A. R., Guillemin, A., Hosey, L., & Varga, M. (2001). The neural organization of discourse: An H2 15O-PET study of narrative production in English and American sign language. Brain, 124, 2028–2044.

Breidbach, O. (1997). Die Materialisierung des Ichs. Zur Geschichte der Hirnforschung im 19. und 20. Jahrhundert. Frankfurt a. M.: Suhrkamp.

Breit S, Reimold M, Reischl G, Klockgether T, Wullner U. (2006) [(11)C]d-threo-methylphenidate PET in patients with Parkinson's disease and essential tremor. J Neural Transm. 113(2):187-193.

Breitenstein C, Daum I, Ackermann H. (1998) Emotional processing following cortical and subcortical brain damage: contribution of the fronto-striatal circuitry. Behav Neurol, 11(1), 29-42.

Breiter HC, Etcoff NL, Whalen PJ, Kennedy WA, Rauch SL, Buckner RL, et al. (1996). Response and habituation of the human amygdala during visual processing of facial expression. Neuron. 17(5):875-887.

Breivik, T, Thrane, PS, Murison, R, Gjermo, P (1996). Emotional stress effects on immunity, gingivitis and periodontitis. Eur J Oral Sci, 104: 327-334.

Brion, S., & Jedynak, C.P. (1972) Troubles du transfer interhémisphérique (callosal disconnection). A propos, de trois observations de tumeurs du corps calleux. Le signe de la main etrangere Rev. Neurol., 126(4), 257–266.

Brodine, AL, Hartshorn, MA (2004). Recognition and management of somatoform disorders. J Prosthet Dent, 91: 268-273.

Brodmann K. (1909). Vergleichende Lokalisationslehre der Grosshirnrinde. Barth, Leipzig.

Brooks SJ, Savov V, Allzén E, Benedict C, Fredriksson R, Schiöth HB (2012). Exposure to subliminal arousing stimuli induces robust activation in the amygdala, hippocampus, anterior cingulate, insular cortex and primary visual cortex: A systematic meta-analysis of fMRI studies. Neuroimage 59: 2962-2973.

Brown, M. W., & Aggleton, J. P. (2001). Recognition memory: what are the roles of the perirhinal cortex and hippocampus? Nature Reviews Neuroscience, 2, 51-61.

Brown, M. W., & Xiang, J. Z. (1998). Recognition memory: neuronal substrates of the judgment of prior occurrence. Progress in Neurobiology, 55, 149-189.

Brownsett, S. L. E., & Wise, R. J. S. (2010). The contribution of the parietal lobes to speaking and writing. Cerebral Cortex, 20, 517–523.

Broyd, S. J., Demanuele, C., Debener, S., Helps, S. K., James, C. J., & Sonuga-Barke, E. J. (2009). Default-mode brain dysfunction in mental disorders: a systematic review. Neurosci Biobehav Rev, 33(3), 279-296. doi: 10.1016/j.neubiorev.2008.09.002 S0149-7634(08)00150-4 [pii]

Bruck A, Virta JR, Koivunen J, Koikkalainen J, Scheinin NM, Helenius H, Nagren K, Helin S, Parkkola R, Viitanen M, Rinne JO (2013). [11C]PIB, [18F]FDG and MR imaging in patients with mild cognitive impairment. Eur J Nucl Med Mol Imaging, 40(10):1567-1572.

Brück C, Kreifelts B, Kaza E, Lotze M, Wildgruber D. (2011) The Impact of Personality on the Cerebral Processing of Emotional Prosody, NeuroImage. 58(1):259-68.

Bruno, M.-A., Vanhaudenhuyse, A., Thibaut, A., Moonen, G., & Laureys, S. (2011). From unresponsive wakefulness to minimally consciouos PLUS and functional locked-in syndromes: Recent advances in our understanding of disorders of consciousness. Journal of Neurology, 258, 1373-1384.

Buccino, G., Binkofski, F., Fink, G.R., Fadiga, L., Fogassi, L., Gallese, V., et al. (2001). Action observations activates premotor and parietal areas in a somatotopic manner: an fMRI study. Euro J Neuroscience 13:400–4.

Buccino, G., Vogt, S., Ritzl, A., Fink, Gr., Zilles, K., Freund, H.-J., et al. (2004a). Neural circuits underlying imitation learning of hand actions: an event-related FMRI study. Neuron 42:323–34.

Büchel C, Dolan RJ. (2000). Classical fear conditioning in functional neuroimaging. Current Oppinion in Neurobiology. 10:219-223.

Buckner, R. L., Andrews-Hanna, J. R., & Schacter, D. L. (2008). The brain's default network: anatomy, function, and relevance to disease. [Research Support, N.I.H., Extramural Research Support, Non-U.S. Gov't Review]. Ann N Y Acad Sci, 1124, 1-38. doi: 10.1196/annals.1440.011

Bullinger, M. & Kirchberger, I. (1998). SF-36. Fragebogen zum Gesundheitszustand. Handanweisung. Göttingen: Hogrefe.

Bundesen, C. (1990). A theory of visual attention. Psychological Review 97, 523-547.

Bush, G., Luu, P., & Posner, M. I. (2000). Cognitive and emotional influences in anterior cingulate cortex. Trends Cogn Sci, 4(6), 215-222. doi: S1364-6613(00)01483-2 [pii]

Bush G, Vogt BA, Holmes J, Dale AM, Greve D, Jenike MA, Rosen BR. (2002) Dorsal anterior cingulate cortex: a role in reward-based decision making. Proc Natl Acad Sci U S A. 99:523-8

Buss , D. M. (1999). Evolutionary psychology: The new science of the mind. Boston: Allyn & Bacon.

Buss, D. M. & Craik, K. H. (1983). The act frequency approach to personality. Psychological Review, 90, 105-126.

Bussey, T. J., Warburton, E. C., Aggleton, J. P., & Muir, J. L. (1998). Fornix lesions can facilitate acquisition of the transverse patterning task: A challenge for "configural" theories of hippocampal function. J Neurosci 18(4): 1622-1631.

Butter, C. M., Rapcsak, S., & Watson, R. T. (1988). Changes in sensory inattention, directional motor neglect and "release" of the fixation reflex following a unilateral frontal lesion: a case report. Neuropsychologia, 26(4), 533-545.

Butterworth, B. (1999). The Mathematical Brain. London: Macmillan.

Butterworth, B., Varma, S. & Laurillard, D. (2011). Dyscalculia: from brain to education. Science, 332, 1049-1053

Buxbaum, L. J. (2001). Ideomotor apraxia: A call to action. Neurocase, 7, 445–458.

Buxbaum, L. J., Johnson, S. H., & Bartlett-Williams, M. (2005). Deficient internal models for planning hand-object interactions in ideomotor apraxia. Neuropsychologia, 43(6), 917–929.

Buxbaum, L. J, & Kalénine, S. (2010). Action knowledge, visuomotor activation, and embodiment in the two action systems. Annals of the New York Academy of Sciences, 1191, 201–218.

Buxbaum, L. J., Kyle, K., & Menon, R. (2005). On beyond mirror neurons: Internal representations subserving imitation and recognition of skilled object-related actions in humans. Cognitive Brain Research, 25(1), 226–239.

Byrne, B. M. (1994). Structural equation modelling with EQS and EQS/Windows: Basic concepts, applications, and programming. Thousand Oaks, CA: Sage.

Byrne, B. M., Shavelson, R. J., & Muthén, B. (1989). Testing for the equivalence of factor covariance and mean structures: the issue of partial measurement invariance. Psychological Bulletin, 105, 456–466.

Cadoret G, Smith AM (1995) Input-output properties of hand-related cells in the ventral cingulate cortex in the monkey. J Neurophysiol 73:2584-90

Calautti C, Leroy F, Guincestre JY & Baron JC. (2001). Dynamics of motor network over-activation after striatocapsular stroke: a longitudinal PET study using a fixed-performance paradigm. Stroke; 32.2534-2542.

Calder AJ, Keane J. Manes F, Antoun N, Young AW. (2000) Impaired recognition and experience of disgust following brain injury. Nat Neurosci. 3(11):1077-1078.

Calder AJ, Keane J, Manes F, Antoun N, Young AW. (2001) Impaired recognition of disgust following brain injury. Nature neuroscience 34: 1077-1078.

Calhoun, V. D., Maciejewski, P. K., Pearlson, G. D., & Kiehl, K. A. (2008). Temporal lobe and "default" hemodynamic brain modes discriminate between schizophrenia and bipolar disorder. [Research Support, N.I.H., Extramural Research Support, Non-U.S. Gov't]. Human Brain Mapping, 29(11), 1265-1275. doi: 10.1002/hbm.20463

Caminiti R, Johnson PB, Galli C, Ferraina S, Bumod Y (1991) Making arm movements within different parts of space; The premotor and motor cortical representation of a coordinate system for reaching to visual targets. J Neurosci 11:1182-1197

Campbell AW. (1905). Histological studies on the localization of cerebral function. University Press, Cambridge.

Campbell, N. A., & Reece, J. B. (2005). Biology (7th Ed.). New York, NY: Benjamin Cummings.

Camus M, Halelamien N, Plassmann H, Shimojo S, O'Doherty J, Camerer C, Rangel A (2000). Repetitive transcranial magnetic stimulation over the right dorsolateral prefrontal cortex decreases valuations during food choices. Eur J Neurosci 30:1980-1988.

Cantagallo, A., Spinazzola, L., Rabuffetti, M., & Della Sala, S. (2010). Verbal commands help the execution of endogenous movements in anarchic hand. Neuropsychological Rehabilitation, 20(3), 406-422.

Cantlon, J. F.; Brannon, E.M., Carter, E.J.; & Pelphrey, K.A. (2006). Functional imaging of numerical processing in adults and 4-year-old children . PLOS Biology, 4, 844-854.

Capitanio, J. P. (2004). Personality factors between and within species. In B. Tierry, M. Singh & W. Kaumanns (Eds.) Macaque societies (pp. 13–33). Cambridge, UK: Cambridge University Press.

Cappelletti, M., Butterworth, B. & Kopelman, M. (2012). Numeracy skills in patients with degenerative disorders and focal brain lesions: a neuropsychological investigation. Neuropsychology, 26, 1-19.

Cappelletti, M., Lee, H.L., Freeman, E.D., & Price, C.J. (2010) The role of right and left parietal lobes in the conceptual processing of numbers. Journal of Cognitive Neuroscience, 22, 331-346.

Caramazza, A. & McCloskey, M. (1987). Dissociations of calculation processes. In G. Deloche and X. Seron ((eds.) Mathematical Disabilities: A Cognitive Neuropsychological Perspective. Hillsdale, N.J.: Erlbaum (pp. 221-234).

Carl, J. R., & Gellman, R. S. (1987). Human smooth pursuit: stimulus-dependent responses. Journal of Neurophysiology, 57(5), 1446-1463.

Carlsson, SG, Johansson, A (2014). The importance of occlusion in clinical dentistry. Danish Dent J, 111: 196-203.

Carlsson, SG, Linde, A, Öhman, A (1980). Reduction of tension in fearful dental patients. J Am Dent Assoc, 101: 638-641.

Carr, L., Iacoboni, M., Dubeau, M.C., Mazziotta, J.C. & Lenzi, G.L. (2003). Neural mechanisms of empathy in humans: A relay from neural systems for imitation to limbic areas. Proc Natl Acad of Sci USA 100: 5497-5502.

Caspers S, Eickhoff SB, Geyer S, Scheperjans F, Mohlberg H, Zilles K, Amunts K. (2008). The human inferior parietal lobule in stereotaxic space. Brain Struct Funct 212, 481-495.

Caspers S, Eickhoff SB, Rick T, von Kapri A, Kuhlen T, Huang R, Shah NJ, Zilles K. (2011). Probabilistic fibre tract analysis of cytoarchitectonically defined human inferior parietal lobule areas reveals similarities to macaques. NeuroImage 58: 362-380.

Caspers S, Geyer S, Schleicher A, Mohlberg H, Amunts K, Zilles K. (2006). The human inferior parietal cortex: cytoarchitectonic parcellation and interindividual variability. NeuroImage 33, 430-448.

Caspers S, Schleicher A, Bacha-Trams M, Palomero-Gallagher N, Amunts K, Zilles K. (2013). Organization of the human inferior parietal lobule based on receptor architectonics. Cereb Cortex 23: 615-628.

Caspers, S., Zilles, K., Laird, A.R., & Eickhoff, S.B. (2010). ALE meta-analysis of action observation and imitation in the human brain. NeuroImage, 50, 1148-1167.

Castelli, F., Glaser, D.E. & Butterworth, B. (2006). Discrete and analogue quantity processing in the parietal lobe: a functional MRI study. Proceedings of the National Academy of Sciences, 103, 4693-4698.

Catani M, Jones DK, Ffytche DH. (2005). Perisylvian language networks of the human brain. Ann Neurol 57, 8-16.

Cattell, R. B. (1946). The description and measurement of personality. New York: World Book.

Cavada C. (2001). The visual parietal areas in the macaque monkey: current structural knowledge and ignorance. NeuroImage 14: 21-26.

Cavada C, Goldman-Rakic PS. (1989a). Posterior parietal cortex in rhesus monkey: I. Parcellation of areas based on distinctive limbic and sensory corticocortical connections. J Comp Neurol 287: 393-421.

Cavinato, M., Volpato, C., Silvoni, S., Sacchetto, M., Merico, A., & Piccione, F. (2011). Event-related brain potential modulation in patients with severe brain damage. Clinical Neurophysiology, 122(4), 719-724.

Cela-Conde, C.J. (2009). Sex-related similarities and differences in neural correlates of beauty. Proceedings of the National Academy of Sciences, 106, 3847-3852.

Cela-Conde CJ, Ayala FJ, Munar E, Maestu F, Nadal M, et al. (2009). Sex-related similarities and differences in the neural correlates of beauty. Proc Natl Acad Sci 106: 3847–3852.

Cervone, D., Shadel, W. G., & Jencius, S. (2001). Social-cognitive theory of personality assessment. Personality and Social Psychology Review, 5, 33-51.

Chang DS, Kang OS, Kim HH, Kim HS, Lee H, Park HJ, Kim H, Chae Y (2012) Preexisting beliefs and expectations influence judgments of novel health information. J Health Psychol 17: 753-763.

Chang, FCT, Scott, TR (1984). Conditioned taste aversions modify neuronal responses to gustatory stimuli. J Neurosci, 4:1850-1862.
Chang LJ, Doll BB, van 't Wout M, Frank MJ, Sanfey AG (2010) Seeing is believing: trustworthiness as a dynamic belief. Cogn Psych 61: 87-105.
Chatterjee, A., Thomas, A., Smith, S. E., Aguirre, G. K. (2009). The Neural Response to Facial Attractiveness. Neuropsychology, 23, 135-143.
Chaudhary, U., Xia, B., Birbaumer, N. (submitted). Brain Computer Interface (BCI) based communication in completely locked-in state (CLIS).
Chen, L. L. & Wise, S. P. (1995). Neuronal activity in the supple- mentary eye field during acquisition of conditional oculomotor associations. Journal of Physiology, 73, 1101–1121.
Chen, Y., Nakayama, K., Levy, D. L., Matthysse, S., & Holzman, P. S. (1999). Psychophysical isolation of a motion-processing deficit in schizophrenics and their relatives and its association with impaired smooth pursuit. Proceedings of the National Academy of Sciences, 96(8), 4724-4729.
Chennu, S., Finoia, P., Kamau, E., Monti, M. M., et al. (2013). Dissociable endogenous and exogenous attention in disorders of consciousness. Neuroimage: Clinical, 3, 450-461.
Chernigovskaya, T.V., Gavrilova, T.A., Voinov, A.V., and Strel'nikov, K.N. (2005). Sensorimotor and cognitive laterality profiles. Human Physiology, 31, 2, 142-149.
Chia, L. G. (1991). Locked-in syndrome with bilateral ventral midbrain infarcts. Neurology, 41, 445-446.
Chiao J.Y., Immordino-Yang M.H. (2013). Modularity and the Cultural Mind: Contributions of Cultural Neuroscience to Cognitive Theory. Perspectives on Psychological Science, 8, 56–61.
Chochon, F., Cohen, L., Van de Moortele, P. and Dehaene, S. (1999). Differential contributions of the left and right inferior parietal lobules to number processing. Journal of Cognitive Neuroscience, 11, 617-630.
Choi SH, Kim YH, Hebisch M, Sliwinski C, Lee S, D'Avanzo C, Chen H, Hooli B, Asselin C, Muffat J, Klee JB, Zhang C, Wainger BJ, Peitz M, Kovacs DM, Woolf CJ, Wagner SL, Tanzi RE, Kim DY (2014). A three-dimensional human neural cell culture model of Alzheimer's disease. Nature, 515(7526):274-278.
Chrousos, GP (1998) Stressors, stress, and neuroendocrine integration of the adaptive response. The 1997 Hans Selye memorial lecture. Ann NY Acad Sci, 851: 311-335.
Churchill SD (2012). Resounding oft he flesh: caring for others by way of „second person" perspectivity. Int J Qualitative Stud Health Well-being 7: 8187.
Churchland MM, Santhanam G, Shenoy KV (2006) Preparatory activity in premotor and motor cortex reflects the speed of the upcoming reach. J Neurophysiol 96:3130-46
Churchland MM, Shenoy KV (2007) Delay of movement caused by disruption of cortical preparatory activity. J Neurophysiol 97:348-59
Churchland, P. S. (1986). Neurophilosophy. Towards a Unified Science of the Mind/Brain. Cambridge, Mass.: MIT Press.
Cipolotti, L., Butterworth, B. & Denes, G. (1991). A specific deficit for numbers in a case of dense acalculia. Brain, 114, 2619-2637.

Cipolotti, L. & Butterworth, B. (1995). Toward a multiroute model of number processing: impaired number transcoding with preserved calculation skills. Journal of Experimental Psychology: General, 124, 375-390.
Cipolotti, L. & Delacycostello, A. (1995). Selective impairment for simple division. Cortex, 31, 433-449.
Cisek P, Crammond DJ, Kalaska JF Neural activity in primary motor and dorsal premotor cortex in reaching tasks with the contralateral versus ipsilateral arm. J Neurophysiol 89:922-942
Cisek P, Kalaska JF (2003) Neural correlates of reaching decisions in dorsal premotor cortex: specification of multiple direction choices and final selection of action. Neuron. 45:801-814, 2005
Clark, GT (2006). Medical management of oral motor disorders: dystonia, dyskinesia, and drug-induced dystonic extrapiramidal reactions. J Calif Dent Assoc, 34: 657-667.
Clarke, A. S., & Boinski, S. (1995). Temperament in nonhuman primates. American Journal of Primatology, 37, 103-125.
Clausen J (2008) Moving minds: ethical aspects of neural motor prostheses. Biotechnology Journal, 3, 1493–1501.
Clausen J (2009) Man, machine and in between. Nature, 457, 1080–1081.
Clerx L, van Rossum IA, Burns L, Knol DL, Scheltens P, Verhey F, Aalten P, Lapuerta P, van de Pol L, van Schijndel R, de Jong R, Barkhof F, Wolz R, Rueckert D, Bocchetta M, Tsolaki M, Nobili F, Wahlund LO, Minthon L, Frölich L, Hampel H, Soininen H, Visser PJ (2013). Measurements of medial temporal lobe atrophy for prediction of Alzheimer's disease in subjects with mild cognitive impairment. Neurobiol Aging, 34(8):2003-2013.
Clow, A, Lambert, S, Evans, P, Hucklebridge, F, Higuchi, K (2003) An investigation into asymmetrical cortical regulation of salivary sIgA in conscious man using transcranial magnetic stimulation. Int J Psychophysiol, 47: 57-64.
Cohen AD, Price JC, Weissfeld LA, James J, Rosario BL, Bi W, Nebes RD, Saxton JA, Snitz BE, Aizenstein HA, Wolk DA, DeKosky ST, Mathis CA, Klunk WE (2009). Basal cerebral metabolism may modulate the cognitive effects of Abeta in mild cognitive impairment: an example of brain reserve. J Neurosci, 29(47):14770-14778.
Cohen, J. (1988). Statistical Power Analysis for the Behavioral Sciences (2. Aufl.). Hillsdale: Lawrence Erlbaum Associates.
Cohen, J. (1988). Statistical power analysis for the behavioural sciences (2nd ed.). Hillsdale, NJ: Lawrence Erlbaum.
Cohen Kadosh, R., Dowker, A., Heine, A., Kaufmann, L. & Kucian, K. (2013). Interventions for improving numerical abilities: present and future. Trends in Neuroscience and Education, 2, 85-93.
Cohen Kadosh, R., Soskic, S., Iuculano, T., Kanai, R. & Walsh, V. (2010). Modulating neuronal activity produces specific and long-lasting changes in numerical competence. Current Biology, 20, 2016-2020.
Cohen, R. A., Grieve, S., Hoth, K. F., Paul, R. H., Sweet, L., Tate, D., Williams, L. M. (2006). Early life stress and morphometry of the adult anterior cingulate cortex and caudate nuclei. [Research Support, Non-U.S. Gov't]. Biol Psychiatry, 59(10), 975-982. doi: 10.1016/j.biopsych.2005.12.016

Colby, P. M. & Sherman, A. (2002). Attachment styles impact on pet visitation effectiveness. Anthrozoös, 15, 150–165.
Cole MW, Yarkoni T, Repovs G, Anticevic A, Braver TS (2012) Global connectivity of prefrontal cortex predicts cognitive control and intelligence. J Neurosci 32: 8988-8999.
Coleman, M. R., Davis, M. H., Rodd, J. M., Robson, T., Ali, A., Owen, A. M., & Pickard, J. D. (2009). Towards the routine use of brain imaging to aid the clinical diagnosis of disorders of consciousness. Brain, 132, 2541-2552.
Coleman, M. R., Rodd, J. M., Davis, M. H., Johnsrude, I. S., Menon, D. K., Pickard, J. D., & Owen, A. M. (2007). Do vegetative patients retain aspects of language comprehension? Evidence from fMRI. Brain, 130, 2494-2507.
Collange J, Fiske ST, Sanitioso R (2009) Maintaining a Positive Self-Image by Stereotyping Others: Self-Threat and the Stereotype Content Model. Soc Cogn27. doi: 10.1521/soco.2009.27.1.138.
Colombo, A., De Renzi, E., & Faglioni, P. (1976). The occurrence of visual neglect in patients with unilateral cerebral disease. Cortex, 12, 221–231.
Condy, C., Rivaud-Pechoux, S., Ostendorf, F., Ploner, C. J., & Gaymard, B. (2004). Neural substrate of antisaccades Role of subcortical structures. Neurology, 63(9), 1571-1578.
Conner, T. S., Barrett, L. F., Tugade, M. M. & Tennen, H. (2007). Idiographic personality: The theory and practice of experience sampling. In R. W. Robins, R. C. Fraley, & R. Kreuger (Eds.), Handbook of Research Methods in Personality Psychology (pp.79 – 98). New York, NY: Guilford Press.
Connolly, P. (1998). Racism, gender identities and young children: Social relations in a multi-ethnic, inner-city primary school. London, UK: Routledge.
Conty L, Dezecache G, Hugueville L, Grèze J (2012) Early binding of gaze, gesture, and emotion: neural time course and correlates. J Neurosci 32: 4531-4539.
Corbetta, M., & Shulman, G. L. (2002). Control of goal-directed and stimulus-driven attention in the brain. Nature Reviews Neuroscience, 3, 201-215.
Corbetta, M., & Shulman, G. L. (2011). Spatial neglect and attention networks. Annu Rev Neurosci., 34, 569–599.
Corbetta M, Tansy AP, Stanley CM, Astafiev SV, Snyder AZ, Shulman GL (2005). A functional MRI study of preparatory signals for spatial location and objects. Neuropsychologia 43: 2041-2056.
Costa, P. T., & McCrae, R. R. (1992). Revised NEO Personality Inventory (NEO-PI-R) and NEO Five-Factor Inventory (NEO-FFI) professional manual. Odessa, FL: Psychological Assessment Resources.
Coull JT, Vidal F, Nazarian B, Macar F (2004) Functional anatomy of the attentional modulation of time estimation. Science 303:1506-8
Coulthard, E., Rudd, A., Playford, E. D., & Husain, M. (2007). Alien limb following posterior cerebral artery stroke: Failure to recognize internally generated movements? Movement disorders, 22(10), 1498-1502.
Cox CL, Uddin LQ, di Martino A, Castellanos FX, Milham MP, Kelly C (2011). The balance between feeling and knowing: affective and cognitive empathy are reflected in the brain's intrinsic functional dynamics. Soc Cogn Affect Neurosci 7: 727-737.

Craik, F. I. M., Hasselmo, M. E., & Davachi, L. (2007). Encoding. In H.L. Roediger, Y. Dudai, & S.M. Fitzpatrick (Eds.), Science of memory: Concepts. New York: Oxford University Press.

Cramer SC. (2008). Repairing the human brain after stroke: I. Mechanisms of spontaneous recovery. Ann Neurol;63:272-287.

Cramer SC & Crafton KR. (2006). Somatotopy and movement representation sites following cortical stroke. Exp Brain Res;168:25-32.

Creutzfeldt, O., Ojemann, G., Lettich, E.. (1989). Neuronal activity in the human lateral temporal lobe. I. Responses to speech. Exp Brain Res 77(3):451-75.

Crick, F. & Koch, C. (2003). A framework for consciousness. Nature Neuroscience 6, 119–126.

Cronbach, L. J., & Meehl, P. E. (1955). Construct validity in psychological tests. Psychological Bulletin, 52, 281-302.

Cruse, D., Chennu, S., Chatelle, C., Bekinschtein, T. A., Fernandez-Espejo, et al. (2011). Bedside detection of awareness in the vegetative state. Lancet, DOI:10.1016/S0140-6736(1011)61224-61225.

Cullen, K. E., & Van Horn, M. R. (2011). Brainstem pathways and premotor control. In Oxford handbook of eye movements (pp. 151-172). Oxford University Press, Oxford.

Cupchik G.C., Vartanian O., Crawley A., Mikulis D.J. (2009). Viewing artworks: Contributions of cognitive control and perceptual facilitation to aesthetic experience. Brain and Cognition, 70, 84–91.

Curran, T. (1999). The electrophysiology of incidental and intentional retrieval: ERP old/new effects in lexical decision and recognition memory. Neuropsychologia, 35, 1035–1049.

Curran, T., & Cleary, A. M. (2003). Using ERPs to dissociate recollection from familiarity in picture recognition. Cognitive Brain Research, 15, 191–205.

d'Acremont M, Schultz W, Bossaerts P (2013) The human brain encodes event frequencies while forming subjective beliefs. J Neurosci 33: 10887-10897.

Dagenbach, D. & McCloskey, M. (1991). The organisation of arithmetical facts in memory: evidence from a brain-damaged patient. Brain and Cognition, 20, 343-366.

Dahlström, L, Lindvall, AM, Milthon, R, Widmark, G (1997). Management of chronic orofacial pain: attitudes among patients and dentists in a Swedish county. Acta Odontol Scand, 55: 181-185.

Daltrozzo, J., Wioland, N., Mutschler, V., & Kotchoubey, B. (2007). Predicting outcome of coma using event-related brain potentials: A meta-analytic approach. Clinical Neurophysiology, 118, 606-614.

Damasio, Antonio. (1994). Descartes'Error. Emotion, Reason, and the Humain Brain. London: Penguin Books.

Damasio A.R., (1998. Emotion in the perspective of an integrated nervous system. Brain Res Rev 26: 83-86.

Damasio, A. R. (2002). Ich fühle, also bin ich. Die Entschlüsselung des Bewusstseins. München: Ullstein Taschenbuch Verlag.

Damasio, H. & Damasio, A. (1980). The anatomical basis of conduction aphasia, Brain, 103 (2), 337-350.

Damasio, H., & Damasio, A. R. (1989). Lesion analysis in neuropsychology (pp. 38-39). New York: Oxford University Press.

Damoiseaux, J. S., Rombouts, S. A., Barkhof, F., Scheltens, P., Stam, C. J., Smith, S. M., & Beckmann, C. F. (2006). Consistent resting-state networks across healthy subjects. [Research Support, Non-U.S. Gov't]. Proc Natl Acad Sci U S A, 103(37), 13848-13853. doi: 10.1073/pnas.0601417103

Dapretto M, Bookheimer SY (1999) Form and content: Dissociating syntax and semantics in sentence comprehension. Neuron. 24:427-432.

D'Aquili, E. G. & Newberg, A. B. (1999). The Mystical Mind: Probing the Biology of Religious Experience. Minneapolis: Fortress Press.

Darwin, C. R. (1859). On the origin of species by means of natural selection, or the preservation of favoured races in the struggle for life. London, UK: John Murray.

Daselaar, S. M., Fleck, M. S., & Cabeza, R. (2006). Triple dissociation in the medial temporal lobes: recollection, familiarity, and novelty. Journal of Neurophysiology, 96, 1902– 1911.

Davachi, L. (2006). Item, context and relational episodic encoding in humans. Current opinion in neurobiology, 16(6), 693–700.

Davachi, L. and Dobbins, I. G. (2008). Declarative Memory. Current Directions in Psychological Science 17(2), 112-118.

Davachi, L., Mitchell, J. P., & Wagner, A. D. (2003). Multiple routes to memory: Distinct medial temporal lobe processes build item and source memories. Proceedings of the National Academy of Sciences of the United States of America, 100, 2157–2162.

Davids S, Lauffer H, Thoms K, Jagdhuhn M, Hirschfeld H, Domin M, Hamm A, Lotze M. (2010) Increased dorsolateral prefrontal cortex activation in obese children during observation of food stimuli. International Journal of Obesity. 34(1):94-104.

Davies, R. R., Graham, K. S., Xuereb, J. H., Williams, G. B., & Hodges, J. R. (2004). The human perirhinal cortex and semantic memory. European Journal of Neuroscience, 20, 2441–2446.

DCSF (Department for Children, Schools and Families). 2008. The Williams Review: Independent Review of Mathematics Teaching in Early Years Settings and Primary Schools. London: DCSF.

De Agostini, M., Kazandjian, S., Cavézian, C., Lellouch, J. and Chokron, S. Visual Aesthetic Preference: Effects of Handedness, Sex and Age-related Reading/Writing Directional Scanning Experience. (2010). Writing Systems Research, 1-9. doi: 10.1093/wsr/wsq006.

De Benedittis, Giuseppe (2002). The healer within. In: Hypnosis International Monographs 6, 2002 (145-155).

de Laat, A, van der Glas, HW, Weytjens, JLF, van Steenberghe, D (1985). The masseteric post-stimulus electromyographic-complex in people with dysfunction of the mandibular joint. Arch Oral Biol, 30: 177-180.

de Leon MJ, Convit A, Wolf OT, Tarshish CY, DeSanti S, Rusinek H, Tsui W, Kandil E, Scherer AJ, Roche A, Imossi A, Thorn E, Bobinski M, Caraos C, Lesbre P, Schlyer D, Poirier J, Reisberg B, Fowler J (2001). Prediction of cognitive decline in normal elderly subjects with 2-[(18)F]fluoro-2-deoxy-D-glucose/poitron-emission tomography (FDG/PET). Proc Natl Acad Sci U S A, 98(19):10966-10971.

De Leon, M. P., Benatti, P., Di Gregorio, C., Losi, L., Pedroni, M., Ponti, G., Genuardi, M., Viel, A., Lucci-Cordisco, E., Rossi, G., & Roncucci, L. (2007). Genotype-phenotype correlations in individuals with a founder mutation in the MLH1 gene and hereditary non-polyposis colorectal cancer. Scand J Gastroenterol 42 (6), 746-53.

de Lussanet MHE, Fadiga L, Michels L, Seitz RJ, Kleiser R, Lappe M (2008) Interaction of visual hemifield and body view in biological motion perception. Eur J Neurosci 27: 514-522.

De Massari, D., Ruf, C.A. , Furdea, A., Matuz, T., van der Heiden, L., Halder, S., Silvoni, S., Birbaumer, N. (2013). Brain communication in the locked-in state. Brain, 136, 1989-2000.

De Renzi, E., & Barbieri, C. (1992). The incidence of the grasp reflex following hemispheric lesion and its relation to frontal damage. Brain, 115(1), 293-313.

De Renzi, E., Cavalleri, F., & Facchini, S. (1996). Imitation and utilisation behaviour. Journal of Neurology, Neurosurgery & Psychiatry, 61(4), 396-400.

De Renzi, E., Scotti, G., & Spinnler, H. (1969). Perceptual and associative disorders of visual recognition. Neurology, 19, 634–642.

De Santi S, de Leon MJ, Rusinek H, Convit A, Tarshish CY, Roche A, Tsui WH, Kandil E, Boppana M, Daisley K, Wang GJ, Schlyer D, Fowler J (2001). Hippocampal formation glucose metabolism and volume losses in MCI and AD. Neurobiol Aging, 22:529–539.

De SS, de Leon MJ, Rusinek H, Convit A, Tarshish CY, Roche A, Tsui WH, Kandil E, Boppana M, Daisley K, Wang GJ, Schlyer D, Fowler J (2001). Hippocampal formation glucose metabolism and volume losses in MCI and AD. Neurobiol Aging, 22(4):529-539.

de Weerth, C., van Geert, P., & Hoitink, H. (1999). Intra-individual variability in infant behavior. Developmental Psychology, 35, 1102–1112. cite

DeCarli C, Frisoni GB, Clark CM, Harvey D, Grundman M, Petersen RC, Thal LJ, Jin S, Jack CR Jr, Scheltens P (2007). Qualitative estimates of medial temporal atrophy as a predictor of progression from mild cognitive impairment to dementia. Arch Neurol, 64(1):108-115.

Decety J, Grézes J. (1999) Neural mechanisms subserving the perception of human actions. TICS. 3(5):172-178.

Decety J, Lamm C (2006). Human empathy through the lens of social neuroscience. ScientificWorldJournal 6: 1146-1163.

Degenhardt, J. (2002). Zwischen Akutversorgung und Hospizarbeit: Die amyotrophische Lateralsklerose. Neurol Rehabil; 8(6): 306-310.

Dehaene, S. (1997). The Number Sense: How the Mind Creates Mathematics. Oxford: Oxford University Press.

Dehaene, S. (2014). Consciousness and the brain. New York: Viking. deutsch: Dehaene, Stanislas. (2014). Denken. Wie das Gehirn das Bewusstsein schafft. München: Knaus.

Dehaene S, Changeux JP, Naccache L, Sackur J, Sergent C (2006). Conscious, preconscious, and subliminal processing: a testable taxonomy. Trends Cogn Sci 10: 204-211.

Dehaene, S. and Cohen, L. (1991). Two mental calculation systems: a case study of severe acalculia with preserved approximation. Neuropsychologia, 29, 1045-1074.

Dehaene, S., Spelke, E., Pinel, P., Stanescu, R. & Tsivkin, S. (1999). Sources of mathematical thinking: behavioural and brain-imaging evidence. Science, 284, 970-974.

Dehaene, S., Tzourio, N., Frank, V., Raynaud, L.,Cohen,, L.,Mehler, J. & Mazoyer, B.(1996), Cerebral activations during number multiplication and comparison: a PET study, Neuropsychologia, 34, 1097-1116.
Delazer, M. (2003). Neuropsychological findings on conceptual knowledge of arithmetic. In A. Baroody and A. Dowker (eds.). The Development of Arithmetical Concepts and Skills. Mahwah, N.J.: Erlbaum.
Delazer, M. and Benke, T. (1997). Arithmetic facts without meaning. Cortex, 33, 697-710.
Dell, G. S., Martin, N., & Schwartz, M. F. (2007). A Case-Series Test of the Interactive Two-step Model of Lexical Access: Predicting Word Repetition from Picture Naming. J Mem Lang, 56 (4), 490-520.
Della Sala, S., Marchetti , C ., & Spinnler, H. (1 994). The anarchic hand: a fronto-mesial sign. In F. Boller & J . Grafman (Eds .) , Handbook of neuropsychology (vol. 9 , pp. 233-255), Amsterdam: Elsevier.
Demeyere, N., Lestou, V., & Humphreys, G. W. (2010). Neuropsychological evidence for a dissociation in counting and subitizing. Neurocase, 16(3), 219-237.
Demeyere, N., Rotshtein, P., & Humphreys, G. W. (2012). The neuroanatomy of visual enumeration: differentiating necessary neural correlates for subitizing versus counting in a neuropsychological voxel-based morphometry study. Journal of Cognitive Neuroscience, 24, 948-964.
Deneen, LJ, Heid, DW, Smith, AA (1973). Effective interpersonal and management skills in dentistry. J Am Dent Assoc, 87: 878-880.
Dennett, D. C. (1994). Philosophie des menschlichen Bewusstseins. Hamburg: Hoffmann und Campe.
DeSmedt, B., Holloway, I. & Ansari, D. (2011). Effects of problem size and arithmetic operation on brain activation during calculation in children with varying levels of arithmetical fluency. Neuroimage, 57, 771-781.
Deubel, H. & Schneider, W. X. (1996). Saccade target selection and object recognition: Evidence for a common attentional mechanism. Vision Research, 36, 1827–1837.
Dewick HC, Hanley JR, Davies AD, Playfer J, Turnbull C. (1991) Perception and memory for faces in Parkinson's disease. Neuropsychologia. 29(8):785-802.
di Pellegrino G, Wise SP (1993) Visuospatial versus visuomotor activity in the premotor and prefrontal cortex of a primate. J Neurosci 13:1227-43
Diana, R. A., Reder, L. M., Arndt, J., & Park, H. (2006). Models of recognition: a review of arguments in favor of a dual-process account. Psychonomic Bulletin and Review, 13(1), 1-21.
Diana, R. A., Yonelinas, A. P., & Ranganath, C. (2007). Imaging recollection and familiarity in the medial temporal lobe: a three-component model. Trends in Cognitive Sciences, 11(9), 379-86.
Diriwächter, R., Valsiner, J., & Sauck, C. (2004). Microgenesis in making sense of oneself: Constructive recycling of personality inventory items. Forum Qualitative Sozialforschung / Forum: Qualitative Social Research, 6, Art. 11.
Dodell-Feder, D., Koster-Hale, J., Bedny, M., & Saxe, R. (2011). fMRI item analysis in a theory of mind task. [Research Support, Non-U.S. Gov't Research Support, U.S. Gov't, Non-P.H.S.]. Neuroimage, 55(2), 705-712. doi: 10.1016/j.neuroimage.2010.12.040
Doering, S, Wolowski, A (2007). Psychosomatik als interdisciplinäres Fach. Zahnärztl Nachr Sachsen-Anhalt, 12: 7.

Döhnel K, Schuwerk T, Meinhardt J, Sodian B, Hajak G, Sommer M (2012). Functional activity of the right temporo-parietal junction and of the medial prefrontal cortex associated with true and false belief reasoning. Neuroimage 60: 1652-1661.

Donegan, N. H., Sanislow, C. A., Blumberg, H. P., Fulbright, R. K., Lacadie, C., Skudlarski, P., Wexler, B. E. (2003). Amygdala hyperreactivity in borderline personality disorder: implications for emotional dysregulation. [Comparative Study Research Support, Non-U.S. Gov't Research Support, U.S. Gov't, P.H.S.]. Biol Psychiatry, 54(11), 1284-1293.

Donges US, Kugel H, Stuhrmann A, Grotegerd D, Redlich R, Lichev V, Rosenberg N, Ihme K, Suslow T, Dannlowski U (2012) Adult attachment anxiety is associated with enhanced automatic neural response to positive facial expression. Neuroscience 220: 149-157.

Dowker, A. (2001). Numeracy recovery: a pilot scheme for early intervention with young children with numeracy difficulties. Support for Learning, 16, 6–10.

Dowker, A. (2005). Individual Differences in Arithmetic: Implications for Psychology, Neuroscience and Education. Hove: Psychology Press.

Dowker, A. (2006). What can brain imaging studies tell us about typical and atypical development? Journal of Physiology Paris, 99, 333-341.

Dowker, A. (2009). What Works for Children with Mathematical Difficulties? The Effectiveness of Intervention Schemes. London: DCSF.

Dowker, A. & Sigley, G. (2010). Targeted interventions for children with arithmetical difficulties. British Journal of Educational Psychology, Monograph Series II:7, 65-81

Drachmann DA (2014). The amyloid hypothesis, time to move on: Amyloid is a down steram result, not a cause of Alzheimer´s disease. Alzheimer´s & Dementia, 10:372-380.

Driver, J., Baylis, G. C., & Rafal, R. D. (1992). Preserved figure-ground segregation and symmetry perception in visual neglect. Nature, 360, 73–75.

Dronkers, N., F., Wilkins, D. P., Van Valin Jr., R., D., Redfern, B. B., & Jaeger, J. J. (2004). Lesion analysis of the brain areas involved in language comprehension. Cognition, 92, 145–177.

Drzezga A, Lautenschlager N, Siebner H, Riemenschneider M, Willoch F, Minoshima S, Schwaiger M, Kurz A (2003). Cerebral metabolic changes accompanying conversion of mild cognitive impairment into Alzheimer's disease: a PET follow-up study. Eur J Nucl Med Mol Imaging, 30(8):1104-1113.

Du S, Tao Y, Martinez AM (2014) Compound facial expressions of emotion. Proc Natl Acad Sci USA 111: E1454-62.

Duan X, Dai Q, Qiyong G, Chen H (2010). Neural mechanism of unconscious perception of surprised facial expression. Neuroimage, 52, 401-407.

Dubois B, Feldman HH, Jacova C, Hampel H, Molinuevo JL, Blennow K, DeKosky ST, Gauthier S, Selkoe D, Bateman R, Cappa S, Crutch S, Engelborghs S, Frisoni GB, Fox NC, Galasko D, Habert MO, Jicha GA, Nordberg A, Pasquier F, Rabinovici G, Robert P, Rowe C, Salloway S, Sarazin M, Epelbaum S, de Souza LC, Vellas B, Visser PJ, Schneider L, Stern Y, Scheltens P, Cummings JL (2014). Advancing research diagnostic criteria for Alzheimer's disease: the IWG-2 criteria. Lancet Neurol, 13(6):614-629.

Dubois B, Pillon B. (1997). Cognitive deficits in Parkinson's disease. J Neurol, 244(1), 2-8.

Dum RP, Strick PL (2002) Motor areas in the frontal lobe of the primate. Physiol Behav. 77:677-82
Dum RP, Strick PL (2005) Frontal lobe inputs to the digit representations of the motor areas on the lateral surface of the hemisphere. J Neurosci. 25:1375-86
Dunbar, R. (1996). Grooming, gossip, and the evolution of language. Cambridge, MA: Harvard University Press.
Duncan J, Owen AM (2000) Common regions of the human frontal lobe recruited by diverse cognitive demands. Trends Neurosci. 23:475-83
Duncan J, Parr A, Woolgar A, Thompson R, Bright P, Cox S, Bishop S, Nimmo-Smith I (2008) Goal neglect and Spearman's g: competing parts of a complex task. J Exp Psychol Gen 137: 131-148, Erratum in: J Exp Psychol Gen 137:261.
Duncan S (1969). Nonverbal Communication. Psychological Bulletin 72: 118-137.
Dunn, J. C. (2004). Remember-know: A matter of confidence. Psychological Review, 111, 524-542.
Dunn, S., Matthews, L. &. Dowrick, N. (2010). Numbers count: developing a national approach to intervention. In I. Thompson, ed. Issues in Teaching Numeracy in Primary Schools (pp. 224–234). Maidenhead: Open University Press.
Düzel, E., Vargha-Khadem, F., Heinze, H. J., & Mishkin, M. (2001). Brain activity evidence for recognition without recollection after early hippocampal damage. Proceedings of the National Academy of Sciences of the United States of America, 98(14), 8101-8106.
Düzel, E., Yonelinas, A. P., Mangun, G. R., Heinze, H. J., & Tulving, E. (1997). Event-related brain potential correlates of two states of conscious awareness in memory. Proceedings of the National Academy of Sciences of the United States of America, 94(11), 5973-5978.
Dworkin B. R. (1993) Learning and Physiological Regulation. University of Chicago Press, Chicago.
Dworkin, B.R. & Miller, N.E. (1986). Failure to replicate visceral learning in the acute curarized rat preparation. Behavioral Neuroscience, 100, 299–314.
Dworkin, SF, Sherman J (2006). Chronic orofacial pain: biobehavioral perspectives. In: D.I. Mostofsky, A.G. Forgione & D.B. Giddon (Eds.) Behavioral dentistry (pp. 99–113). Blackwell Munksgaard, Ames (Iowa).
Dworkin, SF, Turner, JA, Mancl, L, Wilson, L, Massoth, D, Huggins, KH, LeResche, L, Truelove, E (2002). A randomized clinical trial of a tailored comprehensive care treatment program for temporomandibular disorders. J Orofac Pain, 16: 259-276.
Dwyer, F. K., Bennett, P. C. & Coleman, G. J. (2006). Development of the Monash Dog Owner Relationship Scale (MDORS), Anthrozoös, 19, 243-256.
Dziobek, I., Preissler, S., Grozdanovic, Z., Heuser, I., Heekeren, H. R., & Roepke, S. (2011). Neuronal correlates of altered empathy and social cognition in borderline personality disorder. [Research Support, Non-U.S. Gov't]. Neuroimage, 57(2), 539-548. doi: 10.1016/j.neuroimage.2011.05.005
Eacott, M. J., Gaffan, D., & Murray, E. A. (1994). Preserved recognition memory for small sets, and impaired stimulus identification for large sets, following rhinal cortex ablations in monkeys. European Journal of Neuroscience, 6, 1466–1478.
Ebadi, M. (2005). Neuroleptic-Indcued Movement Disorders. In E. Ebadi & R.F. Pfeiffer (Eds.), Parkinson´s disease (pp. 579-622). Florida: CRC Press.
Eccles JS, Wigfield A (2002) Motivational beliefs, values, and goals. Annu Rev Psychol 53: 109-132.

Eger E, Jedynak A, Iwaki T, Skrandies, W. Rapid extraction of emotional expression: evidence from evoked potential fields during brief presentation of face stimuli. Neuropsychologia 2003;41:808-817.

Eichenbaum, H. (2004). Hippocampus: Cognitive processes and neural representations that underlie declarative memory. Neuron 44(1): 109-120.

Eickhoff SB, Pomjanski W, Jakobs O, Zilles K, Langner R (2011). Neural correlates of developing and adapting behavioral biases in speeded choice reactions – An fMRI study on predictive motor coding. Cereb Cortex 21: 1178-1191.

Eidelberg D, Galaburda AM. (1984). Inferior parietal lobule – Divergent architectonic asymmetries in the human brain. Archives in Neurology 41:843-852.

Eisenberger NI, Cole SW (2012) Social neuroscience and health: neurophysiological mechanisms linking social ties with physical health. Nat Neurosci 15: 669-674.

Ekman P & Friesen W (1969). Nonverbal leakage and clues to deception. Psychiatry, 32, 88-106.

Ekman P, Friesen W. (1976) Pictures of facial affect. Consulting psychologists press, Palo Alto

Eldridge, L. L., Knowlton, B. J., Furmanski, C. S., Bookheimer, S. Y., & Engel, S. A. (2000). Remembering episodes: a selective role for the hippocampus during retrieval. Nature Neuroscience, 3 (11), 1149-1152.

Elger, E., Friederici, A. D., Koch, C., Luhmann, H., von der Malsburg, C., Menzel, R., Monyer, H., Rösler, F., Roth, G., Scheich, H. & Singer, W. (2004). Das Manifest. Elf führende Neurowissenschaftler über Gegenwart und Zukunft der Hirnforschung. Gehirn & Geist. Das Magazin für Psychologie und Hirnforschung, (Heft 6), 30-37.

Elias, L.J., Bryden, M.P., Bulman-Fleming, M.B. (1998). Footedness is a better predictor than is handedness of emotional lateralization. Neurpsychologia, 36, 1, 37-43.

Ellert, U. & Bellach, B. M. (1999). Der SF-36 im Bundesgesundheitssurvey – Beschreibung einer aktuellen Normstichprobe. Gesundheitswesen 61, Sonderheft 2, 183-189.

Ellsworth PC & Scherer K (2003). Appraisal processes in emotion. In R. J. Davidson, K. R. Scherer, & H. Goldsmith (Eds.), Handbook of affective sciences (pp. 572_595). Oxford, UK: Oxford University Press.

Engel, G (1977). The need for a new medical model: a challenge for biomedicine. Science, 196: 129-136.

Engler H, Forsberg A, Almkvist O, Blomquist G, Larsson E, Savitcheva I, Wall A, Ringheim A, Långström B, Nordberg A (2006). Two-year follow-up of amyloid deposition in patients with Alzheimer's disease. Brain, 129(Pt 11):2856-2866.

Enns, M. W., Cox, B. J., & Clara, I. (2002). Parental bonding and adult psychopathology: results from the US National Comorbidity Survey. Psychological Medicine, 32, 997-1008.

Epstein, S. (1979). The stability of behavior: I. On predicting most of the people much of the time. Journal of Personality and Social Psychology, 37, 1097-1126.

Epstein, S. (1980). The stability of behavior: II. Implications for psychological research. American Psychologist, 35, 790-806.

Ernst A, Alkass K, Bernhard S, Salehpour M, Perl S, Tisdale J, Possnert G, Druid H, Frisen J. (2014). Neurogenesis in the striatum of the adult human brain. Cell;156:1072-1083.

Ethofer T, Bretscher J, Wiethoff S, Bisch J, Schlipf S, Wildgruber D, Kreifelts B. (2013) Functional responses and structural connections of cortical areas for processing faces and voices in the superior temporal sulcus. Neuroimage. 76:45-56.

Fábián, TK (2012). Mind-body connections. Pathways of psychosomatic coupling under meditation and other altered states of consciousness. Nova Science Publishers, New York. 131-172.

Fábián, TK, Beck, A, Gótai, L, Hermann, P, Fejérdy, P (2012/a). Psychogenic complications of making dentures. Theoretical background, prevention and treatment possibilities. In: T.K. Fábián, P. Fejérdy & P. Hermann (Eds.), Dentures. Types, benefits and potential complications (pp. 199–241). Nova Science Publishers, New York.

Fábián, TK, Csermely, P, Fábián, G, Fejérdy, P (2009/a). Spondyloarthropathies and bone resorption: A possible role of heat shock protein (Hsp70). (Review). Acta Physiol Hungarica, 96: 149-155.

Fábián, TK, Fábián, G, Fejérdy, P (2007/a). Dental Stress. In: G. Fink G (Ed. in chief), Encyclopedia of Stress. Vol. 1. /2-nd enlarged edition/ (pp. 733–736). Oxford: Academic Press, Oxford.

Fábián, TK, Fejérdy, P (2010). Psychogenic denture intolerance. Theoretical background, prevention and treatment possibilities. Nova Science Publishers, New York.

Fábián, TK, Fejérdy, P, Csermely, P (2008/a). Chemical biology of saliva in health and disease. In T. Begley (Ed. In chief), Wiley encyclopedia of chemical biology. (DOI: 10.1002/9780470048672.wecb643). John Wiley & Sons, Hoboken.

Fábián, TK, Fejérdy, P, Csermely, P (2008/b). Salivary genomics, transcriptomics and proteomics: The emerging concept of the oral ecosystem and their use in the early diagnosis of cancer and other diseases. Current Genomics, 9: 11-21.

Fábián, TK, Fejérdy, P, Hermann, P, Fábián, G (in press). Dental Stress. In G. Fink (Ed. in chief), Handbook of Stress / Stress Concepts and Cognition, Emotion and Behavior. Elsevier Inc.

Fábián, TK, Fejérdy, P, Nguyen, MT, Sőti, Cs, Csermely, P (2007/b). Potential immunological functions of salivary Hsp70 in mucosal and periodontal defense mechanisms. Arch Immunol Ther Exp, 55: 91-98.

Fábián, TK, Gáspár, J, Fejérdy, L, Kaán, B, Bálint, M, Csermely, P, Fejérdy, P (2003). Hsp70 is present in human saliva. Med Sci Monitor, 9: BR62-65.

Fábián, TK, Gótai, L, Beck, A, Fábián, G, Fejérdy, P (2009/b). The role of molecular chaperones (HSPAs/HSP70s) in oral health and oral inflammatory diseases: A review. Eur J Inflammation, 7: 53-61.

Fábián, TK, Hermann, P, Beck, A, Fejérdy, P, Fábián, G (2012/b). Salivary defense proteins: Their network and role in innate and acquired oral immunity. Int J Mol Sci, 13: 4295-4320.

Fábián, TK, Hidalgo Wulff, HC (2014). Implant dentistry. Theory and praxis. Nova Science Publishers, New York. 163-168, 169-178.

Fábián, TK, Kovács, KJ, Gótai, L, Beck, A, Krause, WR, Fejérdy, P (2009/c). Photo-acoustic stimulation: Theoretical background and ten years of clinical experience. Contemp Hypnosis, 26: 225-233.

Fábián, TK, Mierzwińska-Nastalska, E, Fejérdy, P (2006). Photo-acoustic stimulation. A suitable method in the treatment of psychogenic denture intolerance. Protet Stomatol, 56: 335-340.

Fábián, TK, Tóth, Zs, Fejérdy, L, Kaán, B, Csermely, P, Fejérdy, P (2004). Photo-acoustic stimulation increases the amount of 70 kDa heat shock protein (Hsp70) in human whole saliva. A pilot study. Int J Psychophysiol, 52: 211-216.

Fadiga L, Fogassi L, Pavesi G, Rizzolatti G. (1995) Motor facilitation during action observation: a magnetic stimulation study. J Neurophysiol. 73:2608-2611.

Fahrenberg, J. (1967). Psychophysiologische Persönlichkeitsforschung. Göttingen: Hogrefe.

Fahrenberg, J. (2008). Gehirn und Bewusstsein. Neurophilosophische Kontroversen. In: S. Gauggel und M. Herrmann (Hrsg.). Handbuch der Neuro- und Biopsychologie (S. 28-43). Göttingen: Hogrefe.

Fahrenberg, J. (2011). Wilhelm Wundt – Pionier der Psychologie und Außenseiter? Leitgedanken der Wissenschaftskonzeption und deren Rezeptionsgeschichte. e-Buch. Dokumentenserver der Universität des Saarlandes. psydok.sulb.uni-saarland.de/volltexte/2011/2901/

Fahrenberg, J. (2012). Wilhelm Wundts Wissenschaftstheorie. – Ein Rekonstruktionsversuch. Psychologische Rundschau, 63 (4), 228-238.

Fahrenberg, J. (2013). Zur Kategorienlehre der Psychologie. Komplementaritätsprinzip. Perspektiven und Perspektiven-Wechsel. Lengerich: Pabst Science Publishers. Dokumentenserver der Universität des Saarlandes: http://psydok.sulb.uni-saarland.de/volltexte/2013/4927/

Fahrenberg, J. (2015, April). Theoretische Psychologie. Zur Systematik der Kontroversen. Lengerich: Pabst Science Publishers.

Fahrenberg, J., Myrtek, M. (2005). Psychophysiologie in Labor, Klinik und Alltag. 40 Jahre Projektarbeit der Freiburger Forschungsgruppe Psychophysiologie – Kommentare und Neue Perspektiven. Frankfurt a.M.: Lang. Dokumentenserver der Universität des Saarlandes: http://psydok.sulb.uni-saarland.de/volltexte/2012/4227/

Fahrenberg, J., Myrtek, M., Pawlik, K. & Perrez, M. (2007). Ambulatory assessment – monitoring behavior in daily life settings. A behavioral-scientific challenge for psychology. European Journal of Personality Assessment, 23, 206-213.

Fairhall S.L., Ishai A. (2007). Neural correlates of object indeterminacy in art compositions. Consciousness and Cognition, doi:10.1016/j.concog.2007.07.005.

Fan Y, Duncan NW, de Greck M, Northoff G (2011). Is there a core neural network in empathy? An fMRI based quantitative meta-analysis. Neurosci Biobehav Rev 3: 903-911.

Fanselow, M. S. (2010). From contextual fear to a dynamic view of memory systems. Trends in cognitive sciences, 14(1), 7-15.

Farrow C, Frith C.D (2002). Experiencing oneself vs another person as being the cause of an action: The neural correlates of the experience of agency. Neuroimage 15: 596–603.

Farwell, L. A., & Donchin, E. (1988). Talking off the top of your head: Toward a mental prosthesis utilizing event-related brain potentials. Electroencephalography and Clinical Neurophysiology, 70, 512-523.

Faugeras, F., Rohaut, B., Weiss, N., Bekinschtein, T. A., Galanaud, D., et al. (2011). Probing consciousness with event-related potentials in the vegetative state. Neurology, 77, 264-268.

Faugeras, F., Rohaut, B., Weiss, N., Bekinschtein, T. A., Galanaud, D., et al. (2012). Event related potentials elicited by violations of auditory regularities in patients with impaired consciousness. Neuropsychologia, 50, 403-418.

Faul, F., Erdfelder, E., Lang, A.-G., & Buchner, A. (2007). G*Power 3: A flexible statistical power analysis program for the social, behavioral, and biomedical sciences. Behavior Research Methods, 39, 175-191.
Ferdinand NK, Mecklinger A, Kray J, Gehring WJ (2012). The processing of unexpected positive response outcomes in the mediofrontal cortex. J Neurosci 32: 12087-12092.
Fernández, G., & Tendolkar, I. (2006). The rhinal cortex – 'gatekeeper' of the declarative memory system. Trends in Cognitive Sciences, 10, 358–362.
Fernandez-Espejo, D., Junqué, C., Vendrell, P., Bernabeu, M., Roig, T., et al. (2008). Cerebral response to speech in vegetative and minimally conscious states after traumatic brain injury. Brain Injury, 22(11), 882-890.
Ferreira, JN. Hoffman, MP (2013). Interactions between developing nerves and salivary glands. Organogenesis, 9: 199–205.
Ferri F, Frassinetti F, Ardizzi M, Costantini M, Gallese V (2012) A sensorimotor network for the bodily self. J Cogn Neurosci 24: 1584-1495.
Fields, HL, Basbaum, AI (1994). Central nervous system mechanisms of pain modulation. In P.D. Wall, R. Melzack (Eds.) Textbook of pain /Third edition/ (pp. 243-257). Churchill Livingstone, Edinburgh.
Filimon, F. (2010). Human cortical control of hand movements: parietofrontal networks for reaching, grasping, and pointing. The Neuroscientist, 16(4), 388-407.
Filimon, F., Nelson, J. D., Huang, R. S., & Sereno, M. I. (2009). Multiple parietal reach regions in humans: cortical representations for visual and proprioceptive feedback during on-line reaching. The Journal of Neuroscience, 29(9), 2961-2971.
Filippopulos, F., Eggert, T., & Straube, A. (2013). Effects of cerebellar infarcts on cortical processing of saccades. Journal of Neurology, 260(3), 805-814.
Fink GR, Frackowiak RS, Pietrzyk U, Passingham RE (1997) Multiple nonprimary motor areas in the human cortex. J Neurophysiol. 77:2164-74
Fischer, B. & Weber, H. (1993). Express saccades and visual attention. Behavioral & Brain Sciences, 16, 553–567.
Fischer, C., Luaute, J., & Morlet, D. (2010). Event-related potentials (MMN and novelty P3) in permanent vegetative or minimally consciouos states. Clinical Neurophysiology, 121, 1032-1042.
Fiske, J, Davis, DM, Frances, C, Gelbier, S (1998). The emotional effects of tooth loss in edentulous people. Brit Dent J, 184: 90–93.
Fiske ST, Cuddy AJ, Glick P (2007) Universal dimensions of social cognition: warmth and competence. Trends Cogn Sci 11: 77-83.
Flechsig, P. (1896). Die Localisation der geistigen Vorgänge insbesondere der Sinnesempfindungen des Menschen. Leipzig: Veit.
Fleeson, W. (2001). Towards a structure- and process-integrated view of personality: Traits as density distributions of states. Journal of Personality and Social Psychology, 80, 1011-1027.
Foerster, O. (1936) Motorische Felder und Bahnen In: Handbuch der Neurologie Bumke H. und Foerster,O Ed. Berlin Springer Verlag
Fogassi L, Gallese V, Buccino G, Craighero L, Fadiga L, Rizzolatti G (2001) Cortical mechanism for the visual guidance of hand grasping movements in the monkey: A reversible inactivation study. Brain 124:571-86
Formisano, R., Pistoia, F., & Sará, M. (2011). Disorders of consciousness: A taxonomy to be changed? Brain Injury, 25(6), 638-639.

Forsberg A, Engler H, Almkvist O, Blomquist G, Hagman G, Wall A, Ringheim A, Långström B, Nordberg A (2008). PET imaging of amyloid deposits in patients with mild cognitive impairment. Neurobiol Aging, 29:1456-1465.

Forster S, Yousefi BH, Wester HJ, Klupp E, Rominger A, Forstl H, Kurz A, Grimmer T, Drzezga A (2012). Quantitative longitudinal interrelationships between brain metabolism and amyloid deposition during a 2-year follow-up in patients with early Alzheimer's disease. Eur J Nucl Med Mol Imaging, 39(12):1927-1936.

Förstl, Hans (Ed.). (20052). Frontalhirn. Funktionen und Erkrankungen. Heidelberg: Springer.

Foti, M. E., Geller, J., Guy, L. S., Gunderson, J. G., Palmer, B. A., & Smith, L. M. (2010). Borderline Personality Disorder: Considerations for Inclusion in the Massachusetts Parity List of "Biologically-Based" Disorders. Psychiatr Q. doi: 10.1007/s11126-010-9154-y

Fox, M. D., Snyder, A. Z., Vincent, J. L., Corbetta, M., Van Essen, D. C., & Raichle, M. E. (2005). The human brain is intrinsically organized into dynamic, anticorrelated functional networks. [Comparative Study Research Support, N.I.H., Extramural Research Support, U.S. Gov't, P.H.S.]. Proc Natl Acad Sci U S A, 102(27), 9673-9678. doi: 10.1073/pnas.0504136102

Fox NC, Freeborough PA, Rossor MN (1996). Visualisation and quantification of rates of atrophy in Alzheimer´s disease. Lancet, 348:94-97.

Fragaszy, D. M., Visalberghi, E., & Fedigan, L. (2004). The complete capuchin. Cambridge: Cambridge University Press.

Fransson, P., & Marrelec, G. (2008). The precuneus/posterior cingulate cortex plays a pivotal role in the default mode network: Evidence from a partial correlation network analysis. Neuroimage, 42(3), 1178-1184. doi: 10.1016/j.neuroimage.2008.05.059 S1053-8119(08)00728-3 [pii]

Fratkin, J. L., Sinn, D. L., Patall, E. A., & Gosling, S. D. (2013). Personality consistency in dogs: A meta-analysis. PLoS ONE, 8, e54907.

Freeman J.B., Rule N.O., Ambady N. (2009). The cultural neuroscience of person perception. In Chiao J.Y. (ed.) Progress in brain research, 178, 191-201.

Freund, H.J. (1987). Abnormalities of motor behavior after cortical lesions in humans. In V.B. Mountcastle, F. Plum, & S.R. Geiger (Eds.), Handbook of Physiology Section 1: The nervous system volume 5: Higher Functions of the brain Part 2 (pp. 763-810). Bethesda Maryland: American Physiological Society.

Freund, H. J. (2001). The parietal lobe as a sensorimotor interface: a perspective from clinical and neuroimaging data. Neuroimage, 14(1), 142-146.

Freund, H.-J., Jeannerod, M., Hallet, M. & Leiguarda, R. (2005). Higher Order Motor Disorders Oxford University Press.

Fridman, E. A., Immisch, I., Hanakawa, T., Bohlhalter, S., Waldvogel, D., Kansaku, K., Wheaton, L., Wu, T., & Hallett, M. (2006). The role of the dorsal stream for gesture production. NeuroImage, 29, 417–428.

Fridriksson, J., Kjartansson, O., Morgan, P. S., Hjaltason, H., Magnusdottir, S., Bonilha, L., & Rorden, C. (2010). Impaired speech repetition and left parietal lobe damage. Journal of Neuroscience, 30 (33), 11057–11061.

Frisoni GB, Fox NC, Jack CR,Jr, Scheltens P, Thompson PM (2010). The clinical use of structural MRI in Alzheimer disease. Nat Rev Neurol, Feb;6(2):67-77.

Friston K (2010). The free-energy principle: a unified brain theory? Nat Rev Neurosci 1-10.

Friston K, Schwartenbeck P, FitzGerald T, Moutoussis M, Behrens T, Dolan RJ (2014) The anatomy of choice: dopamine and decision-making. Philos Trans R Soc Lond B Biol Sci. 2014 Nov 5;369(1655). pii: 20130481. doi: 10.1098/rstb.2013.0481.

Frith U, Frith CD. (2003) Development and neurophysiology of mentalizing. Philos Trans R Soc Lond B Biol Sci. 358(1431):459-73.

Frommelt, Peter und Grötzbach, Holger (Eds.). (1999): Neurorehabilitation. Grundlagen, Praxis, Dokumentation. Berlin, Wien: Blackwell Wissenschafts-Verlag.

Fuchs T (2009) Embodied cognitive neuroscience and its consequences for psychiatry. Poiesis Prax, DOI 10.1007/s10202-008-0068-9.

Fuhr, K, Reiber, T (1995). Klinische Funktionsdiagnostik. In: B. Koeck (Ed.) Funktionsstörungen des Kauorgans (pp. 75-78). Urban & Schwarzenberg, München - Wien – Baltimore.

Fujii N, Mushiake H, Tanji J (2002) Distribution of eye- and arm-movement-related neuronal activity in the SEF and in the SMA and Pre-SMA of monkeys. J Neurophysiol. 87:2158-2166

Fukushima, K., Fukushima, J., Warabi, T., & Barnes, G. R. (2013). Cognitive processes involved in smooth pursuit eye movements: behavioral evidence, neural substrate and clinical correlation. Frontiers in systems neuroscience, 7.

Furdea, A., Ruf, C., Halder, S., De Massari, D., Bogdan, M., Rosenstiel, W., Matuz, T., Birbaumer, N. (2012). A new (semantic) reflexive brain-computer interface: in search for a suitable classifier. Journal of Neuroscience Methods, 203, 233-240.

Fusar-Poli P, Placentino A, Carletti F, Landi P, Allen P, Surguladze S et al (2009). Functional atlas of emotional faces processing: A voxel-based meta-analysis of 105 functional magnetic resonance imaging studies. Journal of Psychiatry & Neuroscience 34: 418-32.

Fuster JM (1990). Prefrontal cortex and the bridging of temporal gaps in.the cycle.perception-action cycle. Ann N Y Acad Sci 608: 318-329.

Gainotti, G., Messerli, P., & Tissot, R. (1972). Qualitative analysis of unilateral spatial neglect in relation to laterality of cerebral lesions. J Neurol Neurosurg Psychiatry, 35, 545–550.

Gallagher HL, Frith CD (2003). Functional Imaging of 'Theory of Mind'. Trends Cogn Sci 7: 77-83.

Gallagher HL, Happé F, Brunswick N, Fletcher PC, Frith U, Frith CD (2000). Reading the mind in cartoons and stories: an fMRI story of 'theory of mind' in verbal and nonverbal tasks. Neuropsychologia 38: 11-21.

Gallegos-Ayala, G., Furdea, A., Takano, K., Ruf, C.A., Flor, H., Birbaumer, N. (2014). Brain communication in a completely locked-in patient using bedside near-infrared spectroscopy. Neurology, 82, 1-3.

Gallese V, Faddiga L, Fogassi L, and Rizzolatti G (1996) Action recognition in the premotor cortex. Brain 119: 593-609

Gardiner, J. M., Java, R. I., & Richardson-Klavehn, A. (1996). How level of processing really influences awareness in recognition memory. Canadian Journal of Experimental Psychology, 50(1), 114–122.

Gardiner, J. M., Parkin, A. J. (1990). Attention and recollective experience in recognition memory. Memory and Cognition, 18, 579-583.

Garibotto V, Borroni B, Kalbe E, Herholz K, Salmon E, Holtoff V, Sorbi S, Cappa SF, Padovani A, Fazio F, Perani D (2008). Education and occupation as proxies for

reserve in aMCI converters and AD: FDG-PET evidence. Neurology, 71(17):1342-1349.
Gauthier I, Logothetis NK (2000) Is face recognition not so unique after all? Cogn. Neuropsych. 17:125-142.
Gaymard, B., Lynch, J., Ploner, C. J., Condy, C., & Rivaud-Pechoux, S. (2003). The parieto-collicular pathway: anatomical location and contribution to saccade generation. European Journal of Neuroscience, 17(7), 1518-1526.
Gaymard, B., Ploner, C. J., Rivaud, S., Vermersch, A. I., & Pierrot-Deseilligny, C. (1998). Cortical control of saccades. Experimental Brain Research, 123(1-2), 159-163.
Gaymard, B., Rivaud, S., & Pierrot-Deseilligny, C. (1993). Role of the left and right supplementary motor areas in memory-guided saccade sequences. Annals of neurology, 34(3), 404-406.
Gazzaniga, M.S., Boen, J.E., Sperr, R.W. (1962). Some functional effects of sectioning the cerebral commissures in man. Proc Acad Ntl Sci Oct 15;48:1765-9.
Gazzaniga, M., LeDoux, J.E. (1978). The Integrated Mind Plenum Press New York and London.
Gebhardt, GF, Sandkühler, J, Thalhammer, JG, Zimmermann, M (1984). Inhibition of spinal cord of nociceptive information by electrical stimulation and morphine microinjection at identical sites in midbrain of the cat. J Neurophysiol, 51: 75-89.
Genkin, A.A. (1960, Summer). A psychoneurological approach to the study of incapacity in mathematics. Paper presented at the Conference on the Problem of Abilities, University of Leningrad. (In Russian.)
Georgopoulos AP, Kalaska JF, Caminiti R, Massey JT (1982) On the relations between the direction of two-dimensional arm movements and cell discharge in primate motor cortex. J Neurosci. 2:1527-37
Geranmayeh, F., Brownsett, S. L., Leech, R., Beckmann, C. F., Woodhead, Z., & Wise, R. J. (2012). The contribution of the inferior parietal cortex to spoken language production. Brain Lang, 121 (1), 47-57.
Gerhardt E. (1940). Die Cytoarchitektonik des Isocortex parietalis beim Menschen. J Psych Neurol 49: 367-419.
Giacino, J. T., Ashwal, S., Childs, N., Cranford, R., Jennett, B., et al. (2002). The minimally conscious state. Definition and diagnostic criteria. Neurology, 58, 349-353.
Gibson JJ (1979) The Ecological Approach to Visual Perception, Hillsdale, NJ, Erlbaum
Gigerenzer, G., Todd, P., & the ABC Group. (1999). Simple heuristics that make us smart. New York, NY: Oxford University Press.
Gillespie, A., Howarth, C., & Cornish, F. (2012). Four problems for researchers using social categories. Culture and Psychology, 18, 391-402.
Gillham, B. & Hesse, K. (2001). Basic Number Screening Test: National Numeracy Strategy Edition: Forms A & B, for Ages 7 to 12 Years. 3rd edition. London: Hodder Education.
Girelli, L. and Delazer, M. (1996). Subtraction bugs in an acalculic patient. Cortex, 32, 547-555.
Glover, S., Rosenbaum, D. A., Graham, J. & Dixon, P. (2004). Grasping the meaning of words. Experimental Brain Research, 154(1), 103-108.
Goel V, Dolan RJ (2003) Explaining modulation of reasoning by belief. Cognition 87: B11-B22.
Goh J.O. & Park D.C. (2009). Culture sculpts the perceptual brain. In Chiao J.Y. (ed.) Progress in brain research, 178, 95-111.

Goldberg G (1985) Supplementary motor area structure and function: Review and hypothesis. Beh Brain Sci 8: 567-616
Goldberg, G., Mayer, N. H., & Toglia, J. U. (1981). Medial frontal cortex infarction and the alien hand sign. Archives of Neurology, 38(11), 683-686.
Goldberg, L. R. (1982). 'From Ace to Zombie: Some explorations in the language of personality'. In C. D. Spielberger & J. N. Butcher (Eds), Advances in Personality Assessment, Vol. 1, pp. 203-234, Erlbaum, Hillsdale.
Goldberg, M. E. (2000). The control of gaze. In E. Kandel, J. H. Schwartz & T. M. Jessel (Eds.) Principles of neural science (4th edn, pp. 782–800), New York: McGraw-Hill.
Goldenberg, G. (1996). Defective imitation of gestures in patients with damage in the left or right hemispheres. Journal of Neurology, Neurosurgery & Psychiatry, 61(2), 176-180.
Goldenberg, G. (2010). The neuropsychological assessment and treatment of disorders of voluntary movement. In J. M. Gurd, U. Kischka, & J. C. Marshall (Eds.), The handbook of clinical neuropsychology (2nd ed., pp. 387–400). Oxford, UK: Oxford University Press.
Goldenberg, G., Hagmann, S. (1998). Tool use and mechanical problem solving in apraxia. Neuropsychologia, 36(7), 581-589.
Goldenberg, G., Hartmann, K., & Schlott, I. (2003). Defective pantomime of object use in left brain damage: Apraxia or asymbolia? Neuropsychologia, 41, 1565–1573.
Goldenberg, G., Hermsdörfer, J., Glindeman, R., Rorden, C. & Karnath, H.O. (2007). Pantomime of tool use depends on integrity of left inferior frontal cortex. Cerebral Cortex, 17 (12), 2769-76.
Goldenberg, G., Karnath, H. O. (2006). The neural basis of imitation is body part specific. The Journal of Neuroscience, 26(23), 6282-6287.
Goldfine, A., Bardin, J., Noirhomme, Q., Fins, J., Schiff, N., & Victor, J. (2013). Reanalysis of "Bedside detection of awareness in the vegetative state: a cohort study". The Lancet, 381, 289-291.
Goldin-Meadow S. (1999) The role of gesture in communication and thinking. Trends in Cognitive Sciences. 3:419-429.
Gonsalves, B. D., Kahn, I., Curran, T., Norman, K. A., & Wagner, A. D. (2005). Memory strength and repetition suppression: multimodal imaging of medial temporal cortical contributions to recognition. Neuron, 47, 751–761.
Goodglass, H., & Kaplan, E. (1963). Disturbance of gesture and pantomime in aphasia. Behavioral & Brain Sciences, 86, 703–720.
Goodman, M., New, A., & Siever, L. (2004). Trauma, genes, and the neurobiology of personality disorders. [Review]. Ann N Y Acad Sci, 1032, 104-116. doi: 10.1196/annals.1314.008
Goschke, T (1996). Wille und Kognition: Zur funktionellen Architektur der intentionalen Handlungssteuerung. In: J. Kuhl & H. Heckhausen (Hrsg.) Motivation, Volition und Handlung (S. 583-663). Enzyklopädie der Psychologie. Serie IV Motivation und Emotion. Band 4. Göttingen: Hogrefe.
Goto S.G., Yee A., Lowenberg K., Lewis R.S. (2013). Cultural differences in sensitivity to social context: Detecting affective incongruity using the N400. Social Neuroscience, 8, 63-74.
Gould E, Reeves AJ, Fallah m, TanapatP, Gross CG, Fuchs E. (1999). Hippocampal neurogenesis in adult Old world primates. Proc Natl Acad Sci USA; 96:5263-5267.

Grabauskas, G, Bradley, R (1998). Ionic mechanisms of GABAA biphasic synaptic potentials in gustatory nucleus of the solitary tract. Ann NY Acad Sci, 855: 486-487.

Grabenhorst F, Rolls ET (2011). Value, pleasure and choice in the ventral prefrontal cortex. Trends Cogn Sci 15:56-67.

Graber, G (1995). Der Einfluss von Psyche und Stress bei dysfunktionsbedingten Erkrankungen des stomatognathen Systems. In B. Koeck (Ed.) Funktionsstörungen des Kauorgans (pp. 50-69). Urban & Schwarzenberg, München - Wien - Baltimore.

Graham, R, Mihaylov, S, Jepson, N, Allen, PF, Bond, S (2006). Determining "need" for a removable partial denture: a qualitative study of factors that influence dentist provision and patient use. Brit Dent J, 200: 155-158.

Grant, B. F., Chou, S. P., Goldstein, R. B., Huang, B., Stinson, F. S., Saha, T. D., Ruan, W. J. (2008). Prevalence, correlates, disability, and comorbidity of DSM-IV borderline personality disorder: results from the Wave 2 National Epidemiologic Survey on Alcohol and Related Conditions. [Research Support, N.I.H., Extramural Research Support, N.I.H., Intramural]. J Clin Psychiatry, 69(4), 533-545.

Gratz, K. L., Tull, M. T., & Gunderson, J. G. (2008). Preliminary data on the relationship between anxiety sensitivity and borderline personality disorder: the role of experiential avoidance J Psychiatr Res (Vol. 42, pp. 550-559). England.

Green, CS, Laskin DM (2000). Temporomandibular disorders: Moving from a dentally based to a medically based model. J Dent Res, 79: 1736–1739.

Greeno, T., Riley, M. & Gelman, R. (1983). Young children's counting and understanding of principles. Cognitive Psychology, 16, 94-143.

Gregg, V. H., & Gardiner, J. M. (1994). Recognition memory and awareness: A large effect of study-test modalities on "know" responses following a highly perceptual orienting task. European Journal of Cognitive Psychology, 6, 131-147.

Gregoriou GG, Borra E, Matelli M, Luppino G. (2006). Architectonic organization of the inferior parietal convexity of the macaque monkey. J Comp Neurol 496 (3): 422-451.

Grézes J, Costes N, Decety J (1999) The effects of learning and intention on the neural network involved in the perception of meaningless actions. Brain. 122:1875-1887.

Griffin, CJ, Harris, R (1975). The regulatory influences of the trigeminal system. In: C.J. Griffin, R. Harris (Eds.) The temporomandibular joint syndrome. The masticatory apparatus of man in normal and abnormal function. /Monographs in oral science, Vol. 4./ (pp. 65-86). Karger, Basel - München - Paris - London - New York – Sydney.

Griffin, D. W. & Bartholomew, K. (1994). The Metaphysics of Measurement: The case of adult attachment. Advances in Personal Relationships, 5, 17-52.

Grill-Spector K, Knouf N, Kanwisher N (2004). The fusiform face area subserves face perception, not generic within-category identification. Nature Neuroscience 7: 555-562.

Grimmer T, Tholen S, Yousefi BH, Alexopoulos P, Förschler A, Förstl H, Henriksen G, Klunk WE, Mathis CA, Perneczky R, Sorg C, Kurz A, Drzezga A (2010). Progression of cerebral amyloid load is associated with the apolipoprotein E ε4 genotype in Alzheimer's disease. Biol Psychiatry, 68(10):879-884.

Grosbras MH, Paus T (2006). Brain networks involved in viewing angry hands or faces. Cereb Cortex 16: 1087-1096.

Gross, J. (2007). Supporting children with gaps in their mathematical understanding. Educational and Child Psychology. 24: 146–156.

Gruber, O., Indefrey, P., Steinmetz, H. and Kleinschmidt, A. (2001). Dissociating neural correlates of cognitive components in mental calculation, Cerebral Cortex, 11, 350-369.

Grunwald, T., Pezer, N., Munte, T.F., Kurthen, M., Lehnertz, K., Van Roost, D., Fernandez, G., Kutas, M., and Elger, C.E. (2003). Dissecting out conscious and unconscious memory (sub)processes within the human medial temporal lobe. Neuroimage 20 Suppl 1, S139-145.

Gruzelier, J, Clow, A, Evans, P, Lazar, I, Walker, L (1998). Mind-body influences on immunity: Lateralized control, stress, individual difference predictors and prophylaxis. Ann NY Acad Sci, 851: 487-494.

Guenther, F. H. (2006). Cortical interactions underlying the production of speech sounds Journal of Communication Disorders, 39 (2006), 350–365.

Guillery RW (2005). Anatomical pathways that link perception and action. Prog Brain Res 149: 235-256.

Guitton, D., Buchtel, H. A. & Douglas, R. M. (1985). Frontal lobe lesions in man cause difficulties in suppressing reflexive glances and in generating goal directed saccades. Experimental Brain Research, 58, 455–472.

Gundlach, H. (1996). Der Willensakt im Reaktionsversuch. Material zur einer Begriffsgeschichte des Willensaktes. In: J. Kuhl & H. Heckhausen (Hrsg.) Motivation, Volition und Handlung (S. 362-409). Enzyklopädie der Psychologie. Serie IV Motivation und Emotion. Band 4. Göttingen: Hogrefe.

Gutchess A.H. & Indeck A. (2009) Culture influences on memory. . In Chiao J.Y. (ed.) Progress in brain research, 178, 137-150.

Guttmann, G. (1972). Einführung in die Neuropsychologie. Bern: Huber.

Guzhova, I, Kislyakova, K, Moskaliova, O, Fridlanskaya, I, Tytell, M, Cheetham, M, Margulis, B (2001). In vitro studies show that HSP70 can be released by glia and that exogenous HSP70 can enhance neuronal stress tolerance. Brain Res, 914: N1, 66-73.

Haaland, K. Y., Harrington, D. L., & Knight, R. T. (1999). Spatial deficits in ideomotor limb apraxia: A kinematic analysis of aiming movements. Behavioral & Brain Sciences, 122, 1169–1182.

Hadland KA, Rushworth MF, Gaffan D, Passingham RE (2003) The anterior cingulate and reward-guided selection of actions. J Neurophysiol. 89:1161-4

Haggard P, Clark S, Kalogeras J (2002) Voluntary action and conscious awareness. Nature Neuroscience 5, 382–385.

Hagner, M. (1996). Zur Geschichte und Vorgeschichte der Neuropsychologie (S. 1-101) In: H. J. Markowitsch (Hrsg.) Grundlagen der Neuropsychologie (S. 1-101). Enzyklopädie der Psychologie. Serie I. Biologische Psychologie. Band 1. Göttingen: Hogrefe.

Hagner, M. (1997). Homo Cerebralis. Der Wandel vom Seelenorgan zum Gehirn. Berlin: Berlin Verlag.

Hahn, E. (2013). Persönlichkeit und Wohlbefinden. Das Zusammenspiel von Anlage und Umwelt in einem erweiterten verhaltensgenetischen Design. Unveröffentlichte Dissertation, Universität Saarbrücken.

Haider, M. (Hrsg.). (1971). Neuropsychologie. Aktuelle Probleme. Bern: Huber.

Hall J, Whalley HC, McKirdy JW, Sprengelmeyer R, Santos IM, Donaldson DI, McGonigle DJ, Young AW, McIntosh AM, Johnstone EC, Lawrie SM (2010). A common neural system mediating two different forms of social judgement. Psychol Med 40: 1183-1192.

Haller, S., Radue, E. W., Erb, M., Grodd, W., & Kircher, T. (2005). Overt sentence production in event-related fMRI. Neuropsychologia, 43, 807-814.

Hällström, T, Halling, A (1984). Prevalence of dentistry phobia and its relation to missing teeth, alveolar bone loss and dental care habits in an urban community sample. Acta Psychiatr Scand, 70: 438-446.

Halsband U (1987) Higher disturbance of movement in monkeys (Macaca mulatta) In: Gantchev GN, editor. Motor Control. Plenum Press, pp. 79-85

Halsband, U. (Ed.)(2004). Mechanismen des Lernens in Trance: funktionelle Bildgebung und Neuropsychologie. In: Hirn und Hypnose. Vol Hykog 21(1+2) 11-38.

Halsband, U. (Ed.) (2004). Vorwort In: Hirn und Hypnose. Vol Hykog 21(1+2) 6

Halsband, U. (2006). Bilingual and multilingual language processing. Journal of Physiology - Paris 99, 355–369.

Halsband U, Freund HJ (1990) Premotor cortex and conditional motor learning in man. Brain. 113:207-22

Halsband, U., Freund, H.-J. (1993). Motor learning. Current Opinion in Neurobiology, 3:940-949.

Halsband, U., Gruhn, S. Ettlinger G. (1985). Unilateral spatial neglect and defective performance in one half of space. International Journal of Neuroscience 28, 173-195.

Halsband, U., Ito, N., Tanji, J. & Freund, H.-J. (1993). The role of premotor cortex and the supplementary motor area in the temporal control of movement in man. Brain, 116:243-266.

Halsband, U., Lange, R. K. (2006). Motor learning in man: A review of functional and clinical studies. Journal of Physiology – Paris, 99, 414–424.

Halsband U, Matsuzaka Y, Tanji J (1994) Neuronal activity in the primate supplementary, pre-supplementary and premotor cortex during externally and internally instructed sequential movements. Neurosci Res. 20:149-155

Halsband U, Passingham RE (1982) The role of premotor and parietal cortex in the direction of action. Brain Res 368-372

Halsband U, Passingham RE (1985) Premotor cortex and the conditions for movement in monkeys (Macaca mulatta). Beh Brain Res 269-276

Halsband U, Schmitt J, Weyers M, Binkofski F, Gruetzner G, Freund HJ. (2001) Recognition and imitation of pantomimed motor acts after unilateral parietal and premotor lesions: a perspective on apraxia. Neuropsychologia. 39:200-16.

Halsell, CB (1998). Differential distribution of amygdaloid input across rostral solitary nucleus subdivisions in rat. Ann NY Acad Sci, 855: 482-485.

Hammersley, M. (2013). The myth of research-based policy and practice. London: Sage

Hammock, E. A., & Young, L. Y. (2005). Microsatellite instability generates diversity in brain and sociobehavioral traits. Science, 308, 1630-1634.

Han S, Mao L, Gu X, Zhu Y, Ge J, Ma Y (2008). Neural consequences of religious belief on self-referential processing. Soc. Neurosci. , 1–15.

Handlin, L., Hydbring-Sandberg, E., Nilsson, A., Ejdebäck, M., Jansson, A., & Uvnäs-Moberg, K. (2011). Short-term interaction between dogs and their owners: Effects on oxytocin, cortisol, insulin and heart rate—An exploratory study. Anthrozoos, 24, 301-315.

Hara, Y. (2015). Brain plasticity and rehabilitation in stroke patients. J Nippon Med Sch; 82(1):4-13.

Hari R, Forss N, Avikainen S, Kirveskari E, Salenius S, Rizzolatti G. (1998) Activation of human primary motor cortex during action observation: a neuromagnetic study. Proc. Nat. Acad. Sci. 95:1561-1569.

Harrington A. & Oepen G. (1989). "Whole Brain" politics and brain laterality research. Eur Arch Psychiatr Neurol Sci, 239, 141-143.

Harris S, Sheth SA, Cohen MS (2008). Functional neuroimaging of belief, disbelief, and uncertainty. Ann. Neurol. 63, 141 – 147.

Harry B, Davis C, Kim J (2012) Subliminal access to abstract face representations does not rely on attention. Conscious Cogn 21: 573-583.

Hart, L. A. (2010). Positive effects of animals for psychosocially vulnerable people: a turning point for delivery. In A.H. Fine (Ed.), Handbook on Animal-Assisted Therapy. Theoretical Foundations and Guidelines for Practice. Third Edition (pp. 59-84), San Diego: Academic Press.

Hartmann, K., Goldenberg, G., Daumüller, M., & Hermsdörfer, J. (2005). It takes the whole brain to make a cup of coffee: The neuropsychology of naturalistic actions involving technical devices. Neuropsychologia, 43, 625–637.

Hartmann, N. (1964). Der Aufbau der realen Welt. Grundriss der allgemeinen Kategorienlehre (3. Aufl.). Berlin: Walter de Gruyter.

He J, Jin X, Zhang M, Huang X, Shui R, Shen M (2013) Anger and selective attention to reward and punishment in children. J Exp Child Psychol 115: 389-404.

He, P., & Kowler, E. (1989). The role of location probability in the programming of saccades: Implications for center-of-gravity tendencies. Vision Research, 29(9), 1165-1181.

Headey, B., Grabka, M. M. (2007). Pets and human health in Germany and Australia: national longitudinal results. Social Indicators Research, 80, 297-311.

Headey, B., Na, F. & Zheng, R. (2008). Pet dogs benefit owners´ health: a ´natural experiment` in China. Social Indicators Research, 87, 481-493.

Heath R. L., Mahmasanni O., Rouhana A., Nassif N. (2005). Comparison of aesthetic preferences among Roman and Arabic script readers. Laterality, 10, 399-411.

Heathcote, A. (2003). Item recognition memory and the receiver operating characteristic. Journal of Experimental Psychology: Learning, Memory, and Cognition, 29, 1210-1230.

Hebb, D.O. (1983). Neuropsychology: retrospect and prospect. Can J Psychol Mar;37(1):4-7.

Heekeren HR, Marrett S, Ruff DA, Bandettini PA, Ungerleider LG (2006). Involvement of human left dorsolateral prefrontal cortex in perceptual decision-making is independent of response modality. Pric Natl Acad Sci USA 103: 10023-10028.

Heggendorn, H, Voght, HP, Graber, G (1979). Experimentelle Untersuchungen über die orale Hyperaktivität bei psychischer belastung, im Besonderen bei Aggression. Schweiz Mschr Zahnheilk, 89: 1148-1161.

Heide, W., Blankenburg, M., Zimmermann, E., & Kömpf, D. (1995). Cortical control of double-step saccades: implications for spatial orientation. Annals of neurology, 38(5), 739-748.

Heide, W., Kurzidim, K., & Kömpf, D. (1996). Deficits of smooth pursuit eye movements after frontal and parietal lesions. Brain, 119(6), 1951-1969.

Heilman, K. M., Bowers, D., Valenstein, E., & Watson, R. T. (1987). Hemispace and hemispatial neglect. In M. Jeannerod (Ed.), Neurophysiological and neuropsychological aspects of spacial neglect (pp. 115–150). Amsterdam, Holland: Elsevier.

Heilman, K. M., Maher, L. M., Greenwald, M. L., & Rothi, L. J. G. (1997). Conceptual apraxia from lateralized lesions. Neurology, 49, 457–464.

Heilman, K.M., Rothi, L.J.G. (2012). Apraxia. In K.M. Heilman & E. Valenstein (Ed.), Clinical Neuropsychology (pp. 214-237, 5th edition). New York: Oxford University Press.

Heilman, K. M., Valenstein, E., Rothi, L. J. G., & Watson, R. T. (2008). Intentional motor disorders and the apraxias. In W. G. Bradley & R. B. Daroff (Eds.), Neurology in clinical practice: Principles of diagnosis and management (pp. 121–132). Philadelphia, PA: Butterworth-Heinemann.

Heine, S. J., Lehman, D. R., Peng, K., & Greenholtz, J. (2002). What's wrong with cross-cultural comparisons of subjective Likert scales?: The reference-group effect. Journal of Personality and Social Psychology, 82, 903-918.

Helmholtz von, H. (1867). Handbuch der Physiologischen Optik, Leipzig, Voss.

Helmholtz, H. von (1878). Die Tatsachen in der Wahrnehmung. Rede gehalten zur Stiftungsfeier der Friedrich-Wilhelms-Universität zu Berlin. In: H. von Helmholtz: Vorträge und Reden II. Braunschweig: Vieweg.

Henik, A., Rafal, R., & Rhodes, D. (1994). Endogenously generated and visually guided saccades after lesions of the human frontal eye fields. Journal of Cognitive Neuroscience, 6(4), 400-411.

Henke, K. (2010). A model for memory systems based on processing modes rather than consciousness. Nature Reviews Neuroscience, 11(7), 523-532.

Henkel LA, Mattson ME (2011) Reading is believing: the truth effect and source credibility. Conscious Cogn 20: 1705-1721.

Henschen, S.E. (1920). Klinische und Anatomische Beitrage zu Pathologie des Gehirns. Stockholm: Nordiska Bokhandeln.

Henseler, I., Regenbrecht, F., & Obrig, H. (2014). Lesion correlates of patholinguistic profiles in chronic aphasia: comparisons of syndrome-,modality- and symptom-level assessment. Brain, 137, 918–930.

Henson, R. (2005). A mini-review of fMRI studies of human medial temporal lobe activity associated with recognition memory. Quarterly Journal of Experimental Psychology B., 58(3-4), 340-360.

Henson, R. N., Cansino, S., Herron, J. E., Robb, W. G., & Rugg, M. D. (2003). A familiarity signal in human anterior medial temporal cortex? Hippocampus, 13, 259-262.

Herbart, J. F. (1825). Psychologie als Wissenschaft neu gegründet auf Erfahrung, Metaphysik und Mathematik. Zweyter, analytischer Theil. Königsberg: Unzer.

Hermes, D, Saka, B, Bahlmann, L, Matthes, M (2006). Behandlungsangst in der Mund-, Kiefer- und Gesichtschirurgie. Mund Kiefer Gesichts Chir, 10: 307-313.

Herpertz, S. C., Dietrich, T. M., Wenning, B., Krings, T., Erberich, S. G., Willmes, K., Sass, H. (2001). Evidence of abnormal amygdala functioning in borderline personality disorder: a functional MRI study. Biological Psychiatry, 50(4), 292-298. doi: 10.1016/s0006-3223(01)01075-7

Herpertz, S., Gretzer, A., Muhlbauer, V., Steinmeyer, E. M., & Sass, H. (1998). [Experimental detection of inadequate affect regulation in patients with self-mutilating behavior]. Nervenarzt, 69(5), 410-418.

Herrmann, C.S., Pauen, M., Min, B.K., Busch, N.A., Rieger, J.W. (2007). Analysis of a choice-reaction task yields a new interpretation of Libet's experiments. Int J Psychophysiol 2008 Feb;67(2):151-7. Epub Nov 22.

Herrmann, E., Hare, B., Cissewski, J., & Tomasello, M. (2011). A comparison of temperament in nonhuman apes and human infants. Developmental Science, 14, 1393–1405.

Hertrich, K, Joraschky, P (1996). Psychotherapie in der zahnärztlichen Praxis: Möglichkeiten der Integration und Kooperation. In H.G. Sergl (Ed.), Psychologie und Psychosomatik in der Zahnheilkunde (pp. 261-279). Urban & Schwarzenberg, München - Wien – Baltimore.

Hessel, A., Schumacher, J., Geyer, M. & Brähler, E. (2001). Symptom-Checkliste SCL-90-R: Testtheoretische Überprüfung und Normierung an einer bevölkerungsrepräsentativen Stichprobe. Diagnostika, 47, 27-39.

Heywood CA, Cowey A. (1992) The role of the "face-cell" area in the discrimination and recognition of faces by monkeys. Philos. Trans. R. Soc. London Ser. B 335: 31-38.

Higuchi, S., Chaminade, T., Imamizu, H. & Kawatoa, M. (2009). Shared neural correlates for language and tool use in Broca's area. Neuroreport, 20 (15), 1376–1381.

Hikosaka, O., & Wurtz, R. H. (1986). Saccadic eye movements following injection of lidocaine into the superior colliculus. Experimental Brain Research, 61(3), 531-539.

Hinde, R. A. (1974). Biological bases of human social behavior. New York: McGraw-Hill.

Hinde, R. A. (1982). Ethology: Its nature and relations with other sciences. Oxford: Oxford University Press.

Hinterberger, T. (2011). The Sensorium: A Multimodal Neurofeedback Environment. Special Issue on Advances in Human-Computer Interaction 2011, Retrieved from: http://www.hindawi.com/journals/ahci/2011/724204/ (31.08.2011).

Hinterberger, T., Kamei, T., Sauer, S. & Kohls, N. (in preparation). Physiological markers of a psychological concept of mindfulness and exceptional experiences.

Hinterberger, T., Schmidt, S.N.L., Kamei, T., Walach, H. (2014). "Decreased Electrophysiological Activity Represents the Conscious State of Emptiness in Meditation" Frontiers in Consciousness Research, 99(5): 1-14. doi: 10.3389/fpsyg.2014.0009

Hinterberger, T., Wilhelm, B., Mellinger, J., Kotchoubey, B., & Birbaumer, N. (2005). A Device for the Detection of Cognitive Brain Functions in Completely Paralyzed or Unresponsive Patients. IEEE Trans. on Biomedical Engineering 52, 211-220.

Hirshman, E., Fisher, J., Henthorn, T., Arndt, J.,& Passannate, A. (2002). Midazolam amnesia and dual-process models of the word-frequency mirror effect. Journal of Memory and Language, 47, 499-516.

Hittmair-Delazer, M., Sailer, V. and Berke, T. (1995). Impaired arithmetical facts but intact conceptual knowledge: a single case study of dyscalculia. Cortex, 31, 139-147.

Hodges, J. R., Bozeat, S., Ralph, M. A. L., Patterson, K., & Spatt, J. (2000). The role of conceptual knowledge in object use evidence from semantic dementia. Brain, 123(9), 1913-1925.

Hoehn, MM, Yahr, MD. (1967). Parkinsonism: onset, progression and mortality. Neurology. 17(5):427-442.

Hoeren M, Kümmerer D, Bormann T, Beume L, Ludwig VM, Vry MS, Mader I, Rijntjes M, Kaller CP, Weiller C. (2014) Neural bases of imitation and pantomime in acute stroke patients: distinct streams for praxis. Brain. 137(Pt 10):2796-810.

Hofsteede, G. (2001). Culture's consequences: Comparing values, behaviors, institutions and organizations across nations. California, CA.: Sage Publications.

Holdstock, J. S., Mayes, A. R., Gong, Q. Y., Roberts, N., & Kapur, N. (2005). Item recognition is less impaired than recall and associative recognition in a patient with selective hippocampal damage. Hippocampus, 15, 203–215.

Holmes, W. & Dowker, A.D. (2013). Catch Up Numeracy: a targeted intervention for children who are low attaining in mathematics. Research in Mathematics Education, 15, 249-265.

Hooker CI, Verosky SC, Germine LT, Knight RT, D'Esposito M (2008). Mentalizing about emotion and its relationship to empathy. 3: Soc Cogn Affect Neurosci 204-217.

Hopf A. (1969). Photometric studies on the myeloarchitecture of the human parietal lobe. I. Parietal region. J Hirnforsch 11: 253-265.

Hopf A, Vitzthum HG. (1957). Über die Verteilung myeloarchitektonischer Merkmale in der Scheitellappenrinde beim Menschen. J Hirnforsch 3: 79-104.

Hoppstädter, M., King, A. V., Frölich, L., Wessa, M., Flor, H., Meyer, P. (2013). A combined electrophysiological and morphological examination of episodic memory decline in amnestic mild cognitive impairment. Frontiers in Aging Neuroscience, 5: 51.

Horwitz, B., Amunts, K., Bhattacharyya, R., Patkin, D., Jeffries, K., Zilles, K. & A.R. Braun (2003). Activation of Broca's area during the production of spoken and signed language: a combined cytoarchitectonic mapping and PET analysis. Neusropsychologia, 41 (14), 1868-1876.

Hoshi E, Sawamura H, Tanji J (2005) Neurons in the rostral cingulate motor area monitor multiple phases of visuomotor behavior with modest parametric selectivity. J Neurophysiol. 94:640-656

Hoshi E, Sawamura H, Tanji J (2005) Neurons in the rostral cingulate motor area monitor multiple phases of visuomotor behavior with modest parametric selectivity. J Neurophysiol. 94:640-56

Hoshi E, Tanji J (2000) Integration of target and body-part information in the premotor cortex when planning action. Nature 408: 466-470

Hoshi E, Tanji J (2004) Differential roles of neuronal activity in the supplementary and presupplementary motor areas: from information retrieval to motor planning and execution. J Neurophysiol. 92:3482-99

Hoshi E, Tanji J (2006) Differential involvement of neurons in the dorsal and ventral premotor cortex during processing of visual signals for action planning. J Neurophysiol 95: 3596-3616

Hoshi E, Tanji J (2007) Distinctions between dorsal and ventral premotor areas: anatomical connectivity and functional properties. Current Opinion in Neurobiol. 17:234-242

Hosseini HSM, Rostami M, Yomogida Y, Takahashi M, Tsukiura T, Kawashima R (2010). Aging and decision making under uncertainty: Behavioral and neural evidence for the preservation of decision making in the absence of learning in old age. Neuroimage 52: 1514-1520.

Howarth, C. (2009). “I hope we won’t have to understand racism one day”: Researching or reproducing ‘race’ in Social research? British Journal of Social Psychology, 48, 407-426.

Hsu, Y. & Serpell, J. A. (2003). Development and validation of a questionnaire for measuring behavior and temperament traits in pet dogs. Journal of the American Veterinary Medical Association, 223, 1293–1300.

Hugdahl, K. (2000). Lateralization of cognitive processes in the brain, Acta Psychologica 105 , 211-235.

Hunt, CC, Paintal, AS (1958). Spinal reflex regulation of fusimotor neurons. J Physiol Lond, 143: 195-212.

Husain, M., Parton, A., Hodgson, T. L., Mort, D., & Rees, G. (2002). Self-control during response conflict by human supplementary eye field. Nature Neuroscience, 6(2), 117-118.

Hutton, S. B. (2008). Cognitive control of saccadic eye movements. Brain and cognition, 68(3), 327-340.

Hynes CA, Baird AA, Grafton ST (2006). Differential Role of the Orbital Frontal Lobe in Emotional Versus Cognitive Perspective-Taking. Neuropsychologia 44: 374-383.

Isaacs, E. B., Edmonds, C. J., Lucas, A. and Gadian, D. G. (2001) Calculation difficulties in children of very low birthweight: a neural correlate. Brain, 124, 1701–1707

Ishikawa, Y, Cho, G, Yuan, Z, Skowronski, MT, Pan, Y, Ishida, H (2006). Water channels and zymogen granules in salivary glands. J Pharmacol Sci, 100: 495-512.

Isomura Y, Ito Y, Akazawa T, Nambu A, Takada M (2003) Neural coding of "attention for action" and "response selection" in primate anterior cingulate cortex. J Neurosci. 23:8002-12

Ito S, Stuphorn V, Brown JW, Schall JD (2003) Performance monitoring by the anterior cingulate cortex during saccade countermanding. Science. 302:120-122

Iuculano, T. & Cohen Kadosh, R. (2014). Preliminary evidence for performance enhancement following parietal lobe stimulation in developmental dyscalculia. Frontiers in Human Neuroscience, 8, 38.

Iversen, G (1989). Geleitwort. In: H. Binder, K. Binder, Autogenes Training, Basispsychotherapeutikum. Deutscher Ärzteverlag, Köln.

Jack CR (2011). Alliance for aging research AD biomarkers work group: structural MRI. Neurobiology of Aging, 32:S48-S57.

Jack CR, Jr., Knopman DS, Jagust WJ, Petersen RC, Weiner MW, Aisen PS, Shaw LM, Vemuri P, Wiste HJ, Weigand SD, Lesnick TG, Pankratz VS, Donohue MC, Trojanowski JQ (2013). Tracking pathophysiological processes in Alzheimer's disease: an updated hypothetical model of dynamic biomarkers. Lancet Neurol, 12(2):207-216.

Jack CR Jr, Lowe VJ, Weigand SD, Wiste HJ, Senjem ML, Knopman DS, Shiung MM, Gunter JL, Boeve BF, Kemp BJ, Weiner M, Petersen RC; Alzheimer's Disease Neuroimaging Initiative (2009). Serial PIB and MRI in normal, mild cognitive impairment and Alzheimer's disease: implications for sequence of pathological events in Alzheimer's disease. Brain, 132(Pt 5):1355-1365.

Jack CR Jr, Petersen RC, O'Brien PC, Tangalos EG (1992). MR-based hippocampal volumetry in the diagnosis of Alzheimer's disease. Neurology, 42(1):183-188.
Jack CR, Jr., Petersen RC, Xu YC, O'Brien PC, Smith GE, Ivnik RJ, Boeve BF, Waring SC, Tangalos EG, Kokmen E (1999). Prediction of AD with MRI-based hippocampal volume in mild cognitive impairment. Neurology, 52(7):1397-1403.
Jack Jr CR, Lowe VJ, Senjem ML, Weigand SD, Kemp BJ, Shiung MM, Knopman DS, Boeve BF, Klunk WE, Mathis CA, Petersen RC (2008). 11C PiB and structural MRI provide complementary information in imaging of Alzheimer's disease and amnestic mild cognitive impairment. Brain,131:665–680.
Jackson A, Mavoori J, Fetz E (2006) Long-term motor cortex plasticity induced by an electronic neural implant. Nature, 444, 56–60.
Jackson PL, Meltzoff AN, Decety J (2006). Neural circuits involved in imitation and perspective-taking. NeuroImage 31: 429-439.
Jacob H, Brück C, Domin M, Lotze M, Wildgruber D. (2014) I can't keep your face and voice out of my head: neural correlates of an attentional bias towards nonverbal emotional cues. Cerebral Cortex. 24(6):1460-73.
Jacobs, R, Serhal, CB, van Steenberge, D (1998). Oral stereognosis: a review of the literature. Clin Oral Invest, 2: 3-10.
Jacobsen T (2006). Bridging the arts and sciences: a framework for the psychology of aesthetics. Leonardo, 39, 155–162.
Jacobsen T. (2010). Beauty and the brain: culture, history and individual differences in aesthetic appreciation. J. Anat., 216, 184–191.
Jacobsen T. (2013) On the electrophysiology of aesthetic processing. In Finger S., Zaidel D.W., Boller F. & Bogousslavsky J., (ed.): Progress in Brain Research, Vol. 204, Amsterdam: The Netherlands, pp. 159-168.
Jacobsen T., Schubotz R.I., Ho¨fel L.,Cramon D.Y.V. (2006). Brain correlates of aesthetic judgment of beauty. NeuroImage, 29, 276 – 285.
Jaeger, G. (2009). Entanglement, Information, and the Interpretation of Quantum Mechanics (1. Edition). Berlin: Springer.
Jagust W, Gitcho A, Sun F, Kuczynski B, Mungas D, Haan M (2006). Brain imaging evidence of Alzheimer´s disease in normal aging. Ann Neurol 59:673-681.
James, W. (1890). Memory. In The Principles of Psychology (pp. 643-689). London: Macmillian and Co.
James, W. (1890). Principles of psychology. New York: Holt, Rinehart & Winston.
Janke, W. & Herrmann, Th. (1971). Apperzeption. Apperzeptionspsychologie. In: J. Ritter et al. (Hrsg.) Historisches Wörterbuch der Philosophie. Band 1. (S. 448-456). Darmstadt: WBG.
Jantz, J. J., Watanabe, M., Everling, S., & Munoz, D. P. (2013). Threshold mechanism for saccade initiation in frontal eye field and superior colliculus. Journal of Neurophysiology, 109(11), 2767-2780.
Jax, S., Buxbaum, L. J., & Moll, A. (2006). Deficits in movement planning and intrinsic coordinate control in ideomotor apraxia. Journal of Cognitive Neuroscience, 18 (12), 2063–2076.
JCGM, Joint Committee for Guides in Metrology. (2008). International vocabulary of metrology – Basic and general concepts and associated terms (VIM) (3rd ed.), Working Group 2 (Eds.), Joint Committee for Guides in Metrology.
Jeannerod, M. (1994). The representing brain. Neural correlates of motor intention and imagery. Behav Brain Sci 17:187–245.

Jeannerod M. (1994) The representing brain: neural correlates of motor intention and imagery. Behav. Brain Sci. 17:197-245.
Jeannerod M, Arbib MA, Rizzolatti G, Sakata H (1995) Grasping objects: the cortical mechanisms of visuomotor transformation. Trends Neurosci. 18:314-320
Jiang Y, Shannon RW, Vizueta N, Bernat EM, Patrick CJ, He S (2009). Dynamics of processing invisible faces in the brain: automatic neural encoding of facial expression information. Neuroimage 44: 269-278.
Jóhannesson, Ó.I., Ásgeirsson, Á.G. & Kristjánsson, Á. (2012). Saccade performance in the temporal and nasal hemifields. Experimental Brain Research. 219(1), 107-120.
Jóhannesson, Ó, Kristjánsson, Á. (2013). Violating the main sequence: asymmetries in saccadic peak velocities for saccades into the temporal versus nasal hemifields. Experimental Brain Research, 227(1), 101-110.
Johnson-Frey, S.H. (2004). The neural bases of complex tool use in humans. Trends in Cognitive Sciences, 8, 71–78.
Joshi AD, Pontecorvo MJ, Clark CM, Carpenter AP, Jennings DL, Sadowsky CH, Adler LP, Kovnat KD, Seibyl JP, Arora A, Saha K, Burns JD, Lowrey MJ, Mintun MA, Skovronsky DM; Florbetapir F 18 Study Investigators (2012). Performance characteristics of amyloid PET with florbetapir F 18 in patients with Alzheimer's disease and cognitively normal subjects. J Nucl Med, 53: 378–384.
Jovchelovitch, S. (2007). Knowledge in context: Representations, community and culture. London, UK: Routledge.
Julius, H., Beetz, A., Kotrschal, K., Turner, D. & Uvnäs-Moberg, K. (2013). Attachment to Pets. New York: Hogrefe.
Jüttemann, G. (2006). (Hrsg.). Wilhelm Wundts anderes Erbe. Ein Missverständnis löst sich auf. Göttingen: Vandenhoeck & Ruprecht.
Kabat-Zinn, J. (2011). Gesund durch Meditation. Full Catastrophe Living. Das vollständige Grundlagenwerk. München: Otto Wilhelm Barth. (American original edition, New York, 1990)
Kabayashi Frank C., Temple E. (2009). Cultural effects on the neural basis of theory of mind In Chiao J.Y. (ed.) Progress in brain research, 178, 213-223.
Kadir A, Almkvist O, Forsberg A, Wall A, Engler H, Langstrom B, Nordberg A (2012). Dynamic changes in PET amyloid and FDG imaging at different stages of Alzheimer's disease. Neurobiol Aging, 33(1):198-204.
Kaeser, T., Baschera, G.M., Kohn, J., Kucian, K., Richtmann, V., Grond, U., Gross, M. & Von Aster, M. (2013). Design and evaluation of the computer-based training program Calcularis for enhancing numerical cognition. Frontiers in Psychology, 4, 489.
Kakei S, Hoffman DS, Strick PL (2001) Direction of action is represented in the ventral premotor cortex. Nat Neurosci 4(10):1020-1025
Kalaska JF, Cohen DA, Hyde ML, Prud'homme M (1989) A comparison of movement direction-related versus load direction-related activity in primate motor cortex, using a two-dimensional reaching task. J Neurosci 9:2080-102
Kalénine, S., Buxbaum, L. J., & Coslett, H. B. (2010). Critical brain regions for action recognition: Lesion-symptom mapping in left hemisphere stroke. Behavioral & Brain Sciences, 133 (11), 3269–3280.

Kampe KKW, Frith CD, Frith U (2003). “Hey John”: Signals conveying communicative intention toward the self activate brain regions associated with “mentalizing”, regardless of modality. J Neuroscience 23: 5258-5263.
Kandel, Eric R. (2012). Psychiatrie, Psychoanalyse und die neue Biologie des Geistes. Frankfurt/Main: Suhrkamp.
Kant I. (1755). Allgemeine Naturgeschichte und Theorie des Himmels Königsberg und Leipzig, bey Johann Friederich Petersen.
Kant, I. (1798/1983). Anthropologie in pragmatischer Hinsicht. Immanuel Kant Werkausgabe in 6 Bänden. Band 6 (S. 395-690). (hrsg. von Wilhelm Weischedel). Darmstadt: Wissenschaftliche Buchgesellschaft.
Kaplan, R. M., & Saccuzzo, D. P. (2008). Psychological testing: Principles, applications, and issues, (7th ed). Belmont, CA: Thompson. Wadsworth.
Karim, A.A., Kammer, T., Lotze, M., Nitsche, M.A., Godde, B., Hinterberger, T., Cohen, L., Birbaumer, N. (2004). Effects of TMS and TDCS on the physiological regulation of cortical excitability in a braincomputer interface. Biomedizinische Technik, 49, Suppl. 1, 55-57.
Karnath, H.-O. (1994). Disturbed coordinate transformation in the neural representation of space as the crucial mechanism leading to neglect. Neuropsychol Rehabil, 4, 147-150.
Karnath H-O. (1997). Spatial orientation and the representation of space with parietal lobe lesions. Philos Trans R Soc Lond B Biol Sci, 352, 1411-14119.
Karnath, H. O., Ferber, S., & Himmelbach, M. (2001). Spatial awareness is a function of the temporal not the posterior parietal lobe. Nature, 411, 950–3.
Karnath, H. O., Perenin, M. T. (2005). Cortical control of visually guided reaching: evidence from patients with optic ataxia. Cerebral Cortex, 15(10), 1561-1569.
Kaufmann, L., Mazzocco, M.M., Dowker, A., Von Aster, M., Göbel, S.M. Grabner, R.H., Henik, A.. Jordan. N.C., Karmiloff-Smith, A.D., Kucian, K., Rubinsten, O., Szucs, D., Shalev, R. & Nuerk, H.C. (2013). Dyscalculia from a developmental and differential perspective. Frontiers in Psychology, 4, 516.
Kaufmann, L., Montanes, P., Jacquier, M., Matallana, D., Eibl, G. & Delazer. M. (2002). About the relationship between basic numerical processing and arithmetics in early Alzheimer's disease - A follow-up study. Brain and Cognition, 48, 398-405.
Kaufmann, L., Vogel, S.E., Starke, M., Kremser, C. & Schocke, M. (2009). Numerical and non-numerical ordinality processing in children with and without developmental dyscalculia: evidence from fMRI.. Cognitive Development, 24, 486-494.
Kawabata H., Zeki S. (2004). Neural correlates of beauty. J Neurophysiol 91:1699-1705.
Kazui, H., Hitagaki, H. & Mori, E. (2000). Cortical activation during retrieval of arithmetical facts and actual calculation: A functional magnetic resonance imaging study. Psychiatry and Clinical Neurosciences, 54, 479-485.
Kemppainen NM, Aalto S, Karrasch M, Nagren K, Savisto N, Oikonen V, Viitanen M, Parkkola R, Rinne JO (2008). Cognitive reserve hypothesis: Pittsburgh Compound B and fluorodeoxyglucose positron emission tomography in relation to education in mild Alzheimer's disease. Ann Neurol, 63(1):112-118.
Kemppainen NM, Aalto S, Wilson IA, Nagren K, Helin S, Bruck A, Oikonen V, Kailajarvi M, Scheinin M, Viitanen M, Parkkola R, Rinne JO (2007). PET amyloid ligand [11C]PIB uptake is increased in mild cognitive impairment. Neurology, 68(19):1603-1606.

Kemppainen NM, Scheinin NM, Koivunen J, Johansson J, Toivonen JT, Nagren K, Rokka J, Karrasch M, Parkkola R, Rinne JO (2014). Five-year follow-up of 11C-PIB uptake in Alzheimer's disease and MCI. Eur J Nucl Med Mol Imaging, 41(2):283-289.

Kendon A. (1983) Gesture and speech: How they interact. In JM Weimann & RP Harrison (Ed.), Nonverbal interaction, Beverly Hills, CA.

Kendon A (1997). Gesture. Annual Review of Anthropology 26: 109-128.

Kennerley SW, Behrens TE, Wallis JD (2011) Double dissociation of value computations in orbitofrontal and anterior cingulate neurons. Nat Neurosci 14: 1581-1589.

Kennerley SW, Dahmubed AF, Lara AH, Wallis JD (2009) Neurons in the frontal lobe encode the value of multiple decision variables. J Cogn Neurosci 21:1162-7

Kennerley SW, Wallis JD (2009) Evaluating choices by single neurons in the frontal lobe: outcome value encoded across multiple decision values. Eur J Neurosci 29: 2061-2073.

Kensinger, E. A., Schacter, D. L. (2006) Amygdala activity is associated with successful encoding of item, but not source, information for positive and negative stimuli. Journal of. Neuroscience, 26, 2564–2570.

Kensinger, E. A., Ullman, M. T., & Corkin, S. (2001). Bilateral medial temporal lobe damage does not affect lexical or grammatical processing: Evidence from amnesic patient HM. Hippocampus, 11(4), 347-360.

Kerns JG, Cohen JD, MacDonald AW 3rd, Cho RY, Stenger VA, Carter CS (2004) Anterior cingulate conflict monitoring and adjustments in control. Science. 303:1023-6

Ketay S., Aron A., Hedden T. (2009). Culture and attention: evidence from brain and behavior. In Chiao J.Y. (ed.) Progress in brain research, 178, 79-92.

Killgore, WD & Yurgelun-Todd, DA (2004). Activation of the Amygdala and Anterior Cingulate during Nonconscious Processing of Sad Versus Happy Faces. NeuroImage 21: 1215-1223.

Kilner JM, Lemon RN (2013) What we know currently about mirror neurons. Curr Biol 23:R1057-62

Kilts CD, Egan G, Gideon DA, Ely TD, Hoffman JM (2003). Dissociable neural pathways are involved in the recognition of emotion in static and dynamic facial expressions. Neuroimage 18: 156-168.

Kim H, Sul JH, Huh N, Lee D, Jung MW (2009) Role of striatum in updating values of chosen actions. J Neurosci 29: 14701-14712.

Kinder M, Lotze M, Davids S, Domin M, Thoms K, Wendt J, Hirschfeld H, Hamm A, Lauffer H. (2014) Imaging in obese children responding to long-term sports therapy. Behavioral Brain Research. 272C:25-31.

King, B. R., Fogel, S. M., Albouy, G., & Doyon, J. (2013). Neural correlates of the age-related changes in motor sequence learning and motor adaptation in older adults. Frontiers in Human Neuroscience, 7 (142), 1-13.

King, J. E., Weiss, A., & Sisco, M. M. (2008). Aping humans: Age and sex effects in chimpanzee (Pan troglodytes) and human (Homo sapiens) personality. Journal of Comparative Psychology, 122, 418-27.

Király, M, Porcsalmy, B, Pataki, A, Kádár, K, Jelitai, M, Molnár, B, Hermann, P, Gera, I, Grimm, WD, Ganss, B, Zsembery, A, Varga, G (2009). Simultaneous PKC and cAMP activation induces differentiation of human dental pulp stem cells into functionally active neurons. Neurochem Int, 55: 323-332.

Klein, Ch. & Stralendorff, I. von (2002). Neuropsychologische Defizite bei ADS: Theorien und Ergebnisse. In: M. Myrtek (Hrsg.) Die Person im biologischen und sozialen Kontext. Göttingen: Hogrefe.

Kleist, K. (1934). Gehirnpathologie Verlag J. Ambrosius Barth,Leipzig

Kluckhohn, C., Murray, H. A., & Schneider, D. M. (1953). Personality in nature, society, and culture. New York, NY: Knopf.

Kluetsch, R. C., Schmahl, C., Niedtfeld, I., Densmore, M., Calhoun, V. D., Daniels, J., Lanius, R. A. (2012). Alterations in default mode network connectivity during pain processing in borderline personality disorder. Arch Gen Psychiatry, 69(10), 993-1002. doi: 1169875 [pii] 10.1001/archgenpsychiatry.2012.476

Klunk WE, Engler H, Nordberg A, Wang Y, Blomqvist G, Holt DP, Bergström M, Savitcheva I, Huang GF, Estrada S, Ausén B, Debnath ML, Barletta J, Price JC, Sandell J, Lopresti BJ, Wall A, Koivisto P, Antoni G, Mathis CA, Långström B (2004). Imaging brain amyloid in Alzheimer's disease with Pittsburgh compound-B. Ann Neurol, 55:306-319.

Koechlin E1, Danek A, Burnod Y, Grafman J (2002) Medial prefrontal and subcortical mechanisms underlying the acquisition of motor and cognitive action sequences in humans. Neuron. 35:371-81

Koenigsberg, H. W., Harvey, P. D., Mitropoulou, V., Schmeidler, J., New, A. S., Goodman, M., Siever, L. J. (2002). Characterizing affective instability in borderline personality disorder. [Comparative Study Research Support, U.S. Gov't, Non-P.H.S. Research Support, U.S. Gov't, P.H.S.]. Am J Psychiatry, 159(5), 784-788.

Koffka, K. (1935). Principles of Gestalt psychology. New York: Harcourt, Brace, & World.

Koivisto M, Henriksson L, Revonsuo A, Railo H (2012). Unconscious response priming by shape depends on geniculostriate visual projection. Eur J Neurosci 35: 623-633.

Koivunen J, Scheinin N, Virta JR, Aalto S, Vahlberg T, Nagren K, Helin S, Parkkola R, Viitanen M, Rinne JO (2011). Amyloid PET imaging in patients with mild cognitive impairment: a 2-year follow-up study. Neurology, 76(12):1085-1090.

Kolb, Bryan / Whishaw, Ian Q. (1996): Neuropsychologie. Heidelberg: Spektrum Akademischer Verlag.

Kossioni, AE, Karzakis, HC (1995). Variation in the masseteric silent period in older dentate humans and in denture wearers. Arch Oral Biol, 40: 1143-1150.

Kotchoubey, B. (2009). Vegetative state. In L. Squire (Ed.), Encyclopedia of Neuroscience (Vol. 10, pp. 61- 66). Amsterdam: Elsevier.

Kotchoubey, B., Kaiser, J., Bostanov, V., Lutzenberger, W., & Birbaumer, N. (2009). Recognition of affective prosody in brain-damaged patients and healthy controls: A neurophysiological study using EEG and whole-head MEG. Cognitive, Affective, and Behavioral Neuroscience, 9, 153-167.

Kotchoubey, B., Lang, S., Mezger, G., Schmalohr, D., Schneck, M., et al. (2005). Information processing in severe disorders of consciousness: Vegetative state and minimally conscious state. Clinical Neurophysiology, 116, 2441-2453.

Kotchoubey, B., Lang, S., Winter, S., & Birbaumer, N. (2003). Cognitive processing in completely paralyzed patients with amyotrophic lateral sclerosis. European Journal of Neurology, 10, 551-558.

Kotchoubey, B., Lotze, M. (2013). Instrumental methods in the diagnostics of locked-in syndrome. Restorative Neurology and Neuroscience, 31, 25-40.

Kotchoubey B., Veser S., Real R., Herbert C., Lang S., Kübler A. (2013). Towards a more precise neurophysiological assessment of cognitive functions in patients with disorders of consciousness. Restorative Neurology and Neuroscience, 31, 473–485.

Kotchoubey, B., Yu T., Mueller F., Vogel D., Veser S., Lang S. (2014). True or false? Activations of language-related areas in patients with disorders of consciousness. Current Pharmaceutical Design, 20, 4239-4249.

Kotrschal, K., Schöberl, I., Bauer, B., Thibeaut, A. M. & Wedl, M. (2009). Dyadic relation-ships and operational performance of male and female owners and their male dogs. Behavioral Processes, 81, 383–391.

Kowler, E., Anderson, E., Dosher, B., & Blaser, E. (1995). The role of attention in the programming of saccades. Vision research, 35(13), 1897-1916.

Krahwinkel, T, Nastali, S, Azrak, B, Willershausen, B (2004). The effect of examination stress conditions on the cortisol content of saliva - a study of students from clinical semesters. Eur J Med Res, 28: 256-260.

Krain AL, Wilson AM, Arbuckle R, Castellanos FX & Milham MP (2006). Distinct neural mechanisms of risk and ambiguity: A meta-analysis of decision-making. Neuroimage 32: 477-484.

Krainik, A., Lehericy, S., Duffau, H., Vlaicu, M., Poupon, F., Capelle, L., ... & Marsault, C. (2001). Role of the supplementary motor area in motor deficit following medial frontal lobe surgery. Neurology, 57(5), 871-878.

Kramer UM, Mohammadi B, Donamayor N, Samii A, Munte, TF (2010). Emotional and Cognitive Aspects of Empathy and Their Relation to Social Cognition--an Fmri-Study. Brain Res 1311: 110-120.

Kraskov A, Philipp R, Waldert S, Vigneswaran G, Quallo MM, Lemon RN (2014) Corticospinal mirror neurons. Philos Trans R Soc Lond B Biol Sci 369:20130174

Krause M, Wendt J, Dressel A, Berneiser J, Kessler C, Hamm A, Lotze M. (2009) Prefrontal function associated with impaired emotion recognition in patients with multiple sclerosis. Behavioural Brain Research. 205:280-5.

Krause, WR (1983). Grundlagen der Biofeedback-Therapie und ihre therapeutischen Anwendungsmöglichkeiten. Z ärztl Fortbild, 77: 493-494.

Krause, WR (1994). Hypnose und Autogenes Training (Selbsthypnose) in der Rehabilitation. Ergänzung. In: J.H. Schultz Hypnose-Technik. Praktische Anleitung zum Hypnotisieren für Ärzte. 9. Auflage - bearbeitet und ergänzt von G. Iversen und W.-R. Krause. (pp.71-79). Gustav Fischer Verlag, Stuttgart - Jena - New York.

Krause, WR (2000). Hypnose und Autogenes Training. Mitteldeutsch Hausarzt, 2: 20-22.

Krauzlis, R.J., Recasting the smooth pursuit eye movement system. (2004). Journal of Neurophysiology, 91, 591-603.

Krebs, R. M., Woldorff, M. G., Tempelmann, C., Bodammer, N., Noesselt, T., Boehler, C. N., & Schoenfeld, M. A. (2010). High-field FMRI reveals brain activation patterns underlying saccade execution in the human superior colliculus. PLoS One, 5(1), e8691.

Krech, D. (1950). Dynamic systems, psychological fields, and hypothetical constructs. Psychological Review, 57, 283-290.

Kreifelts B, Brück C, Ritter J, Ethofer T, Domin M, Lotze M, Jacob H, Schlipf S, Wildgruber D. (2014) They are laughing at me: cerebral mediation of cognitive biases in social anxiety. PlosOne. 9(6):e99815.

Kreyer, G (1989). Advances in dental psychology. Z Stomatol, 86: 123-130.

Kreyer, G (2000). Psychosomatics of the orofacial system. Wien Med Wochenschr, 150: 213-216.
Kristjánsson, Á. (2007). Saccade landing point selection and the competition account of pro- and antisaccade generation: The involvement of visual attention – A review. Scandinavian Journal of Psychology, 48 (2), 97-113.
Kristjánsson, Á. (2011). The intriguing interactive relationship between visual attention and saccadic eye movements. In S. Everling, I.D. Gilchrist & S. Liversedge (eds), The Oxford Handbook on Eye Movements. Oxford: Oxford University Press.
Kristjánsson, Á., Chen, Y. & Nakayama, K. (2001). Less attention is more in the preparation of antisaccades, but not prosaccades. Nature Neuroscience, 4, 1037–1042.
Krüger F, Barbey AK, Grafman J (2009). The medial prefrontal cortex mediates social event knowledge. Trends Cogn Sci 13: 103-109.
Kruger, K. A. & Serpell, J. A. (2010). Animal-Assisted Interventions in mental health. In A. H. Fine (Ed.), Handbook on Animal-Assisted Therapy. Theoretical Foundations and Guidelines for Practice. Third Edition (pp. 33-48), San Diego: Academic Press.
Krutetskii, V.A. (1968). The Psychology of Mathematical Abilities in Schoolchildren. London: University of Chicago Press.
Kübler, A., Birbaumer, N. (2008). Brain-computer interfaces and communication in paralysis: Extinction of goal directed thinking in completely paralysed patients? Clinical Neurophysiology, 119, 2658-2666.
Kübler, A., Kotchoubey, B., Kaiser, J., Wolpaw, J., Birbaumer, N. (2001). Brain-computer communication: unlocking the locked-in. Psychological Bulletin, 127 (3), 358-375.
Kübler, A., Weber, C. Birbaumer, N. (2006). Locked-in - Freigegeben für den Tod? Wenn nur Denken und Fühlen bleiben – Neuroethik des Eingeschlossenseins. Zeitschrift für medizinische Ethik, 52 (1), 57-70.
Kübler, A., Winter, S., Ludolph, A.C., Hautzinger, M., Birbaumer, N. (2005). Severity of depressive symptoms and quality of life in patients with amyotrophic lateral sclerosis. Neurorehabilitation and Neural Repair, 19 (3), 182-193.
Kucian, K., Grond, U., Rotzer, S., Henzi, B., Schönmann, C., Plangger, F., Galli, M., Martin, E. & Von Aster, M. (2011). Mental number line training in children with developmental dyscalculia. Neuroimage 57, 782–795. doi: 10.1016/j.neuroimage.2011.01.070 Pubmed Abstract | Pubmed Full Text | CrossRef Full Text
Kuhl, J. (1996). Wille und Freiheitserleben: Formen der Selbststeuerung. In: J. Kuhl & H. Heckhausen (Hrsg.) Motivation, Volition und Handlung (S. 665-765). Enzyklopädie der Psychologie. Serie IV Motivation und Emotion. Band 4. Göttingen: Hogrefe.
Kuo W-J, Sjöström T, Chen Y-P, Wang Y-H, Huang C-Y (2009) Intuition and deliberation: two systems for strategizing in the brain. Science 324: 519-522.
Kurata K (1993) Premotor cortex of monkeys: set- and movement-related activity reflecting amplitude and direction of wrist movements. J Neurophysiol. 69:187-200
La Berge, S. (2009). Lucid Dreaming: A Concise Guide to Awakening in Your Dreams and in Your Life. Boulder: Sounds True Inc.
LaBar KS, Crupain MJ, Voyvodic JT, McCarthy G (2003). Dynamic perception of facial affect and identity in the human brain. Cereb Cortex 13:1023-1033.

Lacroix, G., Couret, D., Combaz, X., Prunet, B., Girard, N., & Bruder, N. (2011). Transient locked-in syndrome and basilar artery vasospasm. Neurocritical Care. doi: 10.1007/s12028-011-9655-z

Lahlou, S. (1996). Propagation of social representations. Journal for the Theory of Social Behaviour, 26, 157–175.

Lahlou, S. (1998). Penser-manger. Paris, France: Les Presses Universitaires de France.

Lahlou, S. (2001). Functional aspects of social representations. In K. Deaux & G. Philogene (Eds.), Representations of the social: Bridging theoretical traditions (pp.131–146). Oxford: Blackwell.

Laible M, Grieshammer S, Seidel G, Rijntjes M, Weiller C, Hamzei F. (2012). Association of activity changes in the primary sensory cortex with successful motor rehabilitation of the hand following stroke. Neurorehabil Neural Repair; 26:881-888.

Laimgruber, K., Goldenberg, G., Hermsdörfer, J. (2005). Manual and hemispheric asymmetries in the execution of actual and pantomimed prehension. Neuropsychologia, 43, 682–692.

Lamm C, Batson CD, Decety J (2007). The neural substrate of human empathy: Effects of perspective-taking and cognitive appraisal. J Cogn Neurosci 19: 42-58.

Lancaster, GI, Moller, K, Nielsen, B, Secher, NH, Febbraio, MA, Nybo, L (2004). Exercise induces the release of heat shock protein 72 from the human brain in vivo. Cell Stress Chaperones, 9: 276-280.

Langdon R, Coltheart M (2000). The cognitive neurophysiology of delusions. Mind Language 15: 184-218.

Lanius, R. A., Bluhm, R. L., Coupland, N. J., Hegadoren, K. M., Rowe, B., Theberge, J., Brimson, M. (2010). Default mode network connectivity as a predictor of posttraumatic stress disorder symptom severity in acutely traumatized subjects. Acta Psychiatr Scand, 121(1), 33-40. doi: 10.1111/j.1600-0447.2009.01391.x ACP1391 [pii]

Laplane, D., Degos, J. D. (1983). Motor neglect. Journal of Neurology, Neurosurgery & Psychiatry, 46(2), 152-158.

Laplane D, Talairach J, Meininger V, Bancaud J, Orgogozo JM (1977) Clinical consequences of corticectomies involving the supplementary motor area in man J Neurol Sci 34: 310-314

Laskin, DM, Block, S (1986). Diagnosis and treatment of myofacial pain-dysfunction (MPD) syndrome. J Prosthet Dent, 56: 75–85.

Lau HC1, Rogers RD, Haggard P, Passingham RE (2004) Attention to intention. Science 303:1208-10

Laureys, S., Celesia, G. G., Cohadon, F., Lavrijsen, J., León-Carrión, J., et al. (2010). Unresponsive wakefulness syndrome: A new name for the vegetative state or apallic syndrome? BMC Medicine, 8(68).

Lawrence, D.G., Kuypers, H.G. (1968).The functional organization of the motor system in the monkey. I. The effects of bilateral pyramidal lesions. Brain Mar;91(1):1-14.

Lawrence, D.G., Kuypers, H.G. (1968). The functional organization of the motor system in the monkey. II. The effects of lesions of the descending brain-stem pathways. Brain Mar;91(1):15-36.

Lazarus, A. A. (1981). The practice of multimodal therapy : systematic, comprehensive, effective psychotherapy. New York: McGraw-Hill.

Lawrence EJ, Shaw P, Giampietro VP, Surguladze S, Brammer MJ, David AS (2006). The Role of 'Shared Representations' in Social Perception and Empathy: An Fmri Study. NeuroImage 29: 1173-1184.

Lazarus, R. S. (2000). Towards better research on stress and coping. American Psychologist, 55, 665-673.

Lechner, SK, Roessler, D (2001). Strategies for complete denture success: beyond techniqual excellence. Compend Contin Educ Dent, 22: 553-559.

Lee, J.-H., Marzelli, M., Jolesz, F. A., & Yoo, S.-S. (2010). Mind reading: An automated classification of thought processes from imagery fMRI data. Proc. International Conference on Machine Learning and Cybernetics, 2010 (ICMLC), (pp. 3174-3179). Qingdao, China. doi:10.1109/ICMLC.2010.5580708.

Lehner, P. N. (1998). Handbook of ethological methods. Cambridge, UK: Cambridge University Press.

Leigh, R. J. & Zee, D. S. (1999). The neurology of eye movements (3rd edn). Oxford: Oxford University Press.

Leigh, R. J. & Zee, D. S. (2011). The neurology of eye movements (4th edn). Oxford: Oxford University Press.

Lekwuwa, G. U., & Barnes, G. R. (1996). Cerebral control of eye movements I. The relationship between cerebral lesion sites and smooth pursuit deficits. Brain, 119(2), 473-490.

Leon-Carrion, J., Martin-Rodriguez, J. F., Damas-Lopez, J., Barroso y Martin, J. M., & Dominguez-Morales, M. R. (2008). Brain function in minimally conscious state: A quantitative neurophysiological study. Clinical Neurophysiology, 119 (7), 1506-1514.

Lerner, Y., Honey, C. J., Silbert, L. J., & Hasson, U. (2011). Topographic mapping of a hierarchy of temporal receptive windows using a narrated story. Journal of Neuroscience, 31 (8), 2906–2915.

Leslie KR, Johnson-Frey SH, Grafton ST (2004). Functional imaging of face and hand imitation: towards a motor theory of empathy. Neuroimage 21: 601-607.

Leung, K., & Bond, M. H. (1989). On the empirical identification of dimensions for cross-cultural comparisons. Journal of Cross Cultural Psychology, 20, 133-151.

Levine, D., Marziali, E., & Hood, J. (1997). Emotion processing in borderline personality disorders. J Nerv Ment Dis, 185(4), 240-246.

Levy, R., & Goldman-Rakic, P. S. (2000). Segregation of working memory functions within the dorsolateral prefrontal cortex. In Executive Control and the Frontal Lobe: Current Issues (pp. 23-32). Springer Berlin Heidelberg.

Lewin, K. (1936). Principles of topological psychology. New York, NY: McGraw-Hill.

Ley, J. M., Bennett, P. C. & Coleman, G. J. (2008). Personality dimensions that emerge in companion canines. Applied Animal Behaviour Science, 110, 305–317.

Lhermitte, F. (1983). 'Utilization behaviour'and its relation to lesions of the frontal lobes. Brain, 106(2), 237-255.

Lhermitte, F., Pillon, B., & Serdaru, M. (1986). Human autonomy and the frontal lobes. Part I: Imitation and utilization behavior: a neuropsychological study of 75 patients. Annals of neurology, 19(4), 326-334.

Li, W., Moallem, I., Paller, K. A. & Gottfried, J. A. (2007). Subliminal smells can guide social preferences. Psychological Science, 18, 1044-1049.

Li Y, Rinne JO, Mosconi L, Pirraglia E, Rusinek H, DeSanti S, Kemppainen N, Nagren K, Kim BC, Tsui W, de Leon MJ (2008). Regional analysis of FDG and PIB-PET images in normal aging, mild cognitive impairment, and Alzheimer's disease. Eur J Nucl Med Mol Imaging, 35(12):2169-2181.

Liberman, A.M., Cooper, F.S. Shankweiler, D.P., Studdert-Kennedy, M. (1967). Perception of the speech code. Psychol Rev 74:431–61.

Libet, B. (1965). Cortical activation in conscious and unconscious experience. Perspectives in Biology and Medicine 9:77-86

Libet, B. (1985). Unconscious cerebral initiative and the role of conscious will in voluntary action. Cognition 88, 528.

Libet, B. (2004). Haben wir einen freien Willen? In: Geyer, Christian (Ed.): Hirnforschung und Willensfreiheit. Zur Deutung der neuesten Experimente (pp. 268-290). Frankfurt am Main: Suhrkamp.

Lieb, K., Zanarini, M. C., Schmahl, C., Linehan, M. M., & Bohus, M. (2004). Borderline personality disorder. [Research Support, Non-U.S. Gov't Research Support, U.S. Gov't, P.H.S. Review]. Lancet, 364(9432), 453-461. doi: 10.1016/S0140-6736(04)16770-6

Liégeois, F., Morgan, A.T., Stewart, L.H., Helen Cross, J., Vogel, A.P., Vargha-Khadem, F. (2010). Speech and oral motor profile after childhood hemispherectomy. Brain Lang Aug;114(2):126-34. doi: 10.1016/j.bandl.2009.12.004. Epub 2010 Jan 21.

Liepert J, Bauder H, Wolfgang HR, MiltnerWH, Taub E, Weiller C. (2000). Treatment-induced cortical reorganisation after stroke in humans. Stroke; 31:1210-1216.

Liepmann, H. (1920). Apraxia. Ergbn. Ges. Med., 1, 516-54.

Ligier, S, Stenberg, EM (2000) Immune response. In G. Fink (Ed. in chief), Encyclopedia of stress. /vol. 2./ (pp. 523-530). Academic Press, San Diego.

Lindenberg R, Uhlig M, Scherfeld D, Schlaug G, Seitz RJ (2012) Communication with emblematic gestures: Shared and distinct neural correlates of expression and reception. Human Brain Mapp 33: 812-823.

Linehan, M. M. (1993). Cognitive–behavioral treatment of borderline personality disorder. New York: Guilford Press.

Linehan, M. M., Tutek, D. A., Heard, H. L., & Armstrong, H. E. (1994). Interpersonal outcome of cognitive behavioral treatment for chronically suicidal borderline patients. Am J Psychiatry, 151(12), 1771-1776.

Lis, E., Greenfield, B., Henry, M., Guile, J. M., & Dougherty, G. (2007). Neuroimaging and genetics of borderline personality disorder: a review. [Research Support, Non-U.S. Gov't Review]. J Psychiatry Neurosci, 32(3), 162-173.

Lloyd, B. & Duveen, G. (1992). Gender identities and education: The impact of starting school. London: Harvester-Wheatsheaf.

Logothetis NK, Guggenberger H, Peled S, Pauls J (1999) Functional imaging of the monkey brain. Nat. Neurosci. 2: 555-562.

Logothetis N, Pauls J, Augath M et al. (2001). Neurophysiological investigation of the basis of the fMRI signal. Nature, 412, 150–157.

Lotze M, Braun C, Birbaumer N, Anders S, Cohen LG. (2003) Motor learning elicited by voluntary drive. Brain. 126(4):886-872.

Lotze M, Heymans U, Birbaumer N, Veit R, Erb M, Flor H, Halsband, U (2006). Differential Cerebral Activation during Observation of Expressive Gestures and Motor Acts. Neuropsychologia 44: 1787-1795.

Lotze M, Reimold M, Heymans U, Laihinen A, Patt M, Halsband U. (2009) Reduced ventrolateral fMRI response during observation of emotional gestures related to reduced dopamine in the putamen. J Cogn Neuroscience. 21:1321-31.

Luauté, J., Maucott-Boulch, D., Tell, L., Quelard, F., Sarraf, T., et al. (2010). Long-term outcomes of chronic minimally conscious and vegetative states. Neurology, 75, 246-252.

Ludascher, P., Bohus, M., Lieb, K., Philipsen, A., Jochims, A., & Schmahl, C. (2007). Elevated pain thresholds correlate with dissociation and aversive arousal in patients with borderline personality disorder. Psychiatry Res, 149(1-3), 291-296. doi: S0165-1781(06)00047-3 [pii] 10.1016/j.psychres.2005.04.009

Lüdecke, Christel, Sachsse, Ulrich, Faure, Hendrik (Eds.). (2010). Sucht, Bindung, Trauma. Stuttgaart: Schattauer.

Ludolph, A. C., Langen, K. J., Regard, M., Herzog, H., Kemper, B., et al. (1992). Frontal lobe function in amyotrophic lateral sclerosis: A neuropsychologic and positron emission tomographic study. Acta Neurologica Scandinavica, 85, 81-89.

Lüdtke, F. (1911). Kritische Geschichte der Apperzeptionsbegriffe. Zeitschrift für Philosophie und philosophische Kritik, 141, 41-135.

Lulé, D., Häcker, S., Ludolph, A., Birbaumer, N., Kübler, A. (2008). Depression und Lebensqualität bei Patienten mit amyotropher Lateralsklerose. Deutsches Ärzteblatt, 105 (23), 397-403.

Lulé, D., Pauli, S., Altintas, E., Singer, U., Merk, T., Uttner, I., Birbaumer, N., Ludolph, A. (2012). Emotional adjustment in amyotrophic lateral sclerosis (ALS). Journal of Neurology, 259, 334-341.

Lulé, D, Zickler C, Bruno MA, Demertzi A, Pellas F, Laureys S, Kübler A (2009). Life can be worth living in locked-in syndrome. Progress in Brain Research, 177, 339–351.

Luo Q, Holroyd T, Majestic C, Cheng X, Schechter J, Blair RJ (2010) Emotional automaticity is a matter of timing. J Neurosci 30: 5825-5829.

Luppino G, Matelli M, Camarda RM, Gallese V, Rizzolatti G (1991) Multiple representations of body movements in mesial area 6 and the adjacent cingulate cortex: an intracortical microstimulation study in the macaque monkey. J Comp Neurol. 311:463-82

Luria AR (1966) Human Brain and Psychological processes. Harper & Row

Lusseyran, J. (1990). Das Leben beginnt heute (5. Edition. Stuttgart: Klett-Cotta.

Lyons, I.M., Ansari, D. & Beilock, S.L. (2015). Qualitatively different coding of symbolic and nonsymbolic numbers in the human brain. Human Brain Mapping, 36, 475-488.

Maas, H. & Spinath, F. M. (2012). Persönlichkeit und Gesundheit. Eine Zwillingsstudie zur Betrachtung möglicher Mediatoren. Zeitschrift für Gesundheitspsychologie, 20, 129-140.

Macar F, Vidal F, Casini L (1999) The supplementary motor area in motor and sensory timing: evidence from slow brain potential changes. Exp Brain Res. 125:271-80

MacAvoy, M. G., Gottlieb, J. P., & Bruce, C. J. (1991). Smooth-pursuit eye movement representation in the primate frontal eye field. Cerebral Cortex, 1(1), 95-102.

MacDonald AW 3rd, Cohen JD, Stenger VA, Carter CS (2000) Dissociating the role of the dorsolateral prefrontal and anterior cingulate cortex in cognitive control. Science. 288:1835-8

Machado, L., & Rafal, R. D. (2004). Control of fixation and saccades during an anti-saccade task: an investigation in humans with chronic lesions of oculomotor cortex. Experimental Brain Research, 156(1), 55-63.

MacKay, D. G., Stewart, R., & Burke, D. M. (1998). HM revisited: Relations between language comprehension, memory, and the hippocampal system. Journal of Cognitive Neuroscience, 10(3), 377-394.

MacManus I.C. (2005). Symmetry and asymmetry in aesthetics and the arts. European Review, 13, 157-180.

Maier MA, Armand J, Kirkwood PA, Yang HW, Davis JN, Lemon RN (2002) Differences in the corticospinal projection from primary motor cortex and supplementary motor area to macaque upper limb motoneurons: an anatomical and electrophysiological study. Cereb Cortex 12:281-96

Mandler, G. (1980). Recognizing—the judgment of previous occurrence. Psychological Review, 87, 252-271.

Mangels, J. A., Picton, T. W., & Craik, F. I. (2001). Attention and successful episodic encoding: an event-related potential study. Brain Research: Cognitive Brain Research, 11(1), 77-95.

Marchetti, C. & Sala, S.D. (1998). Disentangling the alien and anarchic hand. Cognitive Neuropsychiatry, 3(3), 191-207.

Mark, V. W. (1996). Motor neglect: What do we mean? Neurology, 46(5), 1492–1493.

Markl, A., Yu, T., Vogel, D., Müller, F., Kotchoubey, B., & Lang, S. (2013). Brain processing of pain in patients with unresponsive wakefulness syndrome. Brain and Behavior, 2, doi: 10.1002/brb1003.1110.

Markowitsch, H. J. (1996). Der Netzwerkbegriff – historisch beleuchtet. In: M. Lasar (Hrsg.). Netzwerktheorie. Möglichkeiten für die psychiatrische Wissenschaft S. 9-31). Lengerich: Pabst.

Markowitsch, H, J. (1999). Entstehung und Begründung einer neurowissenschaftlich begründeten Psychologie. Zeitschrift für Psychologie, 207, 383-398.

Mars RB, Jbabdi S, Sallet J, O'Reilly JX, Croxson PL, Olivier E, Noonan MP, Bergmann C, Mitchell AS, Baxter MG, Behrens TE, Johansen-Berg H, Tomassini V, Miller KL, Rushworth MF. (2011). Diffusion-weighted imaging tractography-based parcellation of the human parietal cortex and comparison with human and macaque resting-state functional connectivity. J Neurosci 31: 4087-4100.

Marstaller L, Burianová H. (2015) A common functional neural network for overt production of speech and gesture. Neuroscience. 284:29-41.

Martin, P. & Bateson. P. (2007) Measuring behaviour: An introductory guide (3rd ed). Cambridge: Cambridge University Press.

Marxkors, R, Müller-Fahlbusch, H (1981). Zur Diagnose psychosomatischer Störungen in der zahnarztlich-prothetischen Praxis. Dtsch Zahnarztl Z, 36: 787–790.

Matsumoto K, Suzuki W, Tanaka K (2003) Neuronal correlates of goal-based motor selection in the prefrontal cortex. Science. 301:229-32

Matsuzaka Y, Aizawa H, Tanji J (1992) A motor area rostral to the supplementary motor area (presupplementary motor area) in the monkey: neuronal activity during a learned motor task. J Neurophysiol. 68:653-662

Matsuzaka Y, Tanji J (1996) Changing directions of forthcoming arm movements: neuronal activity in the presupplementary and supplementary motor area of monkey cerebral cortex. J Neurophysiol. 76:2327-2342

Mattingley, J.B., Driver, J. (1997). Distinguishing Sensory and motor deficits after parietal damage: an evaluation of response selection biases in unilateral neglect. In P. Their and H.-O. Karnath (Eds.), Parietal Contributions to Orientationin 3D Space (pp. 309–333). Heidelberg: Springer.

Mattingley, J. B., Husain, M., Rorden, C., Kennard, C., & Driver, J. (1998). Motor role of human inferior parietal lobe revealed in unilateral neglect patients. Nature, 392(6672), 179-182.

Matuz, T., Birbaumer, N., Hautzinger, M., Kübler, A. (2010). Coping with amyotrophic lateral sclerosis: an integrative view. Journal of Neurology, Neurosurgery, and Psychiatry, 81, 893-898.

Maunder, R. G., Hunter, J. J. (2008). Attachment relationships as determinants of physical health. Journal of the American Academy of Psychoanalysis and Dynamic Psychiatry, 36, 11-32.

Mayes, A., Montaldi, D., Migo, E. (2007). Associative memory and the medial temporal lobes. Trends in Cognitive Sciences, 11(3), 126-135.

Mayes, A. R., Holdstock, J. S., Isaac, C. L., Hunkin, N. M., & Roberts, N. (2002). Relative sparing of item recognition memory in a patient with adult-onset damage limited to the hippocampus. Hippocampus, 12, 325–340.

Mazurat, NM, Mazurat, RD (2003/a). Discuss before fabricating: Communicating the realities of partial denture therapy. Part I: Patient expectations. J Can Dent Assoc, 69: 90-94.

Mazurat, NM, Mazurat, RD (2003/b). Discuss before fabricating: Communicating the realities of partial denture therapy. Part II: Clinical outcomes. J Can Dent Assoc, 69: 90-94.

McAdams, D. P. (1985). Power, intimacy, and the life story: Personological inquiries into identity. New York, NY: Guilford.

McCann, SM (2000). Nitric oxide. In G. Fink (Ed. in chief, Encyclopedia of stress. /vol. 3./ (pp. 53-61). Academic Press, San Diego.

McCarthy, G., Nobre, A. C., Bentin, S., & Spencer, D. D. (1995). Language-related field potentials in the anterior-medial temporal lobe: I. Intracranial distribution and neural generators. Journal of Neuroscience, 15, 1080–1089.

McCloskey, M. (1992). Cognitive mechanisms in numerical processing: evidence from acquired dyscalculia. Cognition, 44, 107-157.

McCrae, R. R., Terracciano, A., Realo, A., & Allik, J. (2007a). Climatic warmth and national wealth: Some culture-level determinants of national character stereotypes. European Journal of Personality, 21, 953–976.

McCrae, R. R., Terracciano, A., Realo, A., & Allik, J. (2007b). On the validity of culture-level personality and stereotypes scores. European Journal of Personality, 21, 987–991.

McCrae, R.R., Terracciano, A., & 79 Members of the Personality Profiles of Cultures Project (2005). Personality profiles of cultures: Aggregate personality traits. Journal of Personality and Social Psychology, 89, 407–425.

McKhann GM, Knopman DS, Chertkow H, Hyman BT, Jack CR Jr, Kawas CH, Klunk WE, Koroshetz WJ, Manly JJ, Mayeux R, Mohs RC, Morris JC, Rossor MN, Scheltens P, Carrillo MC, Thies B, Weintraub S, Phelps CH (2011). The diagnosis of dementia due to Alzheimer's disease: recommendations from the National Institute on Aging-Alzheimer's Association workgroups on diagnostic guidelines for Alzheimer's disease. Alzheimers Dement, 7(3):263-269.

McNeil, J.E. and Warrington, E.K. (1993). A modality-specific case of dyscalculia. Journal of Clinical and Experimental Psychology, 15, 415.

McNeil, J.E. & Warrington E.K. (1994). A dissociation between addition and subtraction with written calculation. Neuropsychologia, 32, 717-728.

Mecklinger, A. (2000). Interfacing mind and brain: a neurocognitive model of recognition memory. Psychophysiology, 37, 565–582.

Mecklinger, A. (2006). Electrophysiological measures of familiarity memory. Clincal EEG and Neuroscience, 37, 292–299.

Mehl, M. R., Vazire, S., Ramírez-Esparza, N., Slatcher, R. B., & Pennebaker, J. W. (2007). Are women really more talkative than men? Science, 317, 82.

Meischner-Metge, A. (2003). Wilhelm Wundt und seine Schüler. In: H.-P. Brauns (Hrsg.). Zentenarbetrachtungen. Historische Entwicklungen in der neueren Psychologie bis zum Ende des 20. Jahrhunderts (S. 156-166). Frankfurt a.M.: Peter Lang.

Meltzoff AN, Decety J (2003). What imitation tells us about social cognition: a rapprochement between developmental psychology and cognitive neuroscience. Phil Trans R Soc Lond B 358: 491-500.

Mende, E. M. & Mende, M. (2011). Integratins animals in psychotherapy: the dog as co-therapist in the hypnotherapeutic treatment of trauma – a case report. Contemporary Hypnosis and Integrative Therapy, 28, 8-16.

Menon, G., & Yorkston, E. A. (2000). The use of memory and contextual cues in the formation of behavioral frequency judgments. In A. A. Stone, J. S. Turkkan, C. A. Bachrach, J. B. Jobe, H. S. Kurtzman & V. S. Cain (Eds.) The science of self-report, (pp. 63-79). Mahwah, NJ: Lawrence Erlbaum Associates, Publishers.

Menon, V., Rivera, S.M., White, C.D., Eliez, S., Glover, G.H. and Reiss, A.L. (2000). Functional optimization of arithmetic processing in perfect performers. Cognitive Brain Research, 9, 343-345.

Mériau K, Wartenburger I, Kazzer P, Prehn P, Lammers C, van der Meer E et al (2006). A neural network reflecting individual differences in cognitive processing of emotions during perceptual decision-making. Neuroimage 33:1016-27.

Merten K, Nieder A (2013) Comparison of abstract decision encoding in the monkey prefrontal cortex, the presupplementary, and cingulate motor areas. J Neurophysiol 110: 19-32

Messier J, Kalaska JF (2000) Covariation of primate dorsal premotor cell activity with direction and amplitude during a memorized-delay reaching task. J Neurophysiol. 84:152-65

Mesulam M. M. (1981). A cortical network for directed attention and unilateral neglect. Ann Neurol., 10 (4), 309-325.

Mesulam M (2008). Representation, inference, and transcendent encoding in neurocognitive networks of the human brain. Ann Neurol 64: 367-378.

Mesulam MM, van Hoesen GW, Pandya DN, Geschwind N. (1977). Limbic and sensory connections of the inferior parietal lobule (area PG) in the rhesus monkey: a study with a new method for horseradish peroxidase histochemistry. Brain Res 136: 393-414.

Mesulam, M. M. (1999). Spatial attention and neglect: parietal, frontal and cingulate contributions to the mental representation and attentional targeting of salient extrapersonal events. Phil. Trans. R. Soc. Lond. B, 354 (1387), 1325-1346.

Mesulam, M.M. (1981). A cortical network for directed attention and unilateral neglect. Ann. Neurol. Oct;10(4):309-25.

Metzinger, T. (2005). Bewusstsein. Beiträge aus der Gegenwartsphilosophie. Paderborn: mentis Verlag.
Metzinger, T. (2011). Der Ego-Tunnel: Eine neue Philosophie des Selbst: Von der Hirnforschung zur Bewusstseinsethik (2. Auflage). Berlin: BvT Berliner Taschenbuch Verlag.
Metzinger, Th. (Hrsg.). (1996). Bewusstsein (3. Aufl.). Paderborn: Schöningh.
Meyer, P., Feldkamp, H., Hoppstädter, M., King, A. V., Frölich, L., Wessa, M., & Flor, H. (2013). Using voxel-based morphometry to examine the relationship between regional brain volumes and memory performance in amnestic mild cognitive impairment. Frontiers in behavioral neuroscience, 7.
Meyer, P., Mecklinger, A., Friederici, A. D. (2007). Bridging the gap between the semantic N400 and the early old/new memory effect. NeuroReport, 18, 109-113.
Meyer, P., Mecklinger, A., Friederici, A.D. (2010). On the processing of semantic aspects of experience in the anterior medial temporal lobe. An event-related fMRI study. Journal of Cognitive Neuroscience, 22, 590-601.
Meyer, P., Mecklinger, A., Grunwald, T., Fell, J. Elger, C. E., & Friederici, A. D. (2005). Language processing within the human medial temporal lobe. Hippocampus, 15, 451-459.
Meynert, Th. (1871). Vom Gehirn der Säugetiere. In. S. Stricker (Hrsg.). Handbuch der Lehre von den Geweben der Menschen und Tiere. Leipzig: Engelmann.
Michell, J. (2011). Qualitative research meets the ghost of Pythagoras. Theory & Psychology, 21, 241-259.
Michell, J., (2012). The constantly recurring argument: Inferring quantity from order. Theory & Psychology, 22, 255-271.
Middleton FA, Strick PL. (1996) The temporal lobe is a target of output from the basal ganglia. Proc Natl Acad Sci U S A. 93(16):8683-8687.
Miklósi, Á. (2007). Dog Behaviour, Evolution and Cognition. Oxford: University Press.
Miller G (2012). Alzheimer's research. Stopping Alzheimer's before it starts. Science, 337(6096):790-792.
Millikan, R. (1993). White queen psychology and other essays for Alice. Bradford: MIT Press.
Milner AD, Goodale MA (1995) The visual brain in action. Oxford University press
Minoshima S, Giordani B, Berent S, Frey KA, Foster NL, Kuhl DE (1997). Metabolic reduction in the posterior cingulate cortex in very early Alzheimer's disease. Ann Neurol, 42:85–94.
Mintun MA, LaRossa GN, Sheline YI, Dence CS, Lee SY, Mach RH, Klunk WE, Mathis CA, DeKosky ST, Morris JC (2006). [11C]PIB in a nondemented population: potential antecedent marker of Alzheimer disease. Neurology, 67:446–452.
Minzenberg, M. J., Fan, J., New, A. S., Tang, C. Y., & Siever, L. J. (2007). Fronto-limbic dysfunction in response to facial emotion in borderline personality disorder: an event-related fMRI study. [Research Support, N.I.H., Extramural Research Support, Non-U.S. Gov't Research Support, U.S. Gov't, Non-P.H.S.]. Psychiatry Res, 155(3), 231-243. doi: 10.1016/j.pscychresns.2007.03.006
Mischel, W. (1968). Personality and assessment. New York, NY: Wiley.
Mischel, W. (1977). The interaction of person and situation. In: D. Magnusson, & N. S. Endler (Eds.). Personality at the crossroads: Current issues in interactional psychology, (pp. 333-352). Hillsdale, NJ: Erlbaum.

Mischel, W., Shoda, Y. (1995). A cognitive-affective system theory of personality: Reconceptualizing situations, dispositions, dynamics, and invariance in personality structure. Psychological Review, 102, 246-268.

Mischel, W., Shoda, Y., Ayduk, O. (2007). Introduction to personality: Toward an integrative science of the person (8th ed.). Hoboken, NJ: J. Wiley & Sons.

Mischel, W., Shoda, Y., Mendoza-Denton, R. (2002). Situation-behavior profiles as a locus of consistency in personality. Current Directions in Psychological Science, 11, 50-54.

Mishkin, M., & Ungerleider, L. G. (1982). Contribution of striate inputs to the visuospatial functions of parieto-preoccipital cortex in monkeys. Behavioural Brain Research, 6 (1): 57–77.

Mishkin, M., Ungerleider, L. G., & Macko, K. A. (1983) Object vision and spatial vision: two cortical pathways. Trends Neurosci, 6, 414–417

Mita A, Mushiake H, Shima K, Matsuzaka Y, Tanji J (2009) Interval time coding by neurons in the presupplementary and supplementary motor areas. Nat Neurosci. 12:502-507

Mohler, C. W., & Wurtz, R. H. (1976). Organization of monkey superior colliculus: intermediate layer cells discharging before eye movements. Journal of Neurophysiology, 39(4), 722-744.

Mokrushin, A, Pavlinova, L (2008). Heat shock protein (Hsp70) modifies evoked activity of olfactory cortex cells in vitro and protects them from acute anoxia, from glutamate excitotoxicity and epilepsy. In E. Morel, C. Vinvent (Eds.), Heat Shock Proteins: New research. (pp. 275-297). Nova Science Publisher, New York.

Molenaar, P. C. (2004). A manifesto on psychology as idiographic science: Bringing the person back into scientific psychology, this time forever. Measurement: Interdisciplinary Research and Perspectives, 2, 201–218.

Montaldi, D., & Mayes, A. R. (2010). The role of recollection and familiarity in the functional differentiation of the medial temporal lobes. Hippocampus 20, 1291-1314.

Montaldi, D., Spencer, T. J., Roberts, N., & Mayes, A. R. (2006). The neural system that mediates familiarity memory. Hippocampus, 16, 504–520.

Monti, M. M., Vanhaudenhuyse, A., Coleman, M. R., Boly, M., Pickard, J. D., et al. (2010). Willful modulation of brain activity in disorders of consciousness. New England Journal of Medicine, 362, 579-589.

Moody EJ, McIntosh DN, Mann LJ, Weisser KR (2007). More than mere mimicry? The influence of emotion on rapid facial reactions to faces. Emotion 7: 447-457.

Moore JW, Ruge D, Wenke D, Rothwell J, Haggard P (2010) Disrupting the experience of control in the human brain: pre-supplementary motor area contributes to the sense of agency. Proc Biol Sci 277: 2503-2509.

Moore, R, Birn, H (1990). Phenomenon of dental fear. Danish Dental Journal, 94: 34-41.

Moore, R, Birn, H, Kirkegaard, E, Brodsgaard, I, Scheutz, F (1993). Prevalence and characteristic of dental anxiety in Danish adults. Com Dent Oral Epidemiol, 21: 292-296.

Morbelli S, Perneczky R, Drzezga A, Frisoni GB, Caroli A, van Berckel BN, Ossenkoppele R, Guedj E, Didic M, Brugnolo A, Naseri M, Sambuceti G, Pagani M, Nobili F (2013). Metabolic networks underlying cognitive reserve in prodromal Alzheimer disease: a European Alzheimer disease consortium project. J Nucl Med, 54(6):894-902.

Morecraft RJ, Cipolloni PB, Stilwell-Morecraft KS, Gedney MT, Pandya DN (2004) Cytoarchitecture and cortical connections of the posterior cingulate and adjacent somatosensory fields in the rhesus monkey. J Comp Neurol. 469:37-69

Morecraft RJ1, Van Hoesen GW (1992) Cingulate input to the primary and supplementary motor cortices in the rhesus monkey: evidence for somatotopy in areas 24c and 23c. J Comp Neurol 322:471-489

Morewedge CK, Kahneman D (2010) Associative processes in intuitive judgment. Trends Cogn Sci 14: 435-440

Mori, E., & Yamadori, A. (1982). Compulsive manipulation of tools and pathological grasp phenomenon. Rinshō shinkeigaku = Clinical neurology, 22(4), 329.

Morris JC, Blennow K, Froelich L, Nordberg A, Soininen H, Waldemar G, Wahlund LO, Dubois B (2014). Harmonized diagnostic criteria for Alzheimer's disease: recommendations. J Intern Med, 275(3):204-213.

Morris, RG (2001). 'Theory of Mind' Impairments and Their Relationship to Executive Functioning Following Frontal Lobe Excisions. Brain 124: 600-616.

Morrow, M. J., & Sharpe, J. A. (1995). Deficits of smooth-pursuit eye movement after unilateral frontal lobe lesions. Annals of neurology, 37(4), 443-451.

Mort, D. J., Perry, R. J., Mannan, S. K., Hodgson, T. L., Anderson, E., Quest, R., McRobbie, D., McBride, S., Husain, M. & Kennard, C. (2003). Differential cortical activation during voluntary and reflexive saccades in man. Neuroimage, 18(2), 231-246.

Moschovakis, A. K. (1996). The superior colliculus and eye movement control. Current opinion in neurobiology, 6(6), 811-816.

Mosconi L (2005). Brain glucose metabolism in the early and specific diagnosis of Alzheimer's disease. FDG-PET studies in MCI and AD. Eur J Nucl Med Mol Imaging, 32:486–510.

Mosconi L, Perani D, Sorbi S, Herholz K, Nacmias B, Holthoff V, Salmon E, Baron JC, De Cristofaro MT, Padovani A, Borroni B, Franceschi M, Bracco L, Pupi A (2004). MCI conversion to dementia and the APOE genotype: a prediction study with FDG-PET. Neurology, 63(12):2332-2340.

Mosconi L, Rinne JO, Tsui WH, Murray J, Li Y, Glodzik L, McHugh P, Williams S, Cummings M, Pirraglia E, Goldsmith SJ, Vallabhajosula S, Scheinin N, Viljanen T, Någren K, de Leon MJ (2013). Amyloid and metabolic positron emission tomography imaging of cognitively normal adults with Alzheimer's parents. Neurobiol Aging, 34(1)22-34.

Mosconi L, Tsui WH, De SS, Li J, Rusinek H, Convit A, Li Y, Boppana M, de Leon MJ (2005). Reduced hippocampal metabolism in MCI and AD: automated FDG-PET image analysis. Neurology, 64(11):1860-1867.

Mosconi L, Tsui WH, Herholz K, Pupi A, Drzezga A, Lucignani G, Reiman EM, Holthoff V, Kalbe E, Sorbi S, Diehl-Schmid J, Perneczky R, Clerici F, Caselli R, Beuthien-Baumann B, Kurz A, Minoshima S, de Leon MJ (2008). Multicenter standardized 18F-FDG PET diagnosis of mild cognitive impairment, Alzheimer's disease, and other dementias. J Nucl Med, 49(3):390-398.

Moser, D., Baker, J. M., Sanchez, C. E., Rorden, C., & Fridriksson, J. (2009). Temporal Order Processing of Syllables in the Left Parietal Lobe. The Journal of Neuroscience, 29 (40), 12568-12573.

Motomura, S. (1990). Compulsive manipulation of tools after left anterior cerebral artery infarction. Neurology, Cleveland, Supplement 1, 302.

Moulton, R, Ewen, S, Thieman, W (1957). Emotional factors in periodontal disease. Oral Surg Oral Med Oral Pathol, 5: 833-860.

Mountz, JM. (2007). Nuclear medicine in the rehabilitative treatment evaluation in stroke recovery. Role of diaschisis resolution and cerebral reorganization. Eura Medicophys; 43(2):221-239

Muakkassa KF, Strick PL (1979) Frontal lobe inputs to primate motor cortex: evidence for four somatotopically organized 'premotor' areas. Brain Res. 177:176-182

Müller, U., Fletcher, P. C. & Steinberg, H. (2006). The Origin of Pharmacopsychology: Emil Kraepelin's Experiments in Leipzig, Dorpat and Heidelberg (1882-1892). Psychopharmacology, 184 (2), 131-138.

Müller-Fahlbusch, H, Sone, K (1982). Präprotetische Psychagogik. Dtsch Zahnärztl Z, 37: 703-707.

Munakata, Y, Kasai, S (1992). Contribution of the mucosal tactile information to the mandibular position sense in patients wearing dentures. J Oral Rehabil, 19: 649-654.

Munk, H. (1881). Ueber die Functionen der Grosshirnrinde. Berlin: Hirschwald.

Munoz, D. P., & Everling, S. (2004). Look away: the anti-saccade task and the voluntary control of eye movement. Nature Reviews Neuroscience, 5(3), 218-228.

Munro, RR (1975). Electromyography of the muscles of mastication. In: CJ. Griffin, R. Harris (Eds.), The temporomandibular joint syndrome. The masticatory apparatus of man in normal and abnormal function. /Monographs in oral science, Vol. 4./ (pp. 87-116). Karger, Basel - München - Paris - London - New York - Sydney.

Munte TF, Troger MC, Nusser I et al. (1998). Alteration of early components of the visual evoked potential in amyotrophic lateral sclerosis. Journal of Neurology, 245, 206–210.

Murata A, Fadiga L, Fogassi L, Gallese V, Raos V, Rizzolatti G (1997) Object representation in the ventral premotor cortex (area F5) of the monkey. J Neurophysiol 78: 2226-2230

Murphy ST, Zajonc RB (1993). Affect, cognition, and awareness: Affective priming with optimal and suboptimal stimulus exposures. J Pers Soc Psychol: 64: 723-739.

Murray, E. A. (1996). What have ablation studies told us about the neural substrates of stimulus memory? Seminars in the Neurosciences, 5, 10–20.

Murray, E. A., & Bussey, T. J. (1999). Perceptual-mnemonic functions of the perirhinal cortex. Trends in Cognitive Sciences, 3(4), 142-151.

Murray EA, Davidson M, Gaffan D, Olton DS, Suomi S (1989) Effects of fornix transection and cingulate cortical ablation on spatial memory in rhesus monkeys. Exp Brain Res. 74:173-86

Murray, E. A., Malkova, L., & Goulet, S. (1998). Crossmodal associations, intramodal associations, and object identification. In A. D. Milner (Ed.), Comparative neuropsychology (pp. 51–69). Oxford, UK: Oxford University Press.

Murray-Close, D., & Ostrov, J. M. (2009). A longitudinal study of forms and functions of aggressive behavior in early childhood. Child Development, 80, 828-842.

Nachev, P., Husain, M., & Kennard, C. (2008). Volition and eye movements. Progress in Brain research, 171, 391-398.

Nachev P, Kennard C, Husain M (2008). Functional role of the supplementary and pres-supplementary motor areas. Nat Rev Neurosci 9: 856-869.

Nagasawa, M., Kikusui, T., Onaka, T., & Ohta, M. (2009). Dog's gaze at its owner increases owner's urinary oxytocin during social interaction. Hormones and Behavior, 55, 434-441.

Nakamura K, Roesch MR, Olson CR (2005) Neuronal activity in macaque SEF and ACC during performance of tasks involving conflict. J Neurophysiol. 93:884-908
Nakamura K, Sakai K, Hikosaka O (1998) Neuronal activity in medial frontal cortex during learning of sequential procedures. J Neurophysiol. 80:2671-87
Nakamura K, Sakai K, Hikosaka O (1999) Effects of local inactivation of monkey medial frontal cortex in learning of sequential procedures. J Neurophysiol 82:1063-8
Nakayama Y, Yamagata T, Tanji J, Hoshi E (2008) Transformation of a virtual action plan into a motor plan in the premotor cortex. J Neurosci. 28:10287-97
Nasse, F. (1822). Grundzüge der Lehre von dem Verhältnis zwischen Seele und Leib in Gesundheit und Krankheit. Zeitschrift für psychische Ärzte, 5, (1), 1-35.
Neal JW, Pearson RCA, Powell TPS. (1990a). The ipsilateral cortico-cortical connections of area 7b, PF, in the parietal and temporal lobes of the monkey. Brain Res 524: 119-132.
Neal JW, Pearson RCA, Powell TPS. (1990b). The connections of area PG, 7a, with cortex in the parietal, occipital, and temporal lobes of the monkey. Brain Res 532: 249-264.
Nessler, D., Mecklinger, A., & Penney, T. B. (2001). Event related brain potentials and illusory memories: the effects of differential encoding. Cognitive Brain Research, 10, 283–301.
Nessler, D., Mecklinger, A., & Penney, T. B. (2005). Perceptual fluency, semantic familiarity and recognition-related familiarity: an electrophysiological exploration. Cognitive Brain Research, 22(2), 265-288.
Nestor PJ, Fryer TD, Smielewski P, Hodges JR (2003). Limbic hypometabolism in Alzheimer's disease and mild cognitive impairment. Ann Neurol, 54:343–351.
Neumann, N., & Kotchoubey, B. (2004). Assessment of cognitive functions in severely paralysed and severely brain-damaged patients: Neuropsychological and electrophysiological techniques. Brain Research Protocols, 14, 25-36.
Neumann, O. (1971). Aufmerksamkeit. In: J. Ritter et al. (Hrsg.) Historisches Wörterbuch der Philosophie. Band 1. (S. 635-645). Darmstadt: WBG.
Ngandu T, Lehtisalo J, Solomon A, Levälahti E, Ahtiluoto S, Antikainen R, Bäckman L, Hänninen T, Jula A, Laatikainen T, Lindström J, Mangialasche F, Paajanen T, Pajala S, Peltonen M, Rauramaa R, Stigsdotter-Neely A, Strandberg T, Tuomilehto J, Soininen H, Kivipelto M. A 2 year multidomain intervention of diet, exercise, cognitive training, and vascular risk monitoring versus control to prevent cognitive decline in at-risk elderly people (FINGER): a randomised controlled trial. Lancet. Mar 11. pii: S0140-6736(15)60461-5.
Nickel J, Seitz RJ (2005). Functional clusters in the human parietal cortex as revealed by an observer-independent meta-analysis of functional activation studies. Anatomy and Embryology 210: 463–472.
Niendam TA, Laird AR, Ray KL, Dean VM, Glahn DC, Carter CS (2012) Meta-analytic evidence for a superordinate cognitive control network subserving diverse executive functions. Cogn Affect Behav Neurosci 12: 241-268.
Nierhaus, T. M., D.; Long, X., Villringer, X. (2012). fMRI for the Assessment of Functional Connectivity P. Bright (Ed.) Neuroimaging - Methods Retrieved from http://www.intechopen.com/books/neuroimaging-methods/fmri-for-the-assessment-of-functional-connectivity
Niki H, Watanabe M (1979) Prefrontal and cingulate unit activity during timing behavior in the monkey. Brain Res. 171:213-24

Nobre, A. C., & McCarthy, G. (1995). Language-related Weld potentials in the anterior-medial temporal lobe: II. Effects of word type and semantic priming. Journal of Neuroscience, 15, 1090–1098.
Nomura M, Ohira H, Haneda K, Iidaka T, Sadato N, Okada T, Yonekura Y (2003). Functional association of the amygdala and ventral prefrontal cortex during cognitive evaluation of facial expressions primed by masked angry faces: An event-related fMRI study. Neuroimage, 21, 352-363.
Nordberg A, Carter SF, Rinne J, Drzezga A, Brooks DJ, Vandenberghe R, Perani D, Forsberg A, Langstrom B, Scheinin N, Karrasch M, Nagren K, Grimmer T, Miederer I, Edison P, Okello A, Van Laere K, Nelissen N, Vandenbulcke M, Garibotto V, Almkvist O, Kalbe E, Hinz R, Herholz K (2013). A European multicentre PET study of fibrillar amyloid in Alzheimer's disease. Eur J Nucl Med Mol Imaging, 40, 104-114.
Norensayan A, Gervais WM, Trzesniewski KH (2012) Mentalizing deficits constrain belief in a personal God. PLOS one 7: e36880.
Norman, K., & O'Reilly, R. (2003). Modeling hippocampal and neocortical contributions to recognition memory: a complementary learning-systems approach. Psychological Review, 110 (4), 611-646.
Odendaal, J. & Meintjes, R. (2003). Neurophysiological correlates of affiliative behaviour between humans and dogs. The Veterinary Journal, 165, 296–301.
Ogden, C. K. (1932). Bentham's theory of fictions. New York: Harcourt Brace.
Ohbayashi M1, Ohki K, Miyashita Y (2003) Conversion of working memory to motor sequence in the monkey premotor cortex. Science. 301:233-236
Okello A, Koivunen J, Edison P, Archer HA, Turkheimer FE, Någren K, Bullock R, Walker Z, Kennedy A, Fox NC, Rossor MN, Rinne JO, Brooks DJ (2009). Conversion of amyloid positive and negative MCI to AD over 3 years. An 11C-PIB PET study. Neurology. 73(10):754-760.
Omi, Y. (2012). Tension between the theoretical thinking and the empirical method: Is it an inevitable fate for psychology? Integrative Psychological and Behavioral Science, 46, 118-127.
O'Neill, A., & Frodl, T. (2012). Brain structure and function in borderline personality disorder. [Review]. Brain Struct Funct, 217(4), 767-782. doi: 10.1007/s00429-012-0379-4 Oldham, J. M. (2004). Borderline Personality Disorder: An Overview. The Psychiatric Times, 21(8), 2.
Ong KT, Villemagne VL, Bahar-Fuchs A, Lamb F, Langdon N, Catafau AM, Stephens AW, Seibyl J, Dinkelborg LM, Reininger CB, Putz B, Rohde B, Masters CL, Rowe CC (2015). Aβ imaging with 18F-florbetaben in prodromal Alzheimer's disease: a prospective outcome study. J Neurol Neurosurg Psychiatry, 86(4):431-416.
Ono M, Kubik S, Abernathey CD. (1990). Atlas of the cerebral sulci. Thieme, Stuttgart / New York.
Oram MW, Perrett DI. (1996) Integration of form and motion in the anterior superior temporal polysensory area (STPa) of the macaque monkey. J. Neurophysiol. 76:109-129.
Ornstein R. (1977). The Psychology of Consciousness. New York: Harcourt Brace Jovanovich.
Ossenkoppele R, Tolboom N, Foster-Dingley JC, Adriaanse SF, Boellaard R, Yaqub M, Windhorst AD, Barkhof F, Lammertsma AA, Scheltens P, van der Flier WM,

van Berckel BN (2012). Longitudinal imaging of Alzheimer pathology using [11C]PIB, [18F]FDDNP and [18F]FDG PET. Eur J Nucl Med Mol Imaging, 39(6):990-1000.
Otovic, P., Partan, S. R., Bryant, J. B., & Hutchinson, E. (2014). Let's call a truce ... for now: The silent bared-teeth face expression in mandrills (Mandrillus sphinx) during baseline and post-conflict conditions. Ethology, 120, 1118–1127.
Owen, A. M., Coleman, M. R., Boly, M., Davis, M. H., Laureys, S., & Pickard, J. D. (2006). Detecting awareness in the vegetative state. Science, 313, 1402.
Pagura, J., Stein, M. B., Bolton, J. M., Cox, B. J., Grant, B., & Sareen, J. (2010). Comorbidity of borderline personality disorder and posttraumatic stress disorder in the U.S. population. [Research Support, N.I.H., Extramural Research Support, Non-U.S. Gov't]. J Psychiatr Res, 44(16), 1190-1198. doi: 10.1016/j.jpsychires.2010.04.016
Pandya DN, Seltzer B. (1982). Intrinsic connections and architectonics of posterior parietal cortex in the rhesus monkey. J Comp Neurol 204: 196-210.
Pantke, K. H. (1999). Locked-in: Gefangen im eigenen Körper. Frankfurt: Mabuse-Verlag.
Pantke, K.-H., Birbaumer, N. (2012). Die Lebensqualität nach einem Schlaganfall mit Locked-in Syndrom. Interdisziplinär, 20 (4), 296-300.
Parker GJM, Luzzi S, Alexander DC, Wheeler-Kingshott CAM, Ciccarelli O, Ralph MAL. (2005). Lateralization of ventral and dorsal auditory-language pathways in the human brain. NeuroImage 24: 656-666.
Parsons, S. and J. Bynner. 2005. Does Numeracy Matter More? London: NRDC.
Passingham RE (1993) The Frontal Lobes and Voluntary Action. Oxford Univ Press, Oxford
Passingham RE, Bengtsson SL, Lau HC (2010) Medial frontal cortex: from self-generated action to reflection on one's own performance. Trends Cogn Sci 14:16-21
Passingham RE, Stephan KE, Kotter R (2002) The anatomical basis of functional localization in the cortex. Nat Rev Neurosci 3:606-616
Pau S, Jahn G, Sakreida K, Domin M, Lotze M. (2013) Encoding and recall of finger sequences in experienced pianists compared to musically naïves: a combined behavioural and functional imaging study. Neuroimage. 64:379-87.
Paus T (2001) Primate anterior cingulate cortex: where motor control, drive and cognition interface. Nat Rev Neurosci. 2:417-24
Paus T, Kalina M, Patocková L, Angerová Y, Cerný R, Mecir P, Bauer J, Krabec P (1991)Medial vs lateral frontal lobe lesions and differential impairment of central-gaze fixation maintenance in man. Brain. 114:2051-67
Paus T, Petrides M, Evans AC, Meyer E (1993) Role of the human anterior cingulate cortex in the control of oculomotor, manual, and speech responses: a positron emission tomography study. J Neurophysiol. 70:453-69
Peeters, R.R., Simone, L., Nelissen, K., Fabbri-Destro, M., Vanduffel, W., Rizzolatti, G., & Orban, G.A. (2009). The representation of tool use in humans and monkeys: common and uniquely human features. J. Neurosci., 29 (37), 11523-11539.
Pellegrini, A. D. (2011). "In the eye of the beholder": Sex bias in observations and ratings of students' aggression. Educational Researcher, 40, 281 - 286.
Penfield, W. & Welch, K (1949). The supplementary motor area in the cerebral cortex of man Trans.Am.Neurol.Assn. 74:179-184
Penfield, W., Milner, B. (1958). Memory deficit produced by bilateral lesions in the hippocampal zone. AMA Arch Neurol Psychiatry, May;79(5):475-97.

Peper, M. (2009). Neurobiologische Emotionsmodelle. In G. Stemmler (Hrsg.), Enzyklopädie der Psychologie: Themenbereich C Theorie und Forschung, Serie 4, Band 3: Psychologie der Emotion (S. 21-79). Göttingen: Hogrefe.

Perani, I., Cappa, S., Schnur, T., Tettamanti, M., Collina, S., Rosa, M. M., & Fazio, F. (1999). The neural correlates of verb and noun processing. A PET study. Brain, 122 (12), 2337-2344.

Perelmouter J. & Birbaumer, N. (2000). A binary spelling interface with random errors. IEEE Transactions on Rehabilitation Engineering, 8, 227-232.

Perrin, F., Schnakers, C., Schnabus, M., Degueldre, C., Goldman, S., et al. (2006). Brain response to one's own name in vegetative state, minimally conscious state, and locked-in syndrome. Archives of Neurology, 63 (4), 562-569.

Perugini, M. & Richetin, J. (2007). In the land of the blind, the one-eyed man is king. European Journal of Personality, 21, 977–981.

Pesaran B, Nelson MJ, Andersen RA (2006) Dorsal premotor neurons encode the relative position of the hand, eye, and goal during reach planning. Neuron. 51:125-34

Petersen RC, Stevens JC, Ganguli M, Tangalos EG, Cummings JL, DeKosky ST (2001). Practice parameter: early detection of dementia: mild cognitive impairment (an evidence-based review). Report of the Quality Standards Subcommittee of the American Academy of Neurology. Neurology, 56(9):1133-1142.

Petit L, Courtney SM, Ungerleider LG, Haxby JV (1998) Sustained activity in the medial wall during working memory delays. J Neurosci. 18:9429-37

Petrides M (1986) The effect of periarcuate lesions in the monkey on the performance of symmetrically and asymmetrically reinforced visual and auditory go, no-to tasks. J Neurosci 2054-2063

Peyron, R, Laurent, B, Garcia-Larrea, L (2000). Functional imaging of brain responses to pain. A review and meta-analysis. Neurophysiol Clin, 30: 63-88.

Pfurtscheller, G., Flotzinger, D., Pregenzer, M., Wolpaw, J. R., & McFarland, D. (1996). EEG-based brain computer interface. Medical Progress Through Technology, 21, 11-121.

Phan KL, Wager T, Taylor SF, Liberzon, I. (2002) Functional neuroanatomy of emotion: a meta-analysis of emotion activation studies in PET and fMRI. Neuroimage. 16(2):331-348.

Philipsen, A., Graf, E., Tebartz van Elst, L., Jans, T., Warnke, A., Hesslinger, B., Berger, M. (2010). Evaluation of the efficacy and effectiveness of a structured disorder tailored psychotherapy in ADHD in adults: study protocol of a randomized controlled multicentre trial. [Multicenter Study Randomized Controlled Trial Research Support, Non-U.S. Gov't]. Atten Defic Hyperact Disord, 2(4), 203-212. doi: 10.1007/s12402-010-0046-7

Phillips CG, Porter R (1977) Corticospinal Neurones. Academic Press, London

Phillips ML, Williams LM, Heining M, Herba CM, Russell T, Andrew C, Bullmore ET, Brammer MJ, Williams SCR, Morgan M, Young AW, Gray JA (2004). Differential neural responses to overt and covert presentations of facial expressions of fear and disgust. Neuroimage 21: 1484-1496.

Phillips ML, Young AW, Senior C, Brammer M, Andrew C, Calder AJ, Bullmore ET, Perrett DI, Rowland D, Williams SCR, Gray JA, David AS (1997) A specific neural substrate for perceiving facial expressions of disgust. Nature. 389:495-498.

Piaget R. (1930) Human Speech, Harcourt Brace, New York.

Picard N, Strick PL (1996) Motor areas of the medial wall: a review of their location and functional activation. Cereb Cortex. 6:342-353

Piccione, G., Marafioti, S., Giannetto,C., Di Pietro, S., Quartuccio, M., & Fazio, F. (2014). Comparison of daily distribution of rest/activity in companion cats and dogs. Biological Rhythm Research, 45, 615-623.

Pierrot-Deseilligny, C. H., Ploner, C. J., Müri, R. M., Gaymard, B., & Rivaud-Pechoux, S. (2002). Effects of Cortical Lesions on Saccadic. Annals of the New York Academy of Sciences, 956(1), 216-229.

Pierrot-Deseilligny, C. H., Rivaud, S., Gaymard, B., & Agid, Y. (1991a). Cortical control of reflexive visually-guided saccades. Brain, 114(3), 1473-1485.

Pierrot-Deseilligny, C., Rosa, A., Masmoudi, K., Rivaud, S., & Gaymard, B. (1991b). Saccade deficits after a unilateral lesion affecting the superior colliculus. Journal of Neurology, Neurosurgery & Psychiatry, 54(12), 1106-1109.

Pike KE, Savage G, Villemagne VL, Ng S, Moss SA, Maruff P, Mathis CA, Klunk WE, Masters CL, Rowe CC. (2007). Beta-amyloid imaging and memory in non-demented individuals: evidence for preclinical Alzheimer's disease. Brain, 130:2837– 2844.

Pisella, L., Binkofski, F. C., Lasek, K., Toni, I., Rossetti, Y. (2006). No double-dissociation between optic ataxia and visual agnosia: Multiple sub-streams for multiple visuo-manual integrations. Neuropsychologia, 44 (13): 2734–2748.

Pistoia, F., Sacco, S., Palmirotta, R., Onorati, P., Carolei, A., & Sara, M. (2008). Mismatch of neurophysiological findings in partial recovery of consciousness: A case report. Brain Injury, 22(7-8), 633-637.

Plmer S.E., Schloss K.B., Smmartino J. (2013). Visual aesthetics and human preference. Annu. Rev. Psychol. 2013. 64:77–107.

Pohlack, S. T.*, Meyer, P.*, Cacciaglia, R., Liebscher, C., Ridder, S., Flor, H. (2014). Bigger is better! Hippocampal volume and declarative memory performance in healthy young men. Brain Structure and Function, 219, 255-267. * contributed equally

Polanyi, M. (1969). Knowing and Being. London: Routledge and Kegan Paul.

Pollet, T. V. Tybur, J. M. Frankenhuis, W. E. F., & Rickard, I. J. (2014). What can cross-cultural correlations teach us about human nature? Human Nature, 25, 410–429.

Pomp, AM (1974). Psychotherapy for the myofascial pain-dysfunction syndrome: a study of factors coinciding with symptom remission. J Am Dent Assoc, 89: 629–632.

Porter R and Lemon RN (1993) Corticospinal Function and Voluntary Movement, Oxford, Clarendon

Posner, M. I. & DiGiorolamo, G. J. (2000). Cognitive Neurosciene: Origins and Promise. Psychological Bulletin, 126, (6), 873-889.

Posner, M. I., & Petersen, S. E. (1989). The attention system of the human brain (No. TR-89-1). Washington Univ. St. Louis Mo. Department of Neurology.

Posner, M.I. (1980). Orienting of attention. Quarterly Journal of Experimental Psychology, 32, 3-25.

Powell HW, Parker GJ, Alexander DC, Symms MR, Boulby PA, Wheeler-Kingshott CA, Barker GJ, Noppeney U, Koepp MJ, Duncan JS. (2006). Hemispheric asymmetries in language-related pathways: a combined functional MRI and tractography study. NeuroImage 32: 388-399.

Prestia A, Caroli A, Wade SK, van der Flier WM, Ossenkoppele R, Van Berckel B, Barkhof F, Teunissen CE, Wall A, Carter SF, Schöll M, Choo IH, Nordberg A, Scheltens

P, Frisoni GB (2015). Prediction of AD dementia by biomarkers following the NIA-AA and IWG diagnostic criteria in MCI patients from three European memory clinics. Alzheimers Dement, Jan 31. pii: S1552-5260(14)02890-8.

Preuschoft, S. (1992). "Laughter" and "smile" in Barbary macaques (Macaca sylvanus). Ethology, 91, 200-236.

Preuschoft, S. & van Hooff, J. A. R. A. M. (1995). Homologizing primate facial displays: A critical review of methods. Folia Primatologica, 65, 121-137.

Prévost C, Pessiglione M, Météreau E, Cléry-Melin ML, Dreher JC (2010) Separate valuation subsystems for delay and effort decision costs. J Neurosci 30: 14080-14090.

Price, C. (2000). The anatomy of language: contributions from functional neuroimaging. Journal of Anatomy, 197, 335-359.

Price, C.J., Green, D.W. & von Studnitz, R. (1999). A functional imaging study of translation and language switching. Brain 122 (Pt 12), 2221-2235.

Price, G.R., Mazzocco, M.M. & Ansari, D. (2013). Why mental arithmetic counts: Brain activation during single digit arithmetic predicts high school math scores. Journal of Neuroscience, 33, 156-163.

Prinz, W. (1990). A common-coding approach to perception and action. In: Current approaches—Neumann O, Prinz W. (Eds.). Berlin: Springer. 167–201.

Prochnow D, Brunheim S, Kossack H, Eickhoff SB, Markowitsch HJ, Seitz RJ (2014c). Anterior and posterior subareas of the dorsolateral frontal cortex in socially relevant decisions based on masked affect expressions. F1000 Research 3: 212 [v1; ref status: approved with reservations 1,http://f1000r.es/3wg].

Prochnow D, Brunheim S, Steinhäuser L, Seitz RJ (2014a). Reasoning about the implications of facial expressions: A behavioral and fMRI study on low and high social impact. Brain Cogn 90: 165-173.

Prochnow D, Hoeing B, Kleiser R, Lindenberg R, Wittsack HJ, Schäfer R, Franz M, Seitz RJ (2013a). The neural correlates of affect reading: An fMRI study on faces and gestures. Behav Brain Res 237: 270-277.

Prochnow D, Kossack H, Brunheim S, Müller K, Wittsack H-J, Markowitsch H-J, Seitz RJ (2013b) Processing of subliminal facial expressions of emotion: A behavioral and fMRI study. Soc Neurosci 8: 448-461.

Prochnow D, Steinhäuser L, Brunheim S, Seitz RJ (2014b). Differential emotional state reasoning in young and older adults: Evidence from behavioral and neuroimaging data. J Neurol Psychol 2:8.

Puccinelli N.M., Tickle-Degnen L., Rosenthal R.T. (2006). Stage left, stage right? Position effects on perception of a spokesperson. Advances in Consumer Research, 33, 576-577.

Puce A, Allison T, McCarthy G. (1999) Electrophysiological studies of human face perception. III: Effects of top-down processing on face-specific potentials. Cereb Cortex. 9(5):445-458.

Pulvermueller, F. (1999). Words in the brain's language. Behavioral & Brain Sciences 22, 253–336.

Pulvermueller, F., Shtyrov, Y., & Illmoniemi, R. (2005). Brain Signatures of Meaning Access in Action Word Recognition. Journal of Cognitive Neuroscience, 17 (6), 884-892.

Puvanendran, K., Dowker, A. & Demeyere, N. (submitted). Compensating arithmetic ability with derived fact strategies in Broca's aphasia: a case report.

Qin P, Northoff G (2011). How is our self-related to midline regions and the default-mode network? Neuroimage 57: 1221-1233.

Rafal, R., Henik, A., & Smith, J. (1991). Extrageniculate contributions to reflex visual orienting in normal humans: A temporal hemifield advantage. Journal of Cognitive Neuroscience, 3(4), 322-328.

Rambold, H., Churchland, A., Selig, Y., Jasmin, L., & Lisberger, S. G. (2002). Partial ablations of the flocculus and ventral paraflocculus in monkeys cause linked deficits in smooth pursuit eye movements and adaptive modification of the VOR. Journal of Neurophysiology, 87(2), 912-924.

Ramos Murguialday, A., Hill, J., Bensch, M., Martens, S., Halder, S., Nijboer, F., Schoelkopf, B., Birbaumer, N., Gharabaghi, A. (2011). Transition from the Locked in to the completely Locked-in State: a physiological analysis. Clinical Neurophysiology, 122, 925-933.

Randerath, J., Goldenberg, G., Spijkers, W., Li, Y., & Hermsdörfer, J. (2010). Different left brain regions are essential for grasping a tool compared with its subsequent use. Neuroimage, 53 (1), 171–180.

Ranganath, C. (2010). A unified framework for the functional organization of the medial temporal lobes and the phenomenology of episodic memory. Hippocampus, 20(11), 1263– 1290.

Ranganath, C., Yonelinas, A. P., Cohen, M. X., Dy, C. J., Tom, S. M., & D'Esposito, M. (2003). Dissociable correlates of recollection and familiarity within the medial temporal lobes. Neuropsychologia, 42(1), 2-13.

Rashbass, C. (1961). The relationship between saccadic and smooth tracking eye movements. The Journal of Physiology, 159(2), 326.

Rauch, S. L., Savage, C. R., Brown, H. D., Curran, T., Alpert, N. M., Kendrick, A., Fischman, A. J., & Kosslyn, S. M. (1995). A PET investigation of implicit and explicit sequence learning. Human Brain Mapp, 3, 271-286.

Ravizza, S. M., Delgado, M. R., M. Chein, J. M., Becker, J. T. & Fiez, J. A. (2004). Functional dissociations within the inferior parietal cortex in verbal working memory NeuroImage, 22, 562– 573.

Razran G (1961) The observable unconscious and the inferable conscious in current Soviet psychophysiology: Interoceptive conditioning, semantic conditioning, and the orienting reflex. Psychological Review, 68, 1-147.

Rees G (2007) Neural correlates of the contents of visual awareness in humans. Philos Trans R Soc Lond B Biol Sci 362: 877-886.

Reeves 2nd, JL, Merrill, RL (2007). Diagnostic and treatment challenges in occlusal dysesthesia. J Calif Dent Assoc, 35: 198-207.

Reiman EM, Caselli RJ, Yun LS, Chen K, Bandy D, Minoshima S, Thibodeau SN, Osborne D (1996). Preclinical evidence of Alzheimer's disease in persons homozygous for the epsilon 4 allele for apolipoprotein E. N Engl J Med, 334(12):752-758.

Reinhart RM, Woodman GF (2014) Causal control of medial-frontal cortex governs electrophysiological and behavioral indices of performance monitoring and learning. J Neurosci 34: 4214-4227.

Research Support, N.I.H., Extramural Research Support, Non-U.S. Gov't]. Psychol Med, 40(11), 1759-1765. doi: 10.1017/S0033291709992261

Reuter, B., Kaufmann, C., Bender, J., Pinkpank, T., & Kathmann, N. (2010). Distinct neural correlates for volitional generation and inhibition of saccades. Journal of cognitive neuroscience, 22(4), 728-738.

Revenstorf, Dirk u. Peter, Burkhard (Eds.). (2009). Hypnose in Psychotherapie Psychosomatik und Medizin. Heidelberg: Springer.

Rickard, T. C., Romero, S. G., Basso, G., Wharton, C., Flitman, S. & Grafman, J. (2000) The calculating brain: an fMRI study. Neuropsychologia, 38, 325–335.

Riehle A, Requin J (1989) Monkey primary motor and premotor cortex: single-cell activity related to prior information about direction and extent of an intended movement. J Neurophysiol 61:534-549

Rijntjes M, Hamzei F, Glauche V, Saur D. (2011). Activation changes in sensorimotor cortex during improvement due to CIMT in chronic stroke. Restor Neurol Neurosci; 29:299-320.

Risacher SL, Saykin AJ, West JD, Shen L, Firpi HA, McDonald BC; Alzheimer's Disease Neuroimaging Initiative (ADNI) (2009). Baseline MRI predictors of conversion from MCI to probable AD in the ADNI cohort. Curr Alzheimer Res, 6: 347–361.

Risetti, M., Formisano, R., Toppi, J., Quitadamo, L. R., et al. (2013). On ERPs detection in disorders of consciousness rehabilitation. Frontiers in Human Neuroscience, 7, Article 775.

Rivaud, S., Müri, R. M., Gaymard, B., Vermersch, A. I., & Pierrot-Deseilligny, C. (1994). Eye movement disorders after frontal eye field lesions in humans. Experimental Brain Research, 102(1), 110-120.

Rivera, S.M., Reiss, A.L., Eckert, M.A. & Menon V. (2005). Developmental changes in mental arithmetic: Evidence for increased functional specialization in the left inferior parietal cortex. Cerebral Cortex, 15, 1779-1790.

Rizzolatti G, Arbib MA (1998) Language within our grasp. [Review] Trends Neurosci. 21:188-194.

Rizzolatti, G. Berti A. (1990). Neglect as a neural representation deficit. Revue Neurologique, 146, 626-634.

Rizzolatti G, Camarda R, Fogassi L, Gentilucci M, Luppino G, Matelli M (1988) Functional organization of inferior area 6 in the macaque monkey. II. Area F5 and the control of distal movements. Exp Brain Res. ;71(3):491-507.

Rizzolatti G, Craighero L (2004). The mirror neuron system. Annual Review of Neuroscience 27: 169-192.

Rizzolatti G, Fadiga L, Gallese V, Fogassi L (1996) Premotor cortex and the recognition of motor actions. Brain Res Cogn Brain Res. 3:131-141

Rizzolatti G, Luppino G (2001) The cortical motor system. Neuron 31: 889-901

Rizzolatti, G. Matelli, M. (2003) Two different streams form the dorsal visual system: anatomy and functions. Exp Brain Res, 153, 146–157.

Rizzolatti, G. Sinigaglia, C. (2008). Mirrors in the Brain - How Our Minds Share Actions And Emotions Oxford University Press Oxford New York

Robinson, F. R., Fuchs, A. F. (2001). The role of the cerebellum in voluntary eye movements. Annual review of neuroscience, 24(1), 981-1004.

Robinson, W. S. (1950). Ecological correlations and the behavior of individuals. American Sociological Review, 15, 351–357.

Roepke, S., Vater, A., Preissler, S., Heekeren, H. R., & Dziobek, I. (2012). Social cognition in borderline personality disorder. Front Neurosci, 6, 195. doi: 10.3389/fnins.2012.00195

Rogers, S. L., & Friedman, R. B. (2008). The Underlying Mechanisms of Semantic Memory Loss in Alzheimer's Disease and Semantic Dementia. Neuropsychologia, 46(1), 12–21.

Rohr M, Degner J, Wentura D (2012). Masked emotional priming beyond global valence activations. Cognition & Emotion, 26, 224-244.
Rohracher, H. (1958). Einführung in die Psychologie (6. Aufl.). Wien: Urban & Schwarzenberg.
Roland PE, Meyer E, Shibasaki T, Yamamoto YL, Thompson CJ (1982) Regional cerebral blood flow changes in cortex and basal ganglia during voluntary movements in normal human volunteers. J Neurophysiol 48:467-480
Rolls ET (2006). Brain mechanisms underlying flavour and appetite. Philos Trans R Soc Lond B Biol Sci 361: 1123-1136.
Rorden, C., & Brett, M. (2000). Stereotaxic display of brain lesions. Behavioural neurology, 12(4), 191-200.
Rorschach, H. (1921): Psychodiagnostik. Methodik und Ergebnisse eines wahrnehmungsdiagnostischen Experiments (Deutenlassen von Zufallsformen). Bern: E. Bircher.
Rosca, E.C. (2010). A case of acalculia due to impaired procedural knowledge. Neurological Sciences, 30, 164-170.
Rosenbaum, P. J. & Valsiner, J. (2011). The un-making of a method: From rating scales to the study of psychological processes. Theory and Psychology, 21, 47-65.
Rosenberg-Lee, M., Barth, M. & Menon, V. (2011). What difference does a year of schooling make? Maturation of brain response and connectivity between 2nd and 3rd grades during arithmetic problem solving. Neuroimage, 57, 795-808
Ross, GL, Bentley, HJ, Greene Jr., GW (1953). The psychosomatic concept in dentistry. Psychosom Med, 15: 168-173.
Ross, L. E., & Ross, S. M. (1980). Saccade latency and warning signals: stimulus onset, offset, and change as warning events. Perception & Psychophysics, 27(3), 251-257.
Rossetti, Y., Revol, P., McIntosh, R., Pisella, L., Rode, G., Danckert, J., & Milner, A. D. (2005). Visually guided reaching: bilateral posterior parietal lesions cause a switch from fast visuomotor to slow cognitive control. Neuropsychologia, 43(2), 162-177.
Rossi, Ernest L. (1986). The Psychobiology of Mind-Body-Healing. New York: Norton&Co. Deutsch: Rossi, Ernest L. (1991). Die Psychobiologie der Seele-Körper-Heilung. Neue Ansätze der therapeutischen Hypnose. Essen: Synthesis Verlag.
Rössler, O.E. (1998. Endophysics – The World as an Interface. World Scientiific, Singapore, New Jersey, London, Hong Kong. ISBN 981-02-2752-3.
Rossor, M., Warrington, E. & Cipolotti, L. (1995). The isolation of calculation skills. Journal of Neurology, 242, 78-81.
Roth, Gerhard (2012). Geist, Seele, Gehirn. In: Kandel, Eric R. (20124). Psychiatrie, Psychoanalyse und die neue Biologie des Geistes. Frankfurt/Main: Suhrkamp (9-17).
Rothi, L. J. G., Mack, L., & Heilman, K. M. (1990). Unawareness of apraxic errors. Neurology, 40(suppl 1), 202.
Rothschuh, K. E. (1963). Theorie des Organsimus. Bios – Psyche – Pathos (2. erw. Aufl.). München: Urban & Schwarzenberg.
Rotter, J. B. (1954). Social learning and clinical psychology. New York: Prentice-Hall.

Rotter, J. B. (1981). The psychological situation in social learning theory. In D. Magnusson (Ed.), Toward a psychology of situations: An interactional perspective. Hillsdale, NJ: Lawrence Erlbaum.

Roux F, Wibral M, Mohr HM, Singer W, Uhlhaas PJ (2012) Gamma-band activity in human prefrontal cortex codes for the number of relevant items maintained in working memory. J Neurosci 32: 12411-12420.

Rowe CC, Ackerman U, Browne W, Mulligan R, Pike KL, O'Keefe G, Tochon-Danguy H, Chan G, Berlangieri SU, Jones G, Dickinson-Rowe KL, Kung HP, Zhang W, Kung MP, Skovronsky D, Dyrks T, Holl G, Krause S, Friebe M, Lehman L, Lindemann S, Dinkelborg LM, Masters CL, Villemagne VL (2008). Imaging of amyloid beta in Alzheimer's disease with 18F-BAY94-9172, a novel PET tracer: proof of mechanism. Lancet Neurology, 7:129-135.

Rowe CC, Ellis KA, RimajovaM, Bourgeat P, Pike KE, Jones G, Fripp J, Tochon-Danguy H, Morandeau L, O'Keefe G, Price R, Raniga P, Robins P, Acosta O, Lenzo O, Szoeke C, Salvado O, Head R, Martins, Masters CL, Ames D, Villemagne VL (2010). Amyloid imaging results from the Australian Imaging, Biomarkers and Lifestyle (AIBL) study of aging. Neurobiol Aging, 31, 1275-1283.

Rowe JB, Toni I, Josephs O, Frackowiak RSJ, Passingham RE (2000). The prefrontal cortex: response selection or maintenance within working-memory. Science 288: 1656-1660.

Roy, E. A., Square, P. A. (1985). Common considerations in the study of limb, verbal and oral apraxia. In: E. A. Roy (Ed.), Neuropsychological studies of apraxia and related disorders (pp. 111–162). Amsterdam: North-Holland.

Rozzi S, Calzavara R, Belmalih A, Borra E, Gregoriou GG, Matelli M, Luppino G. (2006). Cortical connections of the inferior parietal cortical convexity of the macaque monkey. Cereb Cortex 16 (10): 1389-1417.

Ruby P, Decety J (2001). Effect of subjective perspective taking during simulation of action: a PET investigation of agency. Nat Neurosci 4: 546-550.

Ruf, C.A., De Massari, D., Furdea, A., Matuz, T., Fioravanti, C. van der Heiden, L., Halder, S., Birbaumer, N. (2013). Semantic classical conditioning and brain-computer interface control: encoding of affirmative and negative thinking. Frontiers in Neuroscience, 7, Article 23.

Rugg, M. D. Coles, M.G. H. (Eds.) (1995). Electrophysiology of mind: Event-related brain potentials and cognition, Oxford psychology series, No. 25. New York: Oxford University Press.

Rugg, M. D., Walla, P., Schloerscheidt, A. M., Fletcher, P. C., Frith, C. D., & Dolan, R. J. (1998). Neural correlates of depth of processing effects on recollection: evidence from brain potentials and positron emission tomography. Experimental Brain Research, 123(1-2), 18-23.

Rumiati, R. I., Zanini, S., Vorano, L., & Shallice, T. (2001). A form of ideatonal apraxia as a selective deficit of contention scheduling. Cognitive Neuropsychology, 18, 617–642.

Ruocco, A. C., Amirthavasagam, S., Choi-Kain, L. W., & McMain, S. F. (2013). Neural correlates of negative emotionality in borderline personality disorder: an activation-likelihood-estimation meta-analysis. Biol Psychiatry, 73(2), 153-160. doi: 10.1016/j.biopsych.2012.07.014 S0006-3223(12)00626-9 [pii]

Rusch, N., Lieb, K., Gottler, I., Hermann, C., Schramm, E., Richter, H., Bohus, M. (2007). Shame and implicit self-concept in women with borderline personality disorder Am J Psychiatry (Vol. 164, pp. 500-508). United States.
Ruschel M, Knösche TR, Friederici AD, Turner R, Geyer S, Anwander A. (2014). Connectivity architecture and subdivisions of the human inferior parietal cortex revealed by diffusion MRI. Cereb Cortex 24 (9), 2436-2438.
Rushworth MFS, Behrens TEJ, Johansen-Berg H. (2006). Connection patterns distinguish 3 regions of human parietal cortex. Cereb Cortex 16: 1418-1430.
Rushworth MF, Hadland KA, Gaffan D, Passingham RE (2003) The effect of cingulate cortex lesions on task switching and working memory. J Cogn Neurosci. 15:338-53
Rushworth MF, Hadland KA, Paus T, Sipila PK (2002) Role of the human medial frontal cortex in task switching: a combined fMRI and TMS study. J Neurophysiol 87:2577-92
Rushworth MF, Walton ME, Kennerley SW, Bannerman DM (2004) Action sets and decisions in the medial frontal cortex. Trends Cogn Sci. 8:410-417
Russo GS, Backus DA, Ye S and Crutcher MD (2002) Neural activity in monkey dorsal and ventral cingulate motor areas: comparison with the supplementary motor area J Neurophysiol 88:2612-29
Ruys KI, Aarts H (2011). I didn't mean to hurt you! Unconscious origins of experienced self-agency over others' emotions. Emotion, 12, 132-141.
Sabat, S. R. (1979). Wundt's Physiological Psychology in retrospect. American Psychologist, 34 (7), 635-638.
Sabatini E, Della Penna S, Franciotti R, Ferretti A, Zoccolotti P, Rossini PM, Romani GL, Gainotti G (2009). Brain Structures Activated by Overt and Covert Emotional Visual Stimuli. Brain Res Bull 79: 258-264.
Saevarsson, S. (2013a). Motor response deficits of unilateral neglect: assessment, therapy, and neuroanatomy. Applied Neuropsychology: Adult, 20(4), 292-305.
Saevarsson, S. (2013b). Prism adaptation theory in unilateral neglect: motor and perceptual components. Frontiers in human neuroscience, 7.
Saevarsson, S., Eger, S., Gutierrez-Herrera, M. (2014). Neglected premotor neglect. Frontiers in human neuroscience, 8.
Saevarsson, S., Halsband, U., & Kristjánsson, Á. (2011). Designing rehabilitation programs for neglect: could 2 be more than 1+1? Applied Neuropsychology, 18 (2), 95-106.
Saevarsson, S., Kristjánsson, Á. (2013). A note on Striemer and Danckert's theory of prism adaptation in unilateral neglect. Frontiers in human neuroscience, 7.
Sakata H, Taira M, Murata A, Mine S (1995) Neural Mechanisms of visual guidance of hand action in the parietal cortex of the monkey. Cereb Cortex 5: 429-438
Saksida, L. M., & Bussey, T. J. (2010). The representational-hierarchical view of amnesia: translation from animal to human. Neuropsychologia, 48(8), 2370–2384.
Salakari MR, Surakka T, Nurminen R, Pylkkänen L. (2015). Effects of rehabilitation among patients with advanced cancer: a systematic review. Acta Oncol; 9:1-11
Samson, A. C., Hempelmann, C. F., Huber, O., & Zysset, S. (2009). Neural substrates of incongruity-resolution and nonsense humor. [Research Support, Non-U.S. Gov't]. Neuropsychologia, 47(4), 1023-1033. doi: 10.1016/j.neuropsychologia.2008.10.028

Samson, A. C., Zysset, S., & Huber, O. (2008). Cognitive humor processing: different logical mechanisms in nonverbal cartoons - an fMRI study. [Comparative Study Research Support, Non-U.S. Gov't]. Soc Neurosci, 3(2), 125-140. doi: 10.1080/17470910701745858

Sanderson, C., Swenson, C., & Bohus, M. (2002). A critique of the American psychiatric practice guideline for the treatment of patients with borderline personality disorder. J Pers Disord, 16(2), 122-129.

Sandson, J., & Albert, M. L. (1984). Varieties of perseveration.Neuropsychologia, 22(6), 715-732.

Sarkar, A., Dowker, A., & Cohen Kadosh, R. (2014). Cognitive enhancement or cognitive cost: Trait-specific outcomes of brain stimulation in the case of mathematics anxiety. The Journal of Neuroscience, 34, 16605-16610.

Sarkissov SA, Filimonoff IN, Preobrashenskaya NS. (1949). Cytoarchitecture of the human cortex cerebri (russ.). Medgiz, Moscow.

Sarlani, E, Balciunas, BA, Grace, EG (2005/a). Orofacial pain - Part I. Assessment and management of musculoskeletal and neuropathic causes. AACN Clin Issues, 16: 333-346.

Sarlani, E, Balciunas, BA, Grace, EG (2005/b). Orofacial pain - Part II. Assessment and management of vascular, neurovascular, idiopathic, secondary, and psychogenic causes. AACN Clin Issues, 16: 347-358.

Sato W, Fujimura T, Kochiyama T, Suzuki N (2013). Relationships among facial mimicry, emotional experience, and emotion recognition. PloS One 8: e57889.

Sato, C, Sato, S, Takashina, H, Ishii, H, Onozuka, M, Sasaguri, K (2010). Bruxism affects stress responses in stressed rats. Clin Oral Investig, 14: 153-60.

Saur, D., Kreher, B. W., Schnell, S., Kuemmerer, D., Kellermeyer, P., Vrya, M.-S., Umarova, R., Musso, M., Glauche, V., Abel, S., Huber, W., Rijntjes, M., Henning, J. , & Weiller, C. (2008). Ventral and dorsal pathways for language. PNAS, 105 (46), 18035–18040.

Saxe, R. R., Pelphrey, K. A. (2009). Introduction to a special section of developmental social cognitive neuroscience. [Introductory Research Support, N.I.H., Extramural Research Support, Non-U.S. Gov't]. Child Dev, 80(4), 946-951. doi: 10.1111/j.1467-8624.2009.01309.x

Saxe, R., Wexler, A. (2005). Making sense of another mind: the role of the right temporoparietal junction. [Clinical Trial Research Support, N.I.H., Extramural Research Support, U.S. Gov't, P.H.S.]. Neuropsychologia, 43(10), 1391-1399. doi: 10.1016/ j.neuropsychologia.2005.02.013

Scangos KW, Stuphorn V (2010) Medial frontal cortex motivates but does not control movement initiation in the countermanding task. J Neurosci. 30:1968-82

Schacter, D. L. (1992). Implicit knowledge: New perspectives on unconscious processes. Proc. Nati. Acad. Sci. USA. 89, 11113-11117.

Schacter, D. L. (1994). Implicit knowledge: new perspectives on unconscious processes. International Review of Neurobiology, 37, 271-284.

Schacter, D. (1999). The seven sins of memory: Insights from psychology and cognitive neuroscience. American Psychologist 54, 182-203.

Schacter, D. L. Addis, D. R. (2007). Constructive memory: Ghosts of past and future. Nature, 445, 27.

Schacter, D. L., Norman, K. A., & Koutstaal, W. (1998). The cognitive neuroscience of constructive memory. Annual Review of Psychology, 49, 289-318.

Schall JD, Stuphorn V, Brown JW (2002) Monitoring and control of action by the frontal lobes. Neuron. 36:309-22

Scheinin NM, Aalto S, Koikkalainen J, Lotjonen J, Karrasch M, Kemppainen N, Viitanen M, Nagren K, Helin S, Scheinin M, Rinne JO (2009). Follow-up of [11C]PIB uptake and brain volume in patients with Alzheimer disease and controls. Neurology, 73(15):1186-1192.

Scheinin NM, Wikman K, Jula A, Perola M, Vahlberg T, Rokka J, Någren K, Viitanen M, Rinne JO (2014). Cortical ^{11}C-PIB uptake is associated with age, APOE genotype, and gender in "healthy aging". J Alzheimers Dis, 41(1):193-202.

Scheltens, D Leys, F Barkhof, D Huglo, H C Weinstein, P Vermersch, M Kuiper, M Steinling, E Ch Wolters, J Valk (1992). Atrophy of medial temporal lobes on MRI in "probable" Alzheimer's disease and normal ageing: diagnostic value and neuropsychological correlates. J Neurol Neurosurgery and Psychiatry, 55:967-972.

Schiller, P. H., True, S. D., & Conway, J. L. (1979). Effects of frontal eye field and superior colliculus ablations on eye movements. Science, 206(4418), 590-592.

Schiller, P. H., True, S. D., & Conway, J. L. (1980). Deficits in eye movements following frontal eye-field and superior colliculus ablations. Journal of Neurophysiology, 44(6), 1175-1189.

Schnakers C., et al. (2009). Detecting consciousness in a total locked-in syndrome: An active eventrelated paradigm. Neurocase, 15, 271-277.

Schnakers, C., Perrin, F., Schabus, M., Majerus, S., Ledoux, D., et al. (2008). Voluntary brain processing in disorders of consciousness. Neurology, 71, 1614-1620.

Schnakers, C., Vanhaudenhuyse, A., Giacino, J., Ventura, M., Boly, M., et al. (2009). Diagnostic accuracy of the vegetative and minimally conscious state: Clinical consensus versus standardized neurobehavioral assessment. BMC Neurology, 9, Article 35.

Schneider, D. J. (2005). The psychology of stereotyping. New York: Guilford Press.

Schoenle, P. W., Witzke, W. (2004). How vegetative is the vegetative state? Preserved semantic processing in VS patients - Evidence from N400 event-related potentials. Neurorehabilitation, 19, 329-334.

Scholz, J., Triantafyllou, C., Whitfield-Gabrieli, S., Brown, E. N., & Saxe, R. (2009). Distinct regions of right temporo-parietal junction are selective for theory of mind and exogenous attention. [Research Support, N.I.H., Extramural Research Support, Non-U.S. Gov't]. PLoS One, 4(3), e4869. doi: 10.1371/journal.pone.0004869

Scholz, O.B. (2008). Die posthypnotische Aufgabe. Abschlußbericht des von der M.E.G. geförderten Forschungsprojektes.

Schredl, M. Erlacher, D. (2004). Lucid dreaming frequency and personality. Personality and Individual Differences 37(7), 1463–1473.

Schulte-Rüther M, Markowitsch HJ, Fink GR, Piefke M (2007). Mirror neuron and theory of mind mechanisms involved in face-to-face interactions: A functional magnetic resonance imaging approach to empathy. J Cogn Neurosci 19: 1354-1372.

Schultz W (2013) Updating dopamine reward signals. Curr Opin Neurobiol 23: 229-238.

Schwartz, M.F., Buxbau, L. J., Montgomery, M. W., Fitzpatrick-DeSalme, E., Hart, T., Ferraro, M., Lee, S. S., & Coslett H. B. (1998). Naturalistic action production following right hemisphere stroke. Neuropsychologia, 37 (1), 51–66.

Schwarz, N. (1999). Self-reports: How the questions shape the answer. American Psychologist, 54, 93–105.

Schweitzer, JM (1964). Oral rehabilitation problem cases. Treatment and evaluation. Vol. 2. C.V. Mosby Company, Saint Louis. 611-625.
Schwichtenberg, J, Doering, S (2008). Success of referral in a psychosomatic-psychotherapeutic outpatient unit of a dental school. Z Psychosom Med Psychother, 54: 285-292.
Scott SH, Sergio LE, Kalaska JF (1997) Reaching movements with similar hand paths but different arm orientations. II. Activity of individual cells in dorsal premotor cortex and parietal area 5. J Neurophysiol 78: 2413-2426
Scoville, W. B., & Milner, B. (1957). Loss of recent memory after bilateral hippocampal lesions. Journal of neurology, neurosurgery, and psychiatry, 20(1), 11.
Searl, J. R. (1992). The Rediscovery of the Mind. Cambridge: MIT Press.
Seghier, M. L. (2013). The Angular Gyrus: Multiple Functions and Multiple Subdivisions. The Neuroscientist, 19 (1), 43-61.
Seib, DR and Martin-Villalba, A. (2014). Neurogenesis in the Normal Ageing Hippocampus: A Mini-Review. Gerontology 2014, Epub online Nov 29.
Seitz, R. J. (2001). Motorisches Lernen: Untersuchungen mit der funktionellen Bildgebung Motor learning: functional neuroimaging studies. Deutsche ZS für Sportmedizin, 52 (12), 343-349.
Seitz RJ, Angel H-F (2012) Processes of believing – a review and conceptual account. Rev Neurosci 23: 303-309.
Seitz RJ, Angel H-F (2014) Psychology of Religion and Spirituality: Meaning Making and processes of believing. Religion, Brain Behavior, DOI:10.1080/2153599X.2014.891249.
Seitz RJ, Franz M, Azari NP (2009) Value judgments and self-control of action: The role of the medial frontal cortex. Brain Res Rev 60: 368-378.
Seitz RJ, Nickel J, Azari NP (2006). Functional modularity of the medial prefrontal cortex: Involvement in human empathy. Neuropsychology 20: 743–751.
Seitz RJ, Schäfer R, Scherfeld D, Friederichs S, Popp K, Wittsack HJ, Azari NP, Franz M (2008). Valuating other people's emotional face expression: A combined fMRI and EEG study. Neuroscience 152: 713-722
Seltzer B, Pandya DN. (1984). Further observations on parieto-temporal connections in the rhesus monkey. Exp Brain Res 55: 301-312.
Sergl, HG (1996). Der Erlebnisraum Mund. In H.G. Sergl (Ed.) Psychologie und Psychosomatik in der Zahnheilkunde (pp. 3-9). Urban & Schwarzenberg, München - Wien - Baltimore.
Serpell, J. A. (1991). Beneficial effects of pet ownership on some aspects of human health and behavior. Journal of the Royal Society of Medicine, 87, 717-720.
Serpell, J. A. (1996). In the company of animals: a study of human-animal relationships. Cambridge: University Press.
Shallice, T., Burgess, P. W., Schon, F., & Baxter, D. M. (1989). The origins of utilization behaviour. Brain, 112(6), 1587-1598.
Shamay-Tsoory S, Aharon-Peretz J, Perry D (2009). Two systems for empathy: a double dissociation between emotional and cognitive empathy in inferior frontal gyrus versus ventromedial prefrontal lesions. Brain 132: 617-627.
Sharpe, J. A., Cheng, P., & Eizenman, M. (2011). Antisaccade generation is impaired after parietal lobe lesions. Annals of the New York Academy of Sciences, 1233(1), 194-199.

Sheline, Y. I., Price, J. L., Yan, Z., & Mintun, M. A. (2010). Resting-state functional MRI in depression unmasks increased connectivity between networks via the dorsal nexus. [Research Support, N.I.H., Extramural]. Proc Natl Acad Sci U S A, 107(24), 11020-11025. doi: 10.1073/pnas.1000446107

Sherrington, Ch. S. (1911). The integrative Action of the Nervous System. London: Henry Frowde.

Shidara M1, Richmond BJ. (2002) Anterior cingulate: single neuronal signals related to degree of reward expectancy. Science. 296:1709-11

Shima K, Aya K, Mushiake H, Inase M, Aizawa H, Tanji J (1991) Two movement-related foci in the primate cingulate cortex observed in signal-triggered and self-paced forelimb movements. J Neurophysiol. 65:188-202

Shima K, Mushiake H, Saito N, Tanji J (1996) Role for cells in the presupplementary motor area in updating motor plans. Proc Natl Acad Sci U S A. 93:8694-8

Shima K, Tanji J (1998) Both supplementary and presupplementary motor areas are crucial for the temporal organization of multiple movements. J Neurophysiol. 80:3247-3260

Shima K, Tanji J (1998) Role for cingulate motor area cells in voluntary movement selection based on reward. Science. 282:1335-8

Shima K, Tanji J (2000) Neuronal activity in the supplementary and presupplementary motor areas for temporal organization of multiple movements. J Neurophysiol. 84:2148-2160

Shimazu H, Maier MA, Cerri G, Kirkwood PA (1998), Lemon RN Macaque ventral premotor cortex exerts powerful facilitation of motor cortex outputs to upper limb motoneurons. J Neurosci. 24:1200-11, 2004 J Neurophysiol. 80:3247-60

Shipley, MT (1982). Insular cortex projections to the nucleus of the solitary tract and brainstem visceromotor nuclei in the mouse. Brain Res Bull, 1982: 139-148.

Shoda, Y., Mischel, W., & Wright, J. C. (1994). Intra-individual stability in the organization and patterning of behavior: Incorporating psychological situations into the idiographic analysis of personality. Journal of Personality and Social Psychology, 67, 674-687.

Shweder, R. A. D'Andrade, R. G. (1980). The systematic distortion hypothesis. In R. A. Shweder (Ed.). Fallible judgment in behavioral research: New directions for methodology of social and behavioral science (Vol. 4, pp. 37–58). San Francisco: Jossey-Bass.

Shweder, R. A. Sullivan, M. A. (1990). The semiotic subject of cultural psychology. In L. A. Pervin (Ed.). Handbook of personality, (pp. 399 - 416). New York, NY: Guilford.

Sierra A, Encinas JM, Maletic-Savatic M. (2011). Adult human neurogenesis: from microscopy to magnetic resonance imaging. Front Neurosci; 5:47

Sieswerda, S., Arntz, A., & Wolfis, M. (2005). Evaluations of emotional noninterpersonal situations by patients with borderline personality disorder J Behav Ther Exp Psychiatry (Vol. 36, pp. 209-225). United States.

Silbersweig, D., Clarkin, J. F., Goldstein, M., Kernberg, O. F., Tuescher, O., Levy, K. N., Stern, E. (2007). Failure of frontolimbic inhibitory function in the context of negative emotion in borderline personality disorder. [Comparative Study Research Support, Non-U.S. Gov't]. Am J Psychiatry, 164(12), 1832-1841. doi: 10.1176/appi.ajp.2007.06010126

Silverman, SI (1961). Oral physiology. Mosby, St Louis. 134, 146.

Silvoni, S., Cavinato, M., Volpato, C., Ruf, C., Birbaumer, N., Piccione, F. (2013). Amyotrophic Lateral Sclerosis progression and stability of brain-computer interface communication. Amyotrophic Lateral Sclerosis and Frontotemporal Degeneration, 14, (5-6), 390-396.

Simon, E. S., Hegarty, A. M., & Mehler, M. F. (1995). Hemispatial and directional performance biases in motor neglect. Neurology, 45(3), 525-531.

Simon, O., Mangin, J. F., Cohen, L., Le Bihan, D., & Dehaene, S. (2002). Topographical layout of hand, eye, calculation, and language-related areas in the human parietal lobe. Neuron 33 (3), 475–487.

Singer T (2006). The neuronal basis and ontogeny of empathy and mind reading: review of literature and implications for future research. Neurosci Biobehav Rev 30: 855-863.

Singer T, Seymour B, O'Doherty J, Kaube H, Dolan RJ, Frith CD (2004). Empathy for pain evolves the affective but not sensory components of pain. Science 303: 1157-1162.

Singer, W. (2001). Consciousness and the binding problem. Annals of the New York Academy of Sciences 929, 123-46.

Sitaram, R., Caria, A., Veit, R., Gaber, T., Rota, G., Kübler, A., Birbaumer, N. (2007b). FMRI Brain-Computer Interface: a tool for neuroscientific research and treatment. Computational Intelligence and Neuroscience. Article ID 82069, doi: 10.1155/2007/82069.

Sitaram, R., Zhang, H., Guan, C., Thulasidas, M., Hoshi, Y., Ishikawa, A., Shimizu, K., Birbaumer, N. (2007a). Temporal classification of multi-channel near-infrared spectroscopy signals of motor imagery for developing a brain-computer interface. NeuroImage, 34, 1416-1427.

Skaret, E, Raadal, M, Berg, E, Kvale, G (1998). Dental anxiety among 18-years-olds in Norway. Prevalence and related factors. Eur J Oral Sci, 106: 835-843.

Skinner, B. F. (1957). Verbal behavior. Englewood Cliffs, NJ: Prentice-Hall.

Skodol, A. E., Bender, D. S. (2003). Why are women diagnosed borderline more than men? [Comparative Study Review]. Psychiatr Q, 74(4), 349-360.

Skodol, A. E., Gunderson, J. G., Pfohl, B., Widiger, T. A., Livesley, W. J., & Siever, L. J. (2002). The borderline diagnosis I: psychopathology, comorbidity, and personality structure. [Research Support, Non-U.S. Gov't Research Support, U.S. Gov't, P.H.S. Review]. Biol Psychiatry, 51(12), 936-950.

Small GW, Ercoli LM, Silverman DH, Huang SC, Komo S, Bookheimer SY, Lavretsky H, Miller K, Siddarth P, Rasgon NL, Mazziotta JC, Saxena S, Wu HM, Mega MS, Cummings JL, Saunders AM, Pericak-Vance MA, Roses AD, Barrio JR, Phelps ME (2000). Cerebral metabolic and cognitive decline in persons at genetic risk for Alzheimer's disease. Proc Natl Acad Sci U S A., 97(11):6037-6042.

Small SA, Chawla MK, Buonocore M, Rapp PR, Barnes CA. (2004). Imaging correlates of brain function in monkeys and rats isolate a hippocampal subregion differentially vulnerable to aging. Proc Natl Acad Sci USA; 101:7181-7186.

Smeraski, CA, Dunwiddie, TV, Diao, L, Finger, TE (1998). Excitatory amino acid neurotransmission in the primary gustatory nucleus of the goldfish Carassius Auratus. Ann NY Acad Sci, 855: 442-449.

Smith, DV, Li, CS, Davis, BJ (1998). Excitatory and inhibitory modulation of taste responses in the hamster brainstem. Ann NY Acad Sci, 855: 450-456.

Smith GE. (1907). A new topographical survey of the human cerebral cortex, being an account of the distribution of the anatomically distinct cortical areas and their relationship to the cerebral sulci. J Anat 41: 237-254.

Smith MC, Smith MK, Ellgring H. (1996) Spontaneous and posed facial expression in Parkinson's disease. J Int Neuropsychol Soc. 2(5):383-391.

Smith MI (2011). Rapid processing of emotional expressions without conscious awareness. Cereb Cortex 22: 1748-1760.

Smith, P. K. (1973). Temporal clusters and individual differences in the behaviour of pre-school children. In R. P. Michael & J. H. Crook (Eds.). Comparative ecology and behaviour of primates, (pp. 751-798). London, U.K.: Academic Press.

Smith, P. K. Connolly, K. J. (1972). Patterns of play and social interaction in preschool children. In N. G. Blurton Jones (Ed.). Ethological studies of child behavior (pp. 65-95). London, U.K.: Cambridge University Press.

Smith, P. K. Connolly, K. J. (1980). The ecology of preschool behaviour. London, U.K.: Cambridge University Press.

Smith, S. M., Fox, P. T., Miller, K. L., Glahn, D. C., Fox, P. M., Mackay, C. E., Beckmann, C. F. (2009). Correspondence of the brain's functional architecture during activation and rest. [Research Support, N.I.H., Extramural Research Support, Non-U.S. Gov't]. Proc Natl Acad Sci U S A, 106(31), 13040-13045. doi: 10.1073/pnas.0905267106

Sojkova J, Driscoll I, Iacono D, Zhou Y, Codispoti KE, Kraut MA, Ferrucci L, Pletnikova O, Mathis CA, Klunk WE, O'Brien RJ, Wong DF, Troncoso JC, Resnick SM (2011). In vivo fibrillar beta-amyloid detected using [11C]PiB positron emission tomography and neuropathologic assessment in older adults. Arch Neurol, 68(2):232-240.

Sokolow, Y. N. (1963). Higher nervous functions: The orienting reflex. Annual Review of Physiology, 25, 545-580.

Soltesz, F. & Szucs, D. (2009). An electro-physiological temporal principal component analysis of processing stages of number comparison in developmental dyscalculia. Cognitive Development, 24, 474-485.

Song Y, Tian M, Liu J (2012) Top-down processing of symbolic meanings modulates the visual word form area. J Neurosci 32: 12277-12283.

Soto, C. J., John, O. P., Gosling, S. D., & Potter, J. (2011). Age differences in personality traits from 10 to 65: Big-Five domains and facets in a large cross-sectional sample. Journal of Personality and Social Psychology, 100, 330-348.

Sperling RA1, Aisen PS, Beckett LA, Bennett DA, Craft S, Fagan AM, Iwatsubo T, Jack CR Jr, Kaye J, Montine TJ, Park DC, Reiman EM, Rowe CC, Siemers E, Stern Y, Yaffe K, Carrillo MC, Thies B, Morrison-Bogorad M, Wagster MV, Phelps CH (2011). Toward defining the preclinical stages of Alzheimer's disease: recommendations from the National Institute on Aging-Alzheimer's Association workgroups on diagnostic guidelines for Alzheimer's disease. Alzheimers Dement, 7(3):280-292.

Sperry, R.W. (1967). Mental unity following surgical disconnections of the hemispheres. New York: Academic Press

Sperry, R.W. (1972). Science and the problem of values. Perspect Biol Med;16(1):115-30. doi: 10.1353/pbm.1972.0017.

Spreng, R. N., Mar, R. A., & Kim, A. S. (2009). The common neural basis of autobiographical memory, prospection, navigation, theory of mind, and the default mode: a quantitative meta-analysis. J Cogn Neurosci, 21(3), 489-510. doi: 10.1162/jocn.2008.21029

Sprengelmeyer R, Rausch M, Eysel UT, & Przuntek H. (1998) Neural structures associated with recognition of facial expressions of basic emotions. Proc Biol Sci. 265(1409):1927-1931.

Stanescu-Cosson, R., Pinel, P., Van de Moortele, P.F., Le Bihan, D., Cohen, L. and Dehaene, S. (2000). Understanding dissociations in dyscalculia: a brain-imaging study of the impact of number size on the cerebral networks for exact and approximate calculation. Brain, 123, 2240-2255.

Steele, H., & Siever, L. (2010). An attachment perspective on borderline personality disorder: advances in gene-environment considerations. [Review]. Curr Psychiatry Rep, 12(1), 61-67. doi: 10.1007/s11920-009-0091-0

Steffanowski, A., Oppl, M., Meyerberg, J., Schmidt, J., Wittmann, W.W. & Nübling, R. (2001). Psychometrische Überprüfung einer deutschsprachigen Version des Relationship Scales Questionaire (RSQ). In M. Bassler, (Hrsg.). Störungsspezifische Therapieansätze – Konzepte und Ergebnisse. S. 320-342, Gießen: Psychosozial.

Stein, D. J., Phillips, K. A., Bolton, D., Fulford, K. W., Sadler, J. Z., & Kendler, K. S. (2010). What is a mental/psychiatric disorder? From DSM-IV to DSM-V. [Editorial

Stein, K. F. (1996). Affect instability in adults with a borderline personality disorder. Arch Psychiatr Nurs, 10(1), 32-40.

Stein, RS (1983). Mutual protective complex of dental restorations. In WR. Laney, JA. Gibilisco (Eds.) Diagnosis and treatment of prosthodontics (pp. 306-326). Lea & Febiger, Philadelphia.

Steinthal, H. (1874). Erwiderung auf Eduard Hitzig. Zeitschrift für Ethnologie, 6, 47-50.

Steinthal, P. (1871). Abris der Sprachwissenschift. Berlin Krager.

Stemmler, G. (1992). Differential psychophysiology: Persons in situations. Heidelberg: Springer.

Stephan KM, Binkofski F, Halsband U, Dohle C, Wunderlich G, Schnitzler A, Tass P, Posse S, Herzog H, Sturm V, Zilles K, Seitz RJ, Freund HJ (1999) The role of ventral medial wall motor areas in bimanual co-ordination. A combined lesion and activation study. Brain. 122:351-68

Steppacher, I., Eickhof, S., Jordanov, T., Kaps, M., Witzke, W., & Kissler, J. (2013). N400 predicts recovery from disorders of consciousness. Annals of Neurology, 73, 594-602.

Stevens, F. L., Hurley, R. A., & Taber, K. H. (2011). Anterior cingulate cortex: unique role in cognition and emotion. J Neuropsychiatry Clin Neurosci, 23(2), 121-125. doi: 10.1176/appi.neuropsych.23.2.121

Stiglmayr, C. E., Grathwol, T., Linehan, M. M., Ihorst, G., Fahrenberg, J., & Bohus, M. (2005). Aversive tension in patients with borderline personality disorder: a computer-based controlled field study Acta Psychiatr Scand (Vol. 111, pp. 372-379). Denmark: Blackwell Munksgaard 2005.

Stoeckel MC, Weder B, Binkofski F, Buccino G, Shah NJ, Seitz RJ (2003). A fronto-parietal circuit for tactile object discrimination: an event-related fMRI study. Neuroimage 19: 1103-114.

Stoerig, P. (2006). Blindsight, conscious vision, and the role of primary visual cortex. Progress in Brain Research 155, 217-234. doi:10.1016/S0079-6123(06)55012-5

Strachan, A. L. (2000). In the brain of the beholder: The neuropsychological basis of aesthetic preferences, The Harvard Brain, 7, 1-10.
Strangman G, Boas DA, Sutton JP. (2002). Non-invasive neuroimaging using near-infrared light. Biological Psychiatry, 52, 679-693.
Strasbaugh, HJ, Levine, JD (2000). Pain. In G. Fink (Ed. in chief) Encyclopedia of stress /Vol. 3/ (pp. 115-118). Academic Press, San Diego.
Sturm, W. (2008) Aufmerksamkeit. In: S. Gauggel und M. Herrmann (Hrsg.). Handbuch der Neuro- und Biopsychologie (S. 329-336). Göttingen: Hogrefe.
Subramanian, S. V., Jones, K., Kaddour, A., & Krieger, N. (2009). Revisiting Robinson: The perils of individualistic and ecologic fallacy. International Journal of Epidemiology, 38, 342–360.
Suda, M, Morimoto, K, Obata, A, Koizumi, H, Maki, A (2008). Emotional responses to music: towards scientific perspectives on music therapy. NeuroReport, 19: 75-78.
Sugawara, N, Shiozawa, I, Masuda, T, Takei, H, Tsuruta, J, Ogura, N, Hasegawa, S (1998). A survey on condition of outpatients at prosthodontics II, University Hospital, Faculty of Dentistry, Tokyo Medical and Dental University. Kokubyo Gakkai Zasshi, 65: 251-259.
Sugiura M, Wakusawa K, Sekiguchi A, Sassa Y, Jeong H, Horie K, Sato S, Kawashima R (2009) Extraction of situational meaning by integrating multiple meanings in a complex environment: a functional MRI study. Hum Brain Mapp 30: 2676-2688.
Sumner P, Nachev P, Morris P, Peters AM, Jackson SR, Kennard C, Husain M (2007) Human medial frontal cortex mediates unconscious inhibition of voluntary action. Neuron 54: 697-711.
Supekar, K., Swigart, A.G., Tenison, C. , Jolles, D.D., Rosenberg-Lee, M., Fuchs, L. & Menon, V. (2013). Neural predictors of individual differences in response to math tutoring in primary-grade school children. Proceedings of the National Academy of Sciences of the United States of America, 110, 8230-8235.
Sussman, A.F., Ha, J.C., Bentson, K.L., & Crockett, C. M. (2013) Temperament in rhesus, long-tailed, and pigtailed macaques varies by species and sex. American Journal of Primatology, 75, 303–313.
Suzuki A, Hoshino T, Shigemasu K, Kawamura M. (2006). Disgust-specific impairment of facial expression recognition in Parkinson's disease. Brain, 129(Pt 3), 707-717.
Suzuki, W. A. (1996). Neuroanatomy of the monkey entorhinal, perirhinal and parahippocampal cortices: Organization of cortical inputs and interconnections with amygdala and striatum. Seminars in the Neurosciences, 8, 3–12.
Svenson O (1996). Decision making and the search for fundamental psychological regularities: What can be learned from a process perspective? Organ Behav Hum Decis Process 65:252-67.
Swoope, CC (1973). Predicting denture success. J Prosthet Dent, 30: 860-865.
Sylvester, R., Josephs, O., Driver, J., & Rees, G. (2007). Visual fMRI responses in human superior colliculus show a temporal–nasal asymmetry that is absent in lateral geniculate and visual cortex. Journal of Neurophysiology, 97(2), 1495-1502.
Szabó, Cs (1998). Regulation of the expression of the inducible isoform of nitric oxide synthase by glucocorticoids. Ann NY Acad Sci, 851: 336-341.

Takagi, M., Zee, D. S., & Tamargo, R. J. (2000). Effects of lesions of the oculomotor cerebellar vermis on eye movements in primate: smooth pursuit. Journal of Neurophysiology, 83(4), 2047-2062.
Tanaka, Y., Yoshida, A., Kawahata, N., Hashimoto, R., & Obayashi, T. (1996). Diagonistic dyspraxia Clinical characteristics, responsible lesion and possible underlying mechanism. Brain, 119(3), 859-874.
Tanji J (1994) The supplementary motor area in the cerebral cortex. Neurosci Res. 19:251-268
Tanji J (1996) New concepts of the supplementary motor area. Curr Opin Neurobiol 6: 782-787
Tanji J (2001) Sequential organization of multiple movements: involvement of cortical motor areas. Annu Rev Neurosci. 24:631-651
Tanji J, Kurata K (1982) Comparison of movement-related activity in two cortical motor areas of primates. J Neurophysiol. 48:633-653
Tanji J, Kurata K, Okano K (1985) The effect of cooling of the supplementary motor cortex and adjacent cortical areas. Exp Brain Res. 60:423-6
Tanji J, Okano K, Sato KC (1987) Relation of neurons in the nonprimary motor cortex to bilateral hand movement. Nature. 327:618-620
Tavalaro, J. (1998). Bis auf den Grund des Ozeans. Freiburg: Herder.
Tehovnik, E. J., Sommer, M. A., Chou, I. H., Slocum, W. M., & Schiller, P. H. (2000). Eye fields in the frontal lobes of primates. Brain Research Reviews, 32(2), 413-448.
Terracciano, A., Abdel-Khalek, A. M., Adám, N., Adamovová, L., et al., (2005). National character does not reflect mean personality trait levels in 49 cultures. Science, 310, 96-100.
Tetley, C. L. & O'Hara, S. J. (2012) Ratings of animal personality as a tool for improving the breeding, management and welfare of zoo mammals. Animal Welfare, 21, 463-476.
Tett, R. P., & Guterman, H. A. (2000). Situation trait relevance, trait expression, and cross-situational consistency: Testing a principle of trait activation. Journal of Research in Personality, 34, 397-423.
Thal DR, Rub U, Orantes M, Braak H (2002). Phases of A beta-deposition in the human brain and its relevance for the development of AD. Neurology, 58:1791–1800.
Thaler DE, Passingham RE (1989) The supplementary motor cortex and internally directed movement. In: Neural Mechaanisms in Disorders of Movement (Ed. A.R.Grossman) Libbey, London, pp. 175-181
Thelen, E., & Smith, L. B. (1993). A dynamic systems approach to the development of cognition and action. Cambridge, MA: MIT Press.
Thiebaut de Schotten M, Dell'Acqua F, Forkel SJ, Simmons A, Vergani F, Murphy DGM, Catani M. (2011). A lateralized brain network for visuospatial attention. Nat Neurosci 14: 1245-1246.
Thierry, B, (2000). Covariation of conflict management patterns across macaque species. In F. Aureli & F. B. M. de Waal (Eds). Natural conflict resolution, (pp. 106-128). Berkeley: University of California Press.
Thierry, B, (2007). Unity in diversity: Lessons from macaque societies. Evolutionary Anthropology, 16, 224-238.
Tholey, P. & Utecht, K. (1997). Schöpferisch träumen (3rd Edition). Eschborn: Klotz.

Thorndike, E. L. (1939). On the fallacy of imputing the correlations found for groups to the individuals or smaller groups composing them. American Journal of Psychology, 52, 122-124.
Tomasello, M. (1999). The Cultural Origins of Human Cognition. Harvard University Press.
Toomela, A. (2010). Modern mainstream psychology is the best? – Noncumulative, historically blind, fragmented, atheoretical. In A. Toomela & J. Valsiner, J. (Eds.). Methodological thinking in psychology: 60 years gone astray? (1 - 26). Charlotte, NC: Information Age Publishers.
Toomela, A. (2011). Travel into a fairy land: A critique of modern qualitative and mixed methods psychologies. Integrative Psychological and Behavioral Science, 45, 21-47.
Torgersen, S., Kringlen, E., & Cramer, V. (2001). The prevalence of personality disorders in a community sample. [Research Support, Non-U.S. Gov't]. Arch Gen Psychiatry, 58(6), 590-596.
Torgerson, C.J., Wiggins, A., Torgerson, D.J., Ainsworth, H., Barmby, P., Hewitt, C., Jones, K., Hendry, V., Askew, M., Bland, M., Coe, R., Higgins, S., Hodgen, J., Hulme, C. &Tymms P. (2011). Every Child Counts: The Independent Evaluation. London: Department for Education.
Toyofuku, A, Kikuta, T (2006). Treatment of phantom bite syndrome with milnacipran - a case series. Neuropsych Dis Treatment, 2: 387-390.
Tragesser, S. L., Robinson, R. J. (2009). The role of affective instability and UPPS impulsivity in borderline personality disorder features J Pers Disord (Vol. 23, pp. 370-383). United States.
Trehub, A. (2007). Space, Self, and the Theater of Consciousness. Consciousness and Cognition 16(2), 310-330.
Treiman R., Allaith Z. (2013). Do reading habits influence aesthetic preference? Read Writ, DOI 10.1007/s11145-012-9424-1.
Tremblay, P., Gracco, V. L. (2010). On the selection of words and oral motor responses: Evidence of a response-independent fronto-parietal network. Cortex, 46 (1), 15–28.
Trulsson, U, Engstrand, P, Berggren, U, Nannmark, U, Brånemark, PI (2002). Edentulousness and oral rehabilitation: experiences from the patients' perspective. Eur J Oral Sci, 110: 417-424.
Trzepacz PT, Yu P, Sun J, Schuh K, Case M, Witte MM, Hochstetler H, Hake A; Alzheimer's Disease Neuroimaging Initiative (2014). Comparison of neuroimaging modalities for the prediction of conversion from mild cognitive impairment to Alzheimer's dementia. Neurobiol Aging, 35(1):143-151.
Tsuchiya N, Kawasaki H, Oya H, Howard MA, Adolphs R (2008). Decoding face information in time, frequency and space from direct intracranial recordings of the human brain. PLoS One 3, e3892, Epub.
Tulving, E., Thomson, D. M. (1973). Encoding specificity and retrieval processes in episodic memory. Psychological Review, 80, 352-373.
Turken AU, Swick D (1999) Response selection in the human anterior cingulate cortex. Nat Neurosci 2:920-924
Turner, JA, Mancl, L, Aaron, LA (2006). Short- and long-term efficacy of brief cognitive-behavioral therapy for patients with chronic temporomandibular disorder pain: A randomized, controlled trial. Pain, 121: 181-194.

Tusche A, Bode S, Haynes J-D (2010) Neural responses to unattended products predict later consumer choices. J Neurosci 30: 8024-8031.

Tzourio-Mazoyer, N., Landeau, B., Papathanassiou, D., Crivello, F., Etard, O., Delcroix, N., Joliot, M. (2002). Automated anatomical labeling of activations in SPM using a macroscopic anatomical parcellation of the MNI MRI single-subject brain. Neuroimage, 15(1), 273-289. doi: 10.1006/nimg.2001.0978

Uher, J. (2008a). Three methodological core issues of comparative personality research. European Journal of Personality, 22, 475-496.

Uher, J. (2008b). Comparative personality research: Methodological approaches. European Journal of Personality, 22, 427-455.

Uher, J. (2011a). Individual behavioral phenotypes: An integrative metatheoretical framework. Why 'behavioral syndromes' are not analogues of 'personality'. Developmental Psychobiology, 53, 521–548.

Uher, J. (2011b). Personality in nonhuman primates: What can we learn from human personality psychology? In A. Weiss, J. King, & L. Murray (Eds.). Personality and Temperament in Nonhuman Primates (pp. 41-76). New York, NY: Springer.

Uher, J. (2013). Personality psychology: Lexical approaches, assessment methods, and trait concepts reveal only half of the story—Why it is time for a paradigm shift. Integrative Psychological and Behavioral Science, 47, 1-55

Uher, J. (2014). Fundamental challenges of contemporary "personality" research. Physics of Life Reviews, 11, 695-696.

Uher, J. (2015a). Conceiving "personality": Psychologists' challenges and basic fundamentals of the Transdisciplinary Philosophy-of-Science Paradigm for Research on Individuals. Integrative Psychological and Behavioral Science, 49(3). DOI: 10.1007/s12124-014-9283-1.

Uher, J. (2015b). Developing "personality" taxonomies: Metatheoretical and methodological rationales underlying selection approaches, methods of data generation and reduction principles. Integrative Psychological and Behavioral Science, 49(3). DOI: 10.1007/s12124-014-9280-4.

Uher, J. (2015c). Interpreting „personality" taxonomies: Why previous models cannot capture individual-specific experiencing, behaviour, functioning and development. Major taxonomic tasks still lay ahead. Integrative Psychological and Behavioral Science, 49(3). DOI: 10.1007/s12124-014-9281-3

Uher, J. (2015d). Agency enabled by the Psyche: Explorations using the Transdisciplinary Philosophy-of-Science Paradigm for Research on Individuals. Annals of Theoretical Psychology, 12, 177-228.

Uher, J. (2016). Exploring the workings of the psyche: Metatheoretical and methodological foundations. Annals of Theoretical Psychology, 13, xx-xx.

Uher, J. (submitted). Principles of measurement and quantification in the physical sciences, life sciences, social sciences and in psychology.

Uher, J., Addessi, E., & Visalberghi, E. (2013a). Contextualised behavioural measurements of personality differences obtained in behavioural tests and social observations in adult capuchin monkeys (Cebus apella). Journal of Research in Personality, 47, 427-444.

Uher, J., Asendorpf, J. B. (2008). Personality assessment in the Great Apes: Comparing ecologically valid behavior measures, behavior ratings, and adjective ratings. Journal of Research in Personality, 42, 821-838.

Uher, J., Asendorpf, J. B., Call, J. (2008). Personality in the behavior of Great Apes: Temporal stability, cross-situational consistency and coherence in response. Animal Behaviour, 75, 99-112.

Uher, J., Werner, C. S., Gosselt, K. (2013b). From observations of individual behaviour to social representations of personality: Developmental pathways, attribution biases, and limitations of questionnaire methods. Journal of Research in Personality, 47, 647–667.

Ullsperger M, Cramon von DY (2001) Subprocesses of performance monitoring: a dissociation of error processing and response competition revealed by event-related fMRI and ERPs. Neuroimage. 14:1387-401

Ullsperger M, Nittono H, von Cramon DY (2007). When goals are missed: dealing with self-generated and externally induced failure. NeuroImage 35: 1356-1364.

Uncapher, M. R., Otten, L. J., & Rugg, M. D. (2006) Episodic encoding is more than the sum of its parts: an fMRI investigation of multifeatural contextual encoding. Neuron, 52, 547–556.

Uncapher, M. R., Rugg, M. D. (2005) Encoding and the durability of episodic memory: a functional magnetic resonance imaging study. Journal of Neuroscience, 25, 7260–7267.

Ungerleider L, Mishkin M. (1982) Two cortical visual systems. In: Analysis of Visual Behaviour. Eds: Ingle D. et al. pp: 549-586. MIT Press.

Ungerleider LG, Haxby JV (1994) „What“and „where “in the human brain. Curr Opin Neurobiol 4: 157-165.

Vaid J., Singh M. (1987). Reading habits influence asymmetries in nonlinguistic perception and production. Presented at tenth annual meeting of the Body for the Advancement of brain, Behavior and Language Enterprises, Niagara Falls.

Vaina, L. M., Goodglass, H., Daltroy, L. (1995). Inference of object use from pantomimed actions by aphasics and patients with right hemisphere lesions. Synthese, 104, 43–57.

Vallar, G. (1997). Spatial frames of reference and somatosensory processing: a neuropsychological perspective. Philosophical Transactions of the Royal Society, London, B, B 352, 1401-1409.

van de Vijver, F. J. R., Leung, K. (1997a). Methods and data analysis of comparative research. In J. W. Berry,Y. H. Poortinga, & J. Pandey (Eds.), Handbook of cross-cultural psychology (2nd ed., Vol. 1, pp. 257-300). Boston: Allyn & Bacon.

van de Vijver, F. J. R., Leung, K. (1997b). Methods and data analysis for cross-cultural research. Newbury Park, CA: Sage.

van de Vijver, F. J. R. Poortinga, Y. H. (1997). Towards an integrated analysis of bias in cross-cultural assessment. European Journal of Psychological Assessment, 13, 29-37.

van de Vijver, F. J. R., Poortinga, Y. H. (2002). Structural Equivalence in Multilevel Research. Journal of Cross-Cultural Psychology, 141, 141-156.

van de Vijver, F. J. R., Tanzer, N. K. (2004). Bias and equivalence in cross-cultural assessment: An overview. European Review of Applied Psychology, 54, 119-135.

van den Stock J, Tamietto M, Sorger B, Pichon S, Grezes J, de Gelder B (2011). Cortico-subcortical visual, somatosensory, and motor activations for perceiving dynamic whole-body emotional expressions with and without striate cortex (V1). Proc Natl Acad Sci USA 108 : 16188-16193.

van der Glas, HW, de Laat, A, Carels, C, van Steenberghe, D (1988). Interactive periodontal and acoustic influences on the masseteric post-stimulus electromyographic complex in man. Brain Res, 444: 284-294.
van der Glas, HW, de Laat, A, van Steenberghe, D (1985). Oral pressure mediate a series of inhibitory and excitatory periods in the masseteric poststimulus EMG complex following tapping of a tooth in man. Brain Res, 337: 117-125.
van Eimeren, L., Grabner, R.H. Koschutnik, K. et al (2010) Structure-function relationships underlying calculation: a combined diffusion tensor imaging and fMRI study. Neuroimage, 52, 358-363.
van Gaal, S., Lamme, V. A. (2012). Unconscious high-level information processing: implication for neurobiological theories of consciousness. [Research Support, Non-U.S. Gov't Review]. Neuroscientist, 18(3), 287-301. doi: 10.1177/1073858411404079
van Gaal, S., Lange de, F. P., & Cohen, M. X. (2012). The role of consciousness in cognitive control and decision making. Front Hum Neurosci, 6, 121. doi: 10.3389/fnhum.2012.00121
van Geert, P. Dijk van, M. (2002). Focus on variability: New tools to study intra-individual variability in developmental data. Infant Behavior & Development, 25, 340-374.
van Harkskamp, N.J. & Cipolotti, L. (2001). Selective impairments for addition, subtraction and multiplication: Implications for the organization of arithmetical facts. Cortex, 37, 363-388.
van Meer MP, Otte WM, van der Marel K et al. (2012). Extent of bilateral neuronal network reorganization and functional recovery in relation to stroke severity. J Neurosci;32:4495-4507
van Veen V, Cohen JD, Botvinick MM, Stenger VA, Carter CS (2001) Anterior cingulate cortex, conflict monitoring, and levels of processing. Neuroimage. 14:1302-8
Vandenberg, R. J., Lance, C. E. (2000). A review and synthesis of the measurement invariance literature: Suggestions, practices, and recommendations for organizational research. Organizational Research Methods, 3, 4-70.
Vandenberghe R, Laere van K, MD, Ivanoiu A, Salmon E, Bastin C, Triau E, Hasselbalch S, Law I, Andersen A, Korner A, MD, Minthon L, Garraux G, Nelissen N, Bormans G, Buckley C, Owenius R, Thurfjell L, Farrar G, Brooks DJ (2010). 18F-Flutemetamol Amyloid Imaging in Alzheimer Disease and Mild Cognitive Impairment A Phase 2 Trial. Ann Neurol, 68:319–329.
Vargha-Khadem, F., Carr, L.J., Isaac,s E., Brett, E., Adams, C., Mishkin, M. (1997). Onset of speech after left hemispherectomy in a nine-year-old boy. Brain Jan; 120 (Pt 1):159-82.
Vargha-Khadem, F., Polkey, C.E. (1992). A review of cognitive outcome after hemidecortication in humans. Adv Exp Med Biol;325:137-51.
Varney, N. R. (1978). Linguistic correlates of pantomime recognition in aphasic patients. Journal of Neurology Neurosurgery & Psychiatry, 41, 564–568.
Vartanian O., Goel V., Lam E., Fisher M., Granic J. (2013). Middle Temporal Gyrus Encodes Individual Differences in Perceived Facial Attractiveness. Psychology of Aesthetics, Creativity, and the Arts, DOI: 10.1037/a0031591.
Venneri, A., McGeown, W. J., Hietanen, H. M., Guerrini, C., Ellis, A. W., & Shanks, M. F. (2008). The anatomical bases of semantic retrieval deficits in early Alzheimer's disease. Neuropsychologia, 46(2), 497-510.

Vidoni, F. (1991). Ignorabismus! Emil du Bois-Reymond und die Debatte über die Grenzen wissenschaftlicher Erkenntnis im 19. Jahrhundert. Frankfurt a. M.: Lang.

Vigneau, M., Beaucousin, V., Herve, P. Y., Duffau, H., Crivello, F., Houde, O., Mazoyer, B. & Tzourio-Mazoyer, N. (2006). Meta-analyzing left hemisphere language areas: Phonology, semantics, and sentence processing. NeuroImage, 30, 1414–1432.

Vignolo, L. A. (1990). Non-verbal conceptual impairment in aphasia. In: F. Boller & J. Grafman (Eds.), Handbook of clinical neuropsychology (pp. 185–206). Amsterdam: Elsevier.

Villain N, Chetelat G, Grassiot B, Bourgeat P, Jones G, Ellis KA, et al., (2012). Regional dynamics of amyloid-beta deposition in healthy elderly, mild cognitive impairment and Alzheimer's disease: a voxelwise PiB-PET longitudinal study. Brain, 135(Pt 7):2126-2139.

Villemagne VL, Burnham S, Bourgeat P, Brown B, Ellis KA, Salvado O, Szoeke C, Macaulay SL, Martins R, Maruff P, Ames D, Rowe CC, Masters CL; Australian Imaging Biomarkers and Lifestyle (AIBL) Research Group (2013). Amyloid β deposition, neurodegeneration, and cognitive decline in sporadic Alzheimer's disease: a prospective cohort study. Lancet Neurol, 12(4):357-367.

Villemagne VL, Pike KE, Chételat G, Ellis KA, Mulligan RS, Bourgeat P, Ackermann U, Jones G, Szoeke C, Salvado O, Martins R, O'Keefe G, Mathis CA, Klunk WE, Ames D, Masters CL, Rowe CC (2011). Longitudinal assessment of Aβ and cognition in aging and Alzheimer disease. Ann Neurol, 69(1):181-192.

Vinard, H, Ravier-Rosenblaum, C (1989). The psychosomatic effects of the sonic environment in the dental office. Rev Odontostomatol (Paris), 18: 101-108.

Vingerhoets, G., Acke, F., Vandemaele, P., & Achten, E. (2009). Tool responsive regions in the posterior parietal cortex: Effect of differences in motor goal and target object during imagined transitive movements. NeuroImage, 47, 1832-1843.

Visalberghi E., Valenzano, D.R., & Preuschoft S. (2006). Facial displays in tufted capuchins. International Journal of Primatology, 27, 1689-1707.

Viskontas, I. V., Knowlton, B. J., Steinmetz, P. N., & Fried, I. (2006). Differences in mnemonic processing by neurons in the human hippocampus and parahippocampal regions. Journal of Cognitive Neuroscience, 18(10), 1654-1662.

Vlaev I, Chater N, Stewart N, Brown GDA (2011). Does the brain calculate value? TICS 15: 546-554.

Vogeley K, Bussfeld P, Newen A, Herrmann S, Happe F, Falkai P, Maier W, Shah NJ, Fink GR, Zilles K (2001) Mind reading: neural mechanisms of theory of mind and self-perspective. Neuroimage 14: 170-181.

Vogeley K, Roepstorff A (2009). Contextualising culture and social cognition. Trends Cogn. Sci. 13, 511 – 516.

Vogt, B. A. (2005). Pain and emotion interactions in subregions of the cingulate gyrus. [Research Support, N.I.H., Extramural Research Support, U.S. Gov't, P.H.S. Review]. Nat Rev Neurosci, 6(7), 533-544. doi: 10.1038/nrn1704

Vogt C, Vogt O. (1919). Allgemeinere Ergebnisse unserer Hirnforschung. J Psychol Neurol 25: 279-461.

Vogt O. (1911). Die Myeloarchitektonik des Isocortex parietalis. J Psychol Neurol 18: 107-118.

Völlm BA, Taylor ANW, Richardson P, Corcoran R, Stirling J, McKie S, Deakin JFW, Elliott R (2006). Neuronal correlates of theory of mind and empathy: A functional magnetic resonance imaging study in a nonverbal task. Neuroimage 29: 90-98.

Vollm, B. A., Taylor, A. N., Richardson, P., Corcoran, R., Stirling, J., McKie, S., Elliott, R. (2006). Neuronal correlates of theory of mind and empathy: a functional magnetic resonance imaging study in a nonverbal task. [Clinical Trial Research Support, Non-U.S. Gov't]. Neuroimage, 29(1), 90-98. doi: 10.1016/j.neuroimage.2005.07.022

von Economo K, Koskinas G. (1925). Die Cytoarchitektonik des Hirnrinde des erwachsenen Menschen. Springer, Wien.

von Korff, M, Balderson, BHK, Saunders, K, Miglioretti, DL, Lin, EHB, Berry, S, Moore, J, Turner, JA (2005). A trial of an activating intervention for chronic back pain in primary care and physical therapy settings. Pain, 113: 323-330.

von Uexküll, J. (1909). Umwelt und Innenwelt der Tiere. Berlin: Springer.

Vos SJ, Verhey F, Frölich L, Kornhuber J, Wiltfang J, Maier W, Peters O, Rüther E, Nobili F, Morbelli S, Frisoni GB, Drzezga A, Didic M, van Berckel BN, Simmons A, Soininen H, Kłoszewska I, Mecocci P, Tsolaki M, Vellas B, Lovestone S, Muscio C, Herukka SK, Salmon E, Bastin C, Wallin A, Nordlund A, de Mendonça A, Silva D, Santana I, Lemos R, Engelborghs S, Van der Mussele S; The Alzheimer's Disease Neuroimaging Initiative, Freund-Levi Y, Wallin ÅK, Hampel H, van der Flier W, Scheltens P, Visser PJ (2015). Prevalence and prognosis of Alzheimer's disease at the mild cognitive impairment stage. Brain. 2015 Feb 17. pii: awv029. [Epub ahead of print].

Vry MS, Tritschler LC, Hamzei F, Rijntjes M, Kaller CP, Hoeren M, Umarova R, Glauche V, Hermsdoerfer J, Goldenberg G, Hennig J, Weiller C. (2015) The ventral fiber pathway for pantomime of object use. Neuroimage. 106:252-63.

Vuilleumier P, Pourtois G (2007). Distributed and interactive brain mechanisms during emotion face perception: evidence from functional neuroimaging. Neuropsychologia 45: 174-194.

Vygotsky, L. S. (1934/1962). Thought and language. Cambridge, MA: MIT Press.

Walker, R., & Findlay, J. M. (1996). Saccadic eye movement programming in unilateral neglect. Neuropsychologia, 34(6), 493-508.

Wallis JD, Miller EK (2003) From rule to response: neuronal processes in the premotor and prefrontal cortex. J Neurophysiol 90:1790-1806

Walton ME, Devlin JT, Rushworth MFS (2004) Interactions between decision making and performance monitoring within prefrontal cortex. Nat. Neurosci. 7 , 1259 – 1265.

Wang J, Fan L, Zhang Y, Liu Y, Jiang D, Zhang Y, Yu C, Jiang T. (2012). Tractography-based parcellation of the human left inferior parietal lobule. NeuroImage 63: 641-652.

Wang Y, Matsuzaka Y, Shima K, Tanji J (2004) Cingulate cortical cells projecting to monkey frontal eye field and primary motor cortex. Neuroreport. 15:1559-63

Wang, X., Merzenich, M.M., Sameshima, K., Jenkins, W.M. (1995). Remodelling of Hand Representation in Adult Cortex Determined by Timing of Tactile Stimulation. Nature 378:71-75.

Ward NS, Brown MM, Thompson AJ, Frackowiak RS. (2003). Neural correlates of motor recovery after stroke: a longitudinal fMRI study. Brain; 126:2476-2496.

Warrington. E.K. (1982). The fractionation of arithmetical skills: a single case study. Quarterly Journal of Experimental Psychology, 34A, 31-51.

Watson, P. D., Voss, J. L., Warren, D. E., Tranel, D., & Cohen, N. J. (2013). Spatial reconstruction by patients with hippocampal damage is dominated by relational memory errors. Hippocampus, 23(7), 570-580.

Weaver, J. (1954). Differentiated instruction in arithmetic: an overview and a promising trend. Education, 74, 300–305.

Weiller, C. (1998). Imaging recovery from stroke. Exp Brain Res;123(1-2).13-17

Weiller, C., Bormann, T., Saur, D., Musso, M., Rijntjes, M. (2011). How the ventral pathway got lost: and what its recovery might mean. Brain Lang, 118, 29-39.

Weinberg, LA (1977). An evaluation of stress in temporomandibular joint dysfunction-pain syndrome. J Prosthet Dent, 38: 192-207.

Weinrich M, Wise SP (1982) The premotor cortex of the monkey. J Neurosci 2:1329-45

Weis, S., Specht, K., Klaver, P., Tendolkar, I., Willmes, K., Ruhlmann, et al. (2004). Process dissociation between contextual retrieval and item recognition. NeuroReport, 15, 2729–2733.

Weiskrantz, L. (1988). Thought Without Language. Oxford: Clarendon Press.

Weisser FB, Bristowe K & Jackson D. (2015). Experiences of burden, needs, rewards and resilience in family caregivers of people living with Motor Neuron Disease / Amyotrophic Lateral Sclerosis: A secondary thematic analysis of qualitative interviews. Palliat Med, Mar 11, Epub ahead of print.

Wells, D. L. (2009). The effects of animals on human health and well-being. Journal of Social Issues, 65, 523-543.

Wells, D. L. Hepper, P. G. (2000). The prevalence of behavior problems reported by owners of dogs purchased from an animal rescue shelter. Applied Animal Behavior Science, 69, 55–65.

Whitehead, A. N. (1929). Process and reality. New York: Harper.

Whitfield-Gabrieli, S., Thermenos, H. W., Milanovic, S., Tsuang, M. T., Faraone, S. V., McCarley, R. W., Seidman, L. J. (2009). Hyperactivity and hyperconnectivity of the default network in schizophrenia and in first-degree relatives of persons with schizophrenia. Proc Natl Acad Sci U S A, 106(4), 1279-1284. doi: 10.1073/pnas.0809141106 0809141106 [pii]

Wildgruber D, Riecker A, Hertrich I, Erb M, Grodd W, Ethofer T, Ackermann H. (2005) Identification of emotional intonation evaluated by fMRI. Neuroimage. 24(4):1233-41.

Wilding, E. L, Herron, J. E. (2006). Electrophysiological measures of episodic memory control and memory retrieval. Clincal EEG and Neuroscience, 37, 315–321.

Wilding, E. L., Rugg, M. D. (1996). An event-related potential study of recognition memory with and without retrieval of source. Brain, 119, 889-905.

Williams, C., Azzopardi, P., & Cowey, A. (1995). Nasal and temporal retinal ganglion cells projecting to the midbrain: implications for “blindsight”. Neuroscience, 65(2), 577-586.

Williams, PL, Warwick, R editors in chief (1980). Gray's anatomy. (36th edition). Churchill and Livingstone, Edinburgh - London - Melbourne - New York. 1980. 529-540, 1060, 1084-1086, 1138-1140, 1271-1272.

Williams ZM, Bush G, Rauch SL, Cosgrove GR, Eskandar EN (2004) Human anterior cingulate neurons and the integration of monetary reward with motor responses. Nat Neurosci. 7:1370-5

Winkielman P, Berridge KC, Wilbarger JL (2005). Unconscious affective reactions to masked happy versus angry faces influence consumption behaviour and judgments of value. Pers Soc Psychol Bull 31: 121-135

Winner B, Kohl Z Gage FH. (2011). Neurodegenerative disease and adult neurogenesis. Eur J Neurosci;33:1139-1151.

Wise SP (1985) The primate premotor cortex: past, present, and preparatory. Annu Rev Neurosci 8:1-19

Wise SP and Murray EA. (2000) Arbitrary associations between antecedents and actions. Trends Neurosci. 23:271-276.

Wittchen, H.-U. & Hoyer, J. (2006). Klinische Psychologie & Psychotherapie. Heidelberg: Springer Medizin Verlag.

Wolf, R. C., Sambataro, F., Vasic, N., Schmid, M., Thomann, P. A., Bienentreu, S. D., & Wolf, N. D. (2011). Aberrant connectivity of resting-state networks in borderline personality disorder. J Psychiatry Neurosci, 36(6), 402-411. doi: 10.1503/jpn.100150

Wontorra, H.M. (2009). Frühe apparative Psychologie. Leipzig: Der Andere Verlag.

Woodward, W. R. (1982). Wundt's Program for the New Psychology: Vicissitudes of Experiment, Theory, and System. In: W.R. Woodward & M. G. Ash (Eds.). The problematic science: Psychology in nineteenth-century thought (pp. 167-197). New York: Praeger.

Woolsey C.N., Settlage P.H., Meyer, D.R., Sencer, W, Pinto Hamuy, T., Travis, A.M. (1952). Patterns of localization in precentral and "supplementary" motor areas and their relation to the concept of a premotor area. Res Pub Assoc Res Nerve Ment Dis, 30:238-64.

Wright, J. C. & Mischel, W. (1987). A conditional approach to dispositional constructs: The local predictability of social behavior. Journal of Personality and Social Psychology, 55, 454-469.

Wright, J. C., & Zakriski, A. L. (2003). When syndromal similarity obscures functional dissimilarity: Distinctive evoked environments of externalizing and mixed syndrome children. Journal of Consulting and Clinical Psychology, 71, 516-527.

Wright, R.J., Martland, J. & Stafford, A. (2006). Early Numeracy: Assessment for Teaching and Intervention, 2nd edition. London: Paul Chapman.

Wundt, W. (1856), Untersuchungen über das Verhalten der Nerven in entzündeten und degenerierten Organen. Dissertation. Heidelberg: Georg Mohr.

Wundt, W. (1862). Beiträge zur Theorie der Sinneswahrnehmung (neubearb. Aufl. von Aufsätzen). Leipzig: Winter.

Wundt, W. (1863). Vorlesungen über die Menschen- und Tierseele (Band 1-2). Leipzig: Voss. (6. Aufl. 1919).

Wundt, W. (1863/1990). Vorlesungen über die Menschen- und Tierseele. Eingeleitet und mit Materialien zur Rezeptionsgeschichte versehen von W. Nitsche (2 Bände). Berlin: Deutscher Verlag der Wissenschaften.

Wundt, W. (1865). Lehrbuch der Physiologie des Menschen (Mit 137 in den Text gedruckten Holzschnitten). (4. Aufl. 1878). Erlangen: Enke.

Wundt, W. (1867). Handbuch der medizinischen Physik. (Mit 244 in den Text gedruckten Holzschnitten). Erlangen: Enke.

Wundt, W. (1874). Grundzüge der Physiologischen Psychologie. Leipzig Verlag W. Engelmann

Wundt, W. (1896). Über die Definition der Psychologie. Philosophische Studien, 12, 9-66.

Wundt, W. (1902-1903). Grundzüge der Physiologischen Psychologie (Band 1-3, 5. Aufl.).
Wundt, W. (1908). Grundzüge der physiologischen Psychologie. Band 1. (6. Aufl.). Leipzig: Engelmann.
Wundt, W. (1910). Grundzüge der physiologischen Psychologie. Band 2. (6. Aufl.). Leipzig: Engelmann.
Wundt, W. (1911). Grundzüge der physiologischen Psychologie. Band 3. (6. Aufl.). Leipzig: Engelmann.
Wundt, W. (1913). Die Psychologie im Beginn des zwanzigsten Jahrhunderts. In: Reden und Aufsätze (S. 163-231). Leipzig: Kröner.
Wundt, W. (1921). Logik. Eine Untersuchung der Prinzipien der Erkenntnis und der Methoden Wissenschaftlicher Forschung. Band 3. Logik der Geisteswissenschaften (4. Aufl.). Stuttgart: Ferdinand Enke.
Yamada M, Decety J (2009). Unconscious affective processing and empathy: An investigation of subliminal priming on the detection of painful facial expressions. Pain, 143, 71-75.
Yamada, J., & Noda, H. (1987). Afferent and efferent connections of the oculomotor cerebellar vermis in the macaque monkey. Journal of comparative neurology, 265(2), 224-241.
Yamagata T, Nakayama Y, Tanji J, Hoshi E (2009) Processing of visual signals for direct specification of motor targets and for conceptual representation of action targets in the dorsal and ventral premotor cortex. J Neurophysiol 102:3280-94
Yang L. Li J., Spaniol J. Hasher L., Wilkinson A.J., et al. (2013). Aging, culture, and memory for socially meaningful item-context associations: an East-West cross-cultural comparison study. PLOS ONE, 8, 1-7.
Yeo BT, Krienen FM, Sepulcre J, Sabuncu MR, Lashkari D, Hollinshead M, Roffman JL, Smoller JW, Zöllei L, Polimeni JR, Fischl B, Liu H, Buckner R. (2011). The organization of the human cerebral cortex estimated by intrinsic functional connectivity. J Neurophysiol 106: 1125-1165.
Yin HH, & Knowlton BJ. (2006) The role of the basal ganglia in habit formation. Nat Rev Neurosci. 7(6):464-476.
Yonelinas, A. P. (2002). The nature of recollection and familiarity: a review of 30 years of research. Journal of Memory and Language, 46, 441-517.
Yonelinas, A. P., Jacoby, L. L. (1995). The relation between remembering and knowing as basis for recognition—effects of size congruency. Journal of Memory and Language, 34, 622–643.
Yoshida K, Saito N, Iriki A, Isoda M (2011) Representation of others' action by neurons in monkey medial frontal cortex. Curr Biol. 21:249-53
Yoshida K, Saito N, Iriki A, Isoda M (2012) Social error monitoring in macaque frontal cortex. Nat Neurosci. 15:1307-12
Yovel, G., Paller, K. A. (2004). The neural basis of the butcher-on-the-bus phenomenon: when a face seems familiar but is not remembered. NeuroImage, 21, 789-800.
Zajonc RB (1980). Feeling and thinking: Preferences need no inferences. Am Psychol 35: 151-175.
Zanarini, M. C., Frankenburg, F. R., Hennen, J., Reich, D. B., & Silk, K. R. (2006). Prediction of the 10-year course of borderline personality disorder. [Research Support, N.I.H., Extramural]. Am J Psychiatry, 163(5), 827-832. doi: 10.1176/appi.ajp.163.5.827

Zeh, T. (2009). Dekohärenz und andere Quantenmißverständnisse. Beitrag zum Didaktik-Workshop Physik an der TU Karlsruhe (unpublished).

Zeig, Jeffrey K. (2001). Erickson Remembered. In: Hypnosis International Monographs 5, 2001. 1-14.

Zetzsche, T., Frodl, T., Preuss, U. W., Schmitt, G., Seifert, D., Leinsinger, G., . . . Meisenzahl, E. M. (2006). Amygdala volume andgossel depressive symptoms in patients with borderline personality disorder. Biological Psychiatry, 60(3), 302-310. doi: S0006-3223(05)01456-3 [pii] 10.1016/j.biopsych.2005.11.020

Zhang, S., Li, C. S. (2012). Functional connectivity mapping of the human precuneus by resting state fMRI. Neuroimage, 59(4), 3548-3562. doi: 10.1016/j.neuroimage.2011.11.023 S1053-8119(11)01304-8 [pii]

Zhang S, Li CS. (2014). Functional clustering of the human inferior parietal lobule by whole-brain connectivity mapping of resting-state functional magnetic resonance imaging signals. Brain Connect 4 (1): 53-69.

Ziche, P. (1999). Neuroscience in its context. Neuroscience and psychology in the work of Wilhelm Wundt. Physis rivista internazionale di storia della scienza, 36 (2), 407-429.

Ziche, P. (2008). Wissenschaftslandschaften um 1900: Philosophie, die Wissenschaften und der nichtreduktive Szientismus. Zürich: Chronos.

Ziehen, Th. (1893). Leitfaden der physiologischen Psychologie in 15 Vorlesungen (2. Aufl.). Jena: Fischer.

Zimmermann, M (2004). Physiologie von Nozizeption und Schmerz. In H.D. Basler, C. Franz, B. Kröner-Hervig & H.P. Rehfisch (Eds.), Psychologische Schmerztherapie (pp. 17-58). Springer, Berlin.

Zinober B and Martlew M. (1985) Developmental change in four types of gesture in relation to acts and vocalization from 10 to 21 months. British J Developmental Psychol. 3: 293-306.

Zukic, S., Mrkonjic, Z., Sinanovic, O., Vidovic, M. & B. Kojic (2012). Gerstmann's Syndrome in Acute Stroke Patients. Acta Inform Med, 20 (4), 242-243

Key Words

Tanji action planning action selection cingulate motor areas higher-order motor areas primary motor cortex premotor cortex pre-supplementary motor area spatial coding supplementary motor area temporal coding voluntary movement	**Lotze** BA 47 Dopaminergic emotional Face Recognition Gesture Mirror neuronal System Putamen social Interaction superior temporal Gyrus temporo-frontal Interaction	**Meyer, Flor** Recognition memory Hippocampus perirhinal cortex fMRI ERPs VBM contextual conditioning semantics aMCI neuropsychological assess-ment
Klann, Binkofski, Caspers anatomical parcellation angular gyrus apraxia IPL language functions multimodal processing spatial neglect supramarginal gyrus tool use verbal working memory	**Seitz, Potthoff** Action Emotion Empathy medial frontal Cortex Neuroimaging Perception Perspective Taking social Interaction Theory of Mind Valuation	**Kotchoubey, Chaudhary, Piccione, Birbaumer** brain-computer interface (BCI) classical conditioning consciousness event-related potentials (ERP) functional magnetic resonance imaging (fMRI) locked-in syndrome (LIS, also complete LIS: CLIS) minimally conscious state (MCS) near-infrared spectroscopy (NIRS) outcome prediction vegetative state (VS, synonym Unresponsive wakefulness Syn-drome UWS)
Rinne aging Alzheimer's disease (AD) brain cognitive reserve cognitive impairment (CI) diagnostic work-up FDG longitudinal amyloid imaging memory complaint MRI PET	**Saevarsson, Kristjánsson** assessment eyes limbs neuroanatomy voluntary movement disor-ders	**D'Souza** ACC affective neuroscience biological markers borderline personality disor-der default mode network emotion regulation fMRI functional connectivity precuneus Theory of Mind
Laihinen restoratio ad integrum, salutogenese plasticity palliative treatment nursing care neurobiology	**Fábián, Beck, Krause, Fejérdy, Hermann, Fábián** autonomic Innervation Pre-vention Brainstem Communication cranial Nerves	**Marandi** aesthetic processing cross-cultural variations fMRI beauty recognition Western-Eastern theory of mind

synapse, positron emission tomography (PET) Barthel index phase of rehabilitation	dental Fear Mind-Body Therapies oral Immunity orofacial Pain salivary Gland	hemisphere specialization symmetry-asymmetry
Dowker Brain development Brain imaging Brain stimulation Dyscalculia Educational interventions Individual differences Mathematical development	**Uher** Configurational comparability/ structural or construct equivalence Cross-species and cross-cultural comparative methodology Limitations of assessment methods Patterning and positioning effects Scientific measurement and quantification Sex/ gender differences and species differences weeper capuchin (*Cebus olivaceus*), mandrill (*Mandrillus sphinx*), toque macaque (*Macaca sinica*), Rhesus macaque (*Macaca mulatta*)	**Buderer, Schreiner, Wohlfahrt** attachment big five canine behavior dog-caretaker relationship dog's behavior problems health Dog Human-animal interaction personality personality traits quality of life
Reventorf direct suggestion DMN Erickson hypnosis indirect induction suggestibility trance depth	**Riebensahm, Scarpinato-Hirt** anosmia declining organic brain dream, metaphor explosive disorder frontal lobe metamorphosis Rapport syndrome therapeutic alliance brain tumor trance	**Hinterberger** Consciousness Dream Event-Related Potentials Neuroscience Objectivity Perception Qualia Self Subjectivity
Fahrenberg Apperzeption/-psychologie Assoziationspsychologie Aufmerksamkeit Bewussteseinspsychologie Lokalisationstheorien Neuropsychologie Wilhelm Wundt	**Freund** Neuropsychology Psychology Neurology brain lesions neurological deficits cognitive deficits bridging specialties single case observation	